国家卫生和计划生育委员会"十三五"规划教材

全国高等学校教材

供本科护理学类专业用

Fundamentals of Traditional Chinese Medicine Nursing

中医护理学基础

双 语

第 **2** 版

主　编　郝玉芳　王诗源

副主编　杨　柳　王春艳　徐冬英

编　者　（按姓氏笔画排序）

马雪玲	▸	北京中医药大学护理学院
王云翠	▸	湖北中医药大学护理学院
王诗源	▸	山东中医药大学护理学院
王春艳	▸	吉林医药学院护理学院
王秋琴	▸	南京中医药大学护理学院
苏春香	▸	北京中医药大学护理学院
杨　柳	▸	福建中医药大学护理学院
杨金花	▸	湖南中医药大学护理学院
周云仙	▸	浙江中医药大学护理学院
单亚维	▸	上海中医药大学护理学院
郝玉芳	▸	北京中医药大学护理学院
徐冬英	▸	广西中医药大学护理学院

编写秘书　苏春香　　▸　北京中医药大学护理学院

人民卫生出版社

·北 京·

图书在版编目（CIP）数据

中医护理学基础：双语：英汉对照 / 郝玉芳，王诗源主编 . —2 版 . —北京：人民卫生出版社，2020.7
ISBN 978−7−117−30111−4

Ⅰ. ①中… Ⅱ. ①郝… ②王… Ⅲ. ①中医学 – 护理学 – 医学院校 – 教材 – 英、汉 Ⅳ. ①R248

中国版本图书馆 CIP 数据核字（2020）第 127229 号

人卫智网	www.ipmph.com	医学教育、学术、考试、健康，购书智慧智能综合服务平台
人卫官网	www.pmph.com	人卫官方资讯发布平台

Fundamentals of Traditional Chinese Medicine Nursing
中医护理学基础（双语）
Zhongyi Hulixue Jichu（Shuangyu）
第 2 版

主　　编：郝玉芳　王诗源
出版发行：人民卫生出版社（中继线 010-59780011）
地　　址：北京市朝阳区潘家园南里 19 号
邮　　编：100021
E - mail：pmph @ pmph.com
购书热线：010-59787592　010-59787584　010-65264830
印　　刷：三河市宏达印刷有限公司（胜利）
经　　销：新华书店
开　　本：850×1168　1/16　　印张：27
字　　数：657 千字
版　　次：2009 年 12 月第 1 版　　2020 年 7 月第 2 版
印　　次：2020 年 8 月第 1 次印刷
标准书号：ISBN 978-7-117-30111-4
定　　价：88.00 元

第六轮修订说明

为了在"十三五"期间，持续深化医药卫生体制改革，贯彻落实《"健康中国 2030"规划纲要》，全面践行《全国护理事业发展规划（2016—2020 年）》，顺应全国高等护理学类专业教育发展与改革的需要，培养能够满足人民群众多样化、多层次健康需求的护理人才。在对第五轮教材进行全面、充分调研的基础上，在国家卫生和计划生育委员会领导下，经第三届全国高等学校护理学专业教材评审委员会的审议和规划，人民卫生出版社于 2016 年 1 月进行了全国高等学校护理学类专业教材评审委员会的换届工作，同时启动全国高等学校本科护理学类专业第六轮规划教材的修订工作。

本轮教材修订得到全国百余所本科院校的积极响应和大力支持，在结合调研结果和我国护理学高等教育的特点及发展趋势的基础上，第四届全国高等学校护理学类专业教材建设指导委员会确定第六轮教材修订的指导思想为：坚持"规范化、精品化、创新化、国际化、数字化"战略，紧扣培养目标，遵循教学规律，围绕提升学生能力，创新编写模式，体现专业特色；构筑学习平台，丰富教学资源，打造一流的、核心的、经典的具有国际影响力的护理学本科教材体系。

第六轮教材的编写原则为：

1. 明确目标性与系统性　本套教材的编写要求定位准确，符合本科教育特点与规律，满足护理学类专业本科学生的培养目标。注重多学科内容的有机融合，减少内容交叉重复，避免某些内容疏漏。在保证单本教材知识完整性的基础上，兼顾各教材之间有序衔接，有机联系，使全套教材整体优化，具有良好的系统性。

2. 坚持科学性与专业性　本套教材编写应坚持"三基五性"的原则，教材编写内容科学、准确，名称、术语规范，体例、体系具有逻辑性。教材须符合护理学专业思想，具有鲜明的护理学专业特色，满足护理学专业学生的教学要求。同时继续加强对学生人文素质的培养。

3. 兼具传承性与创新性　本套教材主要是修订，是在传承上一轮教材优点的基础上，结合上一轮教材调研的反馈意见，进行修改及完善，而不是对原教材进行彻底推翻，以保证教材的生命力和教学活动的延续性。教材编写中根据本学科和相关学科的发展，补充更新学科理论与实践发展的新成果，以使经典教材的传统性和精品教材的时代性完美结合。

4. **体现多元性与统一性**　为适应全国二百余所开办本科护理教育院校的多样化教学需要，本套教材在遵循本科教育基本标准的基础上，既包括有经典的临床学科体系教材，也有生命周期体系教材、中医特色课程教材和双语教材，以供各院校根据自身教学模式的特点选用。本套教材在编写过程中，一方面，扩大了参编院校范围，使教材编写团队更具多元性的特点；另一方面，明确要求，审慎把关，力求各章内容详略一致，整书编写风格统一。

5. **注重理论性与实践性**　本套教材在强化理论知识的同时注重对实践应用的思考，通过教材中的思考题、网络增值服务中的练习题，以及引入案例与问题的教材编写形式等，努力构建理论与实践联系的桥梁，以利于培养学生应用知识、分析问题、解决问题的能力。

全套教材采取新型编写模式，借助扫描二维码形式，帮助教材使用者在移动终端共享与教材配套的优质数字资源，实现纸媒教材与富媒体资源的融合。

全套教材共 50 种，于 2017 年 7 月前由人民卫生出版社出版，供各院校本科护理学类专业使用。

人民卫生出版社

2017 年 5 月

获取图书网络增值服务的步骤说明

❶ ⁃ 扫描封底圆形图标中的二维码，登录图书增值服务激活平台。

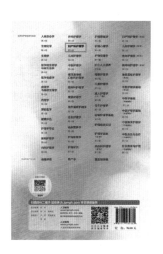

❷ ⁃ 刮开并输入激活码，激活增值服务。

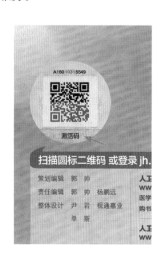

❸ ⁃ 下载"人卫图书增值"客户端。

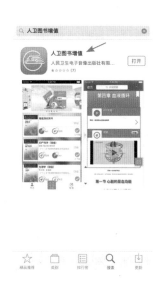

❹ ⁃ 使用客户端"扫码"功能，扫描图书中二维码即可快速查看网络增值服务内容。

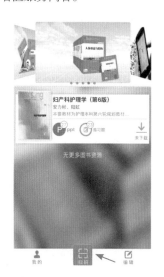

国家卫生和计划生育委员会"十三五"规划教材

全国高等学校本科护理学类专业规划教材

第六轮教材目录

1. 本科护理学类专业教材目录

序号	教材	版次	主审	主编		副主编		
1	人体形态学	第4版		周瑞祥 杨桂姣		王海杰 郝立宏 周劲松		
2	生物化学	第4版		高国全		解 军 方定志 刘 彬		
3	生理学	第4版		唐四元		曲丽辉 张翠英 邢德刚		
4	医学微生物学与寄生虫学	第4版		黄 敏 吴松泉		廖 力 王海河		
5	医学免疫学	第4版	安云庆	司传平		任云青 王 炜 张 艳 胡 洁		
6	病理学与病理生理学	第4版		步 宏		王 雯 李连宏		
7	药理学	第4版		董 志		弥 曼 陶 剑 王金红		
8	预防医学	第4版		凌文华 许能锋		袁 晶 龙鼎新 宋爱芹		
9	健康评估	第4版	吕探云	孙玉梅 张立力		朱大乔 施齐芳 张彩虹 陈利群		
10	护理学导论	第4版		李小妹 冯先琼		王爱敏 隋树杰		
11	基础护理学	第6版		李小寒 尚少梅		王春梅 郑一宁 丁亚萍 吕冬梅		
12	内科护理学	第6版		尤黎明 吴 瑛		孙国珍 王君俏 袁 丽 胡 荣		
13	外科护理学	第6版		李乐之 路 潜		张美芬 汪 晖 李惠萍 许 勤		
14	妇产科护理学	第6版	郑修霞	安力彬 陆 虹		顾 炜 丁 焱 罗碧如		
15	儿科护理学	第6版		崔 焱 仰曙芬		张玉侠 刘晓丹 林素兰		
16	中医护理学	第4版		孙秋华		段亚平 李明今 陆静波		
17	眼耳鼻咽喉口腔科护理学	第4版		席淑新 赵佛容		肖惠明 李秀娥		
18	精神科护理学	第4版		刘哲宁 杨芳宇		许冬梅 贾守梅		
19	康复护理学	第4版		燕铁斌 尹安春		鲍秀芹 马素慧		
20	急危重症护理学	第4版		张 波 桂 莉		金静芬 李文涛 黄素芳		
21	社区护理学	第4版		李春玉 姜丽萍		陈长香		
22	临床营养学	第4版	张爱珍	周 芸		胡 雯 赵雅宁		
23	护理教育学	第4版		姜安丽 段志光		范秀珍 张 艳		
24	护理研究	第5版		胡 雁 王志稳		刘均娥 颜巧元		

序号	教材	版次	主审	主编		副主编			
25	护理管理学	第4版	李继平	吴欣娟	王艳梅	翟惠敏	张俊娥		
26	护理心理学	第4版		杨艳杰	曹枫林	冯正直	周 英		
27	护理伦理学	第2版		姜小鹰	刘俊荣	韩 琳	范宇莹		
28	护士人文修养	第2版		史瑞芬	刘义兰	刘桂瑛	王继红		
29	母婴护理学	第3版		王玉琼	莫洁玲	崔仁善	罗 阳		
30	儿童护理学	第3版	范 玲	崔文香	陈 华	张 瑛			
31	成人护理学（上、下册）	第3版	郭爱敏	周兰姝	王艳玲	陈 红	何朝珠	牟绍玉	
32	老年护理学	第4版	化前珍	胡秀英	肖惠敏	张 静			
33	新编护理学基础	第3版		姜安丽	钱晓路	曹梅娟	王克芳	郭瑜洁	李春卉
34	护理综合实训	第1版		李映兰	王爱平	李玉红	蓝宇涛	高 睿	靳永萍
35	护理学基础（双语）	第2版	姜安丽	王红红	沈 洁	陈晓莉	尼春萍	吕爱莉	周 洁
36	内外科护理学（双语）	第2版	刘华平 李 峥	李 津	张静平	李 卡	李素云	史铁英	张 清
37	妇产科护理学（双语）	第2版		张银萍	单伟颖	张 静	周英凤	谢日华	
38	儿科护理学（双语）	第2版	胡 雁	蒋文慧	赵秀芳	高 燕	张 莹	蒋小平	
39	老年护理学（双语）	第2版		郭桂芳	黄 金	谷岩梅	郭 宏		
40	精神科护理学（双语）	第2版		雷 慧	李小麟	杨 敏	王再超	王小琴	
41	急危重症护理学（双语）	第2版		钟清玲	许 虹	关 青	曹宝花		
42	中医护理学基础（双语）	第2版		郝玉芳	王诗源	杨 柳	王春艳	徐冬英	
43	中医学基础（中医特色）	第2版		陈莉军	刘兴山	高 静	裴秀月	韩新荣	
44	中医护理学基础（中医特色）	第2版		陈佩仪		王俊杰	杨晓玮	郑方道	
45	中医临床护理学（中医特色）	第2版		徐桂华	张先庚	于春光	张雅丽	闫 力	马秋平
46	中医养生与食疗（中医特色）	第2版		于 睿	姚 新	聂 宏	宋 阳		
47	针灸推拿与护理（中医特色）	第2版		刘明军		卢咏梅	董 博		

2．本科助产学专业教材目录

序号	教材	版次	主审	主编		副主编			
1	健康评估	第1版		罗碧如	李 宁	王 跃	邹海欧	李 玲	
2	助产学	第1版	杨慧霞	余艳红	陈 叙	丁 焱	侯 睿	顾 炜	
3	围生期保健	第1版		夏海鸥	徐鑫芬	蔡文智	张银萍		

教材建设指导委员会名单

顾 问	周 军	▸	中日友好医院
	李秀华	▸	中华护理学会
	么 莉	▸	国家卫生计生委医院管理研究所护理中心
	姜小鹰	▸	福建医科大学护理学院
	吴欣娟	▸	北京协和医院
	郑修霞	▸	北京大学护理学院
	黄金月	▸	香港理工大学护理学院
	李秋洁	▸	哈尔滨医科大学护理学院
	娄凤兰	▸	山东大学护理学院
	王惠珍	▸	南方医科大学护理学院
	何国平	▸	中南大学护理学院

| 主任委员 | 尤黎明 | ▸ | 中山大学护理学院 |
| | 姜安丽 | ▸ | 第二军医大学护理学院 |

副主任委员	安力彬	▸	大连大学护理学院
（按姓氏拼音排序）	崔 焱	▸	南京医科大学护理学院
	段志光	▸	山西医科大学
	胡 雁	▸	复旦大学护理学院
	李继平	▸	四川大学华西护理学院
	李小寒	▸	中国医科大学护理学院
	李小妹	▸	西安交通大学护理学院

刘华平	‣	北京协和医学院护理学院
陆　虹	‣	北京大学护理学院
孙宏玉	‣	北京大学护理学院
孙秋华	‣	浙江中医药大学
吴　瑛	‣	首都医科大学护理学院
徐桂华	‣	南京中医药大学
殷　磊	‣	澳门理工学院
章雅青	‣	上海交通大学护理学院
赵　岳	‣	天津医科大学护理学院

常务委员

（按姓氏拼音排序）

曹枫林	‣	山东大学护理学院
郭桂芳	‣	北京大学护理学院
郝玉芳	‣	北京中医药大学护理学院
罗碧如	‣	四川大学华西护理学院
尚少梅	‣	北京大学护理学院
唐四元	‣	中南大学湘雅护理学院
夏海鸥	‣	复旦大学护理学院
熊云新	‣	广西广播电视大学
仰曙芬	‣	哈尔滨医科大学护理学院
于　睿	‣	辽宁中医药大学护理学院
张先庚	‣	成都中医药大学护理学院

本科教材评审委员会名单

指导主委　　　　　　　　尤黎明　　▸　中山大学护理学院

主任委员　　　　　　　　李小妹　　▸　西安交通大学护理学院
　　　　　　　　　　　　崔　焱　　▸　南京医科大学护理学院

副主任委员　　　　　　　郭桂芳　　▸　北京大学护理学院
　　　　　　　　　　　　吴　瑛　　▸　首都医科大学护理学院
　　　　　　　　　　　　唐四元　　▸　中南大学湘雅护理学院

委　　员　　　　　　　　陈　垦　　▸　广东药科大学护理学院
（按姓氏拼音排序）　　　陈京立　　▸　北京协和医学院护理学院
　　　　　　　　　　　　范　玲　　▸　中国医科大学附属盛京医院
　　　　　　　　　　　　付菊芳　　▸　第四军医大学西京医院
　　　　　　　　　　　　桂　莉　　▸　第二军医大学护理学院
　　　　　　　　　　　　何朝珠　　▸　南昌大学护理学院
　　　　　　　　　　　　何桂娟　　▸　浙江中医药大学护理学院
　　　　　　　　　　　　胡　荣　　▸　福建医科大学护理学院
　　　　　　　　　　　　江智霞　　▸　遵义医学院护理学院
　　　　　　　　　　　　李　伟　　▸　潍坊医学院护理学院
　　　　　　　　　　　　李春玉　　▸　延边大学护理学院
　　　　　　　　　　　　李惠玲　　▸　苏州大学护理学院

李惠萍	‣	安徽医科大学护理学院
廖 力	‣	南华大学护理学院
林素兰	‣	新疆医科大学护理学院
刘桂瑛	‣	广西医科大学护理学院
刘义兰	‣	华中科技大学同济医学院附属协和医院
刘志燕	‣	贵州医科大学护理学院
龙 霖	‣	川北医学院护理学院
卢东民	‣	湖州师范学院
牟绍玉	‣	重庆医科大学护理学院
任海燕	‣	内蒙古医科大学护理学院
隋树杰	‣	哈尔滨医科大学护理学院
王 军	‣	山西医科大学汾阳学院
王 强	‣	河南大学护理学院
王爱敏	‣	青岛大学护理学院
王春梅	‣	天津医科大学护理学院
王君俏	‣	复旦大学护理学院
王克芳	‣	山东大学护理学院
王绍锋	‣	九江学院护理学院
王玉琼	‣	成都市妇女儿童中心医院
徐月清	‣	河北大学护理学院
许 虹	‣	杭州师范大学护理学院
许燕玲	‣	上海市第六人民医院
杨立群	‣	齐齐哈尔医学院护理学院
张 瑛	‣	长治医学院护理学院
张彩虹	‣	海南医学院国际护理学院
张会君	‣	锦州医科大学护理学院
张美芬	‣	中山大学护理学院
章泾萍	‣	皖南医学院护理学院
赵佛容	‣	四川大学华西口腔医院
赵红佳	‣	福建中医药大学护理学院
周 英	‣	广州医科大学护理学院

| 秘 书 | 王 婧 | ‣ | 西安交通大学护理学院 |
| | 丁亚萍 | ‣ | 南京医科大学护理学院 |

数字教材评审委员会名单

指导主委	段志光	▸	山西医科大学
主任委员	孙宏玉	▸	北京大学护理学院
	章雅青	▸	上海交通大学护理学院
副主任委员	仰曙芬	▸	哈尔滨医科大学护理学院
	熊云新	▸	广西广播电视大学
	曹枫林	▸	山东大学护理学院
委　员 （按姓氏拼音排序）	柏亚妹	▸	南京中医药大学护理学院
	陈　嘉	▸	中南大学湘雅护理学院
	陈　燕	▸	湖南中医药大学护理学院
	陈晓莉	▸	武汉大学 HOPE 护理学院
	郭爱敏	▸	北京协和医学院护理学院
	洪芳芳	▸	桂林医学院护理学院
	鞠　梅	▸	西南医科大学护理学院
	蓝宇涛	▸	广东药科大学护理学院
	李　峰	▸	吉林大学护理学院
	李　强	▸	齐齐哈尔医学院护理学院
	李彩福	▸	延边大学护理学院
	李春卉	▸	吉林医药学院

李芳芳   ▸   第二军医大学护理学院

李文涛   ▸   大连大学护理学院

李小萍   ▸   四川大学护理学院

孟庆慧   ▸   潍坊医学院护理学院

商临萍   ▸   山西医科大学护理学院

史铁英   ▸   大连医科大学附属第一医院

万丽红   ▸   中山大学护理学院

王桂云   ▸   山东协和学院护理学院

谢　晖   ▸   蚌埠医学院护理学系

许　勤   ▸   南京医科大学护理学院

颜巧元   ▸   华中科技大学护理学院

张　艳   ▸   郑州大学护理学院

周　洁   ▸   上海中医药大学护理学院

庄嘉元   ▸   福建医科大学护理学院

秘　书　　　　　　杨　萍   ▸   北京大学护理学院

范宇莹   ▸   哈尔滨医科大学护理学院

吴觉敏   ▸   上海交通大学护理学院

网络增值服务编者名单

主　编　　郝玉芳　王诗源

副主编　　王春艳　杨　柳　徐冬英

编　者　　（按姓氏笔画排序）

马雪玲　　　　▸　北京中医药大学护理学院

王　黎　　　　▸　北京中医药大学护理学院

王云翠　　　　▸　湖北中医药大学护理学院

王诗源　　　　▸　山东中医药大学护理学院

王春艳　　　　▸　吉林医药学院护理学院

王秋琴　　　　▸　南京中医药大学护理学院

尹永田　　　　▸　山东中医药大学护理学院

乔　雪　　　　▸　北京中医药大学护理学院

孙瑞阳　　　　▸　北京中医药大学护理学院

苏春香　　　　▸　北京中医药大学护理学院

杨　柳　　　　▸　福建中医药大学护理学院

杨晓玮　　　　▸　北京中医药大学护理学院

杨金花　　　　▸　湖南中医药大学护理学院

周云仙　　　　▸　浙江中医药大学护理学院

单亚维　　　　▸　上海中医药大学护理学院

郝玉芳　　　　▸　北京中医药大学护理学院

姜　婧　　　　▸　北京中医药大学护理学院

徐冬英　　　　▸　广西中医药大学护理学院

郭海玲　　　　▸　北京中医药大学东直门医院

主编简介

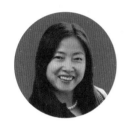

郝玉芳

郝玉芳，护理学博士、教授、博士生导师，北京市护理学重点学科带头人，国家中医药管理局重点学科带头人。北京中医药大学国际循证中医药研究院副院长，北京中医药大学循证护理研究中心主任，JBI循证护理合作中心顾问，RNAO BPSO最佳实践指南研究中心主任。教育部高等学校护理学类专业教学指导委员会委员；全国中医药高等医学教育学会护理教育研究会理事长；残疾人事业发展研究会照护专业委员会副主任委员；北京医学会临床流行病与循证医学分会第三届委员会循证护理学组副组长等。主持和参与各级课题80余项；发表学术论文160余篇（其中SCI文章8篇）；参与了17本教材的编写，主编其中的8本。获北京市高等学校优秀青年骨干教师，校级教学名师称号。其主持的循证护理学课程获国家精品在线开放课程。

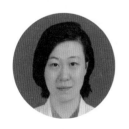

王诗源

王诗源，医学博士、研究生导师。从事中医临床诊疗、中医护理教育、管理及科研工作。发表核心论文70余篇，SCI论文5篇；参与编写国家"十二五""十三五"规划中医类教材6部；主持及参与省部级、厅局级各类课题20余项；获得山东中医药科学技术奖，山东省高校优秀科研成果奖，山东省教学成果奖等多项科研、教学奖励；编写多部护理、科普及医学类专著。

副主编简介

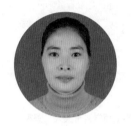

杨柳

杨柳,教授、硕士生导师。曾多次赴丹麦哥本哈根CVU Oeresund大学、香港理工大学等护理学院交流访学。主持或参与国家、省厅级课题10余项;近年来在核心期刊发表学术论文30余篇,SCI收录4篇(JCR I区3篇);获国家专利6项;副主编或参编规划教材及教学参考书10余本;荣获福建省学校教学成果二等奖。现任教福建中医药大学,主讲硕士、本科生中医护理学基础等课程,主要研究方向为中西医结合护理学(肿瘤、康复方向)。

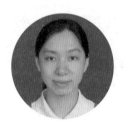

王春艳

王春艳,医学博士、教授、硕士生导师,现任吉林医药学院护理学院副院长、吉林医药学院护理学院护理实训中心主任。主讲中医护理学基础、护理学基础等课程;主编《康复医学基础》,参编《护理心理学》《精神科护理学》等教材;兼任中国老年保健医学研究会精准健康医学分会委员、中国生物物理学会生物微量元素分会委员。

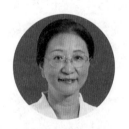

徐冬英

徐冬英,医学博士、硕士研究生导师、广西中医药大学护理学院教授。世界中联护理专业委员会第一届理事会理事,全国高等医学教育学会护理教育分会专家委员会专家。曾到加拿大阿尔伯特大学、英国诺丁汉大学女王医学中心、香港浸会大学作高级访问学者;主持省级、校级科研课题6项,参与国家自然科学基金项目1项;研究方向为中医护理理论与临床应用、中药药性理论与临床应用;代表性学术论著有《三七的药学与临床研究》;主编的教材有国家"十二五"规划教材《壮药学》《专业英语基础》等3部;发表学术论文50余篇,其中SCI 3篇;曾荣获科研成果、教学成果多项。

前 言

按照国家《中医药发展战略规划纲要（2016—2030 年）》以及《中共中央 国务院关于促进中医药传承创新发展的意见》，中医药的发展迎来了千载难逢的历史性机遇。中医护理凭借其独特的理论和实用的护理技术，在预防保健、术后康复和慢性疾病护理中充分体现其"简、便、廉、验、效"的优势。中医护理将中医养生康复方法融入慢性病管理中，不但丰富了护理工作方法、充实了护理健康教育内容，也有力地降低了医疗成本、丰富了中医护理的内涵。中医护理从以疾病为中心转为以健康为中心，加强对疾病预防的重视，不仅与健康中国战略目标高度一致，而且更贴近生活，也更易被人们接受。人民群众对中医护理服务的需求也越来越高。

近几年，国内对中医护理专业人才的需求日益增加，同时国外护理同仁对学习中医护理的需求也在增长。为了满足国内外对中医护理人才和中医护理国际交流与合作的需要，加快中医护理国际化进程，培养出更多具有对外交流能力、有中医特色的高水平护理人才，我们于 2009 年组织专家编写了国内第一本《中医护理学基础》双语教材，这本教材对推动中医护理国际化起到重要的作用。本次教材编写是对上一版教材进行修订，本教材更注重用词的规范性，各章节更加突出实用性和可操作性，同时还进行了多种形式的数字化教育资源的开发。

本教材编写组成员包括护理学、中医学、针灸推拿学专家，各章内容经过多位专家多次审定，保证了其科学性、新颖性、系统性和实用性。

《中医护理学基础》主要介绍中医护理基础理论和基本技能，是中医护理学科的专业基础课程。基础理论方面包括中医基础理论、中药和方剂知识及辨证施护的基础理论。基本技能包括一般护理、针灸、推拿和中医传统护理技术，如拔罐法、刮痧法、熏洗法、热熨法等。具体内容涵盖中医护理学发展简史、中医基础理论概述、经络腧穴概述、中医护理的基本特点和原则、一般护理、中医用药护理及传统的护理技术操作。

本教材可供中西医护理院校护理本科生及涉外方向护理本科生教学使用，对中国传统医学感兴趣的留学生也可用作参考用书。

编写本教材是一项艰巨的工作，编写组付出了很大的努力，但由于经验不足和编者水平有限，仍会存在一些问题，希望大家提出宝贵意见，我们会进一步修订改进。

郝玉芳　王诗源

2019 年 12 月

目 录

Chapter 5

235 **Medication and Nursing of TCM**

第五章

235 **中医用药及护理**

Chapter 1 Introduction

第一章 绪 论

Learning Objectives	学习目标

Mastery

1. To repeat the brief history of TCM nursing.
2. To repeat the famous physicians, works, and relevant theories and techniques of TCM nursing in different historical stages.

Comprehension

To explain connotation and mission of TCM nursing.

识记

1. 能复述中医护理发展简史。

2. 能复述各历史阶段的著名医家、著作、有关中医护理理论与技术观点。

理解

理解中医护理学的任务和范畴。

Case Study

In the Three-State Period (AD 220—280), administer Ni Xun and Li Yan went to see doctor Hua Tuo, both suffering from headache and fever. After diagnosis, Hua Tuo said: "Dispersing method should be used for Ni Xun, while sweating method should be used for Li Yan." Some people didn't understand. Hua Tuo explained that "Ni Xun suffered from exterior excess and the evil qi accumulated in the body, like the accumulated water in the mountain, thus reducing method should be used to disperse the evil pathogen. While Li Yan suffered from interior excess and it was easy to get excessive fire flowing up, just like the earth qi stagnation, thus sweating method should be used to disperse the evil pathogen." Different prescriptions were given to them and both recovered the next day.

Question 1: Two persons with the same symptom were given different medical treatments. What theories or principles is it based on?

Question 2: What are the differences and similarities in nursing for patients with the same kind of symptom but different syndrome-pattern?

In the long process of formation and development of Traditional Chinese Medicine (TCM), ancient Chinese philosophy plays an extremely important role in the ideology system of TCM culture. Ancient physicians melted the ancient philosophy essence into TCM, combined with abundant medical knowledge and clinical experience, formed the unique TCM theory system and have guided the clinical practice over a long period of time. The relationship between TCM and the ancient philosophy is primarily manifested in the original qi theory that explores the origin of the universe, yin-yang theory that observes the nature of life, and five-phase theory that explores the structure of life and its interactions.

Section 1   Connotation and Mission of TCM Nursing

TCM nursing (also called nursing in Chinese medicine) is a subject which is old yet young. Guided by theories of TCM, it adopts the concept of holism and nursing determination based on pattern differentiation. It is a practical science, which combines prevention, health care, rehabilitation and medicine to take care of the sick, the old, the weak, the young and the handicapped, and

导入案例与思考

三国时期，府吏倪寻和李延去找华佗看病，两人都是头痛发热，华佗给二人诊断后说："倪寻应当用下泄的方法治疗，而李延应当用发汗的方法治疗。"有人不解，华佗解释："倪寻外实，邪气滞留体内，就好比山间积水，需要用下的方法来疏导；李延内实，内实就容易实火上冲，就好像地气郁结，需要用发汗的方法来发散。"于是就给二人开了不同的方子，次日两人的病情都有所好转。

问题 1：两人症状相同治法不同，其依据什么中医理论或原则？

问题 2：针对同一症状但不同证型的患者，其护理上有何异同？

中医学历史源远流长，在其思想体系形成和发展的过程中，中国古代哲学占有极其重要的地位。古代医家将当时的哲学思想融入中医学中，结合几千年来与疾病作斗争的诊疗经验，形成了中医学独特的理论体系，并长期指导着临床实践。中医与中国古代哲学的关系，主要体现在中国古代哲学中探索宇宙本源的"元气论"，认识生命本质的"阴阳学说"以及探索生命结构及其关系的"五行学说"。

第一节　中医护理学的概念和任务

中医护理学是中医学的重要组成部分，它是一门既古老、又年轻的学科，有着悠久的历史，是以中医理论为指导，在整体观念指导下，运用辨证施护的方法，结合预防、养生保健、康复等措施，对患者及老、弱、幼、残者加以照料，并施以独特的护理

implements specific nursing techniques to safeguard the health of people. Along with the prosperity of TCM, the theories and techniques of TCM nursing are becoming more and more systematic, concrete and abundant. In the last several decades, under the influence of the transformation of medical mode and rapid progress of the nursing science, modern nursing theories and traditional nursing theories and techniques have been combined together. TCM nursing has thus developed itself into an independent subject.

TCM nursing has rich connotation and unique theories, approaches and techniques. The basic characteristics of TCM nursing is the concept of holism and nursing determination based on pattern, including the basic theory, basic techniques and clinical nursing practice. It consists of knowledge about disease prevention, health care, life cultivation, rehabilitation and so on. The basic theory includes the basic theory of TCM, the knowledge of Chinese Materia medica and prescriptions and the basic theory about nursing determination based on pattern differentiation. The clinical nursing practice includes the general nursing, acupuncture, moxibustion, massage and many other kinds of traditional Chinese nursing techniques such as skin scraping therapy, fumigating and steaming therapy, plastering-ironing therapy, and blood-letting therapy. It also introduces nursing determination based on pattern differentiation on common diseases in internal medicine, surgery, gynecology, pediatrics *etc.*.

This textbook, called *Fundamentals of Nursing Practice in Chinese Medicine*, mainly introduces the basic theories and techniques in TCM nursing.

(Hao Yu-fang)

技术，以促进、维持和恢复人类健康的一门应用学科。随着中医药事业的蓬勃发展，中医护理理论与技术逐步系统化、具体化，内容更加丰富。近几十年，在医学模式转变和护理学飞速发展的影响下，将现代护理学理论与传统的中医护理理论和技术相结合，中医护理学更加完善，逐渐形成为一门独立的学科。

中医护理学内涵丰富，有独特理念、方法和技术。中医护理学的基本特点是整体观念和辨证施护。具体内容分为基础理论、基本技能和临床护理。基础理论方面包括中医基础理论、中药和方剂知识及辨证施护的基础理论。基本技能包括一般护理、针灸、推拿和中医传统护理技术，如拔罐法、刮痧法、熏洗法、热熨法、放血法等，临床护理包括内科、外科、妇科、儿科等临床比较常见病证的辨证施护。

《中医护理学基础》主要介绍中医护理基础理论知识和基本技能，是中医护理学科的专业基础课程。

（郝玉芳）

Section 2　Brief History of TCM Nursing

第二节　中医护理学发展简史

The formation and development of TCM nursing have experienced a long historical period. Since the ancient times, diseases treatment with TCM has incorporated medicine, Chinese materia medica and nursing together. Though TCM nursing science did not develop into an independent subject in the past, abundant knowledge, theories and techniques of TCM nursing can be extracted from various kinds of ancient medical works.

中医护理学的形成和发展，经历了漫长的历史阶段。自古以来，中医治病都是集医、药、护为一体，在历史上虽然没有形成中医护理专门学科，但是我国传统医药学中一直都包含有丰富的护理内容，中医护理学的理论和技术内容散见于历代各种医学著作中。

I. Ancient TCM Nursing

i. Germination Period (Remote Antiquity—21 Century BC)

In ancient times, people accumulated rich experiences on self-protecting in the process of fighting with nature, experiences like using leaves and animal skin to make clothes in order to shield against the chilly weather, using tree branches for fixation after a severe bone fracture, rinsing the wounded area with clean water, covering the wound with materials like grass, soil or leaves, massaging the bruised area, using fire to get warmth *etc.*. These self-protecting methods become the bud of the primeval nursing techniques such as fixation of bone fracture, wound area, massage, moxibustion, *etc.*. People gained knowledge about food compatibility and counteraction by posing experiments on various animals and plants. According to legend, Shen Nong is the founder of Chinese medicine, as it was said in *Tong Jian Wai Ji* (*Tōng Jiàn Wài Jì*, 通鉴外纪): "In ancient times, people knew nothing about herbs and medicine, and if attacked by diseases, they could do nothing. Thus, Emperor Yan started to taste all kinds of herbs for his people. He came across seventy kinds of poison in one day and detoxified all miraculously. Since then, he started to write medical books on disease treatment for his people, and that was the time when Chinese medicine was established". Gradually the oral administration and external application of Chinese herbs became prevalent.

Box 1-1 Learning More

A Well-Known Legend of Shen Nong

The most widely spread story about Shen Nong is Shen Nong tasted hundreds of herbs. In the myths and legends, Shen Nong was described with a head of cow, born with a transparent "crystal belly". Therefore, his organs were visible, and what he ate could be seen from the outside clearly. In ancient times, people knew nothing about farming, but were fed with wild fruits or raw animals' meat, often got poisoned and even died. In order to treat diseases and save lives, Yan Emperor, Shen Nong traveled all over the earth, tasted hundreds of plants to dig out their medicinal properties. "Shen Nong once got poisoned 70 times in a day while tasting various plants to find the edible herbs." In the process of tasting plants, Shen Nong found the herbs that could cure diseases and had the function of health preservation. Thus, he was honored as "saint of herbs" by ancient people.

一、古代中医护理学

（一）萌芽时期（远古～公元前21世纪）

远古时期，人类在与大自然斗争的过程积累中了大量的自我保护经验，如用树叶和兽皮做衣遮体可御风寒，受伤后用树枝干进行骨折后固定，用溪水冲洗伤口，用草茎、泥土、树叶对伤口进行涂裹，对四肢的跌打损伤处进行揉按，用火取暖等，这些成为骨折后固定、伤口处理、按摩、灸法等中医护理技术的萌芽。此外，人们通过对各种动植物的尝试，了解食物宜忌。传说神农氏为医学的创立者，《通鉴外纪》中记载："民有疾病，未知药石，炎帝始味草木之滋，尝一日遇七十毒，神而化之，遂作方书，以疗民疾，而医道立矣。"之后逐渐有了中草药的内服、外敷等。

知识拓展1-1
神农尝百草

有关神农氏的故事，流传最广的就是神农尝百草，神话传说中神农氏是牛头人身，民间还传说神农氏生来就长了一副透明的"水晶肚"，五脏六腑清晰可见，吃下什么东西，从外面都能看得清清楚楚。远古时期，人们还不懂农耕，以采食野生瓜果，生吃动物蚌蛤为生，经常有人误食有毒的食物而中毒、死亡。炎帝神农氏为"宣药疗疾"，救天伤人命，使百姓益寿延年。他跋山涉水，行遍三湘大地，尝遍百草，了解百草之平毒寒温之药性，为民找寻治病解毒良药，"神农尝百草，一日遇七十毒"，他几乎嚼尝过所有植物。神农在尝百草的过程中，识别了百草，发现了具有攻毒祛病、养生保健作用的中药。由此令民有所就，不复为疾病，故先民封他为"药神"。

ii. Period of Xia to Chunqiu (21 Century BC—475 BC)

During the period of Xia to Chunqiu, medicine became an independent subject and the earliest medicine discipline was established. It was written in *Rites of the Zhou Dynasty* (*Zhōu Lǐ*,周礼) that different grades of full-time staff were set up in the medical field, among which named *apprentice* were responsible for patient caring. Since then, people started to realize the importance of personal hygiene and began to participate in environmental and hygiene activities like pollution discharge and deinsectization. They gradually formed the notion of balanced diets and discovered that excessive emotional activities would lead to diseases. It was written in *Rites of the Zhou Dynasty*: "Whenever curing the wound, attack it with five kinds of poison, nurture it with five kinds of gases, treat it with five kinds of medicine and regulate it with five kinds of flavor. As for medicine, the sour nurtures the bone, the spicy nurtures the tendon, the salty nurtures the veins, sweetness nurtures the muscle and greasy nurtures the aperture." It also said, "Emotions like happiness, rage, sadness, joy, love, disgust and lust will damage one's health if excessive" and so on.

iii. From Warring States Period to East Han (475 BC—AD 220)

During the time of Warring States to East Han, *The Yellow Emperor's Inner Classic* (*Huáng Dì Nèi Jīng*, 黄帝内经), *Treatise on Cold Damage and Miscellaneous Diseases* (*Shāng Hán Zá Bìng Lùn*, 伤寒杂病论), *Shen Nong's Classic of the Materia Medica* (*Shén Nóng Běn Cǎo Jīng*, 神农本草经) were published, laying the foundation of TCM theory system. A large amount of content of TCM nursing were scattered across these works.

1. *The Yellow Emperor's Inner Classic* lays the groundwork for the establishment and development of theoretical and clinical system of TCM. *The Yellow Emperor's Inner Classic* is the earliest extant medical classic in China that comparatively expounds the system of TCM. It consists of two books, *Basic Questions* (*Sù Wèn*,素问) and *The Spiritual Pivot* (*Líng Shū*, 灵枢). It systematically expatiates on the theories of human physiology and pathology, as well as diagnosis, prevention and treatment of diseases. It lays a solid foundation for the establishment and development of theoretical and clinical system of TCM. In the aspects of TCM nursing, it expounds

（二）夏至春秋时期（公元前 21 世纪—公元前 475 年）

夏～春秋时期，建立了最早的医学制度。《周礼·天官》中记载，医师之下设有士、府、史、徒等专职人员。"徒"有看护患者的职责。当时开始注意个人卫生习惯、开始有排污、灭虫等环境卫生活动，有了饮食调养意识，也认识到过激的情志活动会导致疾病。《周礼》相关的记载有："凡疗疡，以五毒攻之，以五气养之，以五药疗之，以五味节之。凡药，以酸养骨，以辛养筋，以咸养脉，以甘养肉，以滑养窍"；又云："喜、怒、哀、乐、爱、恶、欲之情，过则伤"等认识。

（三）战国至东汉时期（公元前 475—公元 220 年）

战国至东汉时期，《黄帝内经》《伤寒杂病论》《神农本草经》的相继问世，为中医理论体系的形成奠定了基础。大量的中医护理内容散见于这些医学著作中。

1.《黄帝内经》《黄帝内经》（简称《内经》）是我国现存最早，比较全面、系统阐述中医学理论体系的古典医学巨著，包括《素问》和《灵枢》两部分，系统阐述了人体生理、病理以及疾病的诊断、治疗和预防等内容，形成了中医学独特的理论体系，为中医学理论的形成与发展奠定了坚实的基础。在中医护理学方面，论述了病证护理、饮食护理、生活起居护理、情志护理、养生康复护理、服药护理以及针灸、推拿、导引、热熨、

syndrome nursing, dietary nursing, daily life nursing, emotion nursing, life cultivation and rehabilitation nursing, medication nursing and nursing techniques such as acupuncture and moxibustion, tuina (Chinese medical massage), *dǎo yǐn*, hot compressing and fumigating and steaming therapy, *etc.*. Therefore, *The Yellow Emperor's Inner Classic* also establishes the foundation of TCM nursing.

(1) Daily life nursing: For example, *Basic Questions* points out that for daily life nursing, one should "abide by the rule of yin and yang and the principle of nature, regulate the diet and the living habit and avoid overstrain", which is not only the principle of health cultivation and disease prevention, but also the method of self-nursing. *The Yellow Emperor's Inner Classic* also indicates the concept of "adapting to the variation of seasons and following the rules of nature". It states the law of life cultivation according to seasonal variation and embodies the concept of holism that human beings should be integrated into the nature.

(2) Dietary nursing: In the aspect of dietary nursing, it points out the diet taboos of five visceral diseases that "liver disease patients should avoid pungent food, heart disease patients should avoid salty food, spleen disease patients should avoid acid food and kidney disease patients should avoid bitter food." In the chapter of dieting for illness, it explicates that "patients with spleen trouble should eat steamed rice japonica, beef, jujube and kwai. Patients with heart diseases should have wheat, mutton, apricot and allium japonicum. Patients with kidney diseases should eat soybean, pork, chestnut and leaves of pulse plants; patients with liver problems should have plum, leek. Patients with lung diseases should eat coarse rice, chicken, peach and scallion." In terms of nursing of five visceral diseases, *The Yellow Emperor's Inner Classic* states that "when the spleen is sick, one should neither eat warm or hot food or overeat, nor stay in damp place or wear wet clothes. When the lung is ill, one should neither eat cold food nor wear thin clothes".

(3) Emotional nursing: *The Yellow Emperor's Inner Classic* also highlights mental and psychological nursing which is regarded as an important factor attached to the paroxysm, the progress and prognosis of diseases. It emphasizes that undesirable mental stimulation will cause qi and blood disorder in the body, visceral dysfunction, and induce or exacerbate diseases. For example, "rage causes qi to rise up" "ecstasy causes qi to move slowly" "grief causes qi to be consumed" "fear causes qi to sink" "shock causes qi to disarranged" "obsession causes qi stagnation". Nursing of inter-restriction among emotions and the method of persuasion also are recorded, such as

洗药等护理技术，因此《内经》奠定了中医护理学的基础。

（1）生活起居护理：《素问·上古天真论》指出"法于阴阳，和于数术，食饮有节，起居有常，不妄作劳。"指出要遵循自然界阴阳变化的规律，要按时起卧，劳逸适度。这不仅是养生防病之道，也是日常生活自我调护之理。《内经》之"顺四时而适寒暑"理论，指出了四时养生起居的规律，体现了人与天地相应的整体观。

（2）饮食护理：如在五脏病变饮食的禁忌中指出"肝病禁辛、心病禁咸、脾病禁酸、肾病禁甘、肺病禁苦。"在疾病饮食宜忌中指出"脾病者，宜食粳米饭、牛肉、枣、葵；心病者，宜食麦、羊肉、杏、薤；肾病者宜食大豆黄卷、猪肉、栗、藿；肝病者，宜食麻、犬肉、李、韭；肺病者，宜食黄黍、鸡肉、桃、葱。"对五脏病证的饮食护理，《素问·藏气法时论》中指出"病在脾……禁温食饱食、湿地濡衣""病在肺……禁寒饮食、寒衣"等。

（3）情志护理：《内经》也高度重视情志护理，认为这关系到疾病的发生、发展及预后，强调不良情志刺激可导致人体气血失调，脏腑功能紊乱，而诱发或加重病情，如"怒则气上""喜则气缓""悲则气消""恐则气下""惊则气乱""思则气结"等。《内经》还记载了情志相胜法、说理开导法等情志护理方法。如："悲胜怒，恐胜喜，怒胜思，喜胜忧，思胜恐。"即运用五行之间相生相克原理，

"sorrow overcomes anger" "fear overcomes joy" " anger overcomes thought" "joy overcomes grief" "thought overcomes fear" in *Basic Questions*, which is formed to harmonize the emotions on the basis of inter-restriction and inter-promotion relationship among the seven emotions. One emotion that can restrict the other one can be used to transfer and disturb the other emotion if it becomes excessive enough to damage people's health. The method of persuasion means persuading patients by using correct and wise words to correct their viewpoints, help them to realize the detriments brought by their behavior, relieve their unnecessary worries, boost their confidence in fighting against diseases, follow doctors and nurses' advice to achieve soon recovery.

(4) Observation of illness: The human organ theory in *The Yellow Emperor's Inner Classic* provides a guide for patients' condition observation in TCM nursing. For example, it was recorded in *Basic Question* (*Sù Wèn*, 素问) that "excess of yang qi leads to fever with no sweating, excess of ying qi loads to profuse sweating and chill, excess of both yin and yang lead to chill without sweating."

(5) Nursing techniques: In addition, many special nursing methods are noted in *Yellow Emperor's Inner Classic*, such as acupuncture and moxibustion, *dǎoyǐn*, tuina and hot compressing, which are still applied in the clinical nursing up to the present.

2. *Treatise on Cold Damage and Miscellaneous Diseases* *Treatise on Cold Damage and Miscellaneous Diseases* is the most influential masterwork of clinical medicine in China written by a famous physician Zhang Zhong-jing (AD 150—219) in the late East Han Dynasty (AD 25—220). This work sums up clinical experience of many physicians before the East Han Dynasty (AD 25—220). It not only lays the foundation of the system of treatment based on pattern differentiation in TCM, but also expounds the theory and methods of nursing based on pattern differentiation, and creates a precedent for the clinical nursing based on this system.

(1) Nursing techniques: In the aspect of nursing techniques and its manipulations, *Treatise on Cold Damage and Miscellaneous Diseases* expounds in detail the fumigating and steaming therapy, smoke fumigating therapy, medicated hip bath therapy, needle-cauterizing therapy, spot ironing therapy and feet-soaking therapy. Especially the medicated cluster therapy initiated by Zhang Zhong-jing (AD 150—219), such as the honey suppository and hog's bile enema, fully reflects the

来转移和减轻有害情绪。"告之以其败、语之以其善、导之以其所便、开之以其所苦",即通过说理开导,鼓励患者战胜疾病。

(4)病情观察:《内经》还指导着中医护理的病情观察,例如《素问·脉要精微论》中"阳气有余为身热无汗,阴气有余为多汗身寒,阴阳有余则无汗而寒";《素问·经脉别论》中"饮食饱甚,汗出于胃,惊而夺精,汗出于心。持重远行,汗出于肾。疾走恐惧,还处于肝。摇体劳苦,汗出于脾。"分别讲述了通过观察患者汗液来指导护理。

(5)护理技术:《内经》记载的中医护理技术,包括针灸、导引、推拿、热熨等,至今仍在临床护理中继续使用。

2.《伤寒杂病论》 东汉末年著名医学家张仲景的《伤寒杂病论》,是我国最有影响的一部临床医学巨著。它总结了东汉以前众多医家的临床经验,不仅奠定了中医辨证论治的理论体系,还论述了对疾病的辨证施护的理论和措施,为临床辨证施护开创了先河。

(1)护理技术:《伤寒杂病论》较详细地论述了熏洗法、烟熏法、坐浴法、点烙法、渍脚法等。特别是张仲景首创了药物灌肠法,如"蜜煎导方"及猪胆汁灌肠法,充分反映东汉时期的护理发展水平。在急救护理方面提出了对自缢者的抢救方法,与现代人工呼吸法极其相似。

advanced level of nursing of the East Han Dynasty. In the aspect of emergency nursing, the way to treat the self-hanging person recorded in the book is similar to the modern pneumatogenie.

(2) Medication nursing: In terms of medication nursing, *Treatise on Cold Damage and Miscellaneous Diseases* also expatiates on herbal decocting methods, medicine precautions, effect observation and diet taboos. One can find these nursing requests in attached annotations of many prescriptions in this book, such as *Dà Qīng Lóng Tāng, Wǔ Líng Sǎn, Shí Zǎo Tāng, Dà Chéng Qì Tāng, Gān Cǎo Fù Zǐ Tāng, Fáng Jǐ Huáng Qí Tāng*. For example, in the annotation of *Guì Zhī Tāng*, it notes that "use seven litres (1 ancient litre is equal to 1.5kg) of water to decoct the herbs with weak fire and stop decocting when the decoction becomes three litres, then get rid of the dreg and drink one litre." It requires that after taking the decoction one may "eat one litre hot gruel to help exert the power of the decoction" and "keep warm with quilt for about two hours and mildly sweat all over the body to get better effect", but the diaphoresis "should not be too heavy, or the illness wouldn't be cured." In the aspect of diet taboos, it advises that after taking *Guì Zhī Tāng* one should "keep away from the food that is raw or cold, sticky or slippery, meaty or starchy, pungent or spicy, alcoholic or milky or effluvial."

(3) Dietary nursing: *Treatise on Cold Damage and Miscellaneous Diseases* has a special chapter describing dietary nursing. For example, the taboos for eating bird, beast, fish, worm fruit, vegetable and paddy, the taboos for visceral illness, the taboos for four seasons, the taboos for cold and hot food and the food taboos for pregnant women. It clearly points out that diet should be decided based on pattern differentiation. It indicates that "some food you eat is good for your body, while some is harmful. Appropriate food benefits the body, while harmful food leads to illness." About food sanitation, it warns that "stale meal, rotten meat and olid fish are harmful to the body" "eating too many plums will injure the teeth" "the meat must be rotten and inedible if it floats on water" "the meat with white dots on it is inedible".

Besides, in the aspects of treatment and nursing, *Treatise on Cold Damage and Miscellaneous Diseases* emphasizes on disease prevention and early treatment and preventions from further development of illness. It says "it is better to reinforce the spleen for treatment of a liver disease since the liver disease often affects the spleen."

3. *Shen Nong's Classic of the Materia Medica*
Shen Nong's Classic of the Materia Medica is the earliest pharmacology book existing in China, describes medication nursing. The book categorizes medicine into four natures

（2）服药护理：《伤寒杂病论》对煎药方法，服药注意事项，观察服药后反应及服药期间的饮食宜忌均有详细记载。诸如此类的护理要求，在大青龙汤、五苓散、十枣汤、大承气汤、甘草附子汤、防己黄芪汤等方后注中都有详细记载，还告诫应"如法将息"。如《伤寒论》桂枝汤方后注明在煎煮时应"以水七升，微火煮取三升，去渣，适寒温，一升"，而服药后又应"啜热稀粥一升余，以助药力"，并还应"温覆令一时许，遍身漐漐微似有汗者益佳"。认为出汗，"不可令如水流漓，病必不除"。且在服药后的饮食禁忌方面主张服桂枝汤后要"禁生冷、黏滑、肉面、五辛、酒酪、臭恶等物"。

（3）饮食护理：《伤寒杂病论》针对饮食护理有专篇论述。如对禽兽鱼虫及果实菜谷的禁忌，指出了五脏病食忌、四时食忌、冷热食忌、妊娠食忌等。明确指出了饮食也应辨证，所谓"所食之味，有与病相宜，有与身为害，若得宜则益体，害则成疾。"在饮食卫生方面，已明确告诫"秽饭、馁肉、臭鱼、食之皆伤人""梅多食，坏人齿""猪肉落水浮者，不可食""肉中有米点者，不可食"等。

此外，在治疗与护理上，《伤寒杂病论》强调未病先防和既病防变的观点，如"见肝之病，知肝传脾，当先实脾"等预防医学的思想。

3.《神农本草经》《神农本草经》是我国现存最早的药物学专著，阐述了用药护理内容。书中将药物分为寒、凉、温、热四性，

(cold, cool, warm and hot), and into five flavors (sour, bitter, sweet, spicy and salty). It also establishes the medication principle of "treat cold with hot medicine, treat hot with cold medicine". For medicine with toxic effects, it emphasizes that it should be taken starting with small doses and be gradually increased. The book also mentions the influences that time and method of medicine intake directly have on drug effects. This book works as an important guidance for nursing staff on drug administration, toxic and side effects observation and observations after medicine intake.

4. Hua Tuo Hua Tuo (AD 145—208), a noted physician in the late Han Dynasty and Three Kingdoms period, is the founder of surgery and medical sports. He adopted the essence of the "*dǎo yǐn*" of forerunners and invented the *Wǔ Qín Xì* (five mimic-animal games) which imitated the motions of the five animals: tiger, dear, bear, monkey and bird, is the founder of surgery and medicinal physical training. He held that for keeping fit which required to "have moderate labor but no overstrain, because movement promotes easy digestion and smooth blood circulation. People can avoid diseases by movement just as the door hinge never gets worm-eaten." *Wǔ Qín Xì* exercises are helpful for digestion, promoting qi and blood circulation, reinforcing constitution and decreasing illness. *Wǔ Qín Xì* is the earliest health-care and surgical nursing method in the world that integrates medicine, nursing and physical training together. The other great contribution of Hua Tuo is the invention of *Má Fèi Sàn* (powder for anesthesia) that is used as the general anesthetic in surgery. During the operation, the students of Hua Tuo and the relatives of the patients were guided to do much nursing work. So Hua Tuo can be regarded as the earliest expert of surgical nursing in China.

iv. Wei, Jin, Northern and Southern Dynasties (AD 220—581)

1. The Pulse Classic *The Pulse Classic* (*Mài Jīng*, 脉经) written by Wang Shu-he (AD 201—280) in the Jin Dynasty (AD 265—420), different pulses are regulated and summed up to 24 kinds of pulses. It deeply expounds the theory of pulses, compares the biological and pathological pulse conditions of different visceral organs and analyses the syndromes indicated by the pulses of all kinds of miscellaneous diseases, and diseases of pediatrics and gynecology. It clearly brings forward the theories that examine the pulse should be at *cùn kǒu* (wrist pulse) and each of the six regional pulses corresponds to one of the *zang-fu* organs and the sign of pulse examination reveals the pathological changes of the corresponding organs. It makes the pulse examination become important means of

酸、苦、甘、辛、咸五味，明确了"治寒以热药，治热以寒药"的用药原则；对有毒性作用的药物，强调必须从小剂量开始，逐渐增加剂量；认识到服药的时间和方法直接影响药物效果。该书在用药剂量、毒副作用及用药后效果观察方面对护理人员有重要的指导意义。

4. 华佗 华佗是后汉三国时期的名医，是我国外科和医疗体育的奠基人，他吸取了前人"导引"的精华，模仿虎、鹿、熊、猿、鸟等禽兽的运动姿态，创造了"五禽戏"，奠定了我国外科和传统体育的基础。他认为人体健康，应"欲得劳动，但不当使极耳，动摇则谷得消，血脉流通，病不得生，譬如户枢不朽也"。"五禽戏"可以帮助消化，疏通气血，增强体质，减少疾病，是医疗、护理、体育三位一体的世界上最早的健身保健方法。华佗的另一伟大贡献是发明了麻沸散，并将其作为全身麻醉剂应用在外科手术中，对外科学的发展做出了贡献。在手术治疗过程中指导弟子或家属做了大量护理工作，可以说是我国最早的外科护理专家。

（四）魏晋南北朝时期（公元220—581年）

1.《脉经》 晋代王叔和在其所著《脉经》中将脉象名称规范化，归纳为二十四脉，深入阐述了脉理，并比较了脏腑各部的生理、病理脉象，分析了各种杂病及小儿、妇女的脉证，明确提出了切脉独取寸口及左右手六脉所主脏腑的理论，使诊脉法成为护理临床观察病情时的重要手段。

observing state of illness in clinical nursing.

2. Emergency Formulas stored in One's Sleeve
Emergency Formulas stored in One's Sleeve (*Zhŏu Hòu Bèi Jí Fāng*, 肘后备急方) written by Ge Hong (AD 284—364) in the East Jin Dynasty (AD 316—420) is the integration of emergency, contagion, internal medicine, surgery, gynecology, ophthalmology, otorhinolaryngology, psychoneurosis and traumatology and orthopedics. Many emergency treatments of all these branches noted in this book involve nursing requests. For example, initiating the resuscitation of mouth-to-mouth air injection to save patients with sudden death, points out that heavy bleeding patients caused by the trauma are inhibited from drinking water or taking spicy food and should stay calm, avoiding physical movement and emotional fluctuation. In the prescription for ascites, it notes that "it is good for the patients with ascites to abstain from the salt and they should often eat bean meal, drink soybean milk and eat carp." The book also proposes to use seaweed to cure thyroid diseases, which is the earliest record of using iodine-containing food to cure and prevent thyroid diseases. It suggests using mad dog brain to treat patients bitten by mad dogs, taking the lead in immunization therapy for rabies.

3. Liu Juanzi's Ghost-Bequeathed Formulas
The extant earliest monograph of surgery in China is *Liu Juanzi's Ghost-Bequeathed Formulas* (*Liú Juān Zǐ Guǐ Yí Fāng*, 刘涓子鬼遗方) of the Northern and Southern dynasties (AD 420—589), enriches the connotation of surgery of TCM nursing. It records that one should keep the surroundings sanitary and quiet while pushing back the prolapsed intestines of the patients with abdominal traumatism. Besides, one should also pay attention to keep the herbal paste wet in using external plastering therapy and change the herbal paste when it turns dry. Besides, dietary and emotional nursing are also emphasized for those patients.

v. Sui, Tang Dynasties and the Five Dai Periods (AD 581—960)

1. Treatise on the Origins and Manifestations of Various Diseases *Treatise on the Origins and Manifestations of Various Diseases* (*Zhū Bìng Yuán Hòu Lùn*, 诸病源候论) compiled by Chao Yuan-fang (AD 550—630), a renowned physician of the Sui Dynasty (AD 581—681) describes pathogens, pathological mechanisms, manifestations, diagnoses, prevention and nursing of various diseases and also records many methods of life cultivation and *dǎo yǐn* exercises. For example, in the part of diabetes mellitus, it notes that "this disease is caused by eating too much greasy and tasty food, the patients must

2.《肘后备急方》 东晋葛洪所著《肘后备急方》集中医急救、传染病及内、外、妇、五官、精神、骨伤各科之大成。在书中提出的各科急诊诊治中，已广泛涉及护理要求。如首创了口对口吹气法抢救猝死患者的复苏术；明确提出外伤大出血患者，应禁食水及刺激性食物，患者宜安静，避免活动和情绪波动。又如在"治卒大腹水病方"中说："勿食盐、常食小豆饭，饮小豆汁，鲤鱼佳也"。该书还提出用海藻治疗瘿疾，是世界上用含碘食物治疗与预防甲状腺疾病的最早记载；提出了用疯狗脑敷治被疯狗咬伤的患者，开创了用免疫法治疗狂犬病的先河。

3.《刘涓子鬼遗方》 我国现存最早的一部外科专著，即南北朝时期《刘涓子鬼遗方》，充实了中医外科护理内涵。书中记载，对腹部外伤肠管脱出者，还纳时要注意保持环境卫生、安静，还应注意外敷药的干湿，干后应当立即更换，对这类患者该书还强调饮食护理和情志护理的重要性。

（五）隋唐五代时期（公元 581—960 年）

1.《诸病源候论》 隋朝名医巢元方等所著的《诸病源候论》中有各种疾病的病因、病理、症状、诊断、预防和护理的论述，并有大量的养生导引方法。例如在"消渴候"中记有："此肥美之所发，此人必数食甘美而多肥也。"提出消渴病与过食肥甘美食有关。在外科方面，介绍了外科肠吻合术后的饮食护理。在妇科护理方面，记录了北齐徐之才的"十月养胎法"，强调了妇女妊娠期间的

be always indulging in fatty food." In surgery, this book introduces dietary nursing after the operation of intestinal anastomosis. In gynecology nursing, Xu Zhi-cai (AD 492—572) of the North Qi Dynasty (AD 550—577) summarizes the "cultivating methods for ten pregnant months" which emphasizes diet and daily life nursing and emotion regulation during gestation period. These methods play positive roles in safeguarding the body and mind of pregnant women and protecting the fetus and preventing miscarriage. He also introduces nursing methods for the breast carbuncle during the lactation. It suggests that "using hands to twiddle and squeeze the milk out of the breast and asking other people to help suckle the breast," in order to discharge the stagnated milk and disperse the breast carbuncle. This nursing method is still in use up to the present. In pediatrics, he advocates that on mild and windless days one may take the infant out in the sunlight so as to keep him healthy and endurable to the wind and cold and avoid illnesses.

2. *Important Formulas Worth a Thousand Gold Pieces* it focuses the virtue of the doctor, initiates the method of urethral catheterization, pays more attention to the protection and prevention for women and children.

(1) The virtue of the doctor: In this book, Sun Si-miao (AD 541—682) wrote two papers respectively named "How Does the Divine Doctor Study Medicine" and "the Divine Doctor should be Accomplished and Honest" specially focusing on the virtue of the doctor. He emphasized that the doctor should treat the patients equally without discrimination whether they were poor or wealthy. The doctor should be serious, religious and wholehearted while treating patients. He admonished that the doctor should never regard medical practice as means of capturing lucre. The doctor should also have an elegant appearance and a sense of social responsibility.

(2) The method of urethral catheterization: Sun Si-miao initiated the utilization of thin shallot tube as the catheter to relieve urinary retention. It is more than 1,200 years earlier than the urethral catheterization using rubber tube invented by Frenchmen.

(3) Gynecology and obstetrics nursing: It has detailed descriptions on periods of pregnancy, delivery and puerperium. It emphasizes that pregnant women should live in a quiet and simple environmentand inhibit alcohol and ice, and unsanitary people should be inhibited from entering the delivery room near the time of labor. It points out "After labor, women can't rush around and caregivers should support and watch them carefully. They should avoid being in haste or worrying, because worries can cause dystocia". As for post-labor nursing, it

饮食起居和情志调养，这对于保护孕妇和胎儿身心健康，防止流产具有积极的作用。还介绍了乳痈的护理方法"手助捻去其汁，并令旁人助嘬饮之"，以使淤积的乳汁排出，而使乳痈消散。这一护理方法一直沿用至今。在儿科护理方面，主张应经常在和暖无风的时候抱小儿于阳光中嬉戏，可使孩子身体健康，耐受风寒，不易得病。

2.《千金要方》 论述医德，首创导尿术，重视食疗、妇女与儿童的保健和预防。

（1）专论医德:《千金要方》由唐代孙思邈编撰。该书在"大医习业"与"大医精诚"两篇文章中，强调医家的医德，对患者要不分贫富贵贱、一视同仁，治病要严肃认真、全心全意；告诫医家不可以医疗技术作为获取钱财的手段。在医疗作风方面，须有德有体，仪表要端庄，举止要检点，要有社会责任感。

（2）首创了葱管导尿术：书中详细记载了用细葱管导尿解除患者尿潴留的过程，这一方法比法国人发明的橡皮管导尿术要早1 200多年。

（3）妇产科护理:《千金要方》对孕期、分娩和产褥期均做了详尽的描述。强调妊娠妇女应居处简静，禁酒及冰浆；临产时禁止不洁者进入产房；指出妇人产后不得匆匆忙忙，旁人极须稳审，皆不得预缓预急及忧悒，忧悒则难产；对产后护理指出"女人产后百日以来，极须殷勤，忧畏勿纵心及即便行房。"等。

says "Women need attention and caring during the first hundred days after giving birth, avoid self-indulgent and sexual intercourse." and *etc.*.

(4) Pediatrics nursing: *Important Formulas Worth a Thousand Gold Pieces* collects and summarizes the experiences in children health care before the Tang Dynasty and has made important contributions in pediatrics nursing. For newborns, "firstly it needs to use cotton-wrapped fingers to wipe out the secretion and blood in children's mouth and tongue …" After the newborn is bathed, it needs to apply powder on the armpits and the private parts to avoid rashes. For breastfeeding, there are requirements on frequencies and amounts. Before breastfeeding, the mother should squeeze out overnight milk. It emphasizes that the diet, mental condition as well as physical condition of the mother are closely related to the babies' growth. As the baby grows older, one should appropriately add supplementary food *etc.*.

(5) Dietary nursing: The masterpiece of *Important Formulas Worth a Thousand Gold Pieces* elaborates dietotherapy as well as medicine therapy for treatment of all kinds of diseases. It insists that dietotherapy has precedence over medicine therapy. For example, it suggested the patients to eat animal's liver to treat blurred vision, eat grain husk porridge to prevent and treat beriberi, and take *guālóu* to treat diabetes. For the nursing of diabetes mellitus, Sun Si-miao advocated the importance of diet. He pointed out "the three matters needing attention are alcohol, sexual intercourse and salty or starchy food."

(6) Prevention: His proposition of disease prevention is quite noticeable. It is pointed that "the lofty doctors treat the patients when his disease is still in latent period" and that one should "remember not to spit at random" and "should not share clothes, towel, comb, pillow and mirror with others" so as to prevent contagion.

3. Arcane Essentials from the Imperial Library

Wang Tao (AD 670—755), another famous doctor in the Tang Dynasty, compiled an integrative magnum opus named *Arcane Essentials from the Imperial Library* (*Wài Tái Mì Yào*, 外台秘要), which dissertates nursing measures such as observation of the state of illness, dietary nursing, and daily life regulation of many diseases, including exogenous febrile disease, tuberculosis, malaria, smallpox, cholera. For example, about the observation of the state of patients with phthisis, it is pointed out that "in the afternoon the symptoms of tidal fever, night sweat and flushed face may appear, which are signals of aggravation of illness and usually accompanied with increasing thinness, red-black excrement or ascites". The

（4）儿科护理:《千金要方》收集和总结唐代以前对小儿保健的经验，为儿科临床护理做出了重大贡献。对初生婴儿，"先以绵裹指，拭儿中口及舌上青泥恶血……"；小儿沐浴后，腋窝和阴部要扑上细粉干燥，以防湿疹；在母乳喂养方面，对喂奶的次数和量有一定要求，乳母喂奶前要把宿奶挤掉，强调乳母的饮食、精神状态、健康状态与婴儿的身心发育关系密切；随着婴儿年龄增长，要适当增加辅助食品等。

（5）饮食护理:《千金要方》重视饮食疗法，该书在各种疾病的诊疗中，既有药疗方，又有食疗方，如目不明者用动物肝脏，防治脚气病用谷白皮煎汤煮粥，用瓜蒌治疗糖尿病等。对消渴病的护理提出"所慎者有三：一饮酒，二房事，三咸食及面"的主张，强调了饮食护理对消渴病的重要性。

（6）预防为主的思想：主张"上医医未病之病"，教导人们"常习不唾地"，还提出"凡衣服、巾、栉、枕、镜不宜与人同之"以预防传染病。

3.《外台秘要》 唐代另一著名医家王焘编撰的一部综合性巨著《外台秘要》，论述了伤寒、肺结核、疟疾、天花、霍乱等传染病的病情观察、饮食护理和生活起居等护理措施。如对肺痨患者的病情观察，指出患者午后有可能出现潮热、盗汗、面部潮红，若日益消瘦、大便赤黑色或出现腹水，则是病情加重的象征。该书还详细论述了对黄疸病的病情观察，提出："每日小便里浸少许帛，各书记日，色渐退白则瘥"。另外，还注意到了消渴患者的尿是甜的，对消渴病治疗采用饮

book also has the particular description of observation of jaundice. It mentions that one may "immerse a piece of silk in the urine every day and mark the date on the silk and the gradual fading of the urine-immersed silk means recovering." In addition, the book notices that the urine of the patients with diabetes mellitus is sugary, and diabetes mellitus can be treated by dietotherapy and daily life regulation.

vi. Song, Jin, Yuan Dynasties (AD 960—1368)

After the Song Dynasty (AD 960—1279), the development of paper making industry and typography created favorable conditions for the compilation and generalization of medical masterpieces. Different medical sects created an active atmosphere and contended for their own unique academic views.

1. Medication Nursing *Formulas from Benevolent Sages Compiled during the Taiping Era* (*Tài Píng Shèng Huì Fāng,* 太平圣惠方) is an official herbal masterpiece. It introduces the methods of herb preservation, decoction and oral administration, which still works as guidance for modern medicine storage and usage. For instance, "When decoct... it usually is supposed to be in full attention and apply weak fire to make the soup boil gently for the purpose of taking the medicinal components out of the herb. For purgative herb, it is supposed to add a small amount of water each time and add water frequently. For tonic herb, it is supposed to add a large amount of water with little frequency. One should have the decoction when it is still warm for better absorption. If the soup is cold, it'll induce vomiting. " The book points out the method of medication: "There is a huge difference between the young and the old, the strong and the weak. Some need supplementation and some need purgation. Some are suited for decoction and some are better to take pills. The increment or reduction of medicine must be suitable to the current situation. If the medicine and the illness match, the sickness can be cured. If the disease happens above the chest, one must first eat before taking medicine. If the disease is below the heart and stomach, one must take the medicine first. If the disease is in the four limbs or in the veins, it is suggested to remain empty stomach and take the medicine in the morning..."

2. Dietary Nursing Among the famous "four physicians in the Jin and Yuan dynasties", Li Dong-yuan (AD 1180—1251) created the theory of the spleen and stomach, which attached importance to the regulating and nursing of spleen and stomach. He put forward a series of proposals for nursing these two organs, for example "Don't eat when feeling furious" "Don't have meals when feeling sleepy" "Don't take intense physical activities after

食疗法和饮食起居的禁忌等。

（六）宋金元时期（公元 960—1368 年）

宋代以后，由于造纸业和印刷术的发展，为医药学著作的整理和推广创造了有利条件，医家百家争鸣，各抒己见，中医各科的护理取得长足的进步。

1. **用药护理** 《太平圣惠方》是一部官修中医方剂著作，介绍了中成药保管法、煮药、服药方法，对现代护理的药物保管和使用仍有良好的指导作用。书中记载煮药、服药方法，如"凡煮汤……常令文火小沸，令药出。煮之调和，必须用意。然则利汤欲生，水少而多取；补汤欲熟，多水而少取。服汤宁小热，即易消下，若冷，即令人呕逆。"指出服饵之法"少长殊途，强羸各异，或宜补宜泻，或可汤可丸，加减不失其宜，药病相投必愈。若病在胸膈以上者，先食后服药。病在心腹以下者，先服药而后食。病在四肢血脉者，宜空腹而在旦……"

2. **饮食护理** 著名的金元四大家之一的李杲创立了脾胃学说，重视对脾胃的调养和护理。提出了一系列护理脾胃的主张，如"方怒不可食""勿困中饮食，食后少动作"，重视饮食、劳倦、情志的护理，指出"饮食不节则胃病，胃病则气短，精神少，而生大

a meal", emphasizing the importance of diet, tiredness and emotional nursing. He pointed out that "If one doesn't control his/her diet, it will result in gastritis and further result in the symptoms of shortness of breath, low spirit and high body temperature." "Over-laboring will result in spleen disease and lead to weakness and somnolence, the four limbs flaccidity and diarrhea."

The physicians in the Jin and Yuan Dynasties attached great importance to health cultivation, health care and diet regulation. One representative bookmaking of nutriology of TCM is *Principles of Correct Diet* (*Yǐn Shàn Zhèng Yào*, 饮膳正要). It puts forward taboos of life cultivation, gestation and lactation, as well as many kinds of edible recipes of rare food. It records a lot of medicinal and healthy diet, including soup decoction, dietotherapy, and vegetable food. It summarizes and advances the valuable experience of dietary nursing by inheriting the ancient medical tradition of combination of diet, invigorant and medicine. For each food recorded, the book emphasizes its edible and tonic values related to the medicinal effect. For example, *kǔ dòu Tāng* can be used to "invigorate the kidney, strengthen the waist and knees, warm and coordinate the center qi." The chicken cooked with *shēng dì huáng* can be used to "cure pain of the waist and back, heal deficiency of the marrow and remedy fatigue and lassitude." The crucian carp soup can be used to "treat weakness of the spleen and stomach and heal the patients with chronic diarrhea." These foods can be used to strengthen the body and prolong life, which are delicious food as well as fine medicine for preventing and treating illnesses. The book presents the nursing demand on the sanitation of diet. It advocates that one "shouldn't eat until feeling hungry, should never overeat, shouldn't sleep when being fully satiated, should never eat too much especially in the nighttime, shouldn't eat insanitary or rotten food, should drink moderately, shouldn't get heavily drunk, should pay attention to oral hygiene, should gargle with warm water after meals and should brush the teeth before sleep."

3. Daily Life Nursing *Bao Sheng Yao Lu* (*Bǎo Shēng Yào Lù*, 保生要录) authored by Pu Qian-guan is an early book covering a variety of topics on daily life nursing. It has a relatively detailed description on clothing, eating, sleeping and other topics: "Clothes must be applied according to the weather, meaning that even when it's summer. The clothes shouldn't be too thin, even when it's winter. The clothes shouldn't be excessively warm… When the clothes are soaked by sweat, one should immediately change them." It is said that people can't have heavy consumption of food and drinks and people can't first have hot dishes then follows by cold ones. The dishes

热""形体劳役则脾病，脾病则怠惰嗜卧，四肢不收，大便泄泻"。

金元时期医学家重视养生保健和饮食调护，《饮膳正要》一书中提出了养生避忌、妊娠食忌、乳母食忌、饮食避忌以及各种珍奇食品的食用食谱。记载了大量医疗、保健饮食，包括汤煎、食疗、植物食品等。继承了我国古代食、养、医结合的传统，全书总结并发展了饮食护理中的宝贵经验。该书对每种食品都同时注意到了它的食用、养生与医疗的关系。如用苦豆汤"补下元，理腰膝，温中顺气"；用生地黄鸡"治腰背疼痛，骨髓虚损，身重气乏"；用鲫鱼羹"治脾胃虚弱，泄泻久不瘥者"等。这些食物可使人强壮身体，延年益寿，是预防和治疗疾病的良药，又是鲜美可口的佳肴。该书对饮食卫生提出了护理要求，提倡"先饥后食，勿令过饱""不可饱食而卧，尤其夜间不可多食""勿食不洁或变质之物"；饮酒适量，"不可大醉"；注意口腔卫生，"食毕宜用温水漱口，睡前刷牙"等。

3. 生活起居护理　蒲虔贯所著的《保生要录》是这一时期一本较早也较全面的生活护理专著。该书在衣着、进食、睡眠等方面均有较详尽的论述："衣服厚薄欲得随时合度，是以暑时不可全薄，寒时不可极温……衣为汗湿，即时易之。"认为饮食不可强食强饮，不可先进热食而随餐冷物。进食不可太热太冷，太热则伤胃，太冷则伤筋。应避免偏食，偏食能使脏气不均。其又曰"养生者，形要

can neither be too hot nor too cold. Too hot food damages stomach and too cold food damages muscles. People should avoid dietary bias, which causes the unbalanced viscera qi. It is also said "To keep healthy, one should take mild exercises that don't cause heavy tiredness. It's just like the river, meaning slow flow of springs makes it clear while blockage makes it dirty. To keep healthy, one must maintain the flow of blood, like the smooth flow of river, sit and walk till feeling tired. If one is exhausted, he should take a short break. This is the method of mild exercise."

4. Specific Nursing   *Quintessence of External Medicine* (*Wài Kē Jīng Yì*, 外科精义) written by Qi De-zhi has the special chapter discussing nursing. It firstly brings forward the notions that the surroundings of the ward should be peaceful, and that one should "just visit and greet the patient briefly and not stay long and talk much to make the patient be tired". In Zhang Zi-he's *Confucians' Duties to Their Parents* (*Rú Mén Shì Qīn*, 儒门事亲), anorectal disease nursing has been recorded: "Rectocele is caused by intense heat of the large intestine. It suggested to heat sour paste until being 60% boiled, use it to wash anus when it's still warm, and cover it with bitter herbs, and then the disease will be healed." It demonstrates that sitting bath therapy appeared quite early in Chinese history.

The Complete Compendium of Fine Formulas for Women (*Fù Rén Dà Quán Liáng Fāng*, 妇人大全良方) compiled by Chen Zi-ming (AD 1190—1270) dissertates the dose plan of the pregnant women in their different pregnant months, the nursing methods of prenatal and postpartum, and taboos of food and medicine. For the nursing of pregnant women, the diet of the first five months can be the same with normal people. But for the latter five months, because the fetus is growing much faster, the mother should balance the five flavors to increase her appetite, which still should be kept under control. As for postpartum caring, it emphasizes the importance of abundant rest for the women. Primipara can gently rub their stomach up and down to help restore the womb and decrease postpartum bleeding. They should mainly eat digestible half-liquid food, and avoid undesirable environment and mental stimulation that would affect their physical and mental health.

Key to Diagnosis and Treatment of Children's Diseases (*Xiǎo Ér Yào Zhèng Zhí Jué*, 小儿药证直诀) authored by Qian Yi (AD 1032—1117) proposes that when children are suffering from warm disease, the environment should be kept quiet and "bathing therapy" should be adopted as auxiliary treatment.

小劳，无至大疲。故小流则清，滞则污。养生之人，欲血脉常行，如水之流，坐不欲至倦，行不欲至劳。顿行不已，然后稍缓，是小劳之术也。"

4. **专科护理**   齐德之的《外科精义》中"论将护忌慎法"专篇论述护理，提出病室环境宜安静；规定了"只可方便省问，不可久坐多言，劳倦患者"的探视制度等。张子和的《儒门事亲》中对肛肠疾病的护理记载"脱肛，大肠热甚也，用酸浆水煎三五沸，稍热涤洗三五度，次以苦剂坚之，则愈。"说明我国很早就有了坐浴法。

陈自明的《妇人大全良方》论述了孕妇妊娠按月份服药方法、产前、产后护理、食忌及孕妇药忌。对孕妇的护理，指出妊娠前五个月膳食可与常人相同；后五个月因胎儿发育加快，宜调和五味以增进食欲，但须有节。对产后护理，强调产妇需要充分休息，初产者可用手轻轻自上而下按摩腹部，以促进子宫复原，减少产后出血；饮食以易消化的半流质食物为宜，同时避免影响产妇身心健康的不良环境和精神刺激。

钱乙所著的《小儿药证直诀》主张小儿有热病时，应保持环境安静，以"浴体法"为辅助治疗。

vii. Ming and Qing Dynasties (AD 1368—1840)

In the Ming Dynasty (AD 1368—1644) great progress and prominent achievements are made in technology, culture and many other aspects. There appear many medical inventions and creations of great significance. TCM nursing therefore gets further development and obtains outstanding accomplishments.

Wu You-ke (AD 1582—1652) put forward the idea about the etiology of contagion in his work *Treatise on Warm-Heat Pestilence* (*Wēn Yì Lùn*, 温疫论). He believed that the special pathogens of pestilence were "pestilential qi". Its infection spread through the mouth and nose. Anybody, whether old or young, weak or strong, might contract pestilence once contacting the "pestilential qi". It records the characteristics of many contagions such as black plague, smallpox, diphtheria, the principles and methods of treatment and nursing for pestilence. It is said that it is important to dispel the exogenous evil as early as possible and use the method of purgation to eliminate the pathogens as early as possible. When eliminating the pathogens, one should differentiate the deficiency or excess of the body, assess the degree of the pathogen, and observe the emergency of the illness. In aspect of nursing, it particularly describes the nursing demand for the pestilence. In terms of the dietary nursing of pestilence, it holds that the pestilential pathogen is yang evil which is prone to consume body fluid. About how to complement liquid in time, it brings forward the advice that "when the patients are seriously thirsty and desiring for ice drink, one may satisfy them no matter what season it is." "One may give the patients half of the capacity that they ask for, and give them the rest later on." For the patients with polydipsia caused by inner heat, one may give them "the juice of pear, lotus root, sugar cane and watermelon to meet their needs at intervals". The purpose is to clear heat, relieve thirst and generate liquid.

The Grand Compendium of Materia Medica (*Běn Cǎo Gāng Mù*, 本草纲目) compiled by Li Shi-zhen, a famous physician and pharmacist in the Ming Dynasty, is a significant magnum opus of Chinese pharmacy. Li Shi-zhen picked and processed herbal medicines in person. He not only visited and treated the patients but also decocted the herbs and fed the decoction to the patients, and guided his disciples or the kinfolks of the patients to do the nursing job.

Zhang Jing-yue, another famous doctor, wrote in his work *The Complete Works of Zhang Jing-yue* (*Jǐng Yuè Quán Shū*, 景岳全书) that "the patient with exogenous febrile disease is supposed to follow the diet taboos... One

（七）明清时期（公元 1368—1840 年）

明代在科学技术与文化上有较大的发展，取得多方面突出的成就，出现了很多有重大意义的医学发明与创造，中医护理学也得到进一步发展，并取得了突出的成就。

吴又可在其所著的《温疫论》中，指出引起"疫病"的特殊病因是"戾气"，传染途径是自口鼻而入，无论老少强弱，触之皆病。书中记载了鼠疫、天花、白喉等传染病发病的特点、治疗与护理疫病的原则和方法。在治疗与护理的基本原则上，认为应以"客邪贵乎早逐"，而"早逐"主张早用攻下祛邪法，而祛邪必须"要识人之虚实，度邪之轻重，察病之缓急"；在护理方面详细论述了温疫病的护理要求，如在对温疫病的饮食护理方面，认为温为阳邪，易于伤津耗液，对如何及时补充津液，提出"大渴思饮冰水及冷饮，无论四时，皆可量与"，但"能饮一升，止与半升，宁使少顷再饮"，而对内热烦渴者，应给"梨汁、藕汁、蔗浆、西瓜皆可备不时之需"用以清热止渴生津。

明代著名医药学家李时珍所著《本草纲目》，是一部重要的药物学巨著。李时珍亲自采药、炮炙，不但为患者看病还为患者煎药、喂药，并指导患者家属或弟子对患者实施护理。

名医张景岳在《景岳全书》中写道："凡伤寒饮食有宜忌者，……不欲食，不可强食，强食则助邪。"说明饮食护理的重要性。当时

shouldn't force the patient to eat if he has no appetite, and constrained diet may aid the evil." This illuminates the importance of dietary nursing. At that time there was already the specific cognition that pestilence is a contagious illness. For example, Hu Zheng-xin, a famous physician, said that "the family whose member has contracted plague should steam the clothes of the patient in the container, and then the other members of the family can be free of the plague." This explicitly points out that the clothes of the contagious patients should be disposed with the method of steam sterilizing.

Leng Qian in the Ming Dynasty put forward "sixteen appropriate points for life cultivation" in his book *The Keystone to Prolong and Cultivate Life* (*Xiū Líng Yào Zhǐ*, 修龄要旨), which says that the hair ought to be combed more; the face ought to be washed more; the eyeballs ought to be moved more; the ears ought to be flipped more; the tongue ought to support the maxilla frequently; the teeth ought to knock frequently; the saliva ought to be swallowed frequently; the turbid qi ought to be breathed out frequently; the back ought to be warmed always; the chest ought to be protected always; the abdomen ought to be massaged frequently; the anus ought to be pinched frequently; the extremities ought to sway frequently; the skin ought to be bathed with hands or dry towels frequently; and one should shut the mouth when relieving the bowels. All the above sixteen points are experiential principles for health cultivation. They are still of significant and instructive values for nursing and life cultivation to this day.

Orthodox Lineage of External Medicine Orthodox Lineage of External Medicine (*Wài Kē Zhèng Zōng*, 外科正宗) authored by Chen Shi-gong, records the causes and treatment of abscess and nursing according to pattern differentiation. For example, "After recovery, if one starts to labor too soon, deficiency will happen. If one is engaged in sexual intercourse too soon, his life span will be shortened. If one doesn't avoid exposing from cold and wind, virus relapses." "Although every disease depends on medicine treatment, it also relies on other contraindications and attentions, so one must clean the patient's room … " and *etc.*.

In the Qing Dynasty, after the Opium War, western medicine flooded into China and impacted the development of TCM. The theory of *Warm Diseases* (*Wēn Bìng*, 温病) gradually formed. For example, the famous physician of warm diseases, Ye Tian-shi illuminated the rules of occurrence and advancement of the warm diseases in his masterwork *Treatise on Warm-Heat Diseases* (*Wēn Rè Lùn*, 温热论). He put forward the principle that treatment and nursing should be decided by pattern

对瘟疫是传染性疾病已有明确的认识，如名医胡正心说："凡患瘟疫之家，将初患者之衣于甑上蒸过，则一家不得染"，明确指出传染患者的衣服要用蒸汽消毒法处理。

明代冷谦在《修龄要旨》一书中提出的"养生十六宜"，即发宜多梳、面宜多擦、目宜常运、耳宜常弹、舌宜抵腭、齿宜数叩、津宜数咽、浊宜常呵、背宜常暖、胸宜常护、腹宜常摩、谷道宜常撮、肢节宜常摇、皮肤宜常干沐浴、大小便宜闭口勿言，可谓养生术的经验之谈，至今对护理和养生有着重要的指导价值。

陈实功所著的《外科正宗》记述了痈疽的病源、调治以及外科疾病的辨证施护。如"疮愈之后，劳役太早，乃为赢症，入房太早，后必损寿，不避风寒，复生流毒"；"凡病虽在于用药调理，而又要关于杂禁之法，先要洒扫患房洁净……"等。

在清代，大量西方医学的涌入，冲击了中医药学的发展。由于当时战争频繁，疫病流行，温病学说逐渐形成。如名医叶天士的《温热论》系统阐明了温病发生、发展的规律，提出了温病卫、气、营、血四个阶段辨证论治与辨证施护的纲领。其中，提出对于温病孕妇以"井底泥或蓝布浸冷覆盖腹

differentiation of the four stages of the warm diseases which are named respectively defensive level, qi level, nutrient level and blood level. He said that in terms of the pregnant woman with warm disease, one should "lays the mud from the bottom of a well or the cloth wet by cold water over the abdomen" to protect the fetus. In terms of the senile illness, he suggested that the diet should be of "plain taste" and "alcohol, meat and food with excessively rich taste" should be strictly avoided. In the aspect of emotion, he protested that "one should be sure to be pleased" and "abstain from getting angry" . In the aspect of observation of state of illness, he emphasized observation of the tongue and teeth and the differentiation of macula and anthema. Besides, he insisted on carrying out oral care while estimating the severity of the illness and speculating the prognosis of the illness by observing the tongue appearance. He also put forward the view that "the invigorator or tonic which is suitable for patient just is what he or she badly wants to eat" and advised to use the weighty and strong-flavored food such as meat.

Epidemic diseases became frequent in the Qing Dynasty. Therefore, in terms of the prevention of plagues, besides making the healthy people dose in advance, much more importance was attached to carrying out the measures of seclusion and disinfection. For example, *Cyclopedia of Treatment of the Plagues* (*Zhì Yì Quán Shū*,治疫全书) mentions that "one should not get near to the bed of the contagious patients in case of contracting the dirty evil, should not mourn the dead near his coffin in case of contacting the fetor, should not eat the meals with the family whose member falls into the plague and should not collect the clothes of the contagious dead."

The monograph of essential content about the nursing of illness named *The Nursing of Illness* (*Shì Jí Yào Yǔ*,侍疾要语) written by Qian Xiang, a famous physician in the Qing Dynasty, records dietary nursing, daily life nursing and nursing of the old patients. It records the "*The Ballad of Longevity of Ten Old Men* (*Shí Sǒu Cháng Shòu Gē*, 十叟长寿歌)*" that introduces the experiences of ten centurial old men about prolonging life span, preventing illness and postponing senescence. It holds that one needs to regulate daily life and diet, cultivate temperament, and pay attention to physical exercises to acquire longevity.

II. Modern TCM Nursing

With the development of science and technology, TCM has made great progress in scientization and modernization in recent decades. The TCM and Chinese pharmacology have not only inherited the traditional

上"。对老年病的防护强调颐养，主张饮食当"薄味"，力戒"酒肉厚味"；在情志方面主张"务宜怡悦开怀""戒嗔怒"；在病情观察方面主张温热病要注意观察舌、齿，辨斑疹，而且还指出了在观察舌象、判断病情、推测预后的同时，还应做好口腔护理。他还提出"食物自适者即胃喜为补"的观点，主张使用质重味厚的血肉有情之品。

清代大疫流行频繁，对疫病的预防，除让健康者预服药物外，也非常重视采取隔离消毒的措施，如《治疫全书》说："毋近患者床榻，染其秽污；毋凭死者尸棺，触其恶臭；毋食病家时菜；毋拾死人衣物。"

清代名医钱襄的中医护理学专著《侍疾要语》，记载了饮食护理、生活起居护理和老年患者的护理，其中记录了十位百岁老人延年益寿、防病抗老经验的"十叟长寿歌"，认为要长寿就应该注意起居、饮食、锻炼和情志修养。

二、现代中医护理学

随着科学技术的发展，中医药学近几十年也逐步走向科学化、现代化。中医学和中药学既继承中医传统方法，也结合现代化诊

methods of TCM but also combined the modern diagnostic methods and advanced medical equipment, largely improving therapeutic effect of TCM, which directly leads to the setting up of modern TCM hospitals, strict division of work in health care between doctors and nurses, and formation of a clinical team for TCM nursing. TCM nursing becomes more and more developed and complete under this situation.

i. The Formation of Multi-level, Multi-channel and Multi-form Educational System in TCM Nursing

In the early 1960s, the first training program for TCM nursing was held in Nanjing. Since the middle 1980s, higher vocational nursing education had been set up in universities of Chinese medicine, followed by the baccalaureate nursing education since 1999 and master education since 2003. In 2009, the first Ph.D program in discipline orientation of combination of Chinese and western nursing had been set up in Nanjing University of Chinese Medicine, and nowadays 5 universities of Chinese medicine have been authorized to Ph.D degree-granting. With the development of nursing, professional degree education, which is different from academic degree education, has started to break into the mainstream of master education in nursing. 19 universities of Chinese medicine got permission to enroll students for professional degree education in 2015. Along with full-time education, continuing education and distance education are nationally set up to meet the workforce demand, facilitating the formation of multi-level, multi-channel and multi-form educational system for TCM nursing.

ii. The Construction of Teaching Textbook System

In 1959, the first systematic monograph of TCM nursing, *the Illness TCM nursing* was published in Nanjing, which is the milestone for the development of TCM nursing. Since 1990s, the compiling of teaching textbook for higher TCM nursing education has rapidly expanded. The first systematically published monographs for TCM nursing are a series including the textbooks of *Basic Nursing of Traditional Chinese Medicine, Medical Nursing of Traditional Chinese Medicine, Surgical Nursing of Traditional Chinese Medicine, Gynecological Nursing of Traditional Chinese Medicine*, and *Pediatric Nursing of Traditional Chinese Medicine*, which were published by Xueyuan Press during 1996 to 2000. In 2005, the Institute of National Higher Education of TCM was entrusted by the State Administration of Chinese Medicine to compile 21 books of the New Century Nursing Learning Materials for

断手段和先进的诊疗设备，更加完善了中医诊断和治疗疾病的方法，提高了中医治疗效果。现代化的中医医院相继建成，并开始了严格的医护分工。在综合性医院的中医病房及各中医院，涌现出一支中医护理专业队伍。中医护理学也在此形势下发展，并日益成熟和完善。

（一）多层次、多渠道、多形式的中医特色护理教育体系正在全国范围内逐步形成

20 世纪 60 年代初，中医护理培训班在南京首次举办。20 世纪 80 年代中期开始，北京、南京等多地中医院校开设护理专业，开始招收护理大专学生。1999 年开始招收护理本科学生，2003 年之后各中医院校相继开始招收科学学位护理学硕士研究生。2009 年南京中医药大学率先招收中西医结合护理学博士研究生，目前已有 5 所中医院校护理学院招收博士研究生。2015 年全国 19 所中医药院校护理学院开始招收护理学专业学位硕士研究生。除全日制教育外，全国和各地开展了形式多样的远程教育、继续教育项目（如函授、短期培训等），培养出不同层次的符合临床需求的各类中医护理人才，逐步形成了完善的多层次、多渠道、多形式的中医特色护理教育体系。

（二）教材体系建设日趋完善

1958 年南京出版第一部系统中医护理专著《中医护病学》，标志着中医护理学已走向新时代。1996—2001 年间学苑出版社正式出版了 5 本系列高等中医院校中医护理学教材，分别是《中医护理学基础》《中医内科护理学》《中医儿科护理学》《中医外科护理学》和《中医妇科护理学》。该套教材为当时全国唯一一套正式出版的中医护理高等教育系列教材。2005 年，国家中医药管理局委托全国中医药高等教育学会规划、组织编写了 21 门"十一五"全国高等中医药院校护理专业规划教材，并由中国中医药出版社出版。之后中国中医药出版社、人民卫生

National Universities of TCM, which were published by China Press of TCM.

iii. The Establishment and Increment of Academic Institution

Since 1977, the Chinese Nursing Association and its branches have organized academic activities, such as seminars and training programs, especially after 1980s. One of the important academic conferences held in June 1984, approved for the setting up of Academic Committee in TCM, and Committee in Combination of TCM and Western Nursing, which are the key branches of Chinese Nursing association. In 2002, Chinese Nursing Association in TCM was established supervised by China Association of Chinese Medicine. In the same year, Committee for Higher Education in TCM nursing governed by National Chinese Medicine Higher Education Association was established and had further facilitated the academic activities of TCM nursing. Nursing Committee as one of branch of World Federation of Chinese Medicine Societies was established in 2012, which constructs an international communicating platform for TCM nursing education. The Best Practice Spotlight Organization (BPSO) under Registered Nurses' Association of Ontario (RNAO), a world-famous evidence-based nursing guidelines development organization, established an affiliated RNAO-BPSO Evidence-based Nursing Centre in Beijing University of Chinese Medicine (BUCM) in 2015, which is the first RNAO-BPSO center in China. The Joanna Briggs Institute (JBI), launched in 1996, is the international not-for-profit, research and development center within the Faculty of Health Sciences at the University of Adelaide, South Australia. In June 2015, JBI officially announced BUCM as the third collaborating center in mainland China, which is also the first one dedicated to evidence-based practice in TCM nursing. The center ultimately promotes the evidence translation, practice and dissemination, as well as the standardization of TCM nursing.

iv. The Construction and Promulgation of Standard and Norm

In 1985, Department of Chinese Medicine of the Ministry of Health carried out the *TCM Nursing Practice Routine and Technique Standard*, which stipulates the rules on ward-round and recording for TCM nursing. In May 2013, the *TCM nursing practice guideline for dominant diseases* has been developed and disseminated on a national scale by State Administration of Traditional Chinese Medicine of the People's Republic of China.

出版社及其他多家出版社均出版了系列的"十二五""十三五"规划教材。

（三）学术组织增多，学术活动活跃

1977 年以来，中华护理学会和各地分会先后恢复学术活动，多次召开护理学术交流会，举办各种不同类型专题学习班和研讨班等。1980 年以后，国际学术交流活动日益增多。1984 年 6 月在南京召开了中华护理学会中医、中西医结合护理学术会议，会上宣布成立了中华护理学会中医、中西医结合护理学术委员会，从此中医护理学逐步发展并日渐成熟。2002 年中华中医药学会护理专业委员会成立。2002 年全国中医药高等教育学会护理教育研究会成立，并积极开展中医特色护理教育的学术活动。2012 年世界中医药学会联合会护理专业委员会成立，搭建了中医护理国际交流平台。2015 年，北京中医药大学分别与加拿大安大略注册护士协会（Registered Nurses' Association of Ontario, RNAO）合作成立中国第一家 BPSO 最佳实践指南研究中心（Best Practice Spotlight Organization-Academic，BPSO）；与澳大利亚 JBI（Joanna Briggs Institutions）成立中国大陆第三家 JBI 循证护理合作中心，也是全球第一家从事中医护理的循证护理合作中心。两个国际合作中心的成立，一方面引进全球最佳护理证据，本土化后应用于临床，传播科学证据，使中医护理实践变的更加有效；另一方面促进中医护理标准化、规范化和科学化。

（四）政府部门重视中医护理相关标准和规范的制订

1985 年卫生部中医司下发《中医护理常规和技术操作规范》，对中医护理提出了初步的规范和要求，实行了中医护理查房和书写中医护理病历制度。2013 年 5 月开始，国家中医药管理局医政司出台了系列《优势病种中医护理方案》，并在全国范围的中医医院推广实施。

In 2010, The Ministry of Education announced *Standards for Establishment of Nursing Baccalaureate Program* and *Requirements for Nursing Baccalaureate Education*, which promoted construction and development of nursing education for national medical institutions and provided preconditions of cultivating medical professionals. In 2013, Steering Committee of Nursing Education of the Ministry of Education organized TCM colleges and universities to replenish standards for TCM nursing practices, which has standardized the TCM nursing curricula settings and practices and facilitated talents' normative cultivation in TCM colleges and universities.

v. The New Opportunity and Challenge

With the great strides made in nursing education and practice, the contribution from nursing senior talents facilitates the maturity of TCM nursing profession. Theoretical studies on TCM ancient books, particularly on those nursing knowledge, have promoted the formation of independent TCM nursing theoretical system. In addition, the researches on TCM nursing techniques and the nursing care for chronic diseases and gerontology are strengthened. Attempts are made to reach a combination with western nursing and disseminate the TCM culture. In recent years, the level of academic research of TCM nursing has improved greatly. Internationally academic communication promotes the international influence of TCM nursing.

Furthermore, the *Health Service Development Plan for Traditional Chinese Medicine (2015—2020)*, issued by the State Council of the People's Republic of China, emphasizes the significance of TCM, especially in the field of health preservation, rehabilitation and pension service. While it also highlights the nursing practice with unique TCM characteristics, which brings new challenges to all professionals in this field.

(Hao Yu-fang)

Key Points

1. TCM nursing is a subject which is old yet young. Guided by theories of TCM, it adopts the concept of holism and nursing based on pattern differentiation. It is a practical science, which combines prevention, health care, rehabilitation and medicine together to take care of

---

我国教育部 2010 年出台了《护理专业本科设置标准》和《护理本科教学基本要求》，促进了全国高等医学院校护理专业的建设和发展，为人才培养提供了基本保障。2013 年教育部护理教学指导委员会组织各中医院校制订中医护理模块的补充标准，规范了中医药院校护理专业中医护理课程设置、实践环节等相关内容，促进中医药院校护理人才的规范化培养。

（五）中医护理面临新的机遇与挑战

目前，中医护理队伍正在发展壮大，涌现出一大批富有献身精神、具有中高级职称的专业技术人才。中医护理学术骨干系统挖掘中医护理古籍，梳理中医护理知识与技能，使中医护理理论更加系统、完善，逐渐形成一个独立、完整、系统的科学理论体系；开展中医护理技术规范化研究；积极探索中医护理在慢性病、老年病管理有养生康复方面的作用；尝试与现代护理理念与技术的融合；重视护理人文环境的建设，传播中医护理文化。近几年中医护理的科学研究工作有了新的进展，学术研究氛围日益浓厚，学术水平也不断提高。同时中医护理学的发展，日益受到国际护理界的重视，国际学术交流活跃，扩大了中医护理事业在国际上的影响。

国务院发布《中医药健康服务发展规划》（2015—2020），重点任务包括大力发展中医养生保健服务；支持发展中医特色康复服务；积极发展中医药健康养老服务等。这为中医护理事业的发展带来了新的机遇和挑战。

（郝玉芳）

要点

1. 中医护理学是一门既古老、又年轻的学科，是以中医理论为指导，在整体观念指导下，运用辨证施护的方法，结合预防、养生保健、康复等措施，对患者及老、弱、幼、

patients, the old, the weak, the young and the handicapped, and implements specific nursing techniques to safeguard the health of people.

2. *The Yellow Emperor's Inner Classic* is the earliest extant medical classic in China that comparatively expounds the system of TCM. It consists of two books, *Basic Questions* and *The Spiritual Pivot*. It systematically expatiates on the theories of human physiology and pathology, as well as diagnosis, prevention and treatment of diseases. It lays a solid foundation for the establishment and development of theoretical and clinical system of TCM.

3. *Treatise on Cold Damage and Miscellaneous Diseases* starts the clinical nursing based on pattern differentiation.

4. *Shen Nong's Classic of the Materia Medica* is the earliest pharmacology book existing in China.

5. Hua Tuo, a noted physician in the late Han Dynasty and Three Kingdoms period, is the founder of surgery and medical sports.

6. *The Pulse Classic* makes the pulse examination become important means of observing state of illness in clinical nursing.

7. *Emergency Formulas to Keep Up One's Sleeve* is the integration of every clinical branch of TCM nursing.

8. *Liu Juanzi's Ghost-Bequeathed Formulas* enriches the connotation of surgery of TCM nursing.

9. *Important Formulas Worth a Thousand Gold Pieces* focuses on the virtue of the doctor, initiates the method of urethral catheterization, and pays more attention to the protection and prevention for women and children.

10. *Arcane Essentials from the Imperial Library* records the observation of the state of illness, dietary nursing and *etc.*.

残者加以照料，并施以独特的护理技术，以促进、维持和恢复人类健康的一门应用学科。

2.《黄帝内经》奠定了中医护理学的理论基础。《黄帝内经》是我国现存最早，比较全面、系统阐述中医学理论体系的古典医学巨著，包括《素问》和《灵枢》两部分，系统阐述了人体生理、病理以及疾病的诊断、治疗和预防等内容，为中医学理论的形成与发展奠定了坚实的基础。

3.《伤寒杂病论》开创了辨证施护的先河。

4.《神农本草经》是我国现存最早的药物学专著。

5. 华佗是后汉三国时期的名医，是我国外科和医疗体育的奠基人。

6.《脉经》为中医护理病情观察提供了依据。

7.《肘后备急方》集中医护理临床各科之大成。

8.《刘涓子鬼遗方》充实了中医外科护理内涵。

9.《千金要方》论述医德，首创导尿术，重视食疗、妇女与儿童的保健和预防。

10.《外台秘要》记载传染病的病情观察、饮食护理等护理措施。

Chapter 2 Essential Theory of TCM

第二章 中医基础理论

Learning Objectives	学习目标

Mastery

1. To repeat the basic meaning and content of yin-yang theory and five-phase theory.

2. To repeat the characteristics, functions and relationship among the visceras.

3. To repeat the concept of the meridian, accurately, the composition of the channels and collaterals; to repeat the characteristics of the twelve meridians circulation.

4. To repeat the acu-points classification and methods of acupuncture points locating.

5. To repeat the location, indications of the commonly used acupuncture points.

Comprehension

1. To explain the application of yin-yang and five-phase theory in TCM nursing.

2. To explain the relationship between the five *zang* and the qi, liquid, body and orifices.

3. To explain the concept and function of essence, qi, blood, body fluid.

识记

1. 能复述阴阳学说、五行学说的基本含义和基本内容。

2. 能复述五脏六腑的特点、功能和五脏之间的关系。

3. 能复述经络的概念、经络的组成和十二经脉的循行特点。

4. 能复述腧穴的分类及定位方法。

5. 能复述常用穴位的定位、主治特点。

理解

1. 理解阴阳学说和五行学说在中医护理学中的应用。

2. 理解五脏与志、液、体、窍的关系。

3. 理解精、气、血、津液的概念及功能。

4. To explain the concept, classification and characteristics of TCM etiology; to explain the basic pathomechanism of TCM.
5. To explain the therapeutic effect of acupuncture points.

Application

1. To judge the yin-yang attributes of thing and phenomena correctly.

2. To find viscera of definitely pathological changes according to clinical features.
3. Be able to select appropriate acupuncture points in clinical practice according to the indications of acupuncture points and apply proper methods to locate and manipulate the points.

4. 理解中医病因的概念、分类、特点及中医的基本病机。

5. 理解腧穴的主治作用。

运用

1. 能正确划分事物的阴阳属性和进行五行归类。

2. 能根据临床病理表现判断病变脏腑。

3. 能灵活应用腧穴的定位方法确定常用腧穴的定位，并能够根据穴位的主治特点，灵活选用腧穴。

Case Study

The woman, 49 years old, who has insomnia for many years. Recently she has difficulty in falling asleep at night because of a bad mood. The sleep time lasts 3-4 hours with dreams. She tends to be woke up, and then can't sleep again. With increasing dysphoria, she hence goes to hospital. The present symptoms are: upset, red face, thirst, mouth sores, heat, short and red urine, astringent and pain when urinates, red tongue, yellow tongue coating, and rapid pulse.

Question 1: What is the problem with the heart of the patient according to her upset?

Question 2: Why does the patient appear upset, flushed face, mouth sores, short and red urine meanwhile?

Question 3: What's the principle of treatment and nursing for the patient according to the yin-yang theory?

Theoretical framework of TCM nursing originates from TCM basic theories. This chapter introduces theories of yin-yang, five-phase, visceral manifestation, essence, qi, blood and fluid, etiology and pathomechanism, channels, collaterals and acupuncture points, and their significance and application in nursing.

导入案例与思考

患者，女，49 岁，失眠多年。近日因情绪不佳，每晚入睡困难，睡眠时间 3~4h，多梦易醒，醒后再难入睡，愈发烦躁，遂来院就诊。症见：心烦，面赤，口渴，口舌生疮，身热，小便短、赤、涩、痛，舌尖红，苔黄，脉数。

问题 1：患者心烦体现了心的哪一种功能异常？

问题 2：患者为什么会同时出现心烦、面赤、口舌生疮、小便短赤？

问题 3：针对患者的情况，根据阴阳学说确立的护治原则是什么？

中医护理学的理论基础来自于中医学基础理论。本章节主要介绍中医基础理论中的阴阳学说、五行学说、藏象学说、精气血津液、病因病机和经络腧穴，并简要介绍其在护理学中的指导意义和应用。

Section 1　Yin-Yang Theory

第一节　阴阳学说

Yin-yang theory studies laws of the connotation, movement and change of yin and yang. It is the world outlook and methodology by which people understand and explain the occurrence, development and changes of things and phenomena in nature. When it is used in the medical field by ancient doctors to expound physiological function and pathological changes of human body, and to direct clinical diagnosis, treatment and nursing, yin-yang theory becomes an important and unique component of the theoretical system of TCM throughout all areas.

阴阳学说是研究阴阳的内涵及其运动变化规律，并用以阐释宇宙间万物万象的发生、发展和变化的一种世界观和方法论。阴阳学说引入医学领域，用于阐明人体生理功能和病理变化，指导临床诊断、治疗、预防、护理和康复，形成了中医独特的阴阳学说，成为中医学理论体系的重要组成部分，贯穿于中医学的各个领域。

I. Basic Meaning of Yin and Yang

一、阴阳的基本含义

Originally, the words of yin and yang were used to describe the sides of a mountain that predominately faced away or towards the sun respectively. In other words,

"阴阳"的原始含义是指日光的向背，朝向日光为阳，背向日光则为阴。随着认识的

the side facing the sun pertains to yang while the side facing away from the sun is yin. With the development of understanding, yang is associated with such qualities as warmth, brightness and excitatory while yin is associated with the opposing characteristics like cold, darkness and stillness. Further expansion of this logic leads to an abstractive summarization of yin-yang. The concept of yin-yang is abstracted as a general division of any given thing (including living things, inanimate objects, feelings, actions, *etc.*) into two polar attributes which are related to each other.

Yin and yang can not only stand for opposite things and phenomena, but also serve to analyze two opposite aspects within one thing. Generally speaking, things that bear the properties of being warm, bright, active, rising, excited, dispersive, external and functional pertain to yang, while those that bear properties of being cold, dim, static, descending, suppressive, agglomerate, internal and organic pertain to yin. When the relative attributes of yin and yang are introduced into the medical field, material and function of the human body that bear the properties of being interior, upper, impellent, warm, excited and lifting pertain to yang, while those that bear properties of being exterior, under, tranquil, cool, prohibitive and sedimentary pertain to yin. Table 2-1 shows examples of yin-yang categorization.

深化，阴阳的含义逐渐得到引申，如向日光处温暖、明亮、活跃，背日光处寒冷、晦暗、静止。于是古人就以温暖、寒冷、光明、黑暗、运动、静止等来分阴阳。如此不断引申，阴阳的含义则抽象为自然界相互关联的事物或现象对立双方属性的概括。

阴和阳既可代表相互对立的事物和现象，又可代表同一事物内部相互对立的两个方面。一般而言，凡是温热的、明亮的、运动的、上升的、兴奋的、弥散的、外向的、功能的都属于阳；相对寒冷的、晦暗的、静止的、下降的、抑制的、凝聚的、内守的、物质的都属于阴。阴阳的相对属性引入医学领域，将人体中在外的、在上的和对人体具有推动、温煦、兴奋、升举等作用的物质和功能统属于阳，将在内的、在下的和对人体具有宁静、凉润、抑制、沉降等作用的物质和功能统属于阴。事物和现象的阴阳属性归类举例（表2-1）。

Table 2-1　Examples of Yin-Yang Categorization

Category	Yang	Yin
Time	Day	Night
Space (orientation)	Heaven, upper, out, left, south	Earth, under, in, right, north
Season	Spring, Summer	Autumn, Winter
Temperature	Warm, hot	Cool, cold
Humidness	Dry	Wet
Weight	Light	Heavy
Speed	Fast	Slow
Brightness	Light	Dark
Sex	Male	Female
Motion	Up and out, vigorous	Down and in, subtle
Tissue and organs	Skin, flesh, six-*fu*, lower back	Bone, tendon, five-*zang*, thorax-abdomen
Disease	Acute	Chronic

表 2-1　事物和现象的阴阳属性归类举例

分类	阳	阴
时间	昼	夜
空间（方位）	天，上，外，左，南	地，下，内，右，北
季节	春，夏	秋，冬
温度	温，热	凉，寒
湿度	干燥	湿润
重量	轻	重
速度	快	慢
亮度	明亮	黑暗
性别	雄性	雌性
运动状态	向上，向外，明显的	向下，向内，隐匿的
组织器官	皮肉，六腑，腰背	筋骨，五脏，胸腹
疾病进程	急性	慢性

II. Basic Content of Yin-Yang Theory

Yin-yang theory mainly includes four basic contents of opposition and restriction, interdependence and reciprocity, waning-waxing and balance, and mutual transformation of yin and yang.

i. Opposition and Restriction of Yin-Yang

Opposition and restriction of yin-yang means yin and yang may present the relationship of mutual restriction, control and repulsion. The opposition is manifested in its mutual restraining and opposing actions. For example, warmth and heat can dissipate cold while cold can bring down high temperature. Changes and development of natural phenomena are also the results of such mutual restraining and opposing relations. For example, yang qi is exuberant in summer yet yin qi starts to grow gradually after summer solstice to restrain excessive yang qi,while yin qi is prevailing in winter yet yang qi begins to recover after winter solstice to inhibit cold yin qi. Dynamic changes of yang and yin qi lead to the changes of four seasons with cold, heat, warmth and cool properties.

ii. Interdependence and Reciprocity of Yin-Yang

Interdependence of yin and yang indicates that yin or yang should take the existence of its counterpart as the prerequisite for its own existence, and that neither one can exist alone. For example, the upper pertains to yang and the lower to yin, without the lower there would be no the upper,

二、阴阳学说的基本内容

阴阳学说主要包括阴阳的对立制约、互根互用、消长平衡和相互转化四个方面的内容。

（一）阴阳对立制约

阴阳对立制约，指属性相反的阴阳双方相互斗争、相互制约和相互排斥的关系。阴阳的相互对立，是指阴阳性质的相反，这种相反的特性主要体现为它们之间的相互斗争、相互制约。如温热可以驱散寒冷，寒凉可以清除炎热。阴阳的对立制约，推动着事物的发生、发展和变化，维持着事物发展的动态平衡。如夏季阳气旺盛，但夏至以后，阴气渐生，以制约炎热的阳气；冬季阴寒较盛，但冬至以后，阳气渐复，以制约严寒的阴气，如此，在自然界阴阳相互制约、相互排斥中，形成了四季寒、热、温、凉的气候变化。

（二）阴阳互根互用

阴阳互根，指阴和阳相互依存、互为根本。即阴和阳必须以对方的存在作为自身存在的先决条件，任何一方都不能脱离另一方而单独存在。如上为阳，下为阴，没有上也

and vice versa. Neither yin nor yang can exist separately.

Reciprocity of yin and yang means that the interdependent yin and yang often express the relationship of mutual generation and promotion. Yin keeps inside while yang keeps outside for each other. They make use of each other. Take heaven and earth, cloud and rain for examples, the rising earthly qi can carry the water on the earth up to the heaven and form cloud and mist while the descending heavenly qi can make the cloud and mist in the sky fall onto the earth surface in the form of rain. The reciprocal process of cloud and rain, and earthly qi and heavenly qi is the process of reciprocity of yin and yang.

iii. Waning-Waxing and Balance of Yin-Yang

Waning-waxing and balance of yin-yang means that the two opposite and interdependent sides of yin and yang are not in a state of stillness but in constant change, or in a state of yin waning with yang waxing and yang waning with yin waxing. So they maintain a dynamic balance. Waning-waxing of yin and yang is a form of movement and a process of quantitative change. This change includes forms of the decreasing and increasing change of the two opposite sides of yin and yang (Fig. 2-1).

就无所谓下，没有下也就无所谓上。

阴阳互用，指阴阳双方相互资生、促进和助长。如"阴在内，阳之守也；阳在外，阴之使也"，是指阴为阳守持于内，阳为阴役使在外，阴阳相互为用，不可分离。以天地云雨为例，地气上升，可将地面的水分挟带至天空而形成云雾；天气下降，可将天空的云雾以雨水的形式下降至地面。云和雨，地气与天气的循环往复过程，即为阴阳互用的过程。

（三）阴阳消长平衡

阴阳消长平衡是指阴阳双方不是处于静止的状态，而是始终处于不断地增长和消减运动变化之中，并在运动中维持着动态平衡。阴阳消长是阴阳运动变化的一种形式，是一个量变过程，主要包括此消彼长、此长彼消、此消彼亦消、此长彼亦长四个方面（图 2-1）。

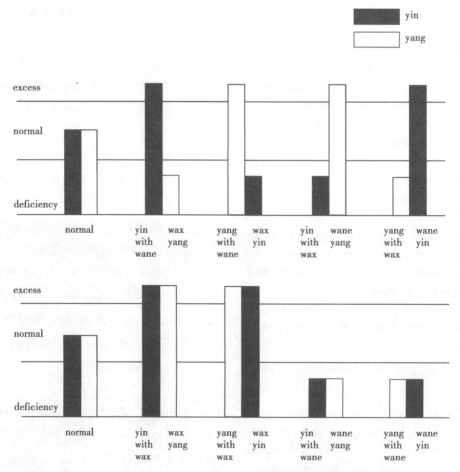

Fig. 2-1 Waning-Waxing of Yin-Yang

图 2-1 阴阳消长示意图

1. One Wane While the Other Wax or One Wax While the Other Wane This means that under the condition of mutual restriction of yin and yang. When one side gets too weak to restrict the other, the other may grow and even get hyperactive. Or when one side gets so strong as to over-restrict the other, the other may decline and even get inferior. Take the weather for example, in the change all the year round from winter to spring and summer, it becomes warm gradually, and this is called "yang waxing while yin waning". In the change from summer to fall and winter, it becomes cold gradually, and this is called "yin waxing while yang waning".

2. One Wane while the Other Wane or One Wax while the Other Wax This means that under the condition of mutual reciprocity of yin and yang, when one side gets too deficient to generate and promote the other, the other may get weak too. Or when one side gets abundant, it may promote growth of the other and make the other strong too. Take the climate and rainfall for example, while the temperature rises in spring and summer, rainfall increases accordingly. It pertains to "yin waxing while yang waxing". While the temperature declines in fall and winter, rainfall cuts down accordingly. It pertains to "yin waning while yang waning". When there is a lack of essence, there is no enough qi. Thus people may feel hungry, weak and dizzy. It pertains to "yang waning while yin waning". When people have some food and water, they may feel better. It pertains to "yang waxing while yin waxing".

iv. Mutual Transformation of Yin-Yang

Mutual transformation of yin and yang means that under certain conditions either yin or yang may transform itself into the other. Yin may turn into yang and yang into yin. It is another form of movement of yin-yang, and also a qualitative change on the basis of waning and waxing of yin-yang which is a quantitative one. They are two inseparable phases in the whole process of development and change of all things in motion. Waning and waxing is the precondition for transformation and transformation is the outcome of waning and waxing.

The transformation of yin and yang always happens under certain conditions. Generally, the attribute of yin or yang could convert into each other only when one thing develops to a certain degree or stage and the proportion of yin and yang of things inside reverses. It is often interpreted as "things will develop in the opposite direction when they become extreme". For example, when yin-cold in winter develops to the extreme, it provides the condition for transformation, and yin-cold weather thus changes to yang-heat weather. When yang-heat in summer develops to the extreme, it also provides the condition for transformation,

1. 此消彼长，此长彼消　指在阴阳双方对立制约的过程中，阴或阳一方衰弱，无力制约对方，从而引起对方的增长，甚至亢奋；或一方因增长而强盛，过度制约对方，从而引起对方的削减，甚至偏衰。以气候变化为例，由冬至春及夏，气候由寒冷逐渐转暖变热，这是"阳长阴消"的过程；由夏到秋及冬，气候由炎热逐渐转凉变寒，这是"阴长阳消"的过程。

2. 此消彼亦消，此长彼亦长　指在阴阳互根互用的过程中，阴或阳一方虚弱，无力资生和促进对方，使对方也随之虚弱，即阴随阳消或阳随阴消；或一方旺盛可助长和促进对方，使对方也随之旺盛，即阴随阳长或阳随阴长。如随着春夏气温的逐渐升高而降雨量逐渐增多，属阴随阳长；随着秋冬气候的转凉而降雨量逐渐减少，属阴随阳消；人饥饿时由于精不足，不能化气，而出现乏力头晕，属阳随阴消；饥饿时补充养分，产生能量，增加气力，则属阳随阴长。

（四）阴阳相互转化

阴阳转化，指在一定的条件下，阴或阳可各自向其相反的方面转化，即阴可转化为阳，阳也可转化为阴。阴阳转化是阴阳运动的又一形式，是在阴阳消长变化的基础上发生的质变。阴阳的消长和转化是运动着的事物发展变化全过程中密不可分的两个阶段，消长是转化的前提，转化是消长的结果。

阴阳转化必须具备一定的条件，一般是阴阳消长变化发展到"物极"阶段，事物内部阴与阳的比例出现颠倒，则该事物的属性发生转化，即所谓"物极必反"。如冬季之阴寒发展到了极致，便具备了转化的条件，阴寒气候就会向阳热方面转化；盛夏之阳热发展到了极致，即具备了转化的条件，阳热气候就会向阴寒方面转化。

thus yang-heat weather changes to yin-cold weather.

Mutual transformation between yin and yang can be not only a gradual change, such as the seasons circulation, the alternation of day and night, but can be a sudden one, such as a sudden cold in hot summer, or a sudden drop of body temperature and limb of appetite of a patient with acute fever, *etc.*.

阴阳相互转化，既可以表现为渐变式，如四季更替，昼夜转化，也可表现为突变式，如夏季酷热天气的骤冷，急性热病患者突然出现体温下降、四肢厥冷等。

III. Application of the Yin-Yang Theory in TCM Nursing

i. Explaining Tissue Structure

The human body, organs, channels and collaterals are organically linked, and can all be attributed by yin and yang according to their location and functional characteristics. In terms of the human body, the upper part pertains to yang while the lower to yin. The body surface pertains to yang while the interior to yin. The back pertains to yang while the abdomen to yin. The lateral sides of the limbs pertain to yang while medial sides to yin. The five *zang* organs pertain to yang while the six *fu* organs to yin. The five *zang* organs can also be divided in terms of yin and yang, namely: the heart and lung which are located in the upper (thorax) pertain to yang while the liver, spleen and kidney which are located in the lower (abdomen) pertain to yin. Moreover, each *zang* organ itself can be further divided into yin and yang aspects. For example, there is heart-yin and heart yang for the heart.

ii. Explaining Physiological Function

The yin-yang theory holds that human life activity and processes are the outcome of the coordination of opposition and unification between yin and yang. Life activities of human beings take material metabolism as the basis. Without life materials (yin), there would be no functional activities (yang). Meanwhile the life activities (yang) constantly promote and generate life materials (yin). During the first half of one's life, it's dominated by the promoting and exciting activities, which can keep the stability of one's growth and development. It pertains to "yin waxing while yang waxing". While during the latter half of one's life, it's dominated by the quiet and suppressive activities, which can help people to live their menopause and aging phase. It pertains to "yang waning while yin waning".

iii. Explaining Pathological Change

TCM regards the imbalance between yin and yang as the root cause of occurrence, development and change of diseases.

The process of occurrence, development and change of diseases is a process of conflict between the

三、阴阳学说在中医护理学中的应用

（一）说明人体组织结构

人体各脏腑经络形体组织，既是有机联系的，又可根据其所在部位、功能特点划分阴阳。就人体部位而言，上为阳，下为阴；体表属阳，体内属阴。就背腹四肢而言，背属阳，腹属阴；四肢外侧为阳，内侧为阴。就脏腑而言，五脏为阴；六腑为阳。五脏之中又可分阴阳，即心肺居上（胸腔），属阳；肝脾肾位下（腹腔），属阴。具体到各脏内部，则又可分阴阳，如心之心阴、心阳等。

（二）说明人体生理功能

阴阳学说认为，人体的正常生命活动和生长壮老已的生命过程，是阴阳双方保持对立统一协调关系的结果。生命活动是以物质代谢为基础的，没有各种生命物质（阴）则无法产生各种生理活动（阳）；而各种生理活动（阳）又不断促进各种生命物质（阴）的新陈代谢。人的前半生以阳气的推动、兴奋作用为主导，阴随阳长，维持人体生长发育的有序稳定；后半生以阴气的宁静、抑制作用为主导，阳随阴消，使人平稳度过更年期和老年阶段。

（三）说明人体病理变化

中医学认为，阴阳失调是各种疾病发生、发展和变化的根本原因。

疾病的发生、发展过程是邪正斗争的过程。正气，是指人体的正常组织结构、生理

healthy qi and the pathogenic qi with either predominance or subordination. The healthy qi generally refers to the normal histological structures, physiological functions, and the ability to resist, stand and repair the damage by diseases. The pathogenic qi generally refers to various factors giving rise to diseases. The healthy qi can be further divided into yang qi and yin fluid while the pathogenic qi can also be classified into two types of yin and yang.

The imbalance between yin and yang mainly expresses as predominance or subordination of one side over the other or the damage to each other (Table 2-2).

1. Predominance of Yin or Yang   It includes yin excess and yang excess, which means that either side of yin or yang is above the normal levels, and thus it brings about diseases and pattern of excessive pathogenic factors.

(1) Predominance of yang brings about heat pattern and the disorder of yin: Yang pathogenic qi is hot, so the predominance of yang brings about heat pattern. Yin

功能，以及机体对疾病损害的抵抗、耐受和修复损伤的能力。邪气，泛指各种致病因素。正气有阴精和阳气之分，邪气有阴邪和阳邪之别。邪气致病，邪正相搏，导致阴阳盛衰变化而发病。

阴阳失调主要表现为阴阳的偏盛、偏衰和互损；用阴阳说明人体病理变化（表2-2）。

1. 阴阳偏盛   即阴盛或阳盛，是属于阴或阳任何一方高于正常水平的病理状态，多为邪气有余的病证。

（1）阳盛则热，阳盛则阴病：阳邪亢盛，性质为热，故出现热证；阳长则阴消，导致

Table 2-2   Explanation of Pathological Change by Yin-Yang

Excess/Deficiency	Meanings	Pathology	Clinical Manifestations
Superiority of yang	Yang is above the normal level	Superiority of yang brings about heat pattern	Fever, profuse sweating, reddish complexion, restlessness, thirst, desire for cold drinks, yellowish-colored sputum, dark-colored urination, constipation, red tongue, yellowish tongue coating, rapid pulse
Superiority of yin	Yin is above the normal level	Superiority of yin brings about cold pattern	Aversion to cold, no sweat, pale complexion, no thirst, desire for warm drinks, thin and watery sputum, loose stool, light-colored tongue, whitish tongue coating, slow or tense pulse
Deficiency of yang	Yang is below the normal level	Deficiency of yang leads to deficiency-cold pattern	Cold limbs, preference for warmth, pale complexion, spontaneous sweating, fatigue, shortness of breath, loose stool, enlarged and light-colored tongue, whitish tongue coating, deep, slow and weak pulse
Deficiency of yin	Yin is below the normal level	Deficiency of yin leads to deficiency-heat pattern	Hot feeling in the soles and palms, afternoon tidal fever, night sweating, red cheeks, thirst, dry mouth and throat, red tongue with little coating, rapid and thready pulse

表2-2   阴阳说明人体病理变化

阴阳盛衰	含义	病理	临床表现
阳偏盛	阳高于正常水平	阳盛则热	发热，大汗，面赤，烦躁，口渴喜冷饮，痰黄，尿赤，便秘，舌红，苔黄，脉数
阴偏盛	阴高于正常水平	阴盛则寒	恶寒，无汗，面白，口不渴，喜热饮，痰液清稀，便溏，舌淡，苔白，脉迟紧
阳偏衰	阳低于正常水平	阳虚则寒	形寒肢冷，喜温，面白，自汗，疲倦，气短，便溏，舌淡胖，苔白，脉沉迟弱
阴偏衰	阴低于正常水平	阴虚则热	五心烦热，午后潮热，盗汗，颧红，口渴，口干，咽干，舌红少苔，脉细数

wanes while yang waxes, which leads to the disorder of yin (Fig. 2-2).

(2) Predominance of yin brings about cold pattern and the disorder of yang: Yin pathogenic qi is cold, so the predominance of yin brings about cold pattern. Yang wanes while yin waxes, which leads to the disorder of yang (Fig. 2-3).

2. Deficiency of Yin or Yang　It includes yin deficiency and yang deficiency, which means that either side of yin or yang is below the normal levels, and thus it brings about diseases and pattern of insufficient healthy qi (Fig. 2-4).

(1) Deficiency of yang leads to cold pattern: When yang-qi of the body is insufficient, it can't restrict yin-qi, and thus leads to deficiency-cold pattern.

(2) Deficiency of yin leads to heat pattern: When

阴液损伤（图 2-2）。

（2）阴盛则寒，阴盛则阳病：阴邪亢盛，性质为寒，故出现寒证；阴长则阳消，导致阳气损伤（图 2-3）。

2. 阴阳偏衰　即阴虚或阳虚，是属于阴或阳任何一方低于正常水平的病理状态，多为正气不足的病证（图 2-4）。

（1）阳虚则寒：人体的阳气不足，阳虚不能制约阴，则阴相对偏盛而出现寒象。

（2）阴虚则热：人体的阴液不足，阴虚不

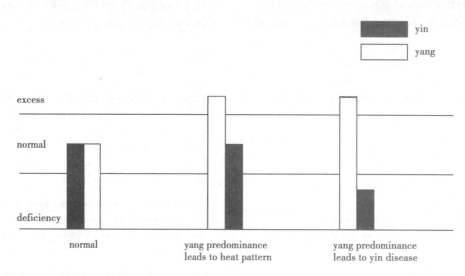

Fig. 2-2　Predominance of Yang
图 2-2　阳偏盛关系示意图

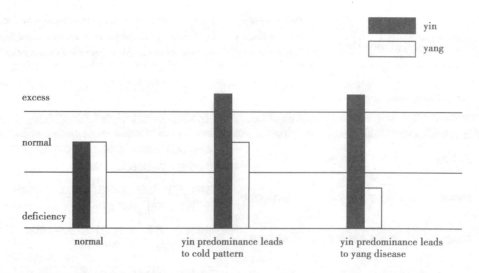

Fig. 2-3　Predominance of Yin
图 2-3　阴偏盛关系示意图

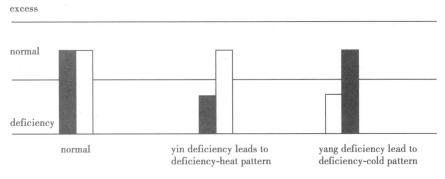

Fig. 2-4   Deficiency of Yin or Yang
图 2-4   阴阳偏衰关系示意图

yin-fluid of the body is insufficient, it can't restrict yang-qi, and thus leads to deficiency-heat pattern.

3. Impairment of Yin or Yang Affecting Each Other   Because of the interdependence and reciprocity of yin-yang, a degree of consumption of any aspect of yin or yang of the organism will usually result in the insufficiency of its opposite, known as the "impairment of yang affecting yin" or the "impairment of yin affecting yang." This will result in deficiency of both yin and yang or the insufficiency of both qi and blood. This is the common process of pathological development in chronic diseases.

iv. Guiding Pattern Differentiation and Nursing Assessment

One must first distinguish yin from yang so as to grasp the essence of the disease and make a correct assessment. For example, in application of the four diagnostic methods of inspection, smelling and listening, inquiring and pulse feeling, the yin and yang attributes of the color and luster of the skin, sound of voice and breath, and pulse condition should be differentiated carefully. In case of inspection, bright complexion pertains to yang while dim complexion to yin. In case of smelling and listening, rapid and strong breathing pertains to yang while shallow and weak breathing to yin. Loud and sonorous voice with talkativeness and restlessness pertains to yang while low and feeble voice with reticence and rest to yin. In case of pulse feeling, viewed from the location, *cùn* site pertains to yang while *chǐ* site to yin. Viewed from the rate, rapid pulse pertains to yang while slow to yin. Viewed from the shape, floating, surging, large, slippery and full pulse pertains to yang while deep, thready, small, unsmooth and choppy pulse to yin.

能制约阳，则阳相对偏盛而出现热象。

3. 阴阳互损   由于阴阳之间互根互用，所以阴阳任何一方虚损到一定程度时，必然导致另一方不足，即所谓"阴损及阳"和"阳损及阴"，最终可导致"阴阳两虚"，气血两虚，此即慢性病常见的病理过程。

（四）指导辨证与护理评估

在辨证与护理评估中，只有辨清阴阳，才能正确分析和判断疾病的本质属性。如在望、闻、问、切四诊合参的过程中，可分辨色泽、声息、脉象等方面的阴阳属性。色泽鲜明者属阳，色泽晦暗者属阴。观察气息，呼吸气粗者属阳，呼吸微弱者属阴。听其声音，语声高亢洪亮，多言躁动者属阳；语声低微，少言沉静者属阴。从脉象部位来分，寸为阳，尺为阴；以迟数分，数者为阳，迟者为阴；以形态分，浮、洪、大、滑者属阳，沉、细、小、涩者属阴。

v. Guiding Clinical Treatment and Nursing

The imbalance between yin and yang is considered as the root cause of the occurrence, development and change of diseases, therefore the basic principle of clinical treatment and nursing should be regulating yin and yang by reinforcing the deficient and reducing the surplus so as to restore the relative balance between yin and yang (Table 2-3).

1. Therapeutic Principle for Relative Superiority of Yin or Yang Predominance of yang results in an excess-heat pattern, which should be treated by restricting yang with cold or cool medications, food, and surroundings, by treating the hot with coldness or "cooling what is hot". Predominance of yin results in an excess-cold pattern, and should be treated by restricting yin with warm or hot medications, food, and surroundings, by treating cold with hot or "heating what is cold".

2. Therapeutic Principle for Relative Inferiority of Yin or Yang In case of deficiency-heat pattern caused by yang hyperactivity due to failure of deficient yin to restrict yang, cold or cool medications and food should not be applied to reduce heat, instead the method of nourishing yin and strengthening water should be used to restrict up-flaring fire caused by hyperactive yang. In case of deficiency-cold pattern caused by excess of yin due to failure of deficient yang to check yin, pungent dispersing medications or food should not be applied to dispel yin-cold, instead the method of strengthening yang

（五）指导疾病治疗与护理

阴阳失调是疾病发生、发展的根本原因，故疾病治疗与护理的基本原则是调整阴阳、补其不足、泻其有余、恢复阴阳的相对平衡（表2-3）。

1. 阴阳偏盛的治则 阳盛则热，属实热证，宜用寒凉药食以制其阳，病室环境宜凉爽，治热以寒，即"热者寒之"。阴盛则寒，属实寒证，宜用温热药食以制其阴，病室宜温暖，治寒以热，即"寒者热之"。

2. 阴阳偏衰的治则 阴虚不能制阳而致阳亢者，属虚热证，一般不能用寒凉药食清其热，须用滋阴壮水法，以抑制阳亢火盛。如果阳虚不能制阴而导致阴盛者，属虚寒证，更不宜用辛温发散药食散其寒，须扶阳益火法，以消退阴翳。此外，根据阴阳互用的关系，还可考虑"阴中求阳，阳中求阴"之法，即在用温阳药时，兼用滋阴药；在用滋阴药时，加用补阳药，以发挥阴阳互用的生化作用。

Table 2-3　The Guideline of Clinical Treatment and Nursing by Yin-Yang

Excess/Deficiency	Pathology	Principle	Nature and Flavor of Herbs and Food
Predominance of yang	Predominance of yang brings about heat pattern	Treating heat with cold	Cool, cold, bitter, sour
Predominance of yin	Predominance of yin brings about cold pattern	Treating cold with heat	Warm, hot, pungent
Deficiency of yang	Deficiency of yang leads to deficiency-cold pattern	Warming yang and restraining yin	Warm, hot, sweet
Deficiency of yin	Deficiency of yin leads to deficiency -heat pattern	Nourishing yin and restraining yang	Cool, cold, sweet

表2-3　阴阳学说指导疾病治疗和护理

阴阳盛衰	病理	护治原则	药食性味
阳偏盛	阳盛则热	热者寒之	寒凉，苦、酸
阴偏盛	阴盛则寒	寒者热之	温热，辛
阳偏衰	阳虚则寒	扶阳抑阴	温热，甘
阴偏衰	阴虚则热	滋阴抑阳	寒凉，甘

and supplementing fire to expel pathogenic yin is adopted. In addition, according to the theory of interdependence of yin and yang, the methods of "seeking yin from yang and seeking yang from yin" may also be considered for treatment of inferiority of yin or yang. When yang-warming medications are used, yin-nourishing medications may be prescribed as a subsidiary method. When yin-nourishing medications are adopted, yang-supplementing medications may be prescribed meanwhile as a subsidiary method. The purpose is to bring into full play of the generating action of mutual reciprocity of yin and yang.

3. Therapeutic Principle for Mutual Impairment of Yin-Yang Because of impairment of yin or yang affecting each other, people should take the principle of complement of both yin and yang. In the case of yin and yang deficiency pattern with yang-deficiency as the predominant one, people should give priority to warming yang-qi, and take account of nourishing yin. While in the case of yin and yang deficiency pattern with yin-deficiency as the predominant one, people should give priority to nourishing yin, and take account of warming yang-qi.

vi. Guiding Health Maintenance and Disease Prevention

Due to both yin-qi and yang-qi of the body as the root of life, adjusting yin and yang is the first principle of health maintenance and disease prevention. People should not only keep the balance of the body, but also keep the harmony between the humanity and nature according to the rule of yin-yang changes. For instance, people can keep healthy by "conserving yang-qi in spring and summer" and "conserving yin-qi in fall and winter". For people with constitution of yang deficiency and yin excess, it should warm yang-qi so as to prevent the occurrence of diseases in winter, which is so-called "treating in summer for diseases tending to occur in winter". For people with constitution of yin deficiency and yang excess, it should nourish yin-qi so as to prevent the occurrence of diseases in summer, which is so-called "caring in winter for diseases tending to occur in summer".

(Wang Qiu-qin)

3. 阴阳互损的治则 阴阳互损导致阴阳两虚，护治时应采用阴阳双补的原则。对阳虚为主的阴阳两虚证，当补阳为主，兼以滋阴；对阴虚为主的阴阳两虚证，当滋阴为主，兼以温阳。

（六）指导养生防病

人体的阴阳，是生命的根本，故养生防病应善于调整阴阳，既要保持人体内部的阴阳协调统一，也要适应自然界的阴阳变化规律，保持人与自然界的协调统一。如"春夏养阳、秋冬养阴"。又如对于阳虚阴盛体质者，需在夏季用温热法预培其阳，则冬不易发病，即所谓冬病夏治；对于阴虚阳亢体质者，需在冬季用凉润法预养其阴，则夏不得发病，即所谓"夏病冬养"。

（王秋琴）

Section 2　Five Phase Theory

第二节　五行学说

Five phase theory studies the connotation, feature and the laws of promotion, restriction, subjugation, and violation

五行学说，是研究木、火、土、金、水五行的含义、特性、生克制化乘侮规律，并

of the five phases: wood, fire, earth, metal and water. It is an ancient Chinese philosophy theory by which people understand and explain the occurrence, development and changes of things and phenomena in nature.

Five phases are not just the materials that the names refer to, but rather metaphors and symbols for describing how things interact and relate to each other. Five phases actually refer to the movement and transformation of these five phases as well as their relationships. In TCM, five-phase theory has had considerable influence in physiology, pathology, diagnosis, treatment and nursing.

I. Basic Meaning of Five Phases

In Chinese language "wǔ" refers to five categories of things in the natural world, namely wood, fire, earth, metal and water, and "xíng" refers to the movement and change, therefore "wǔ xíng" (the five phases) actually refers to the movement and change of the five basic elements.

Ancient Chinese people recognized in their long period of life practice that wood, fire, earth, metal and water were essential materials in human life, so they were called the "five materials". By taking the knowledge of the five materials as the basis, five-phase theory extracts and deduces the attributes of the five phases so as to explain the movement and change of inter-promotion and inter-restriction among all things and phenomena of the nature.

TCM applies the laws of the five phases in characteristic, categorization and promotion-restriction relation to summarize functional attributes of the zang-fu organs, explain the inner relations among the five zang system, expound human physiology, pathology as well as mutual relation between the human body and the outer environment, and guide treatment and nursing based on pattern differentiation for the purpose of prevention and treatment.

II. Characteristic and Categorization of the Five Phases

i. Characteristic of the Five Phases

The characteristics of the five phases were developed by ancient people through extraction and sublimation based on direct observation and simple recognition of the five materials of wood, fire, earth, metal and water. They are generally used to analyze the attributes of various things divided into five materials' categories, and study the interrelations of the five materials. The understanding of the characteristics of the five phases is of more abstract and extensive significance compared with the understanding

用以阐释宇宙万物的发生、发展、变化及相互关系的古代哲学理论。

古代自然哲学的五行学说应用于中医学，以五行的运动变化规律阐释人体生理、病理及其与外在环境的相互联系，进而指导临床诊断、治疗与护理，从而形成了中医独特的五行学说。

一、五行的基本含义

五行中的"五"，指木、火、土、金、水五种物质；"行"，指运动变化。五行，即木、火、土、金、水五种物质及其运动变化。

在长期生活实践中，人们认识到木、火、土、金、水五种物质是人类生活中不可或缺的物质，故称其为"五材"。五行学说是在"五材"说的基础上，将五种物质的属性和相互作用加以抽象描述，用以说明自然界一切事物和现象之间相生、相克的运动变化的一门学说。

中医学运用五行特性、归类以及生克制化规律，来概括脏腑组织的功能属性，阐释五脏系统的内在联系，说明人体的生理、病理及其与外在环境的相互关系等，从而指导辨证论治与辨证施护。

二、五行特性和五行归类

（一）五行特性

五行的特性，是古人在长期生活实践中，对木、火、土、金、水五种物质的直接观察和朴素认识的基础上，进行抽象升华而逐渐形成的理论概念，是用于分析各种事物的五行属性和研究事物之间相互联系的基本依据。对五行特性的认识已超越了五种具体物质的本身，而具有更为广泛、抽象的含义。

of the five phases themselves.

1. Wood　Ancient people stated "wood is characterized by bending and straightening". This means that the stem and branches of trees can bend and strengthen, and can grow upward and outward. Therefore, it is extended that anything that has the function or property of growing, developing and flourishing can be attributed to wood.

2. Fire　It is stated "fire is the flaming upward". This means that fire has the characteristics of warmth, heat and ascending. Therefore, it is extended that anything that has the function or property of warmth, heat and ascending can be attributed to fire.

3. Earth　It is stated "earth is the sowing and reaping". This means that people can grow seed and gain crops on the earth. Therefore, it is extended that anything that has the function or property of generating, holding and receiving can be attributed to earth.

4. Metal　It is stated that "metal is the working of change". This means that metal can follow human's intention to change its shape. Therefore, it is extended that anything that has the function or property of clearing, descending and astringing can be attributed to metal.

5. Water　It is stated "water is the moistening and descending". This means that water has the property of moistening and downward going. Therefore, it is extended that anything that has the function or property of cold or coolness, moistening and downward going can be attributed to water.

ii. The Structural System of the Five Phases

The characteristics of the five phases are the basis for categorization of the five phases. The property and function of a thing is compared with the characteristics of the five phases to decide the property of the thing in the five phases. However, things similar to the five phases in property and function are not the five phases themselves. For example, a thing similar to wood in property pertains to the wood and a thing similar to fire in property pertains to the fire. For another example, the east, where the sun rises, is full of vital energy and similar to growing, developing and flourishing of wood in property, so the east pertains to the wood. The south, where it is hot and plants are flourishing, is similar to burning and up-flaring of fire in property, so the south pertains to the fire.

Taking the correspondence between human and universe as the guidance principle, the five phases as the center, the space structure as the five directions, time structure as the five seasons, and human body structure as the basic framework, the theory of the five phases can serve to categorize all things and phenomena in nature as

1. **木的特性**　古人称"木曰曲直"。曲直，是指树木的枝干能屈能伸，向上向外舒展。引申为凡具有生长、升发、条达、舒畅等性质或作用的事物和现象，均归属于木。

2. **火的特性**　古人称"火曰炎上"。炎上，是指火具有炎热、上升、明亮的特性。引申为凡具有温热、升腾、光明等性质或作用的事物和现象，均归属于火。

3. **土的特性**　古人称"土爰稼穑"。"爰"通"曰"。稼穑，是指土地可播种和收获农作物。引申为凡具有生化、承载、受纳等性质或作用的事物和现象，均归属于土。

4. **金的特性**　古人称"金曰从革"。从革，是指金有刚柔相济之性，可顺从人意，改变其状。引申为凡具有沉降、肃杀、收敛等性质或作用的事物和现象，均归属于金。

5. **水的特性**　古人称"水曰润下"。润下，是指水具有滋润和向下的特性。引申为凡具有寒凉、滋润、向下运行等性质或作用的事物和现象，均归属于水。

（二）五行归类

五行学说是以五行的特性来推演和归类事物和现象的五行属性。事物的五行属性并不等同于木、火、土、金、水五类物质本身，而是将事物的性质和作用，与五行的特性相类比，从而得出事物的五行属性。例如：东方为日出之地，富有生机，与木的升发、生长特性相类，故归属于木；南方气候炎热，植物繁茂，与火的炎上特性相类，故归属于火。

五行学说对事物属性的推演归类以天人相应为指导原则，以五行为中心，以空间结构的五方，时间结构的五季，人体结构的五脏为基本框架，将自然界的各种事物和现象及人体的生理病理现象，按其属性进行归纳，形

well as human physiology and pathology by comparing their properties and functions with the characteristics of the five phases (Table 2-4).

It can be seen from the Table 2-4 that all changing things and phenomena in nature can be categorized into the system of the five phases of wood, fire, earth, metal and water while various tissues and functions of the human body can also be summarized into the five physiological systems centered round the five *zang organs*.

III. Basic Content of Five Phase Theory

Basic content of five phase theory is the law of

成了联系人体内外环境的五行结构系统，用以说明人体及人与自然环境的统一（表2-4）。

由此可见，根据五行特性，自然界千变万化的事物和现象均可归结为木、火、土、金、水的五行系统，人体的各种组织和功能也可归结为以五脏为中心的五个生理系统。

三、五行学说的基本内容

五行学说的基本内容是五行的生克制化

Table 2-4   The Categorization of Things to the Five Phases

		Jué	*zhǐ*	*Gōng*	*Shāng*	*Yǔ*
Nature	Five notes	*Jué*	*zhǐ*	*Gōng*	*Shāng*	*Yǔ*
	Five times	Early morning	Noon	Afternoon	Evening	Midnight
	Five flavors	Sour	Bitter	Sweet	Acrid	Salty
	Five colors	Green	Red	Yellow	White	Black
	Five changes	Germination	Growth	Transformation	Reaping	Storing
	Five climates	Wind	Summer-heat	Dampness	Dryness	Cold
	Five seasons	Spring	Summer	Late summer	Fall	Winter
	Five directions	East	South	Center	West	North
	Five phases	Wood	Fire	Earth	Metal	Water
Human body	Five *zang* organs	Liver	Heart	Spleen	Lung	Kidney
	Five *fu* organs	Gallbladder	Small intestine	Stomach	Large intestine	Urinary bladder
	Five constituents	Tendon	Vessel	Muscle	Skin	Bone
	Five brilliances	Nail	Face	Lip	Fine hair	Hair
	Five emotions	Anger	Joy	Thinking	Sorrow	Fear
	Five sense organs	Eye	Tongue	Mouth	Nose	Ear
	Five secretions	Tear	Sweat	Slobber	Snivel	Spittle
	Five pulse conditions	Wiry	Surging	Moderate	Floating	Deep
	Five voices	Shouting	Laughing	Singing	Crying	Moaning

表2-4   事物属性的五行归类

自然界								五行	人体							
五音	五时	五味	五色	五化	五气	五季	五方		五脏	五腑	五体	五华	五志	五官	五液	五脉	五声
角	平旦	酸	青	生	风	春	东	木	肝	胆	筋	爪	怒	目	泪	弦	呼
徵	日中	苦	赤	长	暑	夏	南	火	心	小肠	脉	面	喜	舌	汗	洪	笑
宫	日西	甘	黄	化	湿	长夏	中	土	脾	胃	肉	唇	思	口	涎	缓	歌
商	日入	辛	白	收	燥	秋	西	金	肺	大肠	皮	毛	悲	鼻	涕	浮	哭
羽	夜半	咸	黑	藏	寒	冬	北	水	肾	膀胱	骨	发	恐	耳	唾	沉	呻

generation, restriction, over-restriction and counter-restriction. Among the five phases, it expounds the holistic unification of mutual relation, coordination and balance among the five phases by normal generation and restriction among them, and clarifies their interaction after the damage to the coordination and balance by abnormal generation and restriction among them.

i. Normal Generation and Restriction among the Five Phases

1. Normal Generation among the Five Phases

It means that one element generates and helps another one sequentially in the five phases. This inter-generating and inter-promoting relation is known as that of generation among the five phases. The order of generation among the five phases is that wood generates fire, fire generates earth, earth generates metal, metal generates water and water generates wood. In the generation relation among the five phases, each element has two sides of "being generated" and "generating". The one generating is termed "mother" while the one being generated is termed "child". Therefore, the generation relationship among the five phases is also called "mother-child relationship". Take the fire as example, the one generating fire is wood and the one that is generated by fire is earth, so fire is the mother of earth and the child of wood.

2. Normal Restriction among the Five Phases

It means that one element restricts and checks another one sequentially in the five phases. This inter-restricting and inter-checking relation is known as that of restriction among the five phases. The order of restriction among the five phases is that wood restricts earth, earth restricts water, water restricts fire, fire restricts metal, and metal restricts wood. In the restriction relation among the five phases, each element has two sides of "being restricted" and "restricting". The one being restricted by another one is its "subordinate" while the one restricting another one is its "dominator". Take the wood as example, the one restricting wood is metal and the one that is restricted by wood is earth, so metal is the dominator and earth is the subordinate of wood.

ii. The Interaction of Five Phases

The interaction of five phases refers to the fact that there is an interaction of inter-generation and inter-restraint under normal conditions, which is illustrated as "there is restriction within generation" and "there is generation within restriction". Each part of the system of the five phases is not isolated from , but closely related to the others. The change of one part may affect the status of the others. Meanwhile it is affected and restrained by the whole structural system of the five phases. Normal

乘侮规律。以五行之间的相生和相克来阐释事物之间的相互联系、协调平衡的整体性和统一性；以五行之间的相乘和相侮来阐释事物之间协调平衡被破坏后的相互影响。

（一）五行相生相克

1. **五行相生** 是指木、火、土、金、水之间存在着有序的递相资生、助长和促进的关系。五行相生的次序是木生火、火生土、土生金、金生水、水生木。在五行的相生关系中，任何一行都有"生我"和"我生"两个方面的关系，生我者为母，我生者为子，所以五行相生关系也称为母子关系。以火为例，由于火生土，故火为土之母，而火由木所生，故火为木之子。

2. **五行相克** 是指木、火、土、金、水之间存在着有序的递相克制、制约的关系。五行相克的次序是木克土、土克水、水克火、火克金、金克木。在五行的相克关系中，任何一行都有"克我"和"我克"两个方面的关系，我克者为我所胜，克我者为我所不胜。以木为例，木克者为土，土为木之所胜；克木者为金，金为木之所不胜。

（二）五行制化

五行制化，指五行之间既相互资生，又相互制约，"生中有克""克中有生"的关系。五行系统结构的各部分都不是孤立的，而是密切相关的，每一部分的变化，都必然影响着其他部分的状态，同时又受着五行系统结构整体的影响与制约。五行制化属于相生与相克相结合的自我调节，维持着事物间的平

generation and restriction among the five phases reflect normal phenomena in nature. It is the relative balance of mutual generation and restriction that maintains normal occurrence and development of all things. The law of the interaction of five phases is that if one element is above the normal level, there will be one element to restrict it.

iii. Abnormal Restriction among the Five Phases

It refers to the following two conditions of over-restriction and counter-restriction.

1. Over-Restriction among the Five Phases

Over-restriction among the five phases refers to the condition in which one element of the five phases excessively restricts its being restricted element. The order of over-restriction is the same as that of restriction among the five phases. But the difference is that restriction among the five phases reflects normal phenomena in nature while over-restriction among the five phases reflects abnormal phenomena in nature. There are usually two causes for over-restriction. One is that one element of the five phases gets very powerful and excessively restricts the element which is supposed normally to restrict, making the element being restricted too weak, such as powerful wood restricts earth. The other is that one element of the five phases gets very weak which makes the element that restricts it relatively stronger, therefore it cannot stand the relatively stronger restriction by the element that is supposed normally to restrict it and gets even weaker, such as wood restricts weak earth.

2. Counter-Restriction among the Five Phases

Counter-restriction among the five phases refers to the condition in which one element of the five phases reversely restricts and bullies the element that restricts it. Counter-restriction among the five phases is an abnormal restriction going in the opposite order of restriction among the five phases, namely: wood counter-restricts metal, metal counter-restricts fire, fire counter-restricts water, water counter-restricts earth, and earth counter-restricts wood. There are usually two causes for counter-restriction. One is that one element of the five phases gets very strong, and it is no longer restricted by the element that normally restricts it, but reversely restricts the element, so this is also called counter-restriction. The other is that one of the five phases gets very weak and makes the element being normally restricted by it relatively stronger, therefore this element is no longer restricted by it, but reversely restricts it.

衡协调，促进稳定、有序的变化与发展。五行制化的规律是五行中一行亢盛时，必然随之有制约，以防止亢而为害，即在相生中有克制，在克制中求发展，循环往复。

（三）五行相乘相侮

五行之间的异常相克现象，称之为相乘、相侮。

1. 五行相乘 乘，乘虚侵袭之意。五行相乘是指五行中某一行对其所胜一行的过度制约或克制。五行之间相乘的次序与相克一致，即木乘土，土乘水，水乘火，火乘金，金乘木，但相克为正常现象，相乘为异常现象。引起相乘的原因有两个方面：一是某一行过于强盛，对其所胜一行克伐太过，导致所胜的一行虚弱，如木旺乘土；二是某一行过于虚弱，难以承受其所不胜一行的正常限度的克制，使其自身更加虚弱，如土虚木乘。

2. 五行相侮 侮，以强凌弱之意。五行相侮是指五行中某一行对其所不胜一行的反向制约和克制。五行相侮的规律以反克推之，即为木侮金、金侮火、火侮水、水侮土、土侮木。引起相侮的原因亦有两个方面：一是某一行过于强盛，非但不受"克我"之行的克制，反而对原来"克我"的一行实施反向克制，如木亢侮金；二是某一行过于虚弱，因而导致"我克"一行相对太过，不仅不能克制"我克"一行，反受其反向克制，如木虚土侮。

IV. Application of Five Phase Theory in TCM Nursing

i. Explaining Physiological Function and Their Relationship

Five-phase theory categorizes the five *zang* organs into the five phases system so as to explain their characteristics of physiological functions according to the attributes of the five phases. For example, wood is characterized by growing and flourishing while liver prefers free flow of qi, so liver pertains to wood. Fire burns and tends to flare up while heart yang warms the whole body, so heart pertains to fire. Earth is characterized by generating while spleen transforms food nutrients and is the source of production of qi and blood, so spleen pertains to earth. Metal is characterized by purifying and astringing while lung-qi is in charge of purification and descending, so lung pertains to metal. Water is characterized by moistening and storage while kidney stores essence and governs liquid metabolism, so kidney pertains to water. Through indirect deduction those things that have physiological relations with the five *zang* organs such as the five *fu* organs, five constituents, five brilliances, five emotions, five orifices, and five secretions can all be attributed to the five phases along with the corresponding *zang organs*.

The relationships of inter-generation and inter-restriction among the five phases can also be used to reflect some intrinsic relationships among the functional activities of the five *zang* organs. Generation among the five phases is used to explain the promotion among the five *zang organs* while restriction among the five phases is used to explain restraint among the five *zang* organs. Besides, the relationship between human beings and the external environment such as four seasons, five climatic factors, and five flavors of food can also be explained by five-phase theory. Thus the application of this theory to physiology lies in explanation of the unity not only among organs and tissues of the human body but also between human and the external environment.

ii. Explaining Pathological Change and Their Inter-Affection

The relationships of abnormal generation and restriction among the five phases can be used to explain inter-affections in pathology among the *zang* organs. Take a liver disease as example, if the liver disease affects the spleen, this is wood over-restricting earth. If a spleen disease involves the liver, this is earth counter-restricting wood. If the liver disease affects the heart, this is mother's disease involving its child. If the liver disease affects the lung, this is wood counter-restricting metal. If the liver disease affects the kidney, this is child's disease involving

四、五行学说在中医护理学中的应用

（一）说明人体生理功能及其相互关系

五行学说将人体的五脏分属于五行，以五行特性来说明五脏的生理功能特点。如肝喜条达，有疏泄的功能，木有生发的特性，故以肝属木；心阳有温煦的作用，火有温热的特性，故以心属火；脾为生化之源，土有生化万物的特性，故以脾属土；肺气主肃降，金有清肃、收敛的特性，故以肺属金；肾有主水、藏精的功能，水有润下、闭藏的特性，故以肾属水。依次类推，与五脏有生理联系的五腑、五体、五华、五志、五窍、五液等也都一并随五脏而归属于相应的五行之中了。

五行学说亦用于阐释人体的脏腑组织之间生理功能的内在联系。五行相生用于说明五脏之间的资生关系，五行相克用于说明五脏之间的制约关系。五行学说推演络绎人体组织结构的功能与相互关系，构建了以五脏为中心的生理病理系统，同时又将自然界的五方、五气、五色、五味等与人体五脏相联系，建立了以五脏为中心的内外环境相联系的五个统一体，体现了天人相应的整体观念。

（二）说明人体病理变化及其相互影响

五行学说可采用五行乘侮和母子相及的规律，说明在病理情况下脏腑之间的相互影响。某脏有病可传至他脏，他脏疾病亦可传至本脏，这种病理上的相互影响称为传变。如肝脏有病，病传至心，为母病及子；病传至肾，为子病及母；病传至脾，为木乘土；病传至肺，为木侮金。其他四脏，以此类推。

its mother. Similarly, diseases of the other *zang* organs can all be explained by the application of laws of generation, restriction, over-restriction and counter-restriction among the five phases.

The five-phase theory can also explain the relationship between diseases of *zang* organs and seasons. *Zang* organs corresponding to the season will be first affected by the pathological qi. That is to say, the liver will be first attacked in spring, the heart will be first attacked in summer, the spleen will be first attacked in late-summer, and the lung will be first attacked in fall, while the kidney in winter. In addition, people should take flexible differentiation according to the reality instead of taking measures on the basis of five-phase theory entirely.

iii. Guiding Clinical Diagnosis and Nursing Assessment

The human body is an organic whole, therefore abnormal changes in functional activities of the *zang* organs and their mutual relationships can be reflected on the external manifestations of complexion, voice, taste and pulse. For example, greenish complexion, preference for sour food and wiry pulse may indicate a liver disease. Reddish complexion, bitter taste in mouth, and surging rapid pulse may indicate a heart disease. Heart disease with darkish complexion may imply that water (kidney) over-restricts fire (heart). Spleen deficiency accompanied by greenish complexion may imply that wood (liver) over-restricts earth (spleen).

iv. Guiding Clinical Treatment and Nursing

1. Deciding Therapeutic Principle and Method According to the promotion relationship among the five phases, the therapeutic principles can be tonifying the mother and reducing the child, and the therapeutic methods can be replenishing water to nourish wood, mutual promotion of metal and water, reinforcing earth to strengthen metal, assisting fire and strengthening earth *etc.*. According to the restriction relationship among the five phases, the therapeutic principles can be checking the strong and strengthening the weak, and the therapeutic methods can be inhibiting wood to assist earth, banking up earth to treat water, assisting metal to subdue wood, reducing the south and tonifying the north *etc.*.

2. Checking Disease Transmission By the generation, restriction, over-restriction and counter-restriction relationships among the five phases, TCM can not only deduce and summarize the law of disease transmission, but also decide measures for disease treatment of prevention. For example, a liver disease may easily affect the spleen, therefore strengthening spleen

五行学说亦可说明五脏发病与季节的关系。五脏外应五时，故五脏一般在其所主之时受邪而发病，即春天多发肝病，夏天多发心病，长夏多发脾病，秋天多发肺病，冬天多发肾病。此外，对于五脏病变的传变，不能完全受五行生克乘侮规律的束缚，临证应结合实际情况灵活分析。

（三）指导诊断与护理评估

人体是一个有机整体，内脏功能活动及其相互关系的异常变化，通常可从色泽、声音、形态、脉象等外部征象反映出来。五行学说把五脏与五色、五味以及脉象变化等，以五行分类归属联系起来，作为诊断疾病的理论基础。如面见青色，喜食酸味，脉见弦象，可初步判断病位在肝；面见赤色，口苦，脉象洪数，是心火亢盛；心气虚弱者，面见黑色，为火虚水乘；脾虚患者，面见青色，为木虚土乘。

（四）指导疾病治疗与护理

1. 确定治则与治法 根据相生规律确定的治则是补母和泻子，治法主要有滋水涵木、金水相生、培土生金、益火补土等。根据相克规律确定的治则包括抑强和扶弱，治法主要有抑木扶土、培土制水、佐金平木、泻南补北等。

2. 控制疾病传变 中医学运用五行生克乘侮关系，既可推断和概括疾病的传变规律，又可确定预防性治疗措施。例如：肝病容易传脾，治疗时可以先健脾，防止肝病传脾。

should be suggested for treatment in order to prevent the transmission of liver disease to spleen.

3. Guiding Emotional Nursing TCM holds that the five emotions of joy, anger, anxiety, thought, and fear originate from the five *zang* organs and among the latter there are relations of generation, restriction, over-restriction and counter-restriction, therefore there are also these relations among the five emotions. By application of the generation, restriction, over-restriction and counter-restriction among the five emotions, the emotional disorders can be regulated and cured. For example, joy is the emotion of heart, which pertains to fire, while fear is the emotion of kidney, which pertains to water. Since water restricts fire, fear can serve to check joy.

The laws of generation and restriction among the five phases are of some significance to guide clinical treatment and nursing. But they are not suitable for all diseases. Flexible application is recommended for concrete conditions in clinical practice.

(Wang Qiu-qin)

3. 指导情志护理 临床以怒、喜、思、悲、恐五情配五脏，运用五行生克乘侮关系，利用不同情志变化的相互抑制作用，达到疾病治疗的目的。例如：喜为心志，属火；恐为肾志，属水。水克火，故恐能胜喜。

五行生克规律对疾病治疗与护理具有一定的指导意义，但并非适用于所有的病证，临床上必须根据具体情况灵活运用。

（王秋琴）

Section 3　Theory of Visceral Manifestation

The theory of visceral manifestation is a theory covering the conception of viscera and manifestations, the morphological structure and physio-pathology of *zang-fu*, as well as the relationship among various *zang-fu organs*, or the relationship among *zang-fu organs* and the organism, essence, qi, blood, body fluid, as well as the natural and social environment.

Zang refers to internal organs inside the body. *Xiang* means image or phenomenon. When combined together, *zang xiang* refers to internal organs and external manifestations of their physiological and pathological state. Therefore, *zang* is the intrinsic base of *xiang* and *xiang* is the external manifestations of *zang*. According to their characteristics of morphological structure and functions, the internal organs can be divided into *zang* organs, *fu* organs and extraordinary *fu* organs. *Zang* organs include heart, lung, spleen, liver and kidney, collectively is called the five *zang* organs. Their common functions are to produce and store essence-qi, meanwhile store spirit, and their characteristics are that "they can be full of essence-qi instead of containing food". *Fu* organs include gallbladder, stomach, small intestine, large intestine, *sanjiao* and urinary

第三节　藏象学说

藏象学说，是研究藏象的概念、脏腑的形态结构与生理病理、脏腑之间以及脏腑与形体官窍、精气血津液、自然社会环境之间相互关系的学说。

藏，是指藏于体内的脏腑；象，是指表现于外的生理、病理现象及与外界相通应的事物或现象。脏腑根据形态结构与功能特点，可分为脏、腑、奇恒之腑。脏，即心、肺、脾、肝、肾，合称为五脏，其共同的生理功能是化生和贮藏精气，并藏神，特点是藏而不泻，满而不实。腑，即胆、胃、大肠、小肠、三焦、膀胱，合称为六腑，其共同的生理功能是受盛和传化水谷，特点是泻而不藏，实而不满。奇恒之腑，即脑、髓、骨、脉、胆、女子胞，因其功能似脏，主贮藏精气，而形态似腑，为中空器官，与五脏、六腑有

bladder, collectively is called the six *fu* organs. Their common functions are to receive, digest and transmit food, and their characteristics are that "they can be full of food instead of storing essence-qi". The extraordinary *fu* organs are brain, marrow, bone, vessel, gallbladder and uterus. Their physiological characteristics are to store the essence-qi, like the five *zang* organs, but their shapes are mostly hollow like the six *fu* organs. Their shapes and functions are distinctly different to five *zang* and six *fu*, thus being called as "extraordinary *fu* organs". Only the five *zang* organs and six *fu* organs are discussed in this section.

The organs of organ manifestations doctrine are not exactly the same as those of modern anatomy or simply organs in anatomy, but refer to physiological functions.

I. Five *Zang* Organs and Six *Fu* Organs

i. Heart and Small Intestine

1. Heart　The major functions of heart are to govern blood vessels and house spirit. Heart and small intestine form interior-exterior relationship through the mutual connection and affiliation of their meridians. Heart is responsible for joy in emotion, sweat in fluid and combing meridians in the body. The mien of heart manifests on face and opens to the tongue. Heart plays a dominant role in the vital activity of the whole body, so it is called the "monarch" and "dominator of *zang* and *fu* organs".

（1）Major functions

1）Governing blood vessels: This includes two aspects of producing blood and circulating blood in vessels.

a. Heart produces blood: Blood is mainly generated from nutritive qi and body fluid, and the action of heart yang is necessary for nutritive qi and body fluid to generate blood or change them into blood.

b. Heart circulates blood: Heart qi can drive and regulate circulation of blood within the vessels. The circulation of blood is closely related to the function of five *zang*, especially the ability of heart to pump out blood. Meanwhile, the pulsating of heart mainly depends upon the driving and regulating function of heart qi. Therefore, if heart qi is sufficient and the function of heart in governing blood vessels is normal, the complexion will be rosy and lustrous, and pulse will be even, moderate and forceful. On the contrary, insufficiency of heart qi will be manifested as palpitation, pale complexion and weak pulse. Or in severe cases there will appear stagnation of qi and blood, obstruction of vessels, chest oppression, stuffiness and stabbing pain, dark and gray complexion, cyanoses of

明显区别，故称奇恒之腑。本节只论述五脏、六腑、五脏关系。

藏象学说中的脏腑，不单纯是一个形态器官，而主要是指一个功能活动系统，故不完全等同于现代解剖学中的脏器。

一、五脏六腑

（一）心与小肠

1. **心**　心的生理功能主要是主血脉和主藏神。心在志为喜，在液为汗，在体合脉，其华在面，在窍为舌。心为"君主之官""五脏六腑之大主"，在人体生命活动中起主宰作用。心与小肠通过经脉相互络属，构成表里关系。

（1）心的主要生理功能

1）主血脉：指心具有生成血液，并推动血液在脉道内运行的生理功能。

a. 主生血：血液主要由营气和津液所化生，而营气和津液在化生血液过程中需要心阳的温煦和气化才能化赤为血液。

b. 主行血：指心气具有推动血液在血脉内运行的作用。血液的运行与五脏功能密切相关，其中心的搏动泵血作用尤为重要，而心脏的搏动，又主要依赖心气的推动和调控作用。心气充沛，心主血脉功能正常，则面色红润而有光泽，脉搏节律均匀、和缓有力。反之，则心悸、面色无华、脉虚无力，甚则气滞血瘀而见心前区憋闷刺痛、唇舌青紫、脉律不齐等。

lips and tongue, and irregular pulse as well.

c. Heart governs vessels: By promoting and regulating the pulsating of heart and systaltic property of vessels, heart qi can keep the expedite condition of blood flow. Vessels, as the house of blood, are the channels containing and transporting blood. Heart, blood and vessels form an airtight circulatory system. The normal flowing of blood in vessels needs the following basic conditions: the sufficiency of heart qi, plenty of blood and expedient situation of vessels, among which the sufficiency of heart qi plays the leading role.

2) Storing spirit: This means heart has the function of dominating mental activities such as psychology and emotion, and life activities of the whole body. When the function of heart in storing spirit is normal, there will appear high spirit, clear consciousness, sharp thinking and acute response. On the contrary, if the function is insufficient, there will appear clinical manifestations of palpitation, amnesia, insomnia, and dreamful sleep. If heart is attacked by phlegm, there will appear coma, dementia, and improper action. When phlegm-fire disturbs the heart, restlessness, delirium and madness will appear, and even endanger the life in severe cases.

The functions of storing spirit and governing blood vessels of heart are closely related. Blood is the major material basis for mental activities, and mental activities can regulate and influence blood circulation. If heart fails to govern blood vessels, such symptoms as insufficiency of heart blood or heat in blood will inevitably lead to disorder of heart spirit. Contrarily, dysfunction of heart in housing spirit may also result in anomaly of blood flow.

(2) Relations of heart with emotion, fluids, constituent and orifice

1) Heart is associated with joy in emotion: Generally speaking, appropriate joy is a reaction of the body to an optimal stimulation, and it is good for heart in governing blood. However, over-joy may make heart spirit injured and lax, leading to clinical manifestations such as poor concentration, even endless joy and mental disorder.

2) Heart is associated with sweat in fluid: Sweat is transformed from body fluid, while body fluid shares the same source of food-essence with blood, and the two can transform themselves into each other. The body fluid, as it permeates into vessels, will become blood. While blood, as it permeates out of the vessels, will become body fluid. Therefore there is a saying that blood and sweat share the same source. Furthermore, blood is governed by heart, therefore when heart blood is abundant, body fluid will be ample and sweat will have its source for production. In addition, heart stores spirit, and the production and

c. 主脉：是指心气推动和调控心脏的搏动和脉管的舒缩，维持脉道通利，血流通畅。"脉为血之府"，是容纳和运输血液的通道。心、血、脉三者构成一个密闭循环的系统。血液在脉中正常运行，以心气充沛、血液充盈、脉管通利为基本条件，其中心气充沛起主导作用。

2）主藏神：指心具有主宰人体生命活动和精神、意识、思维活动的作用。心主藏神功能正常，则精神振作、神志清晰、思维敏捷，对外界信息的反应灵敏。反之，如心血虚，血不养心，可见心悸、健忘、失眠、多梦；痰迷心窍，可见神昏、痴呆、举止失常。

心主藏神与心主血脉的生理功能密切相关。血液是神志活动的物质基础，精神活动能调节和影响血液循环。如果心主血脉功能失常，常可导致神志改变；若心神不安，也可引起血行不畅。

（2）心与志、液、体和窍的关系

1）在志为喜：喜乐愉悦有益于心的功能。但"喜则气缓"，喜乐过度，则又可使心神受伤，神志涣散，甚则出现喜笑不休等神志病变。

2）在液为汗：汗为津液所化生，血与津液又同出水谷精气，且互生互化，津液渗入脉内可生成血液，血液渗出脉外则化为津液，故有"血汗同源"之说；而血又为心所主，心血充盈，津液充足，汗化有源，心又主藏神，汗液生成排泄受心神的调节。

secretion of sweat are regulated by heart spirit.

3) Heart is associated with vessels in constituent and manifests on face: Heart is associated with vessels in constituent as the blood vessels of the whole body are dominated by heart. When heart qi is sufficient, pulse will be moderate and forceful with an even rhythm. If heart qi is insufficient, pulse will be fine and forceless. "It manifests on the face." means the state of the physiological function of heart may be reflected as the changes of color and luster in the face. When heart qi is sufficient and blood vessels are full of blood, pulse will get gentle, strong, and uniform, and face will be rosy and lustrous. If heart qi is insufficient, face will get pale or dark and gloomy. If heart blood is deficient, pulse will get thin and weak, while the face will become lusterless with less brilliant. And if heart blood gets stagnated, pulse will get unsmooth, knotted, or intermittent, while face will get cyanotic.

4) Heart is associated with tongue in orifice: This means tongue is the outer reflection of heart. When the functions of heart in governing blood and housing spirit are normal, tongue will be light red and moist, soft and flexible, with acute sense of taste and fluent speech. If heart qi is deficient, tongue will be pale, enlarged and tender. If heart blood is deficient, tongue will become deep red, thin and shrunken. If heart fire is flaming up, there will be red tongue, even with prickles. If heart blood gets stagnated, tongue will become dark and purplish or with bruises. If heart fails to house the mind, there may be symptoms of curled tongue, stiff tongue with dysphasia or aphasia.

2. Small Intestine Small intestine is located in abdomen. Its upper end connects with stomach, and its lower end connects with large intestine. The major physiological functions of small intestine are to dominate reception and digest chyme, and separate the clear from the turbid.

(1) Small intestine governs reception and digestion of chime: Small intestine accepts chyme sent down by the stomach and holds it for a longer time so spleen qi collaborates with small intestine to facilitate further to digest it into the essence. If small intestine functions abnormally in reception or digestion of chyme, it will result in abdominal distention, diarrhea, loose stool *et al.*

(2) Small intestine governs separation of the clear from the turbid: Small intestine separates its digested food into two parts of essence and waste in the process of further digestion, absorbs the essence and sends the waste down into large intestine. The clear means the essence of water, food and body fluid, and the turbid refers to the food residue and part of the body fluid. During absorbing food, the small intestine also absorbs a great amount of water and sends the waste down into urinary bladder. If

3）在体合脉，其华在面：在体合脉，指全身的血脉都属于心。其华在面，指心脏精气的盛衰，可以从面部的色泽反映出来。若心气旺盛，则脉搏和缓有力、节律均匀，面部红润而有光泽；如心气虚损或心血不足，则脉搏细弱无力，面白无华；若心血瘀阻，则见脉涩、结代，面色青紫等症。

4）在窍为舌：是指舌为心之外候。如心的功能正常，则舌体红活荣润、柔软灵活、味觉灵敏、语言流利。若心气不足，可见舌淡胖嫩；心阴血不足，则舌质红绛瘦瘪；心火上炎则见舌红，甚则生疮；心血瘀阻，则见舌质暗紫，或有瘀斑；心藏神功能异常，则见舌强、语謇等症。

2．小肠 小肠位于腹腔，其上端与胃相接，下端与大肠相连，小肠的生理功能主要是主受盛化物、泌别清浊。

（1）受盛化物：是指小肠接受经胃下传的食糜而盛纳之，食糜在小肠内停留一定的时间，由脾气与小肠共同对其进一步消化和吸收。若小肠受盛化物功能失常，则见腹胀、腹泻、便溏等。

（2）泌别清浊：是指小肠对食糜进一步消化的同时分清别浊。清者，即水谷精微和津液；浊者，即食物残渣和部分津液。小肠吸收水谷精微和大量水分，并将食物残渣下降到大肠，将废液下输膀胱。小肠泌别清浊功能正常，则清浊各走其道。反之，则见便溏、泄泻、小便短少等症。

small intestine functions normally in separation of the clear from the turbid, metabolism of food and drink would be in order. If small intestine functions abnormally in separation of the clear from the turbid, it may lead to mix-up of the clear and the turbid manifesting as sloppy stool, diarrhea and scanty urination.

ii. Lung and Large Intestine

1. Lung　The major functions of lung are governing respiratory qi and qi of the whole body, governing diffusion, purification and down-sending, regulating waterways and connecting with vessels. Lung and large intestine form exterior-interior relationship through connection and affiliation of their meridians. Lung is responsible for grief (worry) in emotion and tears in liquid, related to skin and hair in the exterior, and opens into the nose. Lung is located at the highest position among internal organs and covers the others, thus it is called the "canopy". Because its lobes are delicate and communicate with the outside environment, it is susceptible to invasion of external pathogens and hence there is the name of "delicate viscus".

（1）Main functions

1）Governing qi: Qi of the whole body is governed and managed by the lung, including two aspects of governing respiratory qi and whole body qi.

a. Lung governs respiratory qi: Lung possesses the actions to exhale the turbid qi in the body and inhale the clear air of nature so as to achieve qi exchange between the interior and exterior of the body and maintain the normal metabolisms of the body.

b. Lung governs qi of the whole body: Lung has the actions to govern the production and circulation of qi of the whole body. It includes two aspects as follows:

Lung embodies the production of qi of the whole body, especially the ancestral qi (*zong qi*). The ancestral qi, which forms and accumulates mostly in chest, is mainly produced by the combination of clear air inhaled by lung and food qi transformed and transported by spleen and stomach. Lung governs the flowing of qi in the whole body which mainly embodies in its adjustment function of qi in the whole body. If the function of lung governing qi disorders, the body can't breathe easily, and even cough, asthma and chest distress, or symptoms and disorders like lassitude and fatigue of the body, faint low voice, impeded blood flowing and disturbance of water metabolism may happen. Lung regulates the movement of qi of the whole body. The process of lung's respiratory movement is the upward, downward, inward and outward movement of qi. Thus inhalation and exhalation of lung in rhythm plays an

（二）肺与大肠

1. **肺**　肺的生理功能主要是主气司呼吸，主宣发和肃降，通调水道，朝百脉、主治节。肺在志为悲（忧），在液为涕，在体合皮，其华在毛，在窍为鼻。肺在五脏中位置最高，故有"华盖"之称。肺叶娇嫩，易受外邪，故又有"娇脏"之称。肺与大肠通过经脉相互络属，构成表里关系。

（1）肺的主要生理功能

1）肺主气司呼吸：包括主呼吸之气与主一身之气两个方面。

a. 主呼吸之气：是指肺具有呼出体内浊气，吸入自然界清气，实现人体内外气体交换，从而维持人体新陈代谢正常进行的作用。

b. 主一身之气：是指肺有主持、调节一身之气生成和运行的作用。肺主一身之气的生成，体现于宗气的生成。宗气由肺吸入的自然界清气与脾胃运化的水谷之精气相结合而成。肺主一身之气的运行，体现于对全身气机的调节作用。肺主气功能失常，则见呼吸无力，甚至咳喘胸闷；或见身倦乏力，语声低微，血运不畅及水液代谢障碍等病变。

important role in the movement of qi of the whole body in all directions. Generally speaking, the abnormality of lung in governing qi may manifest as two aspects. One is the disorder of respiratory function, such as difficulty in breathing, shortness of breath, cough with chest oppression. The other is the disorder of lung in governing qi of the whole body, manifesting as lassitude, faint low voice, slack circulation of blood, and disturbance of body fluid metabolism as well.

2) Governing diffusion, dispersion, purification and descent

a. Lung governing diffusion and dispersion implies that lung-qi can diffuse and disperse upwards and outwards, whereas lung governing purification and descent signifies that lung-qi can go downward and keep the respiratory tract pure and clear. The physiological function of lung-qi in dispersion, referring to the function of dispersing and descending inside and downward, mainly embodies three aspects: exhaling turbid qi in the body, dispersing defensive qi to the body surface (to warm the muscle and skin, guard against exogenous pathogens, regulate opening-closing of striae to control the excretion of sweat) and transporting food essence and fluid generated by spleen outward to the surface of the body. Therefore, if lung-qi fails in dispersion, there will appear cough, asthma, intolerance of cold, spontaneous sweating, susceptibility to colds, retention of phlegm, edema, *etc.*.

b. The physiological function of lung-qi in purification and descent also embodies three aspects: inhaling the clear air from nature, next, distributing food essence and fluid generated by the spleen downward and inward to other organs and tissues, and eliminating the foreign body in the lung and respiratory tract so as to keep the respiratory tract intact and smooth. Therefore, if lung-qi fails in this function, there will be shallow breathing, chest oppression, cough with wheezing and panting, or difficulty in urination, retention of phlegm and edema, or constipation. Under the normal physiological conditions, diffusion, dispersion, purification and descent of lung-qi depend upon each other and restrict each other. When lung-qi disperses and descends normally, the respiration will be even and free. Under the pathological conditions, the coordination of the two aspects gets disturbed. There will appear disorders of "failure of lung-qi in dispersion" and "failure of lung-qi in depuration and descent", manifesting as chest distress, cough, panting, retention of phlegm and other morbid fluids.

3) Freeing and regulating waterways: This means lung possesses the actions to dredge and regulate distribution, circulation and excretion of water in the

2）主宣发和肃降

a. 肺主宣发，指肺气具有向上升宣、向外布散的功能，主要体现于以下三个方面：一是呼出体内浊气，完成气体交换；二是宣发卫气，温养肌肤，抵御外邪，调节腠理之开合，控制汗液的排出；三是将脾胃运化的水谷精微及津液布散于周身，润泽皮毛。肺气失宣可见咳喘、畏寒，或自汗、易感外邪；或痰饮、颜面周身水肿等。

b. 肺主肃降，指肺气具有向内向下清肃通降的作用，主要体现在以下三个方面：一是吸入自然界的清气；二是将吸入的清气和脾转输的水谷精微和津液向下、向内布散；三是肃清呼吸道的痰浊等异物，保持呼吸道的洁净、通畅。肺气不降，可见呼吸急促表浅、胸闷、咳喘，或小便不利、痰饮水肿，或便秘等。

3）通调水道：是指肺的宣发和肃降对人体水液代谢具有疏通和调节作用。肺气宣发，

body. Lung-qi not only diffuses the fluid upward and outward to skin and body hair as well as disperses to the body surface, but also diffuses the defensive qi to control the opening and closing of the interstices, freeing and regulating excretion of sweat. At the same time, part of the water can be excreted through respiration. Purification and descent of the lung-qi not only transmits (transports) the water downward to the lower and the internal, but also can transmit the turbid liquid produced by metabolism of the organ into the kidney as the source of urine formation. Meanwhile, it can help push the large intestine to pass stool out with water. Only when lung functions properly in freeing and regulating waterways, the water metabolism can be kept normal. Contrarily if the lung's function of freeing and regulating waterways is disordered, it will lead to accumulation of water manifesting as disorders of water metabolism, dampness, phlegm retention and fluid stagnancy.

4) Linking with all the vessels and governing management and regulation: Qi and blood of the whole body converge in the lung through the meridian vessels. The exchange of Qi is carried out through lung's function of inhaling the clear and exhaling the turbid. By diffusing and descending motion of lung-qi, lung assists heart in promoting blood circulation, and blood richly containing clear qi goes through vessels again to the whole body. Meanwhile, lung governs regulating means that lung can aid heart in regulating qi, blood, fluids and functions of internal organs. Thus lung governs regulating presents a high-level overview of the main physiological function of lung. Therefore when the lung-qi is sufficient, the production and flow of qi will be normal, ensuring smooth blood circulation. On the contrary, if lung qi gets declined and fails to assist heart in promoting blood circulation, blood will not flow smoothly, thus there will appear the signs of qi deficiency and blood stasis marked by chest oppression, palpitation, cyanotic lips and purplish tongue.

(2) Relations of lung with emotion, fluids, constituent and orifice

1) Lung is associated with anxiety in emotion: The major influence of sorrow and anxiety is continuous consumption of qi, so called "grief consumes qi". Lung governs qi, so over sorrow and anxiety may cause deficiency of lung qi manifesting as shortage of breathing. Meanwhile, if lung qi gets deficient, human's tolerance to negative stimulation will decrease, and thus it is more likely to lead to emotions of sorrow and anxiety.

2) Lung is associated with snivel in fluids: Snivel is the nasal discharge, and lung opens at the nose. When essential qi in lung is sufficient, snivel moistens nasal

可将人体的津液布散于皮毛周身，还能布散卫气，主司腠理开合，将代谢后的水液，通过汗孔排出于体外，同时，肺的呼气还可带走一部分水分；肺气肃降，不但可使津液向下布散，还可将代谢后的水液经肾的气化作用下输到膀胱，生成尿液排出于体外，同时，推动大肠传导，通过大便排出一部分水液。肺通调水道功能失调，可导致水液代谢障碍，出现痰饮等。

4）肺朝百脉、主治节：肺朝百脉，是指全身的血液，都通过百脉聚会于肺。通过肺的呼浊吸清，进行气体交换，再通过肺宣发和肃降、助心行血，可将富含养分的血液经过百脉输送到全身。肺主治节是指肺辅助心脏治理调节全身气、血、津液及脏腑生理功能的作用。可见，肺主治节是对肺的主要生理功能的高度概括。若肺气虚衰，不能辅心行血，血液运行迟滞，则可见胸闷心悸，唇青舌紫等症。

（2）肺与志、液、体和窍的关系

1）在志为悲（忧）：悲哀和忧伤使气不断地消耗，即所谓"悲则气消"。由于肺主气，所以过度悲忧易伤肺，则见气短等肺气不足之象。反之，肺气虚衰，人体对外来非良性刺激的耐受性下降，也易于产生悲忧的情绪变化。

2）在液为涕：涕为鼻腔分泌液，而肺开窍于鼻。肺中精气充足，涕液润泽鼻窍而不

cavity and does not flow outward, meanwhile can protect against external pathogens so as to help lung to breathe. If lung is invaded by cold pathogen, it will cause thin nasal discharge. If lung is invaded by heat pathogen, it will cause yellow and stick nasal discharge. If lung is invaded by dryness pathogen, it will cause dry nose.

3) Lung is associated with skin in constituent, manifesting on hair: Skin and hair are on the surface (exterior) of the body, which play the role of shield fighting against invasions of exogenous pathogenic factors. The association between lung and the skin and hair means that lung is able to disperse defensive-qi, make skin and hair rosy and lustrous via transporting essence to them, and play a part in governing the open and close and defensing against attacks of exogenous pathogenic factors. Lung possesses the physiological function of diffusing the defensive qi and transporting the essence of food and drink as well as body fluid onto skin and hair, warming, nourishing and moistening skin and hair, meanwhile regulating body temperature through sweat excreting and resists external pathogens.Therefore, lung is closely related with skin and hair. When lung-qi is sufficient, the function of lung in diffusing defensive qi and transporting essence onto the skin and hair will be normal, then skin will be compact and fine hair be lustrous, body's protection against external pathogens will also be strong. On the contrary, if lung-qi gets declined and fails to diffuse the defensive qi and essence onto the skin and hair, there will occur profuse sweating, being rather easily subject to catching cold, or having haggard skin and hair.

4) Lung opens to the nose: Nose is the passageway for respiration, and attaches directly to the lung, thus nose is connecting with lung. The function of ventilation and smelling of nose must depend on the ability of lung qi. When lung qi diffuses smoothly, nose will be normal in ventilation and smelling, and free from nasal congestion with keen smelling. On the contrary, if lung qi fails in diffusion, it will manifest as nasal obstruction, running nose, sneezing, itching and sore throat, hoarseness, or aphonia. Since lung opens at the nose, external pathogens often invade lung through nose and mouth.

2. Large Intestine　The major function of large intestine is to transform and transport the waste. Large intestine receives the food residue from small intestine by its separation, reabsorbs the extra water in the waste so as to make the waste become solid stool, and then conveys the stool down and discharges it out of the body via the anus. If large intestine functions abnormally in conveyance and transformation of waste, there will be abnormality in quality and quantity of stool and frequency of defecation.

外流，并能防御外邪，有利于肺的呼吸。如风寒犯肺，则鼻流清涕；风热犯肺，则鼻流黄稠涕；燥邪伤肺，则鼻干而无涕。

3）在体合皮，其华在毛：皮毛为一身之表，是抵御外邪侵袭的屏障。肺与皮毛相合，是指肺能宣散卫气、输精于皮毛，使之红润光泽，发挥司开阖及防御外邪侵袭的作用。若肺精、肺气虚损，既可因皮毛失养而见枯槁不泽，又可致卫表不固而见自汗或易感冒。

4）在窍为鼻：鼻为呼吸之气出入的通道，与肺直接相连，故称鼻为肺之窍。鼻的通气和嗅觉功能，必须依赖肺气的作用。肺气宣畅，则鼻窍通利，嗅觉灵敏。肺气失宣，可见鼻塞、流涕、喷嚏等。由于肺开窍于鼻，故外邪侵袭，也常从口鼻而入，引发肺的病变。

2. **大肠**　大肠的主要生理功能是传导糟粕。大肠接受小肠泌别清浊后的糟粕，并吸收多余水分后化为粪便排出体外。若大肠传导功能正常，则大便的质、量、次数正常，若大肠吸收水分过多，则大便干结而致便秘；反之，可见腹泻、便溏。

If large intestine reabsorbs too much water in the food residue, there will be symptoms such as constipation. If water is not properly absorbed, diarrhea, or thinness of stool will occur.

iii. Spleen and Stomach

1. Spleen　The main physiological functions of spleen are to govern transporting and transforming, send up the useful essence and control blood. Spleen and stomach form the exterior-interior relationship through the mutual affiliation and connection of their meridians. Spleen transforms food into essence, thus provides substantial basis for postnatal life activity and production of qi and blood. The spleen and the stomach are thus called "the foundation of acquired constituent" and "the source of qi and blood production". Spleen associates with thought in emotions and slobbers in secretion, dominates muscles and limbs, opens into mouth and manifests on lip.

(1) Major functions

1) Governing transformation and transportation: Spleen can digest food, absorb essence (nutrients) of food and drink, and then transport essence to the whole body. Spleen has two functions: transforming and transporting food and drink, and transforming and transporting body fluid.

a. Transforming and transporting food and drink: Spleen can promote food digestion and essence absorption and further distribute essence. Digestion takes place in gastrointestinal tract, but it must depend on the transformation of spleen to make food transform into essence, and essence again must depend on the transportation of spleen to be absorbed and transported to the whole body, all of which is based on spleen qi. When spleen qi is strong, sufficient transforming from food and drink to essence through digestion and absorption could be achieved, and enough nourishment such as essence, qi, blood and fluid could be produced, so that the organs, meridians and collaterals, four limbs and skeleton, as well as sinews, muscles, skin and body hair could be fully nourished. Contrarily, if spleen's function in transforming and transporting food and drink decreases, there may appear such qi and blood deficient symptoms as abdominal flatulence, sloppy stool, poor appetite, lassitude and emaciation with yellowish complexion.

b. Transporting and transforming body fluid: Spleen has the functions of absorbing and transporting body fluid, which include two aspects. On one hand, spleen qi can transform water into body fluid through its absorption, transforming and transporting functions, and meanwhile, it is distributed to all parts of the body to moisten and nourish the body. On the other hand, it can also timely

（三）脾与胃

1. 脾　脾主要生理功能是主运化、主升清、主统血。脾将水谷化为精微，为人出生后的生命活动和气血生成奠定基础，故脾胃称为"后天之本""气血生化之源"。脾在志为思，在液为涎，在体合肌肉而主四肢，在窍为口，其华在唇。脾与胃通过经脉相互络属，构成表里关系。

（1）脾的主要生理功能

1）主运化：是指脾具有消化吸收食物中的水谷精微并将其传输至全身的生理功能。

a. 运化谷食是指脾气将谷食化为谷精，并将其吸收、转输到全身脏腑的功能。谷食入胃，经胃初步消化后，变为食糜下传于小肠，在脾气的推动、激发作用下，经进一步消化后，其精微部分，再经脾气的转输作用输送到全身，分别化为精、气、血、津液，内养五脏六腑，外养四肢百骸、皮毛筋肉。若脾气虚损，运化谷食功能减退，则可出现腹胀、便溏、食欲缺乏，甚则倦怠乏力，面黄肌瘦等症。

b. 运化水液是指脾对水液的吸收、转输功能。运化水液包括两个方面：一是摄入到人体内的水液，需经过脾的运化传输，气化成津液，布达周身脏腑组织器官，发挥其滋润、濡养作用；二是经过代谢后的水液，亦要经过脾传输，而至肺、肾，通过肺、肾的

transport the surplus water of the body into lung and kidney where the surplus water, through qi transformation of lung and kidney, is transformed into sweat and urine to be discharged out of the body to keep the balance of body fluid metabolism. Therefore, if spleen qi is sufficient, it can not only guarantee the function of transforming and transporting body fluid to be normal, but also prevent pathological products such as excessive water, dampness, phlegm and retained fluid from appearing. If spleen qi is deficient, the function of spleen in transporting and transforming body fluid declines, body fluid stagnates in the certain parts of body, and thus the pathological changes such as retained phlegm, edema, and dampness-turbidity may appear.

2) Governing ascent of the clear: Spleen qi goes upward and thus transports essence of water and food up to heart, lung, head and eyes, meanwhile maintains the positions of internal organs relatively fixed. Spleen can send up essence of water and food up to heart, lung, head and eyes so as to moisten and nourish the clear orifices, meanwhile, nourish the whole body through heart and lung producing qi and blood. If spleen qi fails to raise the clear, then there can appear symptoms of dim complexion, dizziness and vertigo. If spleen loses its power to lift yang qi, there can appear symptoms of abdominal distention with chronic diarrhea. Owing to the ascent of spleen qi, the positions of organs are kept relatively fixed which rely on the essence of water and food coming from transformation and transportation of spleen. If spleen qi is insufficient, it not only cannot send up the clear, but also sink down, resulting in such symptoms of prolapse of internal organs as gastroptosis, hysteroptosis and chronic diarrhea with prolapse of the rectum.

3) Governing control of blood: Spleen governs the action of keeping blood circulating within meridian vessels and preventing it from leaking. When spleen qi is strong and healthy, it can control blood circulating within meridian vessels without escaping and bleeding. Contrarily, if spleen is too insufficient to transform and transport, securing and governing function of qi and blood will be deficient, then it will cause bleeding.

(2) Relations of spleen with emotion, fluids, constituent and orifice

1) Spleen is associated with thought in emotion: Over thinking may lead to qi stagnation and melancholy, thus it will influence the functions of spleen in transformation and transportation, and sending up the clear, then there may appear symptoms of poor appetite, distension and stuffiness of the epigastrium, dizziness and vertigo. Therefore, there is the saying that "over thinking leads to qi stagnation and melancholy".

气化作用，化为汗、尿等而排出体外，以维持人体水液代谢的协调平衡。若脾气虚，运化水液功能减退，则水液停滞于局部，即可产生痰饮、湿浊、水肿等病变。

2）主升清：是指脾具有将水谷精微上输于心、肺、头面，通过心、肺作用化生气血，以濡养全身的作用。脾气的运动特点以上升为主，对维持内脏位置的相对稳定、防止其下垂具有重要作用。若脾不升清，可见面色无华、头晕目眩、腹胀、慢性泄泻等症。若脾气虚损，无力升举，则可导致内脏下垂，如胃下垂、子宫脱垂、久泻脱肛等。

3）主统血：是指脾具有统摄血液在经脉内运行，防止逸出脉外的功能。脾气强健，统摄有权，血液才不会逸出于脉外而出血；反之，脾的运化功能减退，则气血虚亏，气的固摄功能减退，则导致出血。

（2）脾与志、液、体和窍的关系

1）在志为思：思虑过度，导致气滞与气结，影响脾的运化和升清功能，出现食欲缺乏，脘腹胀闷，头目眩晕等症，即所谓"思则气结"。

2) Spleen is associated with saliva in fluids: Saliva is the secretion in mouth. When spleen functions normally in transformation, transportation and rising of the clear, body fluid will go up to the mouth, forming sufficient saliva to help to swallow and digest food. If there is disorder of spleen and stomach, it will lead to acute increase of excretion of saliva drooling out of mouth.

3) Spleen is associated with muscles in constituent, governing four limbs: When spleen functions normally in transformation and transportation, muscles and four limbs can get enough nourishment of the food essence, which is the source of qi and blood. Then muscles will be well developed, thick and strong, and four limbs will be nimble and forceful. If spleen's function in transformation and transportation gets disordered, it will lead to the inadequate intake of the transformation into qi and blood, and muscles and four limbs will lose their nourishment, causing extenuation of muscles and flaccidity and weakness of limbs, even atrophy.

4) Spleen is associated with mouth in orifice, manifesting on lips: When spleen qi is sufficient in transformation and transportation, appetite, taste and color of lips will be normal. If spleen fails in normal transformation and transportation, there will appear poor appetite, abnormal sensations of tastelessness, greasy, sweet tastes of mouth or abnormal color of lips such as purple and pale with no luster.

2. Stomach　Stomach is responsible for receiving, digesting and transforming water and food. Stomach is concerned with descending and stomach qi is normal when there is harmonious down-bearing.

(1) Stomach governs intaking and decomposing (of food): Stomach would receive the food first and then preliminarily transform them into chyme for further digestion and absorption. The dysfunction of stomach in receiving and transforming food and drink will be characterized by loss of appetite, abdominal distention and pain, food stagnation or acid regurgitation and polyorexia, while its normal function will bring about a good appetite.

(2) Stomach governs descending and dredging of stomach qi: This means stomach is characterized by descending stomach qi. It's normal for stomach qi to descend. Food enters stomach, after being received, transformed and preserved for a while, then it would be reduced to chyme. Then the chyme is forced downward into intestine by stomach qi to be further digested and absorbed. Small intestine would separate the refined matter from the feces. The refined matter would be distributed to the whole body by the transformation and transport of spleen, while

2）在液为涎：涎为口津，是唾液中较清稀的部分。脾的运化和升清功能正常，则津液上行于口，但不溢出于口外而为涎，有助于食物的吞咽和消化。若脾胃不和，则导致涎液分泌急剧增加，出现口涎自出等现象。

3）在体合肌肉、主四肢：脾气健运，气血生化有源，才能保持肌肉丰满，四肢健壮有力。若脾失健运，气血化源不足，肌肉失养，则可致肌肉瘦削无力，甚至痿软不用。

4）在窍为口、其华在唇：脾气强健，则饮食、口味、唇色才能正常。若脾失健运，则可见食欲缺乏、口淡无味、口腻、口甜等异常感觉，或唇色异常，如青紫、苍白无华等。

2. 胃　胃的生理功能主要是受纳和腐熟水谷，主通降。胃以降为和。

（1）受纳和腐熟水谷：是指胃有接受和容纳食物，并初步消化，使水谷变成食糜，有利于进一步消化吸收的功能。如胃的受纳、腐熟功能失常，则表现为食欲缺乏、胃脘部胀满疼痛、饮食停滞，或吞酸嘈杂、消谷善饥等。

（2）主通降：是指胃有通利下降的功能及特性。食物经过胃的受纳腐熟并保留一定时间后，必须下降到小肠，泌别清浊，其清者，经脾的运化输布周身，浊者继续下降到大肠，形成糟粕排出到体外。若胃失和降，可见脘腹胀满或疼痛、口臭、大便秘结等症；胃气不降，反而上逆，则可见恶心、呕吐、嗳气及呃逆等症。

the feces would descend to large intestine and finally be transported out in wastes. If stomach (qi) fails in dredging and descending, and stomach qi gets stagnated, it will lead to epigastric distention or pain, gingivitis and foul breath, and constipation. If the descending function is abnormal, there may be such symptoms of adverse rising of the stomach qi as nausea, vomiting, acid regurgitation and hiccup.

iv. Liver and Gallbladder

1. Liver The major functions of liver are governing the free flow of qi, and storing the blood. Liver and gallbladder form the exterior-interior relationship through the affiliation and connection of their meridians. Liver is characterized by ascent and movement of qi, and liver qi tends to be flourishing and free from obstruction, therefore liver has the name of "unyielding viscus".

(1) Major functions

1) Governing the free flow of qi: Liver dredges the routes and regulates the movement of qi so as to ensure smooth flow of qi, blood, body fluid, and to regulate functions of spleen and stomach in transformation and transportation, secretion and excretion of bile, emotional activities, as well as ejaculation of men and menstruation of women. The major effects of dredging and regulating are as follows:

a. Promoting circulation of blood and body fluid: If qi flows normally, blood will circulate soundly. On the contrary, if qi gets stagnated, blood and body fluid will get stagnated. Liver can regulate and dredge the activity of ascending, descending, inward and outward movement of qi. If liver functions normally in governing the free flow of qi, circulation of blood and distribution of body fluid will be smooth. On the contrary, if liver qi gets stagnated, it will lead to disturbance of blood and body fluid circulation. For example, longtime stagnation of qi will lead to blood stagnation or tumor. If liver qi rises adversely, it will force blood to go upward and lead to bleeding like hematemesis and hemoptysis, even faint and unconsciousness. Besides, the abnormality of liver in governing the free flow of qi may also lead to disturbance of body fluid metabolism causing pathological changes of water dampness and retention of phlegm and fluid.

b. Promoting transformation and transportation of spleen and stomach: On the one hand, when liver functions normally and qi flows freely and smoothly, spleen qi can raise the clear, and stomach qi can direct the turbid downward, then foodstuff can be properly digested, absorbed and excreted. As liver functions abnormally, it will not only affect spleen in sending up the clear manifesting as dizziness and vertigo in the upper part and diarrhea in the lower part of the body, but also affect stomach in sending down the turbid manifesting as hiccup and eructation in the upper, epigastric

（四）肝与胆

1. **肝** 肝胆生理功能主要是主疏泄和主藏血。肝在体合筋，其华在爪，在窍为目，在志为怒，在液为泪。肝喜条达而恶抑郁，被称为"刚脏"。肝与胆通过经脉相互络属，构成表里关系。

（1）肝的主要生理功能

1）主疏泄：指气具有疏通、畅达全身气机的作用，具体表现在以下四个方面。

a. 促进血液和津液的运行输布：气行则血行，气滞则血瘀；气行则水行，气滞则水停。肝主疏泄的功能正常，气机调畅，则血与津液运行通利。若肝气郁滞，则可形成血瘀，或肿块，或生成水、湿、痰、饮等病理产物；血随气逆，则可致吐血、咯血，甚则猝然昏倒、不省人事。

b. 促进脾胃的运化和胆汁的分泌排泄：肝主疏泄功能正常，脾胃才能升清降浊有序，食物方能得以正常的消化吸收和排泄。肝失疏泄，可导致脾胃升降失常，脾不升清，则见腹胀、纳呆、眩晕、腹泻；胃气不降，则见呕逆、嗳气、脘腹胀满、便秘。肝主疏泄正常，肝脏生成、分泌胆汁，以助消化则正常；如肝失疏泄，则胆汁生成排泄障碍，可

distention and fullness in the middle, and constipation in the lower. On the other hand, when liver functions normally in governing free flow of qi, bile will be normally secreted and excreted, thus it is conducive to spleen's transformation and transportation and stomach's decomposition. If liver qi gets depressed, it will affect the secretion and excretion of bile, resulting in pathological changes of distension, fullness and pain in the hypochondrium, bitter taste in the mouth, indigestion, and even jaundice when bile overflows to skin.

c. Regulating mental activity: If liver functions excessively in transformation and transportation with hyperactivity of qi, it will lead to irritability and headache. If liver functions insufficiently in governing the free flow of qi, liver qi will be stagnated, giving rise to depression, melancholy and sentimentality.

d. Regulating men's ejaculation and women's menstruation: When liver functions normally, qi movement will be free and smooth, men's ejaculation will be smooth and proper, and women's menstrual cycle will be regular as well. Contrarily, if liver's function gets abnormal, qi movement will get disordered, then ejaculation will become unsmooth and improper, and menstrual cycle will become disturbed and obstructed.

2) Storing blood: Liver can store the blood, regulate blood volume and prevent bleeding. It can be expressed in three aspects. Firstly, liver can store certain amount of blood to check yang qi of liver to prevent its over-rise, and thus to maintain the normal process of flow of liver qi. Next, liver can regulate the amount of blood demanded by every tissue according to the physiological conditions of the body. As a person is in movement, his blood will circulate through the meridians and collaterals, and as he is at rest, his blood will return to the liver. Thirdly, the function of liver storing a certain amount of blood helps to hold blood within the vessels to prevent it from losing unduly. Therefore, if liver fails to store blood, it will not only lead to shortage of liver blood and over rise of yang qi manifesting as dizziness, numb limbs and tense tendon, scanty and light-colored menses, amenorrhea, irascibility, and susceptibility to rage, but also may result in various kinds of bleeding.

(2) Relations of liver with emotion, fluids, constituent and orifice

1) Liver is associated with anger in emotion: Anger is an expression when emotion changes, and it pertains to liver. On one hand, over anger easily injures the liver, leading to abnormal dredging and regulating function of the liver with liver qi hyperactivity and blood ascending adversely along with rising of qi , red face and eyes, vexation and irritability, even haematemesis, nose bleeding, sudden coma, and unconsciousness. On the other hand,

见胁肋胀满疼痛、口苦、纳食不化等症。若胆汁外溢于皮肤，则见黄疸。

c. 调畅情志：如果肝气升发太过，可见急躁易怒、头胀头痛等症。若肝气疏泄功能不及，肝气郁结，可见情绪低沉、抑郁寡欢、多疑善虑等症。

d. 调节男子排精和妇女行经：肝的疏泄功能正常，气机调畅，则男子排精通畅、有度，女子月经正常通畅；反之，则男子排精失畅、无度，女子月经不调，经行不畅。

2）主藏血：是指肝脏具有贮藏血液、调节血量和防止出血的生理功能。它表现在三个方面：一是肝脏贮藏一定的血量，以涵敛肝阳，防止其生发太过；二是肝脏根据机体需要，调节血量分配，人动则血运于诸经，人静则血归于肝脏；三是肝藏血的功能有助于血液收摄在血脉之中，可以防止出血。因此，肝不藏血既可见肝血虚少的目暗昏花、筋脉拘急、妇女月经量少、闭经等，还可见肝阳生发太过的急躁易怒等，又可见各种出血证。

（2）肝与志、液、体和窍的关系

1）在志为怒：怒是情绪激动时的一种情志变化，肝主疏泄，阳气主发，为肝之用。一方面，怒可以伤肝，导致疏泄失常，肝气亢奋，血随气涌，可见面红目赤，甚则可见吐血、衄血、猝然昏倒、不省人事。另一方面，肝失疏泄，也可致情志失常，表现为情

if liver fails to dredge and regulate qi and blood flow, it will also lead to improper emotions, manifesting as depression or impetuousness and irritability.

2) Liver is associated with tear in fluid: When qi and blood of liver are harmonious, tear can moisten eyes and will not flow out. On the contrary, if liver blood gets deficient, dry and uncomfortable feelings in the eye will appear. In case of invasion of wind and fire in the liver meridian, red eyes and aversion to light and epiphora will appear, and in case of dampness-heat in liver meridian, too much secretion in eyes will occur.

3) Liver is associated with tendons in constituent, manifesting on the nails: *Jin* in TCM is often translated as tendon yet it refers to both ligament and sinew. If liver blood gets deficient, tendons will lose their nourishment, while the numbness of limbs, and even tremors of hand and foot will appear. If heat damages liver meridian, impairment of liver-yin, loss of nourishment in tendons, and such wind-like shaking symptoms as convulsion of four limbs, stiff and hard neck, and opisthotonus will appear.

4) Liver is associated with eyes in orifice: If liver blood is insufficient, eyes will be dry and uncomfortable with blurred vision or night blindness. Liver fire will cause redness, swelling, hotness and pain of eyes, and excessive liver yang due to liver yin deficiency may cause dizziness and vertigo.

2. Gallbladder　The major function of gallbladder is to store and excrete bile. When liver functions normally in governing the free flow of qi, and the secretion and excretion of bile is proper, the digestion and absorption of food will be normal. On the contrary, if liver functions abnormally, and the secretion and excretion of bile is obstructed, it will affect the digestion and absorption of foodstuff, while there may appear distending pain in the hypochondrium, abdominal distention, poor appetite, nausea and vomit. If bile goes adversely upward, there may occur bitter taste in the mouth, or vomiting with bitter liquid yellowish and green in color. If bile spreads out from the bile tract, there may appear jaundice all over the body such as skin, face, and eyes.

v. Kidney and Urinary Bladder

1. Kidney　The major functions of kidney are storing essence, governing water and governing qi reception. Kidney and urinary bladder form the exterior-interior relationship through mutual connection and affiliation of their meridians. Kidney stores the innate essence, which is the origin of life, so it is called "the foundation of congenital (prenatal) constitution".

绪抑郁，或急躁易怒。

2）在液为泪：泪由肝之阴血所化。肝之气血调和，则泪液濡润目而不外溢。若肝阴血不足，则两目干涩；如肝经风热，则可见两目红赤，羞光流泪；肝经湿热，则见目眵增多，迎风流泪。

3）在体合筋，其华在爪：筋包括韧带和肌腱。如肝血虚少，血不养筋，可见肢体麻木、屈伸不利，甚则手足震颤；若热邪燔灼肝经，劫夺肝阴，筋脉失养，则可见四肢抽搐、颈项强直、角弓反张等动风之象。

4）在窍为目：肝的经脉上连目系，目的视物辨色功能依赖肝血的濡养和肝气的疏泄。若肝之阴血不足，则可见两目干涩，视物昏花或夜盲；肝火上炎，则可见两目红肿热痛；肝阴虚而阳亢，可见头晕目眩。

2. 胆　胆的生理功能主要是贮藏和排泄胆汁。肝疏泄正常，胆汁生成、排泄正常，水谷消化吸收则正常。如肝疏泄功能失常，胆汁不能正常生成和排泄，则可见胁痛腹胀、食欲缺乏、恶心、呕吐；胆汁上逆，则可见口苦、呕吐黄绿苦水等；若胆汁外溢肌肤，则见身、尿、目俱黄的黄疸症状。

（五）肾与膀胱

1. 肾　肾的主要生理功能是主藏精，主水，主纳气。肾藏先天之精，为生命之本原，故称为"先天之本"。肾在体合骨，生髓，其华在发，在窍为耳及二阴，在志为恐，在液为唾。肾与膀胱通过经脉相互络属，构成表里关系。

(1) Major functions

1) Storing essence: Kidney stores essential qi. It prevents qi from escaping, promotes individual growth, development and reproduction, and modulates visceral activities of the whole body. Kidney is the root for storage, being in charge of storing essence.

a. The essence stored in kidney includes "congenital essence" and "acquired essence". The congenital essence comes from the reproductive essence of one's parents and provides the original substance to compose embryo, also called "reproductive essence". The acquired essence comes from the water and food essence transformed and transported by spleen and stomach. After birth, the water and food essence is stored in every *zang-fu* organs, so is called "visceral essence". After supporting the functions of every *zang-fu* organ, the residual part of visceral essence is transported into kidney to supplement and nourish the congenital essence. The congenital essence and the acquired essence are combined with each other to form kidney essence. Kidney essence is the material basis for generation of kidney qi.

b. The physiological effects of essential qi in kidney are mainly to promote the growth, development as well as reproduction and modulate activities of the whole body. There is a life law of birth, growth, prime, aging and death in human body, and the whole process of life is influenced by qi of kidney essence. When essential qi is sufficient, the growth, development and reproduction will be normal and sound. Contrarily, if essential qi gets deficient, there could be poor development in children, while early senility, hyposexuality, amenorrhea and sterility in adult. So taking good care of essential qi is of great importance for maintaining health, preventing premature senility, and prolonging life.

c. Kidney essence can transform into kidney qi, and kidney qi can present with physiological effects of two respects of kidney yin and kidney yang. Kidney yin has the effect of moistening, calming and inhibiting; while kidney yang warming, propelling and exciting. Kidney yin and kidney yang restrict each other and depend on each other to maintain the balance of yin and yang of every *zang-fu* organ. In case of kidney yin deficiency, there may appear internal heat with restlessness in palms, soles and chest, sore and weak feeling of waist and knees, tinnitus, dizziness, nocturnal seminal emission, red tongue with lack of moisture *etc.*. If kidney yang is deficient, there may occur cold body and limbs, cold pain and weakness of waist and knees, clear urine with increased volume, or inhibited urination, enuresis, sexual hypofunction and

（1）肾的主要生理功能

1）肾主藏精：指肾为封藏之本，对精气具有贮存、封藏作用。

a. 肾所藏的精包括"先天之精"和部分"后天之精"。先天之精，来源于父母的生殖之精，主要藏于肾，是构成胚胎发育的原始物质，又称为"生殖之精"。后天之精，来源于脾胃运化生成的精微物质，藏于五脏六腑，又称为"脏腑之精"。各脏腑之精在完成各脏腑生理功能后多余的部分输送至肾，以充养"先天之精"。"先天之精"和"后天之精"互相融合构成"肾精"。

b. 肾中精气的生理功能主要是促进人体的生长、发育和生殖，并调控全身各脏腑生理活动。人的整个生、长、壮、老、已的生命过程，都由肾中精气的盛衰主管和调节。肾中精气旺盛，人的生长、发育和生殖能力较强。肾中精气虚衰，在幼年，可见小儿发育障碍；在成年人，可见早衰现象，还可致性功能减退、闭经、不孕等。因此，保养肾中精气，对养生保健、预防早衰、延年益寿具有重要意义。

c. 肾精化生肾气，肾气又可分为肾阴、肾阳。肾阴具有凉润、宁静、抑制等作用，肾阳具有温煦、推动、兴奋等作用。肾阴、肾阳相互制约、相互协调，共同维持并调控着各脏腑阴阳的平衡。若肾阴虚，则现五心烦热、腰膝酸软、耳鸣、眩晕、遗精、舌红少津等症；若肾阳虚，则见形寒肢冷、腰膝酸困、冷痛、小便清长、遗尿、性欲低下、水肿、舌质淡等症。

edema as well as pale tongue.

2) Governing water: Kidney controls and regulates the distribution and excretion of water in the body so as to balance water metabolism. The whole process of water metabolism is concerned with a series of physiological activities of several organs; however the essential qi in the kidney plays a controlling and regulating role. If the steaming and transformation of essential qi in kidney get disordered, it will lead to disorders of production and discharge of urine, resulting in pathological phenomena of inhibited urination, edema, enuresis and urinary incontinence.

3) Governing qi reception: Kidney receives the fresh air inhaled by lung so as to keep the depth of respiration. The respiratory function of body is governed by lung, but it must be achieved through the absorption and storage of kidney qi to keep a certain depth. There is the saying "Lung is the governor of qi and kidney is the root of qi." Lung governs exhalation of qi and kidney governs absorption of qi. When essential qi in kidney is sufficient and with ability to receive qi, the respiration will be even and harmonious. On the contrary, if essential qi in kidney gets deficient and with no power to receive qi, then lung qi cannot go down, but will float upward, manifesting as pathological phenomena of tachypnea, dyspnea on exercise, or dyspnea with prolonged expiration, and decompensation.

(2) Relations of kidney with emotion, fluids, constituent and orifice

1) Kidney is associated with fear in emotion: Great fear makes qi sink. If a person is in a state of great fear, the kidney qi will fail to go up and conversely go downward, thus kidney qi cannot normally spread, and the symptoms of incontinence of urination and stool will occur.

2) Kidney is associated with spittle in fluids: Too much or prolonged excretion of the spittle will be apt to consume kidney essence. So health preservation specialists suggest that one should touch the palate with tongue for a while until spittle is full of the mouth, then swallow it down to nurture the essential qi in kidney, this is so called "drinking nourishing nectar".

3) Kidney is associated with bone in constituent, generating marrow, and manifesting on hair: When kidney essence is sufficient, bone will be strong and firm with teeth solidity, so tooth is called the surplus of bone. If kidney essence gets deficient, bone marrow will be short, and the bone will have less nourishment. Then there may appear stunt, weak bone with no strength and delayed closure of the fontanel in children, weak waist and knees, and inability to walk in adults, and fragile and weak bone subject to fracture, flexible teeth in the elderly people.

2）肾主水：是指肾气具有主持和调节体内津液的输布和排泄，维持津液代谢平衡的作用。在整个水液代谢过程中，涉及多个脏腑一系列活动，而肾气及肾阴肾阳通过对各脏腑之气及其阴阳的资助和促进作用，主司和调节着机体水液代谢的各个环节。若肾气的蒸腾气化功能失常，可引起小便不利、水肿、遗尿、尿失禁等病理变化。

3）肾主纳气：是指肾有摄纳肺所吸入的清气，保持呼吸深度的生理功能。人体的呼吸虽然由肺来主司，但肺所吸入的清气，必须下达到肾，靠肾的封藏作用才能摄纳潜藏，保持呼吸深度。故有"肺为气之主，肾为气之根，肺主出气，肾主纳气"的说法。肾中精气充盛，摄纳有权，则呼吸均匀和调；若肾中精气不足，摄纳无权，则肺失肃降，可出现呼吸表浅，动则气喘，呼多吸少等症。

（2）肾与志、液、体和窍的关系

1）在志为恐：恐则气下，肾气不能向上布散而下泄，则出现二便失禁等。

2）在液为唾：唾为唾液中较稠厚的部分，由肾精化生，若舌抵上腭，待津唾满口后，咽而不吐，则能回滋肾精；若唾多或久唾，则易耗伤肾中精气。

3）在体合骨，生髓，其华在发：肾精充盛，骨髓充足，骨骼得养，则骨坚劲有力，牙齿坚固。齿与骨同由肾精充养，故又称"齿为骨之余"。若肾精不足，骨髓空虚，骨骼失养，在小儿可见生长发育迟缓、骨软无力、囟门迟闭；在成人可见腰膝酸软、足痿不能行走；在老年人则易发生骨折、牙齿松动。肾其华在发，肾气强盛，则头发浓密乌

When kidney qi is abundant, hair will be dense and jet black with luster. Contrarily, as kidney qi gets deficient, hair will lose its nourishment, leading to grey with falling off, and dry with no luster.

4) Kidney is associated with the ear and two yin organs (genital and anus) in orifice: When essential qi in kidney is sufficient, marrow sea will get nourished and hearing will be sharp. On the contrary, if essential qi in kidney gets deficient, marrow sea will lose its nourishment, leading to blunt hearing, tinnitus, or even deafness. Two yin organs are genital and anus. The genital has the function of urination and reproduction, and the anus is the passage to discharge feces. The reproduction function of human beings depends upon the abundance of the essential qi. The discharge of urine and feces is closely related to qi transformation of kidney. Therefore there is the saying "kidney is in charge of urine and feces" and "kidney opens at the two yin organs".

2. Urinary Bladder The major function of urinary bladder is to store and discharge urine. Urine is produced from water under qi transformation of kidney, and then poured into bladder for storage. If kidney qi is sufficient, and bladder closes and opens orderly, then the function of storing and discharging urine will be normal. If the essential qi fails in transformation due to deficiency, urinary bladder will also have difficulty in qi transformation, leading to obstruction of urination, and even the retention of urine. If kidney qi fails in fixation due to deficiency, the urinary bladder will be unable to control, and symptoms such as frequent urination, enuresis, and urinary incontinence will appear.

vi. Pericardium and *Sanjiao*

1. Pericardium Pericardium in TCM is referring to the outer membrane that encloses heart, whose function is to protect heart by undertaking pathogens invading heart. In the theory of visceral manifestation, heart, the monarch organ, is so important that it can never be invaded by any pathogens. Therefore, pericardium serves as the frontier protection for heart, which often manifests as disorders of consciousness, as heart fails to store the spirit. In warm diseases by external pathogens, warm pathogen invades inward, leading to coma, high fever, delirium and other symptoms of disturbed heart spirit. These manifestations are often summarized as heat entering pericardium. Actually, if pericardium is affected, its clinical manifestation will be identical to those of heart disorders. Therefore, similar treatment methods based on similar pattern differentiation are often applied in the management of pericardium and heart diseases.

2. *Sanjiao* *Sanjiao*, or three *jiao*, refers to upper,

黑而有光泽；肾气衰弱，头发花白脱落，失去光泽。

4）在窍为耳及二阴：肾精充足，髓海得养，则耳的听觉功能正常；肾中精气虚衰，髓海空虚，则可见听力减退，或见耳鸣、耳聋。二阴，即前阴和后阴。前阴具有排尿及生殖功能；后阴是排泄粪便的通道。人的生殖功能依赖于肾中精气的充盛，而尿液和粪便的排泄也与肾的气化密切相关，故称"肾司二便""肾开窍于二阴"。

2. **膀胱** 膀胱的主要生理功能为贮尿和排尿。肾气充足，膀胱开合有度；若肾气虚，气化失常，引起膀胱的气化不利，则见小便不利，甚或癃闭；若肾气虚，固摄失常，引起膀胱失于约束，则见尿频、尿急、遗尿或尿失禁。

（六）心包与三焦

1. **心包** 心包是心脏外面的包膜，其功能为保护心脏，代心受邪。心为君主之官，邪不能犯，所以若外邪侵心，心包络当先受病，其临床表现主要是心藏神的功能异常。如在外感温热病中，因温热之邪内陷，出现神昏、高热、谵语等心神受扰的症状，称为"热入心包"。事实上，心包受邪所出现的病证，即心之病证，心和其他脏腑一样，亦可受邪。

2. **三焦** 三焦是上、中、下三焦的合称。

middle and lower *jiao*. As for the Chinese character *jiao*, there are still controversies about its explanation. Some experts think that *jiao* means an organ, some say it is about the food-ripening function, while others argue it means segments, referring to the three sections that the human body can be divided into: upper, middle and lower *jiao*. There are three kinds of *sanjiao*. One is one of the six *fu* organ, one is a concept of simple regions, and another is the meaning of differentiation.

The major functions of *sanjiao* as one of the six *fu* organs are water passages. The functions of the second are governing qi movement and water passages. The last are three different pathological stages of warm diseases.

关于"焦"的含义，历代医家认识不一。有的认为"焦"为体内脏器，是有形之物；有的认为"焦"指能腐熟变化水谷的功能；有的认为"焦"谓人体有上、中、下三节段也。三焦概念有六腑之三焦、部位之三焦与辨证之三焦的不同。

六腑之三焦的主要功能是疏通水道，运行津液；部位之三焦的主要功能是通行诸气，运行水液；辨证之三焦是温病发生发展过程中由浅及深的三个不同病理阶段。

II. Relationship between *Zang* Organs

1. Relationship between Heart and Lung

The relationship between heart and lung is mainly manifested in two respects of blood circulation and respiratory movement. Blood circulation is dependent upon the propelling of heart qi, and also upon the assistance of lung qi. Lung connects with vessels to assist heart in circulating blood, thus keeping normal blood circulation. If lung qi gets insufficient or lung is invaded by cold, and thus lung fails in assisting the heart to circulate blood, it will lead to stasis of heart blood with obstructed circulation of blood, manifested as palpitations, purple tongue, unsmooth pulse, *etc.*. Lung controls respiration, inhaling the clear and exhaling the turbid, so as to maintain the normal respiratory movement, while heart governs circulation of blood. Only when blood circulates normally, and lung gets its nourishment of blood, the lung's function of controlling respiration can keep normal. If heart qi gets weak and fails to circulate blood, blood circulation will be unsmooth, then it may affect lung in controlling respiration, resulting in chest distress, cough, panting, *etc.* (Fig. 2-5).

2. Relationship between Heart and Spleen

The relationship between heart and spleen is mainly manifested by two respects of generation and circulation of blood. Heart governs blood circulation to provide nourishment of blood for spleen to maintain its normal function of transformation and transportation. Spleen governs transformation and transportation, being the source for generation of qi and blood. When spleen qi is sound in transformation and transportation, generation of blood will possess its source, then blood will be kept abundant. So clinically insufficiency of heart-blood or disorder of heart-spirit affects the function of spleen,

二、五脏之间的关系

1. **心与肺** 心与肺的关系，主要是心主血与肺主气之间的关系，体现在气和血两方面。心主血脉，心血载气维持肺主气功能的正常进行。肺主气，肺朝百脉，辅心行血，是血液正常运行的必要条件。若肺气不足，可影响心的行血功能，易致心血瘀阻，表现为心悸、舌紫、脉涩等症；反之，若心血瘀阻也可影响肺的呼吸功能，导致肺气不宣，出现胸闷、咳喘、气促等症（图2-5）。

2. **心与脾** 心与脾的关系，主要体现在血液的生成和运行上的相互协调。心血赖脾气健运以化生，而脾的转输功能又赖心血滋养和心阳推动；血液在脉中正常运行，有赖于心气的推动与脾气的统摄。只有心脾两脏功能正常，相互为用，才能保持正常的生血与行血。若脾气虚弱，化源不足，或统血无权，血液妄行，均可导致心血不足；若心血不足，无以滋养脾，则致脾气虚弱。最终均

while dysfunction of spleen or failure of spleen to command blood also leads to disorder of heart, bringing on simultaneous disorder of both spleen and heart with the symptoms of dizziness, palpitation, insomnia, poor appetite, tiredness, apathy, pale complexion, *etc.* (Fig. 2-6).

3. The Relationship between Heart and Liver

The relationship between heart and liver is signified by circulation of blood and regulation of mental activities. Heart governs blood, and is the motivation of blood circulation, while liver stores blood, and is a very important factor in the storage and regulation of blood. So heart and liver coordinate with each other in blood circulation. Heart governs the mind and regulates mental activities, while liver governs dredging and dispersing and adjusts emotional activities. They are closely related to each other in maintaining mental and emotional activities. Clinically insufficiency of liver-blood and deficiency of heart-blood may affect each other, leading to deficiency of both liver-blood and heart-blood, manifested as blood deficiency of heart and liver, qi depression of heart and liver, exuberance of heart fire and liver fire, *etc.* (Fig. 2-7).

可形成心脾两虚之证，临床常见眩晕、心悸、失眠、食少、体倦、精神萎靡、面色无华等（图 2-6）。

3. 心与肝　心与肝的关系，主要表现在行血与藏血以及精神调节两个方面。心主行血，肝藏血，二者相互配合，共同维持血液的正常运行。心藏神，主宰精神、意识、思维及情志活动，肝主疏泄，调畅气机，调节情志，二者相互为用，共同维持正常的精神情志活动。心与肝在病理上相互影响，主要表现为心肝血虚、心肝气郁、心肝火旺等证（图 2-7）。

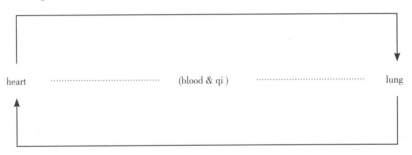

Fig. 2-5　The Relationship Between Heart and Lung

图 2-5　心与肺生理功能关系示意图

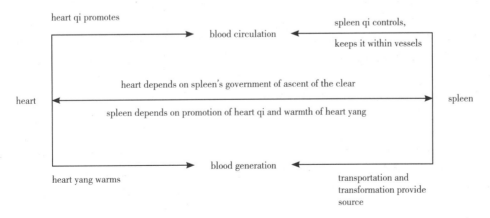

Fig. 2-6　The Relationship Between Heart and Spleen

图 2-6　心与脾生理功能关系示意图

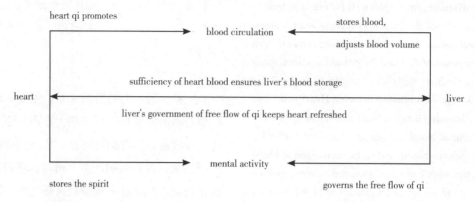

heart qi promotes → blood circulation ← stores blood, adjusts blood volume

heart ←→ liver

sufficiency of heart blood ensures liver's blood storage

liver's government of free flow of qi keeps heart refreshed

→ mental activity ←

stores the spirit

governs the free flow of qi

Fig. 2-7　The Relationship Between Heart and Liver
图 2-7　心与肝生理功能关系示意图

4. The Relationship between Heart and Kidney

The relationship between heart and kidney is mainly manifested as follows:

(1) Coordination between water and fire: Heart pertains to fire in the five phases and is located in the upper energizer, while kidney pertains to water in the five phases and is located in the lower energizer. Heart fire (heart yang) has to descend to the kidney to warm kidney-yang and prevent abnormal flow of water, while kidney water (kidney yin) has to ascend to nourish heart-yin and prevent hyperactivity of heart-yang. Such coordination between the upper and the lower can keep the balance and coordination of physical functions between heart and kidney.

(2) Essence and spirit promoting each other: Heart stores spirit, which can control essence. Kidney stores essence, which can generate spirit. Spirit and essence depend upon each other. Essence is the material basis of spirit, and spirit is the external expression of essence. Therefore, essence and spirit can promote each other.

(3) Harmony between heart yang and kidney yang: Heart is located in the upper energizer, and pertains to yang. Heart yang is the most important factor just like the emperor dominating all the activities. Kidney is located in the lower energizer, and kidney yang can promote the function of heart-yang. If kidney-yang is sufficient, heart yang will be kept abundant. If heart yang is sufficient, kidney can function well. Therefore, harmony between heart yang and kidney-yang can lead to coordination between heart and kidney.

Pathological influence between heart and kidney is mainly manifested as discordance between heart and kidney, yin deficiency and fire hyperactivity, yang deficiency of heart and kidney, deficiency of essence and spirit, *etc.* (Fig. 2-8).

5. The Relationship between Lung and Liver

4. **心与肾**　心与肾的关系，主要表现为"心肾相交"，具体体现在以下三方面：

（1）水火既济：心居上焦属阳属火，肾居下焦属阴属水。心火（阳）须下降于肾，使肾水不寒；肾水（阴）须上济于心，使心火不亢。另外，肾阴上济依赖肾阳的鼓动；心火下降需要心阴的凉润。心与肾水火升降互济，维持了两脏之间生理功能的协调平衡。

（2）精神互用：心藏神，肾藏精，精能化气生神，神能统精驭气。精是神的物质基础，神是精的外在表现。故积精可以全神，神清可以驭精。

（3）君相安位：心为君火，肾为相火（命火）。君火在上，如日照当空，为一身之主宰；相火在下，为神明之臣辅。命火秘藏，则心阳充足；心阳充盛，则相火潜藏守位。君火相火，各安其位，则心肾上下交济。

心与肾在病理上相互影响，主要表现为水不济火，阴虚火旺，心肾阳虚，或精亏神逸等病理变化（图 2-8）。

5. **肺与肝**　肺与肝的关系，主要体现在

The relationship between lung and liver is signified by the regulation of qi and blood circulation. Lung-qi functions to descend and depurate while liver-qi functions to elevate and disperse. Liver and lung, by means of ascent and descent, restrain each other and depend on each other so as to maintain the normal flow of qi in the whole body. In addition, liver stores blood while lung governs qi in the whole body, controls respiration and regulates qi activity, which need nourishment of blood. Meanwhile, blood circulation depends on the promotion of qi. Therefore, lung and liver coordinate with each other in regulating qi activity. Dysfunction of lung and liver can clinically lead to abnormal flow of qi and blood (Fig. 2-9).

6. The Relationship among Lung, Spleen and Kidney The relationships among the lung, spleen and kidney are signified by the generation of qi and metabolism of body fluid, the respiratory activity, as well as the interdependence of kidney and spleen.

(1) Lung, spleen and kidney are jointly involved in the generation of qi and metabolism of body fluid. Lung is

气机升降和气血运行方面。肝气以升发为宜，肺气以肃降为顺。肝升肺降，相互协调，共同维持人体气机的正常升降运动。肝藏血，肺主气，肺调节全身之气的功能需要得到血的濡养，肝向周身输送血液又必须依赖于气的推动。两脏对气血的运行有一定的调节作用。肺与肝在病理上主要表现为气机升降失常和气血运行不畅（图 2-9）。

6. 肺、脾与肾 肺、脾、肾三脏的关系主要体现在气的生成、津液代谢、阴阳互资、呼吸运动以及先后天互助等方面。

（1）肺、脾、肾共同参与了气的生成与津液代谢。肺吸入自然界清气与脾运化的谷气

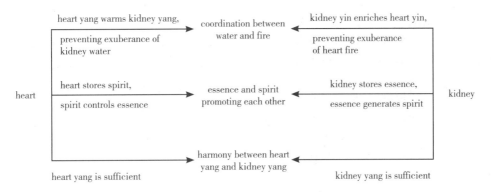

Fig. 2-8　The Relationship Between Heart and Kidney
图 2-8　心与肾生理功能关系示意图

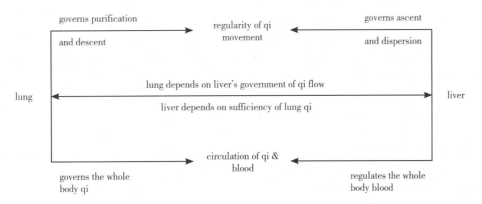

Fig. 2-9　The Relationship Between Lung and Liver
图 2-9　肺与肝生理功能关系示意图

responsible for inhaling fresh air and spleen for absorbing food nutrients through transportation and transformation. The accumulation of fresh air and food nutrients in the chest eventually transforms into the pectoral qi (*zōng qì*, 宗气). The pectoral qi and healthy qi from kidney essence become all qi in body. Lung governs water passage and is located on the top, spleen controls water and body fluid and is the hub of metabolism of body fluid, while kidney maintains the normal distribution and excretion of water and is the lower source. Therefore, the coordination of lung, spleen and kidney maintains the normal transportation and transformation of water and body fluid.

(2) Lung and kidney work together to accomplish the respiratory activity. Lung governs qi and controls respiration, while kidney stores essence and receives qi and kidney. Lung and kidney work together to keep a deep breath. The kidney yin and kidney yang are the base of yin and yang of five *zang*-organs, which can support lung yin and lung yang and descent lung qi. Meanwhile, lung-yin and lung-yang can promote kidney-yin and kidney-yang.

(3) Kidney is the congenital base of life while spleen is the acquired base of life. The relationship between spleen and kidney is in fact the inter-independence between the congenital and acquired bases of life.

The interplay of lung, spleen and kidney is manifested as little generation of qi, abnormal metabolism of body fluid, abnormal breathing, deficiency of yin and yang, dysfunction of digestion, *etc.*. If spleen functions abnormally, water-dampness may be produced internally, which can often affect lung to result in failure of lung in diffusion and descent. It is called that "spleen is the source of water-dampness, while lung is the storage containers of water-dampness" in TCM (Fig. 2-10).

7. The Relationship between Liver and Spleen

The relationship between liver and spleen involves two aspects: digestion and blood circulation. Liver governs dredging and dispersing, regulates the ascending and descending activities of spleen-qi and stomach-qi, and secrets bile, which is beneficial to the transportation and transformation of spleen. Spleen governs the transportation and transformation of food nutrients which are transformed into blood to nourish liver. Spleen controls blood, and spleen qi holds blood to prevent its escape from the vessels. If liver blood is sufficient, liver proper will get its nourishment, then liver's function in governing free flow of qi will be normal, qi dynamic will be smooth, and thus blood will be free from obstruction. Liver and spleen cooperate with each other to guarantee both smooth blood flow and non-escape of blood from the vessels. If liver and spleen get injured, the control and

汇为宗气，宗气与肾精所化的元气合为一身之气；肺主行水，为水之上源；脾主运化水饮，为津液代谢的枢纽；肾为水脏，为水之下源，三者相互配合，共同维持津液正常输布与排泄。

（2）肺与肾阴阳互资，共同维持呼吸运动。肾阴肾阳为五脏阴阳之根本，能资助肺阴肺阳，肺气肃降，肺阴肺阳亦能资助肾阴肾阳；肺主气而司呼吸，肾藏精而主纳气，二者配合共同维持呼吸的深度。

（3）脾与肾先后天相互资助。肾为先天之本，脾为后天之本，脾运化水谷，先天温养激发后天，后天补充培育先天。

三脏病理上相互影响，主要表现为气的生成不足、津液代谢失调、呼吸异常、阴阳虚损、消化功能失调等。若脾失健运，聚湿生痰，影响肺的宣降而痰嗽喘咳，故称"脾为生痰之源，肺为贮痰之器"（图 2-10）。

7. 肝与脾　肝与脾的关系，主要表现在饮食消化和血液运行两个方面。肝主疏泄，调畅气机，协调脾胃升降，并分泌排泄胆汁，促进脾胃运化；脾主运化正常，气血生化有源，肝体得以濡养而有利于肝之疏泄。脾气健运，生血有源，统血有权，使肝有所藏；肝血充足，藏泻有度，血量得以有效调节，气血才能运行无阻。二者共同维持血液的正常运行。肝与脾在病理上的相互影响，主要表现为饮食运化和血液运行失常，出现纳呆、腹胀、便溏、出血、贫血等（图 2-11）。

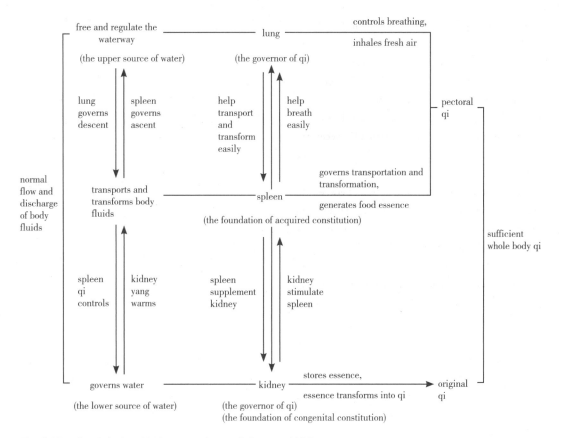

Fig. 2-10   The Relationship Between Lung, Spleen and Kidney

图 2-10   肺、脾、肾生理功能关系示意图

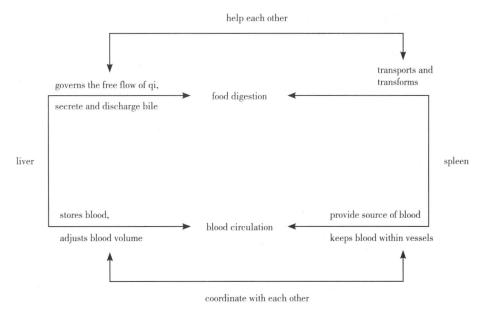

Fig. 2-11   The Relationship Between Liver and Spleen

图 2-11   肝与脾生理功能关系示意图

storage of blood will become disordered, manifested as anorexia, abdominal distension, loose stools, bleeding, anemia, *etc.* (Fig. 2-11).

8. Relationship between Liver and Kidney

8. 肝与肾　肝与肾的关系，主要表现在精

The relationship between liver and kidney is mainly marked by mutual transformation between essence and blood, and interdependence of storage and discharge.

(1) Same origin of essence and blood: Liver stores blood, and kidney stores essence. Sufficient blood in liver makes it possible for kidney to store the essence and abundant essence in kidney provides necessary nourishment for liver. Therefore blood and essence promote each other and transform into each other.

(2) Mutual promotion and restraint between yin and yang: Kidney-yin and kidney-yang are the foundation of yin and yang of five *zang* organs. Kidney-yin nourishes liver-yin, and both can constrain hyperactivity of liver-yang, while kidney-yang can promote liver-yang to warm liver-yin to prevent cold and stagnation of liver blood. Thus the inter-promotion between liver and kidney is vital to life activities.

(3) Mutual promotion in dredging, dispersing and storage: Liver governs dredging and dispersing, and kidney is responsible for storage. Dredging and dispersing of liver qi makes it possible for kidney to promote and store qi, while storage of kidney-qi prevent liver to over-dredge and over-disperse. Both organs coordinate with each other in dredging, dispersing and storage in order to regulate ovulation, menstruation and discharge of seminal fluid.

Pathologically, mutual influence between liver and kidney mainly involves dysfunction of essence and blood, yin and yang, dredging, dispersing and storage, *etc.* (Fig. 2-12).

血同源、阴阳互滋互制以及藏泄互用等方面。

（1）精血同源：肝藏血，肾藏精，精血皆由水谷精微化生和充养，且能相互资生，故称"精血同源"。肝血依赖肾精的滋养，肾精又依赖肝血的不断补充。

（2）阴阳互滋互制：肾阴与肾阳为五脏阴阳之本，肾阴滋养肝阴，共同制约肝阳，则肝阳不亢；肾阳资助肝阳，共同温煦肝脉，防止肝脉寒滞。肝肾阴阳之间互制互用维持了肝肾之间的协调平衡。

（3）藏泄互用：肝主疏泄，肾主封藏，肝气疏泄可促使肾气开阖有度，肾气闭藏可制约肝气疏泄太过。疏泄与封藏，相辅相成，调节女子排卵、月经来潮和男子排精。

肝与肾在病理上的相互影响，主要表现在精血失调、阴阳失调和藏泄失司等方面（图 2-12）。

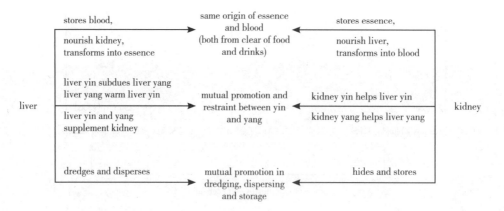

Fig. 2-12 The Relationship Between Liver and Kidney
图 2-12 肝与肾生理功能关系示意图

(Wang Qiu-qin)　　　　　　　　　　　　　　　　　（王秋琴）

Section 4　Essence, Qi, Blood and Body Fluid

The essence, qi, blood and body fluid are the basic substances that constitute the human body and maintain its life activity. They are produced by the functional activities of the viscera, channels, tissues and organs. Therefore, they are closely related to the viscera, channels, tissues and organs physiologically and pathologically.

I. Essence

i. Concept of Essence

The essence is a type of refined nutritious substances in the body. In a broad sense, it means the refined nutritious substances transformed by qi and constituting the human body and maintaining its life activity, including qi, blood, body fluid, marrow, and the essence of food and drinks. In a narrow sense, it refers to the reproductive essence stored in the kidney with function of producing offspring, being the basic substance of promoting growth, development and reproductive function of the human body.

ii. Function of Essence

The essence has functions of multiplying offspring, promoting growth and development, transforming itself into marrow and blood, nourishing and moistening the viscera, as well as producing qi and spirit.

1. Producing Offspring　The reproductive essence originates from the combination of congenital and acquired essence. It stores in kidney and constitutes essential qi of kidney. With its gradual abundance, marked by full development and mature body till a certain period of youth when reproduction-stimulating essence named "*tiān guǐ*" is generated, the individual will have the ability to produce offspring.

2. Moistening and Nourishing Human Body　The essence has the function of moistening and nourishing. If the essence is sufficient, the viscera, tissues, sense organs and orifices can all get necessary nourishment to perform their normal physical functions.

3. Producing Qi　The congenital essence can generate original qi (*yuán qì*,元气). The foodstuff qi, which is transformed from the foodstuff essence, combines with the fresh air inhaled by the lung to form the acquired qi of the body. Qi promotes and regulates the metabolism of human body constantly to maintain its life activity.

4. Transforming into Marrow and Blood　The

第四节　精气血津液

精、气、血、津液是构成人体和维持生命活动的基本物质，是由脏腑、经络及组织器官功能活动所化生，因此，精、气、血、津液与脏腑经络及组织器官之间在生理、病理上关系非常密切。

一、精

（一）精的概念

精是体内的一种精微物质，具有广义和狭义之分，广义之精，泛指由气而化生的构成人体和维持生命活动的精微物质，包括气、血、津液、髓以及水谷精微等；狭义之精是指藏于肾中具有繁衍后代作用的生殖之精，是促进人体生长发育和生殖功能的基本物质。

（二）精的功能

人体之精具有繁衍生命、促进生长发育、生髓化血、濡养脏腑、生气化神等作用。

1. 繁衍生命　指由先天之精与后天之精合化而成的生殖之精，藏于肾中，组成肾中精气，随着肾中精气的不断充盛、形体逐渐发育成熟，到一定年龄便产生了"天癸"，从而具备了繁衍生命的功能。

2. 濡养脏腑　人体之精能濡养全身脏腑组织形体器官。脏腑之精充盈，肾精充盛，脏腑组织得以充养，则各种生理功能方能正常发挥。

3. 精能化气　先天之精可以化生先天之气（元气），水谷之精可以化生谷气，再加上由肺吸入的自然清气，构成一身之气。气不断地推动和调控人的新陈代谢，维系生命活动。因此，精是气化生之本原。

4. 生髓化血　肾藏精，精生髓，髓分为

kidney stores essence that can transform itself into marrows including brain marrow and bone marrow. The brain marrow can nourish the brain. So if it is sufficient, the human body will have consciousness and an agile mind， as well as fluent language. The bone depends upon nourishment of the marrow. If kidney essence is sufficient, the bone marrow will be abundant, the skeleton will be firm and powerful and the teeth will be strong without falling off. If kidney essence is deficient, it will affect the production of the marrow, and then the brain will be insufficient marked by dizziness, vertigo, amnesia and retarded intelligence, and the skeleton will lose its nourishment, leading to looseness, even loss of teeth. The essence produces marrow, which is one of the sources for blood production. Sufficient essence in the kidney provides necessary nourishment for the liver and then blood will be replenished. If essence is sufficient, then the blood will be rich, contrarily if essence is insufficient, then the blood will be poor, and vice versa. Therefore there is a saying "essence and blood share the same source".

5. Producing Spirit The essence is the substantial basis for mental activity. Only when the essence is sufficient can the spirit be sound, which is the basic assurance of life existence. On the contrary, shortage of the essence will lead to weariness of spirit, and depletion of the essence will cause loss of spirit.

II. Qi

TCM holds that qi is one of the most basic materials of the world and constant movement of qi produces all things in the universe.

i. Concept of Qi

Qi is a kind of active and refined substance that is in constant motion, but cannot be seen. Qi constitutes the human body and maintains its life activity.

Qi is the basic material constituting the human body. It is stated in *Basic Questions* "the human body is generated by qi of the heaven and earth". *Precepts for Physicians (Yī Mén Fǎ Lù,* 医门法律) *says* that gathering of qi gives rise to life while dispersion of qi puts an end to life.

Qi is the basic material maintaining life activity. All life activities of the human body are produced by qi transformation. Therefore, qi is the most important material for life activity, which is seen as the root of life.

Qi is a kind of active and essential substance that

脑髓和骨髓。脑髓能够养脑，故脑髓充盈，则意识清楚、思维灵敏、语言清晰等。骨髓养骨，故肾精充足、骨髓充满，则骨骼坚固、牙齿牢固而不脱落。若肾精亏虚，不能生髓，则髓海不足、头昏眩晕、健忘、智力减退、骨骼失养、牙齿松动易脱落。精生髓，髓化血。肾精充盈则肝有所养，血有所充，精足则血旺，精亏则血虚，反之亦然，故有"精血同源"之说。

5. **精能化神** 精是神的物质基础。只有积精，才能全神，这是生命健康的根本保证。反之，精亏则神疲，精亡则神散。

二、气

中医学认为气是构成世界的最基本物质，自然界的一切事物都是由气的运动变化而产生的。

（一）气的概念

人体之气是构成人体和维持生命活动的基本物质之一，具有活力很强、不断运动、且无形可见的特性。

气，是构成人体的最基本物质。《素问》曰"人以天地之气生"，《医门法律》曰"气聚则形成，气散则形亡。"

气，又是维持人体生命活动的最基本物质。人的全部生命活动都是在气的作用下得以进行。所以，气对人的生命活动至关重要，被视为人体生命的根本。

气，是具有很强活力并不断运动、且无

constantly circulates inside the body, whose characteristics express the aspects of invigorating and promoting functions of the viscera, as well as circulation of essence, blood and body fluid. Qi cannot be seen, but can be observed indirectly from activity of the viscera. Therefore, the motion and change of qi can be used to explain life activity of the human body in TCM.

ii. Movement of Qi

The movement of qi is referred to as "qi mechanism" or "qi dynamic" sometimes. The moving style of qi can be usually classified into four types, namely ascending, descending, exiting and entering. Ascending is a sort of motion of qi from the lower to the upper. Descending is from the upper to the lower. Exiting is from the interior to the exterior. Entering is from the exterior to the interior. With regard to the human body, the movement of qi should keep balance in ascending, descending, exiting and entering, while in terms of each *zang* and *fu* organ, it may lay particular stress on a certain type. For example, among the five *zang* organs, ascending is the main aspect of liver and spleen, while descending is the leading respect of heart and lung. As far as the six *fu* organs are concerned, the gallbladder is in charge of ascending, while most of the others are apt to descend. As a whole, the movement of qi keeps a coordinative balance in ascending, descending, exiting and entering. For instance, the liver governs ascending and the lung governs descending, while the spleen qi ascends the essence and the stomach qi descends the turbid, so as to maintain the normal life activity.The ascending, descending, exiting and entering of qi can regulate the physiological function to attain the relative equilibrium. The state of coordinative balance without qi obstruction is known as "free flow of qi". On the contrary, if the motion of qi gets obstructed, or fails to be harmonious, it will then be called "disorder of qi movement".

iii. Function of Qi

Qi of the human body is the source to maintain life activity, and the power of physiological functions of the viscera, channels, tissues and other organs. Generally speaking, actions of qi in life activity can be summarized as the following six aspects.

1. Propelling　Qi, with its vitality and motion, may propel growth and development of the human body, invigorate physiological functions of the viscera, channels, tissues and other organs, and promote the formation and circulation of liquid substances such as blood and body fluid. When qi within the body is abundant, the physiological functions are normal and strong. If qi is deficient, it may result in the hypofunction of the viscera as

形可见的精微物质。气所具有的活力和不断运动特性主要表现在激发和推动脏腑功能以及精血津液的运行等方面；气无形可见，但可以从脏腑生理活动中间接观察到。因此，中医学以气的运动变化来阐释人的生命活动。

（二）气的运动

气的运动称作"气机"，其基本形式是升、降、出、入。升，即气向上的运动；降，即气向下的运动；出，即气由内向外的运动；入，即气由外向内的运动。就人整体而言，升、降、出、入必须保持平衡，但具体到某一个脏腑则各有所偏重。如五脏之中肝、脾以升为主，心、肺以降为主；六腑之中除胆气主升外，多以和降为顺。从整体来看，升、降、出、入之间是协调平衡的。如肝主升发与肺主肃降，脾主升清与胃主降浊等，从而维持正常的生命活动。气的升、降、出、入运动能够调节人的生理功能，使其达到相对协调平衡的状态。

（三）气的功能

人体之气既是维持生命活动的物质基础，又是脏腑经络和组织器官功能活动的动力。气在人的生命活动中的作用有六个方面：

1. 推动作用　气以其自身活力和运动，激发和推动人的生长发育以及脏腑经络和组织器官的生理功能，促进和推动血、津液等液态物质的生成及运行。若体内之气充沛，则功能健旺；若体内之气虚弱，则脏腑功能减退、精血津液代谢失常，甚至生长发育

well as metabolic disorders of essence, blood, body fluid, even retarded growth and development.

2. Warming The warming function of qi means that qi produces energy, which enables human body to maintain a stable temperature, helps the viscera, channels, body and organs to maintain normal physiological activities, and contributes to the normal circulation and distribution of blood and body fluid. If qi fails to warm due to its deficiency, such symptoms as cold limbs, intolerance of cold, hypofunction and sluggish circulation of essence, blood and body fluid will occur.

3. Defending The defending function of qi means that qi can guard the body surface and resist invasion of exogenous pathogens or drive the pathogens out. When the defending function of qi is normal, the human body won't be easily invaded by pathogens, or even if invaded by pathogens, the person will be seldom diseased, and even though when he is suffering, he will be cured easily. If the defending function of qi gets weakened, the resistant ability will decline gradually, and exogenous pathogens will take advantage of the insufficiency to attack the body, resulting in illness.

4. Controlling The controlling function of qi means that qi has the action to control the liquid materials, such as blood, body fluid and sperm so as to prevent them from losing unduly. If the controlling function of qi is weakened, it will lead to loss of liquid materials inside the body in large quantities. For example, failure of qi to control blood may cause bleeding. Failure of qi to control body fluid may lead to polyhidrosis, polyuria or aconuresis, slobbering or salivation. Failure of qi to control sperm may result in prospermia or spermatorrhea. In addition, such conditions as diarrhea, prolapse of the rectum, leukorrhagia and threatened abortion are mostly related with failure of qi in controlling.

5. Transforming The transforming function means that qi can produce and promote changes of various materials and energy through the motion of qi. If qi transformation is out of order, it will affect digestion and absorption of foodstuffs, normal conversion of essence, qi, blood and body fluid, and discharge of sweat, urine and stool, leading to various pathological changes and metabolic disturbance.

6. Nourishing The nourishing function of qi mainly refers to nourish the body surface through the defensive qi flowing in the muscular striae, to transport nutrients so as to moisten and nourish the tissues and organs through the channel qi, and to nourish the whole body through the nutritive qi transforming into blood. If it is weak, it will lead to infirmity of the whole body.

迟缓。

2. 温煦作用 是指气可以产生热能的作用。气的温煦作用可使人体维持相对恒定的体温，有助于各脏腑、经络、形体、官窍进行正常的生理活动，有助于精血津液的正常施泄、循行和输布。若气虚而失于温煦，则四肢不温、畏寒怕冷、功能低下、精血津液等运行迟缓。

3. 防御作用 是指气既能护卫肌表，防御外邪入侵，同时也可以驱除侵入人体内的病邪。气的防御作用强盛，则邪气不易入侵；或虽有邪气侵入也不易发病；即使发病也容易治愈。若气的防御作用减退，则机体抗病能力就会下降，外邪易乘虚而入，使机体罹患疾病。

4. 固摄作用 是指气对血液、津液、精液等液态物质具有固护、统摄、约束，以防止其无故流失的作用。若气虚而固摄作用减弱，可导致体内液态物质大量流失。如气不摄血则出血；气不摄津则多汗、多尿或小便失禁、口流涎唾；气不摄精则遗精滑泄。此外，大便泄利、脱肛、妇女白带过多及孕妇滑胎失固等病证多与气失固摄有关。

5. 气化作用 是指气具有通过运动而产生和促进各种物质和能量变化的功能。如果气化失常，则影响食物的消化吸收，影响精气血津液之间的正常转化，影响汗、尿及粪便的排泄，形成各种代谢失常的病变。

6. 营养作用 主要指卫气对体表组织的充养，经络之气输送营养，濡润组织器官的作用。营气化生血液，以营养全身。若气的营养作用减弱，可导致虚弱病证。

III. Blood

i. Concept of Blood

The blood is a red liquid material circulating within the vessels and possessing the nourishing and moistening functions. It is one of the basic materials constituting the human body and maintaining life activity. Essence of cereal and kidney is the basis of blood metaplasia, which can be changed into blood through a series of gasification process with the function of spleen, stomach, heart, lung, kidney and other organs.

ii. Function of Blood

1. Nourishing and Moistening If blood is sufficient, the viscera can get enough nourishment, marked by ruddy and shining complexion, strong muscle, lustrous hair and skin, sharp senses, and free movement. If blood is deficient, its function will decline, manifested by pale complexion, dizziness, vertigo, withered hair or even loss of hair, rough skin, numbness or impaired movement of limbs, scanty menstruation, delayed menstruation, or even amenorrhea in women.

2. Providing Material Basis for Mental Activity The blood is the main material basis for mental activities, which is based on the nourishment of blood. If blood is sufficient, people will be full of vitality, quick in mind, alert in consciousness, keen in response, and free in movement. If blood is deficient, and blood flows unsmoothly, there will appear a series of mental disorders such as insomnia with dreaminess, fidget, amnesia, absent-mindedness, dispiritedness, even delirium, mania, and unconsciousness.

IV. Body Fluid

i. Concept of Body Fluid

Body fluid is a general term for normal liquids within the body, which mainly exists in the viscera and body tissues. In addition, normal secretions also belong to the category of body fluid. It is one of the basic materials constituting the human body and maintaining life activity.

Body fluid can be subdivided into two parts of thin fluid (*jin*, 津) and thick liquid (*yè*, 液). Generally speaking, the lucid and thin type with more fluidity, mainly spreading onto the skin, muscles and orifices, and seeping into the vessels as a component part of blood to play the moistening and nourishing function, is called *jin*, while the dense and thick type with less fluidity, mainly

三、血

（一）血的概念

血是指循行于脉中，具有营养与滋润作用的红色液态物质，是构成人体和维持生命活动的基本物质之一。水谷精微和肾精是血液化生的基础。它们在脾胃、心、肺、肾等脏腑的共同作用下，经过一系列的气化过程，而得以化生为血液。

（二）血的功能

1. 具有营养和滋润作用 血液充盛，脏腑得养，则面色红润、肌肉壮实、毛发和皮肤润泽、感觉灵敏、运动自如。若血液亏虚，营养和滋润作用减弱，则多见面色苍白无华、头晕目眩、毛发干枯脱落、皮肤粗糙、肢体麻木或屈伸不利、妇女月经减少、迟至，甚或闭经等。

2. 血是精神活动的物质基础 血，是人体精神活动的主要物质基础。血液充盈则人的精神振奋、思维敏捷、神智清晰、感觉灵敏、活动自如。若血液亏虚，血脉失于调和流畅，可出现不同程度的神志病变，表现为失眠多梦、烦躁健忘、神志恍惚、精神萎靡，甚至谵妄、狂乱或不省人事等。

四、津液

（一）津液的概念

津液是体内一切正常水液的总称，包括脏腑形体官窍的内在体液及其正常的分泌物。津液是构成人体和维持生命活动的基本物质之一。

津液可分为津和液两部分。一般而言，津性状较清稀，流动性较大，主要布散于体表皮肤、肌肉和孔窍，并可渗入血脉，而成为血的组成部分，能起到滋润作用；液性状较稠厚，流动性较小，主要灌注于骨骼、关节、脏腑、髓脑以及皮肤等组织，能起到濡

pouring into the skeleton, joint, viscera, brain and skin to play the nourishing and lubricating function, is called *yè*.

The thin and thick fluids are of no difference in nature, and can mutually supply and convert during the process of metabolism, so they are often collectively named as body fluid.

ii. Functions of Body Fluid

Body fluid is extensively distributed in the viscera, sense organs, orifices, body constituent and limbs. The function of body fluid can be summarized as the following four aspects:

1. Moistening and Nourishing Body fluid contains not only a great deal of moisture, but also various nourishing substances, with moistening and nourishing function for the whole body.

2. Transforming and Regulating Body fluid is one of the important components of blood. The body fluid can combine with the nutritive qi to transform into blood. Besides blood concentration can be regulated through the exuding and inleak of body fluid from the vessels.

3. Regulating Yin-Yang Body fluid pertains to yin, and has the function of regulating yin and yang, moderating cold and hot, and keeping equilibrium of body temperature through being sweated more in hot days, and urinated more in cold days.

4. Excreting Waste Through the metabolic process, the body excretes metabolite out of the body in time in ways of urine, sweat and feces, thus the normal physiological activity can be kept.

(Ma Xue-ling)

养和滑润作用。

生理上津和液互生互化，统称为"津液"。

（二）津液的功能

津液广泛分布于脏腑官窍及形体肢节，具有四个功能：

1. **滋润与濡养** 津液不仅拥有大量水分，而且含有多种营养物质，对全身起着滋润与濡养作用。

2. **充养血脉** 津液是血液的重要组成部分，可以与营气结合化生血液，通过渗出、渗入血脉还可以调节血液浓度。

3. **调节阴阳** 津液性质属阴，对机体有调节阴阳、协调寒热、平衡体温的作用。气候炎热或体内发热时，津液化为汗液向外排泄以散热，而天气寒冷或体温低下时，津液因腠理闭塞而不外泄，如此可维持人体体温相对恒定。

4. **排泄废物** 津液通过代谢过程，能将机体各部的代谢产物借排泄尿、汗、粪等途径适时地排出体外，从而保证机体生理活动的正常进行。

（马雪玲）

Section 5　Pathogenic Factor and Pathomechanism

I. Pathogenic Factor

Pathogenic factors refers to the cause of diseases, mainly including the externally-contracted six pathogenic factors, seven emotions, improper diet, overstrain and

第五节　病因病机

一、病因

病因，是指引起人体发生疾病的原因，又称致病因素，主要包括六淫、七情、饮食劳逸、痰饮和瘀血等，其中痰饮和瘀血是脏

over ease, phlegm retention and blood stasis, of which the latter two are pathological outcome of disorder of *zang-fu* organs.

i. Externally-Contracted Six Pathogenic Factors

The externally-contracted six pathogenic factors are a collective term for six kinds of exogenous pathogens of wind, cold, summer-heat, dampness, dryness and fire. Under normal conditions, wind, cold, summer-heat, dampness, dryness and fire as "six climatic factors", are normal climatic changes in nature that do not cause diseases. Only when the climatic change is abnormal or the resistance of body becomes weak will the six climatic factors become pathogens, causing the body to fall ill. The six climatic factors are then called the externally-contracted six pathogenic factors.

Generally speaking, the pathogenic characteristics of the externally-contracted six pathogenic factors are as follows:

(1) Exogenous nature: The externally-contracted six pathogenic factors usually invade the body through body surface, or through mouth and nose, or through both simultaneously, therefore, diseases caused by them are known as "exogenous diseases".

(2) Seasonal nature: The pathomechanism of the externally-contracted six pathogenic factors is often connected with seasons and environmental conditions. For example, wind pattern often occurs in spring, while summer-heat pattern in summer, dampness pattern in late summer, dryness pattern in autumn, and cold pattern in winter.

(3) Regional nature: The pathomechanism of the externally-contracted six pathogenic factors is often connected with living environment. For example, prolonged stay in a damp environment may lead to the invasion of dampness, and high temperature may lead to the invasion of dryness-heat or fire.

(4) Incorporate nature: Each of the externally-contracted six pathogenic factors may cause disease alone or together. For example, wind and cold can invade the body and cause common cold. Dampness and heat can cause diarrhea, while wind, cold and dampness can cause arthralgia syndrome.

(5) Transforming nature: In the pathological process, the nature of a syndrome caused by the six pathogenic factors may change under certain conditions. For example, cold may turn into heat after entering the interior of body. After long stay in the body, summer-heat dampness may change into dryness to consume yin.

1. Wind　Wind prevails in spring, but it may occur

腑病理产物形成的病因。

（一）六淫

六淫，即风、寒、暑、湿、燥、火六种外感病邪的统称。风、寒、暑、湿、燥、火，在正常的情况下称为"六气"，是自然界六种不同的气候变化。正常的六气不使人致病，只有气候异常变化或人体抵抗力降低时，六气才能成为致病因素，侵犯人体发生疾病，这种情况下的六气称为"六淫"。

六淫致病，具有下列几个特点：

（1）外感性，其发病途径多侵犯肌表，或从口鼻而入，或两者同时受邪，故称之为"外感病"。

（2）季节性，多与季节气候有关。如春季多风病，夏季多暑病，长夏多湿病，秋季多燥病，冬季多寒病等。

（3）地域性，多与居住环境有关。如久居潮湿之地常有湿邪为病，高温环境作业又常有燥热或火邪为病等。

（4）相兼性，六淫邪气既可单独侵袭人体，又可夹杂致病。如风寒感冒，湿热泄泻，风寒湿痹等。

（5）转化性，六淫在发病过程中，在一定条件下其证候性质可发生转化。如：寒邪入里化热，暑湿日久化燥伤阴等。

1. 风邪　风为春季主气，但四季皆有风。

in any other season. Wind pathogen mostly invades the body from the surface to cause exogenous diseases. TCM holds that wind pathogen is a very important pathogenic factor in causing exogenous diseases.

The nature and pathogenic characters of wind pathogen are as follows:

(1) Wind is a yang pathogen, and is characterized by dispersing. Wind pathogen tends to move constantly, possessing a nature of dispersal, upward and outward movement, and thus belongs to yang. The dispersal nature means that when it invades the body it tends to loosen the striae of skin and muscles, and open the pores. Wind pathogen is apt to invade the upper portion of body (head and face) and body surface, and thus results in headache, sweating, and aversion to wind.

(2) Wind is characterized by constant movement and rapid change. Constant movement implies that diseases caused by wind pathogen possess the feature of migration. For example, in the arthralgia syndrome mainly caused by invasion of wind, arthralgia is migratory, and is also called migratory arthralgia or wind arthralgia. Rapid change denotes that diseases caused by wind pathogen are characterized by sudden attack and quick transformation. For instance, urticaria is characterized by cutaneous pruritus, changeable in location and rising one after another.

(3) Wind is characterized by shaking, so dizziness, tremor, limb convulsion, opisthotonos and other shaking symptoms are mainly caused by wind.

(4) Wind is the first and foremost factor in the causes of disease. Wind, a leading exopathic factor, is the precursor of exogenous pathogens causing disease, and other pathogens usually follow wind to invade the body. For example, wind-cold, wind-heat and wind-dampness may attack the body exogenously.

2. Cold　　Cold is prevalent in winter. There is a difference between exogenous cold and endogenous cold. Exogenous cold means that cold pathogen attacks the body from outside. In diseases caused by exogenous cold, there is a difference between cold-attack and cold-stroke. A case in which cold pathogen attacks the body surface and depresses the defensive-yang is known as a "cold-attack", while a case in which cold pathogen directly invades the interior and damages the visceral yang-qi is called "cold-stroke". Endogenous cold is the pathological state generating from the failure of yang-qi to warm the body due to its deficiency. While exogenous cold is different from endogenous cold, they are mutually influencing

风邪外袭多从皮毛腠理而入，从而产生外风病证。中医学认为风邪为外感发病的一种极为重要的致病因素。

风邪的性质和致病特点如下：

（1）风为阳邪，其性开泄，易袭阳位：风邪善动不居，具有升发、向上、向外的特性，故属于阳邪。其性开泄，是指易使腠理疏泄开张。故风邪常侵袭人体上部（头面）和肌表，出现头痛、汗出、恶风等症状。

（2）风性善行数变：善行，是指风邪致病具有病位行无定处的特性而言。如风气偏盛的"风痹"或"行痹"具有病位游移，时发时止的特点。数变，是指风邪致病具有发病迅速和变幻无常的特性而言。如风疹之皮肤瘙痒、发无定处、此起彼伏的特点。

（3）风性主动："动"是指风邪致病具有动摇不定的特点，故凡临床所见眩晕、震颤、四肢抽搐，甚则颈项强直，角弓反张等摇动性症状，即多数动风病变。

（4）风为百病之长：风邪为六淫病邪中主要的致病因素，是外邪致病的先导，其他病邪多依附于风而侵犯人体。如：外感风寒、风热、风湿等。

2. **寒邪**　　寒为冬季主气。寒邪为病有外寒、内寒之分，外寒是指寒邪外袭，其致病又有伤寒、中寒之别。寒邪伤于肌表，郁遏卫阳，称为"伤寒"；寒邪直中于里，伤及脏腑阳气，则为"中寒"。内寒则是机体阳气不足，失去温煦的病理反应。外寒与内寒虽有区别，但它们又互相联系，互相影响。阳虚内寒之体，容易感受外寒；而外寒侵入人体，积久不散，又常能损及人体阳气，导致内寒。

each other and related with each other. A patient with endogenous cold due to deficiency of yang is predisposed to an invasion of exogenous cold pathogen. Exogenous cold pathogen invading and lingering in the body is apt to damage yang-qi, causing endogenous cold.

The nature and pathogenic characters of cold pathogen are listed in the following:

(1) Cold is a yin pathogen, and is apt to damage yang-qi. Cold is an expression of excessive yin-qi, belonging to yin. Invasion of cold pathogen is thus apt to damage yang-qi of the body. For example, as cold pathogen attacks the exterior, defensive-yang will get depressed, marked by aversion to cold. If cold directly invades the spleen and stomach, it can damage spleen-yang and result in epigastric pain with a cold feeling, vomiting, and diarrhea.

(2) Cold is characterized by stagnation and obstruction. Invasion of the body by cold pathogen may cause stagnation of qi and blood in the channels, giving rise to pain.

(3) Cold is characterized by contraction and constriction. When cold pathogen invades the body, it may depress qi movement, and constrict and tighten the striae, channels and tendons. If cold pathogen attacks the body surface, it may make the pores and striae close up, resulting in depression of defensive-yang, thus chills, fever and no sweating may occur. If cold pathogen invades and stays in blood vessels, the flow of qi and blood will stagnate, and the vessels will contract. Therefore, pain in the head and trunk, with a tense pulse might appear. If cold pathogen invades the channels and joints, the channels and tendons will tighten and contract, and there may appear spasm and pain of the limbs and joints and impaired movement.

3. Summer-Heat Summer-heat prevails in summer, and it comes from transformation of fire and heat. It is remarkable in seasonal nature in that it only appears in summer. Summer-heat is a pure exogenous pathogen, and there is no such things as endogenous summer-heat.

The nature and pathogenic character of summer-heat pathogen are as follows:

(1) Summer-heat is a yang pathogen characterized by burning heat. Summer-heat comes from transformation of the fiery hotness of summer. As fiery hotness belongs to yang, summer-heat is a yang pathogen. Invasion of the body by summer-heat pathogen often results in high fever, fidget and thirst, flushed face and surging pulse.

(2) Summer-heat is characterized by rising and dispersion, and is apt to consume body fluid and qi. Rising and dispersion means summer-heat tends to go upward and outward. Invasion of the body by summer-heat tends to make the striae of the skin and the muscles open,

寒邪的性质及致病特点如下：

（1）寒为阴邪，易伤阳气：寒为阴气盛的表现，其性属阴，故寒邪致病，最易损伤人体阳气。如寒邪袭表，卫阳被遏，可见恶寒；寒邪直中脾胃，脾阳受损，可见脘腹冷痛、呕吐、腹泻等症。

（2）寒性凝滞：凝滞，即凝结阻滞之意。寒邪伤人可使人之经脉气血凝滞，运行不畅而见疼痛。

（3）寒性收引：收引，即收缩牵引之意。寒邪侵入人体，可使气机收敛，腠理、经络、筋脉收缩而挛急。如寒邪侵袭肌表，毛窍腠理闭塞，卫阳被郁，不得宣泄，可见恶寒、发热、无汗；寒客血脉，则气血凝滞，血脉挛缩，可见头身疼痛、脉紧；寒客经络关节，筋脉拘急收引，则见肢节屈伸不利、拘挛作痛。

3. 暑邪 暑为夏季主气，乃火热所化。暑邪有明显的季节性，独见于夏季。暑邪纯属外邪，无内暑之说。

暑邪的性质及致病特点如下：

（1）暑为阳邪，其性炎热：暑为夏季的火热之气所化，火热属阳，故暑为阳邪。暑邪伤人，多出现壮热、烦渴、面赤、脉洪等症。

（2）暑性升散，伤津耗气：升散，即上升发散之意。暑邪伤人，易使腠理开泄而多汗。出汗过多则耗伤津液，津液亏损，即可出现口渴喜饮、尿赤短少等。在大量汗出的同时，

resulting in heavy sweating. Too much sweating consumes body fluid, and a shortage of body fluid may in turn lead to thirst, deep yellow and scanty urine. When heavy sweating occurs, qi will escape with release of body fluid, resulting in qi deficiency. This may then lead to shortness of breath, lassitude, collapse or loss of consciousness.

(3) Summer-heat often combines with dampness. In summer, it is often rainy and moist, and heat evaporates dampness, increasing the level of humidity in the air. Summer-heat, therefore, often combines with dampness pathogen to attack the body. Besides fidget and thirst, there usually appears lassitude with a heavy sensation of the limbs, chest stuffiness, nausea, vomiting and loose and sticky stools.

4. Dampness　Dampness is prevalent in late summer. The period when summer is changing into autumn is the time of a year with the highest humidity. There is a difference between exogenous and endogenous dampness. Exogenous dampness is a pathogenic factor invading the body from outside because of damp climate, being caught in the rain, or living in a damp condition. Endogenous dampness is a pathological state when water-dampness accumulates internally, which is usually caused by failure of the spleen in transportation. Exogenous dampness and endogenous dampness are different, but they often affect each other in outbreak of disease. Exogenous dampness that invades the body usually affects the spleen, making the spleen fail in transportation, and thus causes formation of dampness internally. However, a patient with retention of water-dampness internally because of deficiency of spleen yang is predisposed to invasion of exogenous dampness.

The nature and pathogenic character of dampness pathogen are as follows:

(1) Dampness is characterized by heaviness, turbidity and sinking downward. Heaviness means a disease caused by dampness pathogen usually has symptoms of a heavy sensation in the head, general lassitude, aching and a heavy feeling in the limbs. Turbidity means the disease caused by dampness pathogen presents with filthy and foul discharges or secretions, such as a dirty complexion with pus hypersecretion in the eyes, turbid urine, massive leukorrhea in female, or eczema with filthy purulent fluid. Sinking downward means the symptoms caused by dampness pathogen mostly appear in the lower part of the body, such as leukorrhea, stranguria with turbid urine, and diarrhea or dysentery.

(2) Dampness is characterized by viscosity and stagnation. This appears in two ways. First, in symptoms, invasion by dampness pathogen mostly leads to sticky

往往气随津泄而致气虚，出现气短乏力，甚则突然昏倒、不省人事。

（3）暑多挟湿：暑季多雨而潮湿，热蒸湿动，使空气的湿度增加，故暑邪为病，常兼挟湿邪以侵犯人体，在发热烦渴的同时，常兼见四肢困倦、胸闷呕恶、大便溏泻不爽等症。

4. 湿邪　湿为长夏主气，夏秋之交，为一年中湿气最盛的季节。湿邪为病有外湿、内湿之分。外湿多由于气候潮湿、涉水淋雨、居处潮湿等外在湿邪侵袭人体所致。内湿多由于脾失健运、水湿停聚而生。外湿和内湿虽有不同，但在发病中又常相互影响。伤于外湿，湿邪困脾，脾失健运，则湿从内生；而脾阳虚损，水湿不化，也易招致外湿的侵袭。

湿邪的性质及致病特点如下：

（1）湿性重浊而趋下，易袭人之阴位。重，即沉重或重着之意，常指湿邪为病，多见头身困重，四肢酸懒沉重等症状。浊，即秽浊，指分泌物或排泄物秽浊不清。如面垢眵多，大便溏泻，小便浑浊，妇女白带过多，湿疹浸淫等病。趋下，是指湿邪为病，其症状多见于下部，如带下、淋浊、泄利等症。

（2）湿性黏滞。黏，即黏腻；滞，即停滞。湿性黏滞主要表现在两方面：一是湿病

and greasy discharges and secretions. Next in course, a disease caused by dampness pathogen usually has a long course, relapses repeatedly, and is lingering and difficult to cure. Dampness arthralgia, eczema, and dampness-warm disease are such examples.

(3) Dampness is a yin pathogen, apt to damage yang-qi and hinder qi movement. The nature of dampness is similar to that of water, and thus it is a yin pathogen. When invading the body, dampness pathogen is most likely to damage yang-qi. When dampness pathogen invades the spleen and causes hypofunction of spleen-yang, leading to failure in transformation and transportation that cause water and moist to stay in the body, it will then give rise to diarrhea, oliguria and edema. When attacking the body and staying in the viscera and channels, dampness pathogen is apt to depress qi movement leading to disharmony of qi in ascending and descending, and obstruction of the channels, there will appear chest oppression, epigastric distention, dysuria with scanty urine and dyschesia.

5. Dryness Dryness is prevalent in autumn. The climate in autumn is dry, and the atmosphere is lacking of moisture. As a result, dryness diseases often occur. Dryness attacks the body mostly through the mouth and nose to damage the defensive system of the lung. Dryness can be divided into warm-dryness and cool-dryness. In early autumn, summer heat lingers, and dryness combines with warm-heat to invade the body, leading to a warm-dryness disease. In late autumn, early winter cold appears, and dryness and cold usually associate with each other to attack the body, leading to cool-dryness disease.

The nature and pathogenic character of dryness pathogen are as follows:

(1) Dryness is characterized by aridity and apt to consume body fluid. Exogenous dryness pathogen is an aridity pathogen, so when invading the body, it is most likely to consume body fluid, resulting in various dry symptoms and signs, such as dry mouth and nose, thirst, dry rough and chapped skin, dry hair, scanty urine, and constipation.

(2) Dryness is easy to impair the lung. The lung is a "delicate organ" with a desire for moisture and an aversion to dryness. The lung governs qi and controls respiration, which relates externally to the skin and hair, and opens into the nose. Therefore, a dryness pathogen invading the body via the mouth and nose is most likely to consume lung-fluid, making the lung fail in diffusing and descending with such symptoms as dry cough with little sputum, or sticky sputum that is difficult to be coughed out, blood-tinged

症状在分泌物及排泄物方面多黏腻不爽；二是湿邪为病多病程较长或反复发作，缠绵难愈，如湿痹、湿疹、湿温病等。

（3）湿为阴邪，易损伤阳气，阻遏气机：湿性重浊，其性类水，故为阴邪。其侵犯人体，最易伤脾阳，导致脾阳不振，运化无权，水湿停聚，发为泄泻、尿少、水肿等症。湿邪侵及人体，留滞于脏腑经络，最易阻遏气机，使其升降失常，经络阻滞不畅，出现胸闷脘痞，小便短涩，大便不爽等症。

5. 燥邪　燥为秋季主气。此时气候干燥，水分亏乏，故多燥病。燥邪感染途径，多从口鼻而入，侵犯肺卫。燥邪为病又有温燥、凉燥之分：初秋有夏热之余气，燥与温热结合而侵犯人体，则多见温燥病证；深秋又有近冬之寒气，燥与寒邪结合侵犯人体，故多见凉燥病证。

燥邪的性质及致病特点如下：

（1）燥性干涩，易伤津液：燥邪为干涩之病邪，故外感燥邪最易耗伤人体的津液，造成阴津亏虚的病变，而出现种种津亏干涩的症状和体征，如口鼻干燥、咽干口渴、皮肤干涩甚则皲裂、毛发不荣、小便短少、大便干结等症。

（2）燥易伤肺：肺为娇脏，喜润而恶燥。肺主气司呼吸，外合皮毛，开窍于鼻，故燥邪伤人，多从口鼻而入，伤及肺津，影响肺的宣发肃降功能，出现干咳少痰，痰液胶黏难咯或痰中带血以及喘息胸痛等症。

sputum, asthma and chest pain.

6. Fire　Fire and heat are both generated from yang in nature and may be collectively called fire-heat. Though they are similar, there are still differences between them. Warm is the lesser of heat, and strong heat results in fire. Warm and heat such as wind-heat, summer-heat, and dampness-heat, mostly come from the outside, while fire such as flaring up of the heat-fire and hyperactivity of liver-fire, usually generates inside.

There is difference between exogenous and endogenous diseases caused by fire and heat. Exogenous diseases mainly originate from direct invasion of warm-heat pathogen exogenously. Endogenous diseases often develop from hyperactivity of yang-qi due to insufficient of yin and yang as well as qi and blood of *zang-fu* organs. In addition, invasion of the body by wind, cold, summer-heat, dampness, dryness, and fire that are exogenous pathogens or violent emotional stimulations may all give rise to fire under certain conditions. Therefore there is a saying that "the five climatic pathogens generate fire" and "the five emotional pathogens generate fire".

The nature and pathogenic characters of fire pathogen are as follows:

(1) Fire is a yang pathogen characterized by burning heat. Yang is characterized by restlessness and upward going, so fire is a yang pathogen that flares up. Invasion of the body by fire often leads to high fever, fidget and thirst, sweating, and a surging and rapid pulse.

(2) Fire is characterized by flaring up, so diseases caused by fire pathogen mostly have symptoms in the upper part of the body, such as in the head and face. Fire pathogen invading the body often goes upward to disturb the heart-spirit, marked by fidget with insomnia, mania, and even coma and delirium. If heart fire flares up, it will lead to a red tongue tip and mouth or tongue ulcers. If stomach-fire flares up, it will result in toothache with swollen gums. If liver-fire flares up, it will cause red eyes with swelling and pain.

(3) Fire is likely to consume fluid and qi. Fire pathogen invading the body is most likely to result in loss of body fluid, thus symptoms of thirst with a desire for drink, dryness in the throat and tongue, deep yellow urine scanty in volume, and constipation often appear. Fire pathogen is most likely to consume healthy qi. So diseases caused by fire pathogen may have the symptoms of general weakness such as shortness of breath, reluctance to talk *etc.*.

(4) Fire is apt to stir up wind and cause bleeding. Fire pathogen invading the body often burns and impairs the liver channel to consume yin-fluid, which in turn deprives

6. 火（热）邪　火热为阳盛所生，故火热常可并称。但火与温热，同中有异，温为热之渐，火为热之极，温热多属外淫，如风热、暑热、湿热之类病邪；而火常由内生，如心火上炎、肝火亢盛等。

火热为病亦有内外之分，属外感者，多是直接感受温热邪气之侵袭；属内生者，则常由脏腑阴阳气血失调，阳气亢盛而成。此外，感受风、寒、暑、湿、燥等各种外邪，或精神刺激，在一定条件下皆可化火，故有"五气化火""五志化火"之说。

火邪的性质及致病特点如下：

（1）火为阳邪，其性炎热：阳主躁动而向上，火热之性，燔灼焚焰，升腾上炎，故属于阳邪。因此，火热伤人，多见高热、烦渴、汗出、脉洪数等症。

（2）火性炎上：火邪致病，证候多表现在人体的上部，如头面部位。如火热阳邪常可上炎扰神，出现心烦失眠、狂躁妄动、神昏谵语。若心火上炎，则见舌尖红、口舌生疮；胃火炽盛，可见牙龈肿痛；肝火上炎，常见目赤肿痛。

（3）火易耗气伤津：火邪为患，最易耗伤津液，故常兼有口渴喜饮、咽干舌燥、小便短赤、大便秘结等津伤症状。火邪最能损伤人体的正气，故火邪致病，还可兼见少气懒言、肢倦乏力等气虚之症。

（4）火易生风动血：火热之邪侵袭人体，往往灼伤肝经，劫耗阴液，使肝经失养而

the nourishment of tendons. As a result, it leads to internal stirring of liver-wind, called "extreme heat producing wind" marked by high fever, coma and delirium, convulsive limbs, upward staring of the eyes, rigid neck and opisthotonus. Meanwhile, fire pathogen may accelerate blood circulation, burn and impair the vessels, force blood to flow out of the vessels and contribute to bleeding.

(5) Fire is likely to cause pain and swell of the body surface. Invasion of fire pathogen into the blood system may accumulate in local areas, corrode muscles and putrefy blood, resulting in carbuncles and abscesses marked by redness, swelling, hotness and pain, even maturation and ulceration.

ii. Seven Emotions

The seven emotions refer to joy, anger, grief, thinking, sorrow, fear and fright that are the psychological states of the body and different reflections of the body to objective things. Under normal conditions, they generally do not cause diseases. Only those sudden, intense or prolonged emotional stimulations beyond the regulatory range of physiological activities of the body can cause disturbances of qi movement and disorders of yin-yang and qi and blood of the viscera, resulting in the onset of disease. As they mainly cause endogenous diseases, they are also known as the "seven emotional pathogens of endogenous diseases".

1. Relation between the Seven Emotions and Qi, Blood and *Zang-fu* Organ　TCM holds that emotional activities are closely related to the *zang-fu* organs, and functional activities of the organs depend on the driving and warming functions of qi, and the nourishment of blood. The five *zang* organs are in charge of five emotions separately, i. e., the heart is associated with joy, the liver with anger, the spleen with thought, the lung with grief, and the kidney with fear. Different emotional changes have different impacts on the visceral organs, and changes in qi and blood and the visceral organs also influence emotional changes.

2. Pathogenic Characteristic of the Seven Emotions　There are differences between the seven emotions and externally-contracted six pathogenic factors in terms of pathogenicity. The externally-contracted six pathogenic factors invade the body through the skin or mouth and nose leading to exterior syndrome initially. An endogenous injury by the seven emotions, however, directly affects the relative viscus, causing disorder of qi movement in the viscus, disturbance of qi and blood, resulting in a variety of diseases.

(1) Direct injury to the viscus: Anger damages the

"热极生风"，表现为高热、神昏谵语、四肢抽搐、目睛上视、项背强直、角弓反张等。同时，火热之邪，可以加速血行，灼伤脉络，甚则迫血妄行，而致各种出血。

（5）火易致肿疡：火热之邪入于血分，可聚于局部，腐蚀血肉，发为痈肿疮疡，表现为红肿热痛，甚则化脓溃烂。

（二）七情

七情即喜、怒、忧、思、悲、恐、惊七种情志变化，是机体的精神情绪状态。七情是人体对客观事物的不同心理反映，在正常情况下，一般不会使人致病。只有突然、强烈或长期持久的情志刺激，超过了人体的生理活动调节范围，使人体气机紊乱，脏腑阴阳气血失调，才会导致疾病的发生，由于它主要造成内伤病，故又称"内伤七情"。

1. 七情与内脏气血的关系　中医学认为人的情志活动与内脏有密切的关系，而内脏的功能活动要靠气的推动、温煦和血的濡养。五脏主五志，即心主喜，肝主怒，脾主思，肺主忧，肾主恐。不同的情志变化对内脏有不同的影响，而内脏气血的变化，也会影响情志的变化。

2. 七情内伤的致病特点　七情致病不同于六淫。六淫侵袭人体，从皮肤及口鼻而入，发病多见表证。而七情内伤，则直接影响相应的内脏，使脏腑气机内乱，气血失调，导致疾病发生。

（1）直接伤及内脏：怒伤肝，喜伤心，思

liver, excessive joy damages the heart, excessive thinking damages the spleen, grief damages the lung and fear damages the kidney. Since the heart governs the spirit, which is the master of five *zang* and six *fu* organs, if the heart-spirit is damaged, it will involve other viscera. The heart governs blood and stores the spirit. The liver governs free flow of qi and stores blood. The spleen governs transformation and transportation, being located in the middle-jiao as the hub of qi movement in ascending and descending, and the source for generation of qi and blood. Therefore, diseases caused by emotional pathogens are commonly related with the heart, liver and spleen, and with disturbances of qi and blood.

(2) Influence on qi movement of the viscera: Different emotional fluctuating may cause different changes of qi movement of the viscera. For instance, "anger causes qi to rise, excessive joy causes qi to slacken, grief causes qi to be consumed, fear causes qi to sink, fright causes qi to be chaotic, excessive thinking causes qi to knot".

(3) Tendency to induce emotional diseases, which are associated with abnormal emotional symptoms, mainly including: the disease induced by emotional stimulus (depression, epilepsy, *etc.*) and induced by symptoms (psychosomatic diseases, such as chest pain and dizziness), and other causes but with abnormal emotional symptoms (diabetes, cancer, chronic liver disease *etc.*).

(4) Abnormal emotional fluctuation may aggravate or deteriorate the disease. For example, over rage may result in liver-yang going upward suddenly, leading to dizziness, abrupt coma or faint, hemiplegia and facial paralysis.

iii. Improper Diet

Food and drink are essential materials for the body to obtain nourishment and maintain vital activities. However, an immoderate, insanitary or unbalanced diet may be an important pathogen leading to diseases. Food and drink mainly depend on digestion of the spleen and stomach, therefore improper diet mainly damages the spleen and stomach, leading to disorders of ascending and descending of qi, and accumulation of dampness, production of phlegm, generation of heat, or other diseases.

1. Immoderate Diet It is important to take moderate food and drink properly. Either starvation or overeating may lead to diseases. Starvation may result in a reduction of the source of production of qi and blood. If it lasts for a long time, it will result in deficiency of qi

伤脾，忧伤肺，恐伤肾。由于心主神志，为五脏六腑之大主，心神受损可涉及其他脏腑。心主血藏神，肝主疏泄藏血，脾主运化而位于中焦，是气机升降的枢纽，又为气血生化之源。故情志所伤的病证，以心、肝、脾三脏和气血失调为多见。

（2）影响脏腑气机：由于导致各种情志变化的刺激因素不同，脏腑气机的变化也不一样，常表现为与各种情志相关的特殊的气机变化。如："怒则气上，喜则气缓，悲则气消，恐则气下，惊则气乱，思则气结"。

（3）多发为情志病：情志病，是指发病与情志刺激有关，具有情志异常表现的病证。主要包括因情志刺激而发的病证（郁证、癫、狂等）；因情志刺激而诱发的病证（胸痹、眩晕等身心疾病）；其他原因所致但具有情志异常表现的病证（消渴、恶性肿瘤、慢性肝胆疾病等）。

（4）影响病情变化：情志异常波动，可使病情加重，或迅速恶化。如有眩晕病史的患者，若过度恼怒，肝阳上亢，常发生头晕目眩，甚则突然昏厥，或昏仆不语、半身不遂、口眼歪斜等。

（三）饮食所伤

饮食是人体摄取营养，维持生命活动所不可缺少的物质。但若饥饱失宜、饮食不洁及饮食偏嗜，又是导致疾病发生的重要原因。饮食主要靠脾胃消化，故饮食不节主要伤及脾胃，而使脾胃升降失常，并可聚湿、生痰、化热或变生他病。

1. **饮食不节** 饮食以适量为宜，过饥、过饱或饥饱无常均可发生疾病。饥即摄食不足，气血生化乏源，久则气血衰少而为病。过饱即饮食摄入过量，超过了脾胃的消化、

and blood and cause diseases. Overeating and fullness may cause stagnation of food and drink, if it exceeds the limit of digestion, absorption, and transportation and transformation of the spleen and stomach. As a result, epigastric or abdominal distention with pain, foul belch and acid regurgitation, anorexia, vomiting, and diarrhea with foul and stinking stools will occur.

2. Insanitary Diet   Intake of unhealthy dirty food may cause a variety of gastrointestinal diseases, marked by abdominal pain, vomiting, diarrhea and dysentery. Some parasitic diseases are marked by abdominal pain, parorexia and sallow complexion with emaciation. If poisonous or stale foods are taken, acute abdominal pain, vomit and diarrhea may occur, or in severe cases it may lead to coma or death.

3. Diet Partiality   Diet should be properly arranged to meet the nutrition requirements of the body. An improper diet may easily lead to a deficiency of certain nutrients, or superiority or inferiority of either yin or yang, and hence cause diseases. For example, excessive intake of raw or cold foods may easily damage spleen yang, leading to internal cold dampness, resulting in abdominal pain and diarrhea. Over intake of greasy or spicy foods or indulgence in alcohol may lead to dampness heat and phlegm, stagnation of qi and blood, thus, bleeding, hemorrhoids, carbuncles and sores may occur.

iv. Maladjustment of Work and Rest

Improper work and rest include overstrain and over-ease. Appropriate work and physical exercise help the body to maintain normal circulation of qi and blood, and at the same time to build up the physique. Proper rest helps to dispel tiredness and restore energy of both the body and mind while prolonged over-work or over-ease may induce diseases.

1. Overstrain   Overstrain refers to over toil including three aspects: physical overstrain, mental overstrain and sexual overstrain.

(1) Physical overstrain refers to a too long period of physical work leading to diseases. Overstrain of the body consumes qi, leading to deficiency of qi and strength. Manifestations are feebleness, lassitude, reluctance to talk, listlessness, mental exhaustion, shortness of breath and sweating with motion.

(2) Mental overstrain refers to too much mental work and thinking that damage the spleen and heart. Mental overstrain consumes heart blood and damages spleen qi, and leads to the heart spirit losing its nourishment, manifesting as palpitation, amnesia, insomnia and dream-disturbed sleep. In addition, it may also lead to failure of the spleen in transportation and transformation, manifesting

吸收和运化能力，可导致脘腹胀满、嗳腐泛酸、厌食呕吐、泻下臭秽等症。

2. 饮食不洁   进食不洁的食物，可引起多种胃肠道疾病，出现腹痛、吐泻、痢疾等，或引起寄生虫病，临床见腹痛、嗜食异物、面黄肌瘦等症。若进食腐败变质的有毒食物，常出现剧烈腹痛、吐泻等中毒症状，重者可出现昏迷或死亡。

3. 饮食偏嗜   饮食全面可起到营养人体的作用。若饮食偏嗜，则易引起部分营养物质缺乏或机体阴阳的偏盛、偏衰，从而引发疾病。如偏嗜生冷，则易损伤脾阳，内生寒湿，发生腹痛泄泻等症；偏嗜肥甘厚味，或嗜酒无度，易致湿热痰浊内生、气血壅滞，可见痔疮下血、痈疮等病证。

（四）劳逸失度

劳逸失度，包括过度劳累和过度安逸两个方面。正常的劳动和体育锻炼，有利于气血流通，增强体质；必要的休息可以消除疲劳，恢复体力和脑力。而过度劳累，或过度安逸，易诱发疾病。

1. 过劳   过劳是指过度劳累，包括劳力过度、劳神过度和房劳过度三个方面。

（1）劳力过度是指较长时间的体力劳动过度而发病。劳力过度则伤气，久则气少力衰。表现为四肢困倦、少气懒言、乏力、精神疲惫、动则气喘、汗出等症。

（2）劳神过度是指脑力劳动过度，思虑太过，劳伤心脾而言。劳神过度，耗伤心血、损伤脾气，可出现心神失养的心悸、健忘、失眠、多梦及脾不健运的纳呆、腹胀、便溏等症。

as poor appetite, abdominal distention, and loose stools.

(3) Sexual overstrain implies intemperance in sexual activities or excess sexual intercourse. It consumes kidney essence, resulting in aching and weakness of the waist and knee joints, dizziness, tinnitus, lassitude and listlessness, spermatorrhea, premature ejaculation, impotence and menstrual disorders.

2. Over-Ease　Over-ease refers to lack of labor or exercise. Proper physical exercise everyday is good for circulation of qi and blood. Over-ease may damage qi causing qi and blood deficiency and stagnation, manifesting as listlessness, general weakness, poor appetite, palpitation, dyspnea, and sweating with motion, or obesity with the overstuffed, weak resistance against the disease, and being subject to invasion of exopathic pathogens.

v. Phlegm Rheum and Blood Stasis

Phlegm rheum and blood stasis are the pathological outcomes during the course of disease. Once they are formed, they may act as new pathogenic factors causing a variety of diseases. Being step-pathogens, they belong to pathogens of pathological products.

1. Phlegm Rheum

(1) Definition: Phlegm rheum is the pathological product of water metabolism disorder. Generally speaking, phlegm is thick and turbid, and rheum (fluid retention) is thin and clear.

Phlegm not only implies sputum that is coughed up and visible, but also includes turbid phlegm that is in scrofula, subcutaneous nodules, or stagnating in the viscera and tissues that cannot be discharged. The latter is known as "invisible phlegm" that can be determined by the syndrome caused by it in clinic.

Rheum means body fluid accumulation in a certain area of the body. According to the place where it accumulates and the symptoms it causes, it has different names such as "phlegm rheum" "pleural rheum" "subcutaneous rheum" and "thoracic rheum".

(2) Formation: Stagnant phlegm and fluid form because of water metabolism disturbances from dysfunction of the lung, spleen, kidney and *sanjiao* in qi movement. This condition is usually caused by an invasion of externally-contracted six pathogenic factors, improper diet or the seven emotions. Dampness accumulates to form water. Water stores up to form stagnant fluid. Stagnant fluid coagulates to form phlegm. After formation, stagnant fluid usually stays in the stomach, intestines, hypochondrium, chest, and subcutaneous areas while phlegm follows the ascending and descending of qi to go to the whole body leading to a variety of illnesses.

（3）房劳过度是指性生活不节、房事过度而言。房事过频则肾精耗伤，出现腰膝酸软、眩晕耳鸣、精神萎靡，或男子遗精、滑泄、阳痿，女子月经不调、带下等病证。

2. 过逸　过逸是指过度安逸，缺乏劳动和运动。适当活动，则气血流畅，若过逸则伤气，使气血不足，流通不畅，表现为精神不佳、肢体软弱、食少乏力、动则心悸、气喘、汗出，或发胖臃肿，抗病能力低下，易受外邪侵袭。

（五）痰饮、瘀血

痰饮、瘀血都是在疾病过程中所形成的病理产物。这些病理产物形成后，又作为新的致病因素引发多种病证，故属于病理产物形成的致病因素，为继发性病因。

1. 痰饮

（1）痰饮的含义：痰和饮都是水液代谢障碍所形成的病理产物。一般以较稠浊的称为痰，较清稀的称为饮。

痰不仅是指咯吐出来的有形可见的痰液，还包括瘰疬、痰核和停滞在脏腑经络等组织中而不能排出的痰浊，临床上可通过其所表现的证候来确定，这种痰称为"无形之痰"。

饮即水液停留于人体局部者，因其所停的部位和症状不同而有不同的名称，有"痰饮""悬饮""溢饮""支饮"的区分。

（2）痰饮的形成：痰饮多由外感六淫、饮食及七情内伤等，使肺、脾、肾及三焦等脏腑气化功能失常，水液代谢障碍，以致水液停滞而成。湿聚为水，水积则为饮，饮凝为痰。痰饮形成后，饮多留积于肠胃、胸胁及肌肤，而痰则随气升降，无处不到，形成多种病证。

(3) Characteristics of disorders caused by phlegm rheum

1) Blocking qi and blood circulation: Stagnant phlegm rheum is substantial pathological products. If they block channels, they may block the circulation of qi and blood. If stagnating in the viscera, they may lead to dysfunction of the viscera and abnormal qi movement.

2) Influencing water metabolism: When phlegm rheum stagnates in the viscera, they may cause dysfunction of the viscera and abnormal qi movement and metabolism of water.

3) Being prone to disturb heart-spirit: Heart-spirit should keep clear and bright to maintain its normal function. As stagnant phlegm rheum is turbid product, when they rise upward following qi movement, they may confuse the heart and disturb the spirit.

4) Causing various and changeable diseases: Phlegm rheum may follow the flow of qi to go to every part of the body, inward to the viscera and outward to subcutaneous tissues, resulting in many miscellaneous diseases.

2. Blood Stasis

(1) Definition: Blood stasis refers to stagnated blood within the body, including sluggish or stagnated blood within the viscera and vessels or extravagated blood not eliminated yet.

(2) Formation: There are two main aspects involved in the formation of blood stasis. One is due to circulatory retardation caused by various factors including qi deficiency, qi stagnation, blood-cold and blood-heat. Qi is the commander of blood, thus deficient or stagnated qi cannot promote the normal circulation of blood, resulting in stagnant blood. Other causes for stagnant blood include cold pathogen invading the blood vessels, making the vessels contract and spasm, and heat pathogen invading the blood vessels and mingling with blood. The other is extravasated blood in the body caused by various traumas, deficiency of qi failing to control blood, and abnormal flow of blood due to heat inside the body.

(3) Characteristics of disorders caused by stagnant blood

1) Blocking qi movement and blood circulation: Blood can convey qi. As stagnant blood is formed, it will contribute to disorder of qi movement. Qi can promote blood circulation. As qi movement is disordered, it will lead to obstructed blood circulation.

2) Influencing generation of new blood: As the stagnant blood blocks in the interior, it will cause disturbance of qi movement and blood circulation, leading to visceral dysfunction from losing their nourishment which may influence generation of new blood.

（3）痰饮的致病特点

1）阻滞气血运行：痰饮为有形之邪，若阻滞于经络，可致气血运行失畅；若停滞于脏腑，可使脏腑气机升降失常。

2）影响水液代谢：痰饮停滞于脏腑，可导致脏腑功能失调，气化不利，水液代谢障碍。

3）易蒙蔽心神：心神以清明为要。痰饮为浊物，若随气上逆，易蒙蔽清窍，扰乱心神。

4）致病广泛，变幻多端：痰饮可随气流行，内至脏腑，外至肌肤，产生各种错综复杂的病证。

2. 瘀血

（1）瘀血的含义：瘀血，指体内血液停滞，包括血行不畅停滞在脏腑、经脉内的血液以及逸出脉外尚未消散之血。

（2）瘀血的形成：瘀血的形成，主要有两方面：一是由于气虚、气滞、血寒、血热等原因，使血行不畅所致。气为血帅，气虚或气滞，不能推动血液的正常运行；或寒邪客于血脉，使经脉挛缩拘急，血液凝滞不畅；或热入营血，血热搏结等，均可形成瘀血。二是因内外伤、气虚失摄或血热妄行等原因造成离经之血，未能及时消散而停留体内，形成瘀血。

（3）瘀血的致病特点

1）阻滞气机，影响血脉运行：血能载气，瘀血形成后，必定导致气机失畅；气能行血，气机失畅，进而引起血行不畅。

2）影响新血生成：瘀血内阻，气血运行失畅，脏腑失于濡养，功能失常，可影响新血的生成。

3) Fixed location of diseases with many and varied patterns: When stagnant blood stays in a certain part of the body, it will not easily be dispelled in a short time manifesting as characteristics of relatively fixed location. The different locations of stagnant blood are of different pathological manifestations. The most common characteristics are stabbing pain, bump, bleeding, cyanosis, cyanotic tongue with petechia, and intermittent, thin, unsmooth, or knotted pulse.

II. Pathomechanism

Pathomechanism refers to the fundamental mechanism of the onset, development and progress of the disease.

TCM holds that diseases are complicated and changeable, but their pathological processes generally fall into several types of struggle between the healthy qi and the pathogenic qi, imbalance of yin and yang, disorder of qi and blood, disorder of metabolism of body fluid and so on.

i. Superiority or Inferiority of the Healthy Qi and the Pathogen

Superiority or inferiority of the healthy qi or the pathogen refers to the success or failure of the fight between the body resistance and the pathogenic factors after the pathogen invades the body.

1. Struggle between the Healthy Qi and the Pathogen and the Change of Deficiency or Excess As the healthy qi grows will the pathogen decline, and as the pathogen grows will the healthy qi decline.

Excess in this case means that the pathogenic qi is excessive. It is often seen in the early or middle stage of exogenous diseases, and in the disorders caused by stagnation of phlegm, foodstuff, blood or water. Pathogenic qi is excessive and the healthy qi is not subdued thus the struggle between the healthy qi and the pathogenic is acute. Such clinical symptoms as high fever, mania, speaking lustily, coarse breathing, abdominal pain aggravated on pressure, retention of urine and stool, and forceful pulse, will be seen under the category of excess syndrome.

Deficiency implies that the healthy qi is deficient. This usually occurs in patients with a weak physique, or in the late stage of a disease, or in a chronic disease. The healthy qi gets deficient and fails to fight against the pathogenic qi, which causes hypofunction or consumption of qi, blood, body fluid. The manifestations are listlessness, lassitude, wan and thin appearance, palpitation, shortness

3）病位固定，病证繁多：瘀血常停留在人体某一部位，不易及时消散，表现出病位相对固定的特征。瘀血停留的部位不同，表现出的病证各异，最常见的共同特征是刺痛、肿块、出血、发绀、舌紫暗有瘀斑、瘀点、脉细涩结代等。

二、发病机制

发病机制即病机，是指疾病发生、发展与变化的机理。

中医学认为尽管疾病种类繁多，表现错综复杂，但究其根本，都不外乎邪正盛衰、阴阳失调、气血失常、津液代谢障碍等方面。

（一）邪正盛衰

邪正盛衰是指在疾病过程中，机体正气与致病邪气之间相互斗争中所发生的盛衰变化。

1. 邪正盛衰与虚实变化 正气增长则邪气消退，而邪气增长则正气消减。

实，指邪气盛，常见于外感病的初、中期以及痰、食、血、水等滞留所引起的病证。邪气亢盛而正气未衰，正邪斗争激烈，表现为壮热、狂躁、声高气粗、腹痛拒按、二便不通、脉实有力等反应剧烈的实证。

虚，指正气不足，多见于素体虚弱或疾病后期以及多种慢性病证。正气已虚，无力与邪气抗争，导致功能衰退，耗伤人体气血津液，表现为神疲体倦、面容憔悴、心悸、气短、自汗、盗汗、五心烦热或畏寒肢冷，脉虚无力等病证。

of breath, spontaneous or night sweating, dysphoria with a feverish sensation in the palms and soles, aversion to cold with cold limbs, and feeble pulse.

2. Struggle between the Healthy Qi and the Pathogen and Conversion of Disease During the course of a disease, the struggle between healthy qi and pathogen may result in either a superiority of the healthy qi with a decline of the pathogenic qi or a superiority of the pathogenic qi with a deficiency of the healthy qi. In the former, the disease takes a turn to recovery, and in the latter, the disease gets deteriorated or the patient died. If the healthy qi and the pathogenic qi are evenly matched, the chronic or persistent trend will be manifested.

(1) Superiority of the healthy qi with decline of the pathogenic qi: In the struggle between the healthy qi and the pathogenic qi, if the healthy qi is sufficient, then the pathogenic qi will have difficulty in growing, and the disease will be cured. For example, in exogenous diseases, when the healthy qi is sufficient to fight against the pathogenic qi, through diaphoresis which can relieve the exterior and eliminate pathogens, the defensive and the nutritive qi will be harmonized, and hence the disease will be cured.

(2) Superiority of the pathogenic qi with deficiency of the healthy qi: In the course of the disease, if the pathogenic qi is excessive and healthy qi is deficient, the condition of the patient will tend to deteriorate. If the healthy qi collapses and pathogenic qi gets rampant, yin and yang will separate from each other, the healthy qi activities of the body will stop and the patient will die.

In addition, if the healthy qi and the pathogenic qi keep in a stalemate or the healthy qi is deficient while the pathogenic qi lingers, or the pathogen is eliminated while the healthy qi is not restored yet, the disease will develop from acute to chronic, or even leave sequelae.

ii. Imbalance of Yin and Yang

The imbalance of yin and yang is a pathological state in which either yin fails to control yang or yang fails to control yin, or exuberance of yin with decline of yang, or exuberance of yang with decline of yin results from a loss of their relative balance due to action of pathogenic qi on the body.

1. Abnormal Exuberance of Yin or Yang This refers to a pathological state of the body that either side of yin and yang gets as predominant as to make the other suffer. It belongs to an excess syndrome because "exuberance of pathogenic qi leads to excess".

(1) Abnormal exuberance of yang is a pathological state, during the process of a disease, presenting itself

2. 邪正盛衰与疾病转归 在疾病过程中，或为正胜邪退，疾病趋于好转而痊愈，或为邪胜正衰，疾病趋于恶化，甚或死亡。若正邪力量相持不下，则疾病趋向迁延或慢性化。

（1）正胜邪退：是指在疾病过程中，正气充实，邪气难于发展，疾病向好转和痊愈方向发展的一种病理变化。例如由六淫所致的外感病，若正气充足，抗邪有力，一经发汗解表，则邪祛表解，调和营卫，疾病痊愈。

（2）邪胜正衰：是指在疾病过程中，邪气强盛，正气虚衰，机体无力抗邪，病情就会趋向恶化，若正气衰竭，邪气独盛，阴阳离决，生命活动亦告终止而死亡。

此外，若出现正邪相持或正虚邪恋，邪去而正气不复的情况，则常常是许多疾病由急性转为慢性，或留下某些后遗症，或慢性病经久不愈的主要原因之一。

（二）阴阳失调

阴阳失调，是指机体在病因的作用下，导致阴阳双方失去相对平衡，形成阴阳偏盛、偏衰，或阴不制阳、阳不制阴的病理状态。

1. 阴阳偏盛 是指人体阴阳双方中的某一方的病理性亢盛状态，属"邪气盛则实"的实证。

（1）阳偏盛是指机体在疾病过程中，所出现的阳气偏盛、功能亢奋、热量过剩的病理

exuberance of yang qi, hyperactive function and surplus heat. A superiority of yang often manifests itself as high fever, flushed face, red eyes, restlessness, red tongue with yellow and dry coating, abdominal distending pain which is aggravated on pressure, tidal fever, and delirium. Predominating yang makes yin suffer, so accompanying symptoms of yin deficiency such as thirst with a desire for cold drink, constipation, and scanty urine may also appear.

(2) Abnormal exuberance of yin is a pathological state during the process of a disease in which yin-qi is prevailing with dysfunction or hypofunction, shortage of thermogenesis and pathological accumulation of metabolic products. A superiority of yin often manifests itself as cold excess syndrome with symptoms of cold body and limbs, pale tongue, abdominal pain with a cold feeling aggravated on pressure, and loose stools. Since predominating yin makes yang suffer, yang deficiency symptoms of aversion to cold, listlessness, and lying with the body curled up may also appear.

2. Abnormal Debilitation of Yin or Yang This refers to a pathological state of the body that either side of yin and yang gets too weak. It belongs to a deficiency syndrome because "despoliation of essential qi leads to deficiency".

(1) Abnormal debilitation of yang is a pathological state during the process of a disease with impaired or deficient yang qi, hypofunction, and shortage of thermogenesis. The causative factors are congenital defects, dietary ignorance, overstrain, or damage of yang-qi due to a protracted disease. Clinically it often shows a deficiency cold syndrome manifesting as aversion to cold, cold limbs, restlessness, lying with the body curled up, abdominal pain responsive to warmth and pressure, loose stools, clear and plethoric urine, and slow and forceless pulse.

(2) Abnormal debilitation of yin is mostly due to damage of yin by yang-pathogens, consumption of yin by fire resulting from extreme emotional changes, or injury of yin due to a protracted disease that results in consumption of essence, blood and body fluid, and hyperfunction of deficiency nature due to relative hyperactivity of yang because of failure of yin to check yang. Clinically it usually presents with a deficiency heat syndrome. The manifestations are heat sensation in the palms, soles and chest, steaming bones, tidal fever, flushed face, emaciation, night sweating, dry throat and mouth, red tongue with little coating, and thready, rapid forceless pulse.

3. Mutual Impairment of Yin and Yang The mutual affection of yin and yang means that deficiency of either yin or yang may involve the counterpart, resulting in

状态，主要是指"邪气盛则实"的实证。其多表现为壮热、面红、目赤、烦躁不安、舌红、苔黄燥，或腹部胀满、腹痛拒按、潮热、谵语等。由于阳盛则阴病，故阳偏盛还可兼见口渴、喜冷饮、大便秘结、小便短少等阴伤症状。

（2）阴偏盛是指机体在疾病过程中，所出现的阴气偏盛、功能障碍或减退、产热不足，以及病理性代谢产物积聚的病理状态。其多表现为形寒、肢冷、舌淡、脘腹冷痛拒按、大便溏泻等寒实证。由于阴盛则阳病，故阴偏盛还可兼见畏寒、神疲倦卧阳虚症状。

2. 阴阳偏衰 是指人体阴阳双方中的一方虚衰不足的病理状态，属"精气夺则虚"的虚证。

（1）阳偏衰是指机体在疾病过程中所出现的阳气虚损、功能减退或衰弱，温煦不足的病理状态，或多由于先天禀赋不足，或后天饮食失养和劳倦内伤，或久病损伤阳气所致。其多表现为畏寒肢冷、神疲倦卧、腹痛喜温喜按、大便稀溏、小便清长、脉迟无力等虚寒证。

（2）阴偏衰是指机体多由于阳邪伤阴，或因五志过极，化火伤阴，或因久病耗伤阴液所致精、血、津液等物质亏耗，以及阴不制阳，导致阳相对亢盛，功能虚性兴奋的病理状态。临床表现为五心烦热、骨蒸潮热、面红升火、消瘦、盗汗、咽干口燥、舌红少苔、脉细数无力等虚热证。

3. 阴阳互损 是指阴或阳任何一方虚损的基础上，病变发展影响到相对的另一方，

a pathological state of deficiency of both yin and yang.

(1) Yin impairment affecting yang: This implies that, because of shortage of yin-fluid, there appears yang deficiency, forming a pathological state of deficiency of both yin and yang, but with yin deficiency being more serious. For instance, in deficiency of kidney-yin, there is dizziness and vertigo, and soreness and weakness in the lower back and knees. It may lead to kidney-yang deficiency manifested by dizziness or impotence or cold limbs.

(2) Yang impairment affecting yin: This implies that, because of deficiency of yang-qi, yin deficiency appears, forming a pathological state of deficiency of both yin and yang, with yang deficiency standing out. For instance, in edema due to yang deficiency there may appear accompanying symptoms of yin deficiency such as emaciation, dysphoria, or chronic convulsion.

4. Mutual Exuberant of Yin or Yang　Yin or yang becomes so extreme that it condenses internally and rejects its counterpart externally, rendering a condition that yin and yang are unable to hold together. Thus there appears the pathological phenomenon of real cold with pseudo-heat or real heat with pseudo-cold. It includes two respects: exuberant yin blocking yang and exuberant yang blocking yin.

(1) Exuberant yin repelling yang: This is a pathological state that exuberant yin-cold pathogens accumulate internally and force yang qi to go outside. It is clinically characterized by reddened complexion, dysphoria with heat sensation, thirst and large pulse. Therefore, it is called a real cold syndrome with pseudo-heat symptoms.

(2) Exuberant yang repelling yin: This is a pathological state that excessive yang-heat accumulates deeply and internally, while yang-qi fails to go externally to the limbs and rejects yin externally. It is clinically characterized by the signs of pseudo-cold such as cold limbs, and deep and hidden pulse. Therefore, it is called a real heat syndrome with pseudo-cold symptoms.

5. Collapse of Yin or Yang　Depletion of yin or yang is a pathological state of critical illness caused by a sudden massive loss of yin-fluid or yang-qi of the body.

(1) Yang collapse is a pathological state of sudden failure of bodily functions caused by a sudden exhaustion of yang-qi. It is a critical syndrome with manifestations of profuse sweating, cold skin and limbs, listlessness, and faint pulse hardly felt.

(2) Yin collapse is a pathological state of collapse of bodily function caused by a sudden and massive loss or consumption of yin-fluid. The clinical manifestations

形成阴阳两虚的病理状态。

（1）阴损及阳：是指由于阴液亏损，累及阳气生化不足或无所依附而耗散，形成了以阴虚为主的阴阳两虚病理状态。如肾阴不足，出现头晕目眩、腰膝酸软，会同时兼见阳痿、肢冷等肾阳虚的症状。

（2）阳损及阴：是指由于阳气虚损，从而在阳虚的基础上又导致了阴虚，形成了以阳虚为主的阴阳两虚的病理状态。如阳虚水泛的水肿，可同时兼见消瘦、心烦等阴虚症状。

4. **阴阳格拒**　是由于某些原因引起阴或阳的一方偏盛至极，因而壅遏于内，将另一方排斥格拒于外，使阴阳之间不相维系，出现真寒假热或真热假寒等复杂的病理现象。它包括阴盛格阳和阳盛格阴两方面。

（1）阴盛格阳：是指阴寒之邪壅盛于内，逼迫阳气浮越于外的一种病理状态。临床上出现面红、烦热、口渴、脉大等真寒假热之象。

（2）阳盛格阴：是指阳热内盛，深伏于里，阳气被遏，郁闭于内，不能外达于肢体而格阴于外的一种病理状态。临床上出现四肢厥冷、脉象沉伏等真热假寒之象。

5. **阴阳亡失**　机体阴液或阳气突然大量地亡失，导致生命垂危的病理状态。

（1）亡阳：是指机体的阳气发生突然性大量脱失，而致全身功能突然衰竭的病理状态。临床表现为大汗淋漓、肌肤手足厥冷、蜷卧、神疲、脉微欲绝等危重证候。

（2）亡阴：是指由于机体阴液发生突然性大量消耗或丢失，而致全身功能严重衰竭的

of this critical syndrome are short and rapid breathing, thirst, warm limbs, and hyperhidrosis with a tendency to collapse.

iii. Disorder of Qi and Blood

Disorders of qi and blood include pathological states of insufficiency of qi or blood, disturbance in circulation or physiological function of qi or blood, and disturbance in relationship between qi and blood that are caused by struggle between the healthy qi and the pathogenic, or disturbance of visceral functions.

1. Disorder of Qi　Disorders of qi mainly refer to qi deficiency due to poor production of qi or over consumption of qi, functional insufficiency of qi, and disturbance of qi movement as well.

(1) Qi deficiency: It is the condition of insufficient body qi and pathological state of qi dysfunction. Clinically its manifestations are lassitude, listlessness, spontaneous sweating, and being apt to catch cold.

(2) Disorder of qi movement: It refers to the abnormal movements of qi, which can be summarized into five respects including qi stagnation, qi counterflow, qi sinking, qi blockage and qi desertion.

1) Qi stagnation, which refers to unsmooth or obstructed flow of qi, is clinically marked by stuffiness, distension and pain.

2) Qi counterflow, which refers to hyper-ascending or hypo-descending or transversely adverse movement of qi, is clinically marked by nausea, vomiting, hiccup, eructation irritability, oven hematemesis, and syncope.

3) Qi sinking, which refers to hypo-ascending or hyper-descending of qi, is clinically marked by dizziness and vertigo, tinnitus, deafness, down-bearing sensation of the lower abdomen, frequent desire for defecation, or prolapse of the rectum, hysteroptosis and gastroptosis.

4) Qi blockage, which refers to failure of qi to exit and accumulation of qi in the interior, is clinically marked by sudden syncope, unconsciousness, cold limbs, dyspnea, and cyanotic face and lips.

5) Qi desertion, which refers to outside escape of qi due to its failure in holding itself inside, is clinically marked by critical signs of pale complexion, continuous sweating, open mouth with closed eyes, general paralysis, flaccid hands, incontinence of urine and stool.

2. Disorder of Blood　Disorders of blood mainly refer to the pathological state of deficiency of blood caused by poor generation of blood or over consumption of blood, hypofunction of blood in nourishing and

病理状态。临床表现为喘渴烦躁、手足虽温而汗多欲脱的危重证候。

（三）气血失常

由于正邪斗争的盛衰，或脏腑功能的失调，导致气或血的不足、运行失常和各自生理功能及其相互关系的失常而产生的病理状态。

1. **气的失常**　是指气的生化不足或耗散过多而致气的不足，或气的功能减退，以及气机失调的病理状态。

（1）气虚：指一身之气不足及其功能低下的病理状态。临床表现精神疲乏、全身乏力、自汗、易于感冒等。

（2）气机失调：是指气的升降出入失常而引起的气滞、气逆、气陷、气闭、气脱等病理变化。

1）气滞，指气的流通不畅、郁滞不通的病理状态，临床最常见的表现为闷、胀、痛。

2）气逆，指气升之太过，或降之不及，以脏腑之气逆上为特征的一种病理状态，临床表现为恶心、呕吐、嗳气、呃逆、急躁易怒，甚至吐血、昏厥等病证。

3）气陷，指气的上升不足或下降太过，以气升举无力而下陷为特征的一种病理状态，表现为头晕眼花、耳鸣耳聋、小腹坠胀、便意频频，或见脱肛、子宫脱垂、胃下垂等病变。

4）气闭，指气机闭阻，外出严重障碍，以致清窍闭塞，出现昏厥的一种病理状态，表现为突然昏厥、不省人事、四肢欠温、呼吸困难、面唇青紫等病情较急症状。

5）气脱，指气不内守，大量向外亡失，以致功能突然衰竭的一种病理状态，临床多表现为面色苍白、汗出不止、口开目闭、全身软瘫、手撒、二便失禁等危重征象。

2. **血的失常**　是指血的生化不足或耗伤太过而致血虚，或血的濡养功能减退，以及血的运行失常的病理状态。

disordered circulation of blood.

(1) Deficiency of blood: This is a pathological state of shortage of blood or hypofunction of blood. There will appear serious general or local asthenic presentations of pale and lusterless complexion, lips and nails, dizziness, amnesia, listlessness, lassitude, emaciation, palpitation, insomnia, dry and discomfort feeling of eyes, and blurred vision.

(2) Disorder of blood flow: This means a pathological change of blood stasis, or accelerated flow of blood, or bleeding due to frenzied flow of blood. Blood stasis:

1) When blood stagnates in the viscera, channels or a local part, it will cause local pain either being fixed or forming into masses in severe cases.

2) Acceleration of blood flow: The common presentations of this condition are flushed complexion, red tongue, rapid pulse, dysphoria, even bleeding and coma.

3) Bleeding: This mainly includes hematemesis, hemoptysis, hemafecia, hematuria, hypermenorrhea, epistaxis, gingival bleeding and hematohidrosis.

3. Disorder of Qi and Blood Simultaneously This refers to a pathological state due to destruction of the interdependent relationship between qi and blood.

(1) Qi stagnation and blood stasis: It is a pathological state in which qi stagnancy and blood stasis coexist. Obstruction of qi flow may lead to disturbance of blood flow, and blood stasis will further deteriorate qi stagnancy.

(2) Failure of qi to control blood: It is a pathological state of various bleeding due to qi deficiency with hypofunction in controlling blood, leading to escape of blood out of the vessels.

(3) Qi deficiency and blood stasis: It is a pathological state that deficient qi fails to drive blood to circulate, resulting in blood stasis. This disorder takes qi deficiency as its basis.

(4) Deficiency of both qi and blood: It is mostly caused by gradual injury of both qi and blood due to consumption in a prolonged illness, qi depletion following early bleeding, or lack of source for blood production because of qi deficiency. This is a pathological state in which qi deficiency and blood deficiency coexist.

(5) Qi collapse following blood desertion: Since blood is the mother of qi, and conveys qi, a large amount of bleeding such as traumatic hemorrhage, metrorrhagia or massive postpartum hemorrhage in women will make qi loose its attachment, and thus escape and deplete accordingly.

（1）血虚：是指血液不足，或血的功能减退的病理状态。出现全身或局部的虚弱表现，如面色、爪甲淡白无华，头晕健忘，神疲乏力，形体消瘦，心悸失眠，手足麻木，两目干涩，视物昏花等。

（2）血行失常：是指在疾病过程中，血液运行瘀滞不畅，或血液运行加速，甚至血液妄行，逸出脉外而出血的病理变化。

1）血瘀：如血液瘀滞于脏腑、经络等某一局部，不通则痛，可出现局部疼痛，固定不移，甚至形成癥积肿块等。

2）血行迫疾：常表现为面赤舌红、脉数、心烦，甚至出血、神昏等病证。

3）出血：主要有吐血、咯血、便血、尿血、月经过多，以及鼻衄、齿衄、肌衄等。

3. 气血关系失调　是指气与血相互依存、相互为用的关系破坏而产生的病理状态。

（1）气滞血瘀：是指气滞和血瘀同时存在的病理状态。气的运行阻滞，可以导致血液运行的障碍，而血液瘀滞又必将进一步加重气滞。

（2）气不摄血：是指因气的不足，固摄血液的功能减弱，血不循经，逸出脉外，导致各种出血的病理状态。

（3）气虚血瘀：是指气虚无力推动血行，致使血液瘀滞的病理状态。气虚血瘀是以气虚为基础的。

（4）气血两虚：多因久病消耗，渐致气血两伤；或先有失血，气随血脱；或先因气虚，血液生化无源而日渐衰少等所致气虚与血虚同时存在的病理状态。

（5）气随血脱：由于血为气母，血能载气，在大量出血的同时，气也随着血的流失而耗脱的病理状态。如外伤出血、妇女崩漏、产后大失血等。

iv. Disorder of Body Fluid Metabolism

Disorders of body fluid metabolism refer to the pathological state of retention of fluids in the body or shortage of body fluid because the formation, distribution and excretion of body fluid are disordered.

1. Shortage of Body Fluid It is mostly due to consumption of body fluid caused by invading exogenous heat pathogens of yang, or fire transformed from excessive emotional disturbance, or profuse sweating, serious vomiting and diarrhea, polyuria, heavy bleeding or over administration of acrid and dry remedies. Shortage of body fluid implies a pathological state that there appear a series of dry and puckery symptoms because the viscera, sense organs and orifices cannot be sufficiently moistened and nourished due to shortage of body fluid.

2. Retention of Water This is a summarization of the pathological state of retention of water dampness and phlegm resulting from the disturbance of body fluid in distribution and excretion.

As the lung qi fails to diffuse and disperse, the body striae will close, and then the excretion of sweat will be disordered. If the urinary bladder fails to close and open normally, the urine will not be discharged out of body. If the qi transforming action of kidney yang is declined, it will cause disturbance of production and excretion of urine, leading to illness with retention of water.

3. Disorder of Body Fluid and Qi-Blood Simultaneously There may appear the following several pathological changes.

(1) Water retention with qi obstruction: This is a pathological state that water stagnates and accumulates in the body to block qi movement. For example, if phlegm and stagnant fluids accumulate in the lung, there may appear chest depression, cough, and inability of lying flat with dyspnea. If water-dampness stays in the middle-jiao, it may lead to failure of the clear qi to ascend and failure of turbid qi to descend, with manifestations of distension and fullness in the epigastrium and abdomen, belching, and poor appetite. If water fluids overflow to the limbs, there may appear heaviness and distending pain of the limbs.

(2) Qi exhaustion following fluid loss: It is a pathological state of sudden exhaustion of yang-qi because of massive loss of body fluid and thus qi escapes out of the body along with the fluid. It is mostly caused by burning of fluid by high fever, or consumption of fluid due to profuse sweating, serious vomiting and diarrhea, and polyuria, leading to qi exhaustion following fluid loss.

(3) Fluid exhaustion and blood dryness: This is a pathological state that body fluid and blood become deficient at the same time. For example, high fever,

（四）津液代谢失常

津液代谢失常是指津液的生成、输布、排泄失常，引起体内津液不足，或在体内滞留的病理变化。

1. 津液不足 是指多由外感阳热病邪，或五志化火，消灼津液；或多汗、剧烈吐泻、多尿、失血，或过用辛燥之物等引起津液的亏少，导致脏腑、组织官窍失于濡润滋养而干燥枯涩的病理状态。

2. 水液停聚 水液停聚是对津液的输布、排泄障碍，导致水湿痰饮积聚的病理状态。

当肺气失于宣发布散，汗液排泄障碍；或膀胱的开合作用失常，不能使尿液排出体外。如果肾阳的气化功能减退，尿液的生成和排泄障碍，则必致水液停留而为病。

3. 津液与气血关系失调 可出现如下几种病理变化：

（1）水停气阻：水液停聚于体内，导致气机阻滞的津液代谢障碍的病理状态。如痰饮阻肺，可见胸满咳嗽、痰多、喘促不能平卧等病证；水湿停留中焦，可见脘腹胀满、嗳气食少症；水饮泛溢四肢，可见肢体沉重、胀痛不适等症。

（2）气随津脱：指由于津液大量亡失，气随津液外泄，致使阳气暴脱的病理状态。多由高热伤津，或大汗出，或严重吐泻、多尿等，耗伤津液，气随津脱所致。

（3）津枯血燥：指津液和血同时出现亏损不足的病理状态。如高热大汗、大吐、大

polyhidrosis, heavy vomiting and serious diarrhea may present with restlessness, dry and squamous skin with itching feeling.

(4) Fluid consumption and blood stasis: It is a pathological state of obstructed circulation of blood due to shortage of body fluid. If body fluid is consumed massively due to high fever, burns and scalds in large areas, or severe vomiting, diarrhea and sweating, clinically it usually presents with dark purplish complexion, ecchymoses in the skin, dark purplish tongue, or with petechiae and ecchymoses.

v. Five Endogenous Pathogen

The five endogenous pathogens are the disorders of yin and yang of the viscera, and anomalies of qi, blood and body fluid. They refer to the five pathologic changes similar to those caused by exogenous wind, clod, dampness, dryness and fire (heat).

1. Wind Stirring Internally　This is also called endogenous wind, liver wind or stirring of liver wind internally due to failure of the liver in governing free flow of qi. It may be classified into the following four types.

(1) Liver yang transforming into wind: Its clinical manifestations are numbness of the limbs, tremor, vertigo with a tendency to fall down, or wry mouth with distorted eyes, or hemiplegia in a mild case, or sudden coma and unconsciousness in a severe case.

(2) Extreme heat producing wind: Its clinical manifestations are high fever, coma, delirium, spasm of the limbs, staring eyes straightly upward, and opisthotonus.

(3) Stirring of wind due to yin deficiency: Its clinical manifestations are peristalses of the hands and feet.

(4) Blood deficiency generating wind: Its clinical manifestations are coma, numbness of the limbs, tremor of tendons and muscles, constriction of the hands and feet.

2. Production of Cold Internally　This is endogenous cold that is mostly associated with decline of the spleen and kidney yang. It is a pathological state that deficiency-cold is produced internally or yin-cold spreads all over the body, which is caused by decline of yang-qi with hypofunction of warming and qi transforming.

Deficiency of yang qi leads to internal production of deficiency-cold. There are mainly three respects of manifestations: first, yang qi has declined and failed to warm the body, there appear intolerance of cold and cold limbs. Secondly, the function of qi transformation decreases, thus it leads to disturbance of fluid metabolism with accumulation of pathological products such as phlegm, stagnant fluid, and water-dampness. Thirdly, yang-qi fails to steam and vaporize yin, thus body fluid cannot be transformed into

泻后等表现为心烦、肌肤甲错、皮肤瘙痒等病变。

（4）津亏血瘀：指因津液亏损而导致血液运行瘀滞不畅的病理状态。如因高热、大面积烧烫伤，或大吐、大泻、大汗等，表现面质紫暗、皮肤紫斑、舌体紫暗，或有瘀点、瘀斑等血瘀表现。

（五）内生五邪

内生"五邪"，是脏腑阴阳失调，气、血、津液代谢异常所产生的类似风、寒、湿、燥、火（热）五种外邪致病特征的病理变化。

1. **风气内动**　简称"内风"，多是肝失调畅出现的一系列病理现象，故又称为肝风或肝风内动。它分为四类：

（1）肝阳化风：临床表现轻则肢体麻木、震颤、眩晕欲扑，或为口眼㖞斜，或为半身不遂；重则血随气逆于上，出现猝然昏倒、不省人事等。

（2）热极生风：又称热甚动风。临床表现以高热、神昏谵语、四肢抽搐、目睛上吊、角弓反张等症。

（3）阴虚风动：临床表现为手足蠕动等症。

（4）血虚生风：临床表现为肢体麻木、筋肉跳动、手足拘挛等症。

2. **寒从中生**　即是内寒，多与脾肾阳气虚衰有关，是指机体阳气虚衰，温煦气化功能减退，虚寒内生，或阴寒之邪弥漫的病理状态。

阳气不足，虚寒内生，主要表现在三个方面：一是阳气不足，机体失于温煦，如畏寒肢冷等；二是气化功能减退，津液代谢障碍导致病理产物在体内聚积，如痰饮、水湿等；三是阳不化阴，蒸化无权，津液不化，如尿频清长、痰涎清稀等。

qi, with such symptoms as frequent, lucid and profuse urine, and lucid sputum and slobber.

3. Internal Generation of Turbid Dampness This is endogenous dampness, which mostly lies in disorder of the spleen in transformation and transportation. It is a pathological state of internal generation and accumulation of water, dampness, phlegm and stagnant fluid, which is caused by disturbance of distribution and excretion of body fluid. The major manifestations are of two respects. First, the dampness is characterized by heaviness, turbidity, and viscosity, and being apt to hinder qi movement, thus, there may appear chest distress, abdominal distention and discomfort of defecation. Secondly, dampness is a turbid-yin material, therefore internal blockage of dampness pathogen may further affect functional activities of the lung, spleen and kidney.

4. Dryness from Fluid Consumption This is endogenous dryness. It is a pathological state of a series of dry and aningeresting symptoms because the tissue organs of the body lose their moisture caused by shortage of fluid in the body.

The development of endogenous dryness is mostly due to consumption of yin-fluid in a prolonged illness, or shortage of yin-fluid resulting from heavy sweating, serious vomiting, or diarrhea, or massive loss of blood and essence, consumption of fluid by exuberant heat in the process of some exogenous febrile diseases. There appear a series of dry symptoms such as dry skin, dry mouth and throat, dry stools and constipation.

5. Generation of Fire-Heat Internally This is endogenous fire or heat. It is a pathological state of internal fire with hyperactive function of the body, which is caused by exuberance of yang, or yin deficiency with yang hyperactivity, or transformation of fire from emotional disturbance. The pathogeneses are as follows:

(1) Fire transformed from exuberance of yang-qi: If yang-qi gets too hyperactive, it will transform into fire to make abnormal excitement of functional activity.

(2) Fire produced from stagnation of pathogens: This includes two types. One is that the invading pathogenic wind, cold, dampness and dryness generate fire through a long period of stagnation during the pathological process. For example, cold pathogen leads to production of fire by stagnation. The other is that the pathological products such as phlegm-dampness, stagnant blood and foodstuff retention make generation of fire by a long period of stagnation.

(3) Fire produced by extreme emotions: This is a pathological state of generation of fire resulting from yang exuberance, or a long period of depression of qi movement

3. 湿浊内生 即是"内湿"，主要与脾的运化功能失常有关，指因体内津液输布、排泄障碍，导致水湿痰饮内生并蓄积停滞的病理状态。表现在两个方面：一是由于湿性重浊黏滞，多易阻滞气机，出现胸闷、腹胀、大便不爽等症；二是湿为阴浊之物，湿邪内阻，可进一步影响肺、脾、肾等脏腑的功能活动。

4. 津伤化燥 即是"内燥"，是指体内津液不足，导致人体各组织器官失于濡润而出现一系列干燥枯涩症状的病理状态。

内燥病变的形成多由久病耗伤阴津，或大汗、大吐、大下；或亡血、失精；或某些外感热性病过程中所致热盛伤津、阴液亏少等。临床表现为肌肤干燥、口燥咽干、大便燥结等一系列干燥失润的症状。

5. 火热内生 即是"内火"，又称"内热"，是指阳盛有余，或阴虚阳亢，或五志化火等而致的火自内扰，功能亢奋的病理状态。其病机如下：

（1）阳气过盛化火：指阳气过于亢奋，亢烈化火，使功能活动异常兴奋的病理性的阳亢。

（2）邪郁化火：包括两个方面：一是外感风、寒、湿、燥等病邪，如寒邪化热、湿郁化火等，郁久而化热化火；二是体内的病理性产物，如痰湿、瘀血、饮食积滞等，郁久而化火。

（3）五志过极化火：是指由于精神情志刺激或气机郁结，影响脏腑气血阴阳，导致脏腑阳盛，气郁日久而从阳化火所形成的病理

caused by abnormal psychological and emotional stimuli That affect qi and blood and yin-yang of the viscera.

(4) Yin deficiency resulting in vigorous fire: This is a pathological state of internal production of deficiency-fire, which is caused by yang hyperactivity with failure of deficient yin to restrict yang due to great injury of yin-fluid. It is most common among persons with either chronic or prolonged illness. For example, gingival swelling and pain, sore throat, steaming bones, and flushed cheek due to yin deficiency are all the outcome of flaring of deficiency-fire.

(Ma Xue-ling)

状态。

（4）阴虚火旺：是指阴液大伤，阴不制阳，阴虚阳亢，虚热内生的病理状态。其多见于慢性久病之人，如阴虚而引起的牙龈肿痛、咽喉疼痛、骨蒸颧红等均为虚火上炎所致。

（马雪玲）

Section 6　Channel, Collateral and Acupuncture Point

第六节　经络腧穴

I. Channel and Collateral

一、经络

i. Concept of the Channel and Collateral

Channels and collaterals, or "*Jing Luo*" in Chinese, are the pathways running through the body that transport qi and blood, and link the internal *zang-fu* organs with the surface and other parts of the body. "*Jing*", the Chinese name for "channel" means "path" "route", or "longitudinal main line". The term "*Jing*" refers to the channels in general and comprises the main part of the channel system. The channels travel at deeper level of the body and perform an extremely important role of linking and integrating the interior with the exterior and the upper with the lower. "*Luo*", the Chinese name for "collateral" means "network", refers to the smaller branches of the channels. The collaterals run superficially and enmesh the body horizontally like a network. The channel system connects internally with *zang-fu* organs and externally with the tendons, muscles and skin. Channels and collaterals assume the responsibility of circulating qi and blood, communicating so as to connect all the viscera, organs, orifices, skin, muscles, tendons and bones to form an integral organic whole.

（一）经络的概念

经络是人体运行全身气血、联络脏腑肢节、沟通表里上下内外的通路，是人体组织结构的重要组成部分。经，有"路径""通道"的意思，就是纵行的主线，是经络系统中的主干，深而在里，贯通上下，沟通内外；络，有"网络"的意思，是经络别出的细小分支，浅而在表，纵横交错，网络全身。经络系统在内连属于脏腑，在外连属于筋肉、皮肤。经脉和络脉共同担负着运行气血，联络沟通等作用，把人体所有的脏腑、器官、孔窍以及皮肉筋骨等组织联结成一个统一的有机整体。

ii. Composition of the Channel System

The channel system is composed of the channels, collaterals and affiliated muscle channels and cutaneous regions that link the main channels with the surface of the body. The channels mainly include twelve regular

（二）经络系统的组成

人体的经络系统由经脉和络脉及其连属部分所组成，经脉可分为十二正经、奇经八脉和十二经别。络脉有别络、浮络和孙络之

channels, eight extraordinary vessels and twelve divergent channels. The collaterals mainly include fifteen collaterals, superficial collaterals and minute collaterals. Besides there are also twelve channel musculatures and twelve skin areas that connect the twelve channels with tendons, muscles and skin (Fig. 2-13).

1. Twelve Regular Channels   The twelve regular channels are the dominant part in the channel system, which pertain to the *zang-fu* organs internally and connect to the extremities and joints externally. The twelve regular channels include three yin channels of hand, three yang channels of hand, three yin channels of foot and three yang channels of foot. They are the major pathways for qi and blood circulation.

The twelve channels have their own starting and terminating points, running regions, connecting orders, certain regularities in distribution and course in the limbs and trunk. They have direct connection and affiliation relationships with *zang-fu* organs within the body, and have external-internal relationships among themselves. The twelve channels are the necessary passages for qi and

分。另有十二经筋和十二皮部，是十二经脉与筋肉和体表的连属部分，共同组成经络系统，成为不可分割的整体（图2-13）。

1. **十二经脉**   是经络系统的主体，在内属络于脏腑，在外联络四肢、头面和躯干，是气血运行的主要通道，又称十二正经，包括手三阴经、手三阳经、足三阳经、足三阴经。

十二经脉有一定的起止、循行部位和交接顺序，在肢体的分布和走向有一定的规律，与体内脏腑有直接的络属关系，相互之间有表里关系。

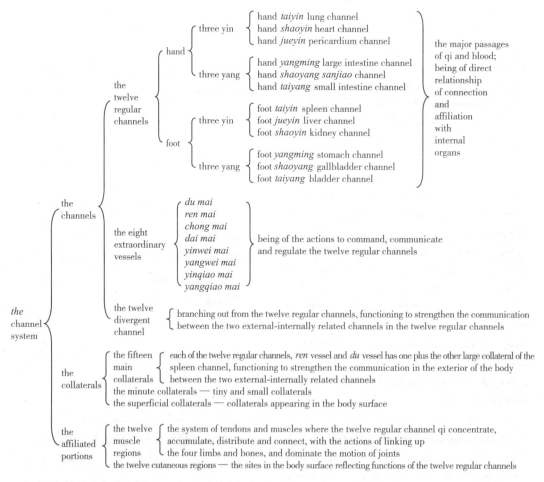

Fig. 2-13   The Channel System
图2-13   经络系统简表

blood circulation.

(1) Nomenclature of the twelve regular channels: The nomenclature of the twelve regular channels is based on three factors, which are hand or foot, yin or yang, and *zang* or *fu* organs. Hand or foot refers to the channel running on the upper or lower limbs respectively along their external pathways. The channels run on the upper limbs are named hand channels, while those run on the lower limbs are named foot channels. The second factor, yin or yang indicates the channel's yin or yang property and the amount of yin qi or yang qi it carries. Yin channels travel on the medial side of the body, while yang channels on the lateral side. The yin and yang are then further divided into three yin and three yang categories in order to differentiate the amount of yin qi or yang qi of the channels. The channels that carry the most abundant yin qi are called *taiyin*. The channels that carry the lesser amount of yin qi are called *shaoyin*. The ones that carry the least yin qi are called *jueyin*. Similarly, the channels that carry the most abundant yang qi are called *yangming*. The channels that carry lesser amount of yang qi are called *taiyang*. The ones that carry the least amount of yang qi are called *shaoyang*. The third factor, *zang* or *fu* organs indicate the *zang* or *fu* organ to which the channel pertains.

(2) Distribution of the twelve regular channels on the surface of the body: The superficial pathways of twelve regular channels are distributed symmetrically on the head, the trunk and the four limbs.

The terms for the orientation of the human body used in locating the distribution of channels and acupuncture points are not the same as those used in modern anatomy. For example, the palmar side of the upper limb, or the flexional side, is called the medial side. The dorsal side or the extensional side of the upper limb is called the lateral side. The side of the lower limb closer to the midline is called the medial side, while the side of the lower limb away from the midline is called the lateral side.

The twelve channels in the body basically run vertically. With an exception of the foot yangming stomach channel, all yin channels run on the medial side of the limbs and chest-abdominal parts of the trunk, and all yang channels run on the lateral side of the limbs and back parts of the trunk. The hand channels run in the upper limbs, and foot channels run in the lower limbs.

In the four limbs, yin channels run on the medial side and yang channels on the lateral side. There are three yin channels on the medial side, thus there are three yang

（1）十二经脉的名称：十二经脉的名称由手足、阴阳和脏腑三部分组成。手足，表示经脉的外行路线分别分布于上肢或下肢，行于上肢的称为手经，行于下肢的称为足经。阴阳，表示经脉的阴阳属性和阴气、阳气的多少。阴经循行于肢体的内侧，阳经循行于肢体的外侧。阴气最盛为太阴，其次为少阴，再次为厥阴；阳气最盛为阳明，其次为太阳，再次为少阳。脏腑，表示经脉所连属的脏腑。

（2）十二经脉在体表的分布：十二经脉在体表左右成对分布于头面、躯干和四肢，称为外行部分。

经络腧穴分布定位的方位术语与现代解剖学不完全相同。比如：将上肢的掌侧称为内侧，上肢的背侧称为外侧；将下肢向正中线的一侧称为内侧，远离正中线的一侧称为外侧。

十二经脉在体表的分布大多是纵行的。除足阳明胃经外，阴经均行于四肢内侧及躯干的胸腹面，阳经均行于四肢外侧及躯干的背面。手经行于上肢，足经行于下肢。

在四肢部，阴经分布在内侧面，阳经分布在外侧面，内侧分三阴，外侧分三阳。上

channels on the lateral side. On the medial side of upper limb, *taiyin* channel runs in the anterior, *jueyin* channel in the middle, and *shaoyin* in the posterior. On the lateral side of upper limb, *yangming* runs in the anterior, *shaoyang* channel in the middle, and *taiyang* channel in the posterior. On the medial side of lower limb, in the region 8 cun below the medial malleolus, *jueyin* channel runs in the anterior, *taiyin* channel in the middle, and *shaoyin* channel in the posterior, while in the region 8 cun above the medial malleolus, *taiyin* channel runs in the anterior, *jueyin* channel in the middle and *shaoyin* channel in the posterior. On the lateral side of lower limb, *yangming* channel runs in the anterior, *shaoyang* channel in the middle and *taiyang* channel in the posterior.

In the head and face, *yangming* channels run in the face, *taiyang* channels run in the zygomatic regions, vertex and posterior side of the head, while *shaoyang* channels run on both lateral sides of the head. But not all yin channels arrive at the neck and chest. Some of them run in the deeper parts of the head and face or even to the vertex. Among them, the hand *shaoyin* heart channel and the foot *jueyin* liver channel run up to the eye connector, and the foot *jueyin* liver channel meets the *du mai* at the vertex. The foot *shaoyin* kidney channel runs up to the root of the tongue, and the foot *taiyin* spleen channel connects with the root of the tongue and scatters its collaterals over the lower surface of the tongue.

In the trunk, the three yang channels of hand run in the scapular regions. Among the three yang channels of foot, *yangming* channel runs in the ventral part (chest and abdomen), *taiyang* channel runs in the dorsal part (back side), and *shaoyang* channel runs on the lateral sides. The three yin channels of hand all run out from the axillae. All of the three yin channels of foot run in the ventral part (Table 2-5).

(3) The exterior-interior relationship of the twelve regular channels: The twelve regular channels connect to *zang-fu* organs. Among them, yin channels pertain to *zang* organs and connect to *fu* organs. The yang channels pertain to *fu* organs and connect to *zang* organs. The twelve regular channels form six pairs of exterior-interior relationship (Table 2-5).

(4) Running direction and connection of the twelve regular channels: The three yin channels of hand in the twelve channels run from the internal viscera of the thoracic cavity to the ends of fingers, and connect with the three yang channels of hand there. The three yang channels of hand run from the ends of fingers to the head and face, and connect with the three yang channels of foot there. The three yang channels of foot run from the head

肢内侧为太阴经在前，厥阴经在中，少阴经在后；上肢外侧为阳明经在前，少阳经在中，太阳经在后；下肢内侧，内踝尖上 8 寸以下为厥阴经在前，太阴经在中，少阴经在后；内踝尖上 8 寸以上则太阴经在前，厥阴经在中，少阴经在后；下肢外侧为阳明经在前，少阳经在中，太阳经在后。

在头面部，阳明经行于面部；太阳经行于面颊部、头顶及头后部；少阳经行于头侧部。诸阴经并不都是皆到颈部、胸中而还，其中手少阴心经、足厥阴肝经均上达目系，足厥阴肝经与督脉会于头顶部，足少阴肾经上抵舌根，足太阴脾经连舌本、散舌下，均行达头面之深部或巅顶。

在躯干部，手三阳经行于肩胛部；足三阳经则阳明经行于前（胸、腹面）；太阳经行于后（背面）；少阳经行于侧面。手三阴经均从腋下走出，足三阴经均行于腹面（表 2-5）。

（3）十二经脉的属络表里关系：十二经脉内属络于脏腑，其中阴经属脏络腑为里，阳经属腑络脏为表，组合成六对"表里相合"关系。十二经脉的表里关系还通过经别和络脉的表里沟通而得到加强（表 2-5）。

（4）十二经脉的走向与交接规律：十二经脉的走向是手三阴经从胸腔内脏走向手指端，与手三阳经交会；手三阳经，从手指走向头面部，与足三阳经交会；足三阳经，从头面部走向足趾端，与足三阴经交会；足三阴经，从足趾走向腹部和胸部，在胸部内脏与手三

Table 2-5　Nomenclature and Classification of the Twelve Channels

	yin channel (pertains to *zang* organ)	yang channel (pertains to *fu* organ)		running route (yin channel on the medial side, yang channel on the lateral side)
hand	*taiyin* lung channel	*yangming* large intestine channel	upper limb	anterior line
	jueyin pericardium channel	*shaoyang sanjiao* channel		middle line
	shaoyin heart channel	*taiyang* small intestine channel		posterior line
foot	*taiyin* spleen channel	*yangming* stomach channel	lower limb	anterior line
	jueyin liver channel	*shaoyang* gallbladder channel		middle line
	shaoyin kidney channel	*taiyang* bladder channel		posterior line

表 2-5　十二经脉名称分布表

	阴经 （属脏）	阳经 （属腑）		循行部位 （阴经行内侧、阳经行外侧）
手	太阴肺经	阳明大肠经	上肢	前缘
	厥阴心包经	少阳三焦经		中线
	少阴心经	太阳小肠经		后缘
足	太阴脾经	阳明胃经	下肢	前缘
	厥阴肝经	少阳胆经		中线
	少阴肾经	太阳膀胱经		后缘

and face to the ends of toes, and connect with the three yin channels of foot there. The three yin channels of foot run from the ends of toes to the abdomen and thorax, and connect with the three yin channels of hand in the viscera of the thoracic cavity. In this way, the hand channels connect at the hand and the foot channels connect at the foot, while yang channels connect at the head, and yin channels connect at the viscera in the thoracic cavity. Thus the twelve channels form a circulatory cycle in which "yin and yang channels communicate with each other".

There are three models of connection in the twelve channels.

1) The exterior-interiorly related yin and yang channels connect with each other at the ends of limbs. There are altogether six pairs of exterior-interiorly related yin and yang channels. Among them, the exterior-interiorly related three yin channels of hand and three yang channels of hand connect at the ends of upper limbs, and the exterior-interiorly related three yin channels of foot and three yang channels of foot connect at the ends of

阴经交会。如此，手经交于手，足经交于足，阳经交于头，阴经交于胸腹内脏，十二经脉就构成了"阴阳相贯，如环无端"的循环路径（图 2-14）。

十二经脉的交接有三种方式：

1）相为表里的阴经与阳经在四肢末端交接。相为表里的阴经与阳经共六对，都在四肢末端交接。其中相为表里的手三阴经与手三阳经交接在上肢末端，相为表里的足三阳经和足三阴经交接在下肢末端。

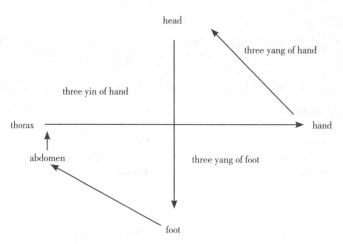

Fig. 2-14   Running Direction and Connection of the Twelve Regular Channels
图 2-14   十二经脉走向交接规律

lower limbs.

2) The yang channels of hand and foot with the same name connect in the head and face. There are three pairs of yang channels of hand and foot with the same name. For example, hand *yangming* large intestine channel and foot *yangming* stomach channel connect at the side of nose wing. hand *taiyang* small intestine channel and foot*Taiyang* bladder channel connect at the inner canthus. And hand *shaoyang sanjiao* channel and foot *shaoyang* gallbladder channel connect at the outer canthus.

3) Yin channels of foot and hand connect in the thorax. The yin channels of foot and hand are also called "channels with different names". There are three pairs of them. They connect in the viscera of the thoracic cavity. For example, foot *taiyin* spleen channel and hand *shaoyin* heart channel connect in the heart. foot *shaoyin* kidney channel and hand *jueyin* pericardium channel connect in the chest. foot *jueyin* liver channel and hand *taiyin* lung channel connect in the lung (Fig. 2-14).

(5) Flow of qi in the twelve regular channels: The twelve channels are the main pathways for circulation of qi and blood. They communicate with each other from the head to the foot, connecting in a fixed order. The flow of qi and blood within them also follows a definite order.

Since qi and blood of the whole body are produced by foodstuff essence through transformation and transportation of the spleen and stomach, the flow of qi and blood within the twelve channels starts from the hand *taiyin* lung channel that originates from the middle energizer, in turn it flows to the foot *jueyin* liver channel, then it runs back to and starts again from the Hand *taiyin* lung channel. It is thus communicated from the head to the foot, and there is no end. The Fig. 2-15 shows its flow

2）同名手足阳经在头面部交接。同名的手足阳经有三对，都在头面部交接。如手阳明大肠经与足阳明胃经交接于鼻翼旁，手太阳小肠经与足太阳膀胱经交接于目内眦，手少阳三焦经与足少阳胆经交接于目外眦。

3）足手阴经在胸部交接。足手阴经，又称"异名经"，也有3对，交接部位皆在胸部内脏。如足太阴脾经与手少阴心经交接于心中；足少阴肾经与手厥阴心包经交接于胸中；足厥阴肝经与手太阴肺经交接于肺中。

（5）十二经脉流注次序：十二经脉是人体气血运行的主要通道，它们首尾相贯、依次衔接，因而脉中气血的运行也是循经脉依次传注的。

由于全身气血皆由脾胃运化的水谷之精化生，故十二经脉气血的流注从起于中焦的手太阴肺经开始，依次传至足厥阴肝经，然后再传手太阴肺经，首尾相贯，如环无端（图 2-15）。

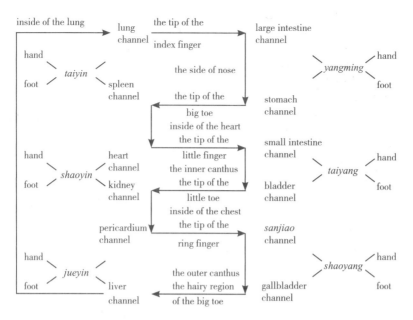

Fig. 2-15　Flow of Qi in the Twelve Regular Channels
图 2-15　十二经脉流注次序图

order.

2. Eight Extraordinary Vessels Eight extraordinary vessels are separate and different from the main channels, including *Ren Mai, Du Mai, Chong Mai, Dai Mai, Yin Wei Mai, Yang Wei Mai, Yin Qiao Mai* and *Yang Qiao Mai*. The eight extraordinary vessels are called "extraordinary" because they have no direct connection and pertaining relationships with *zang-fu* organs, and have no exterior-interior relationships. They have the actions to govern, communicate and regulate qi and blood within the twelve regular channels.

3. Twelve Divergent Channels The twelve divergent channels are the channels branching out from the twelve regular channels. They originate respectively from the four limbs and run through the deeper parts of the body cavity and reach up the superficial parts of the neck. The divergent channels of the yang channels branch out from their channel-proper and still return to the channel-proper after running through the body internally. While the divergent channels of the yin channels branch out from their channel-proper, after running through the interior of the body, however, they join their external-internally related yang channels. The functions of the twelve divergent channels are mainly to strengthen the communication between the two external-internally related channels in the twelve regular channels. They also supplement certain weakness of the regular channels since they can reach some organs and components where the regular channels do not reach.

4. Fifteen Main Collaterals The fifteen main

2. 奇经八脉 奇经八脉包括任脉、督脉、冲脉、带脉、阴维脉、阳维脉、阴跷脉、阳跷脉。奇经八脉与十二经脉不同，与体内脏腑没有直接的络属关系，相互之间也没有表里关系，故称为奇经。它们有统率、联络和调节十二经脉中气血的作用。

3. 十二经别 十二经别是从十二经脉别出的正经，属于经脉范围。它们分别起自四肢，循行于体腔脏腑深部，上出于颈项浅部。阳经的经别从本经别出而循行体内后，仍回到本经；阴经的经别从本经别出而循行体内后，却与相为表里的阳经相合。十二经别的作用，主要是加强十二经脉中相为表里的两经之间的联系，由于它通达某些正经未循行到的器官与形体部位，因此能补正经之不足。

4. 十五络脉 十二经脉在四肢部各分出

collaterals are the larger and major collaterals. Each of the twelve channels, *Ren Mai* and *Du Mai* has one and there is the other large collateral of the spleen channel. All these are collectively called the "fifteen main collaterals". The major functions of the fifteen main collaterals are to strengthen the communication in the exterior of the body between the two external-internally related channels, to supplement the regular channels by reaching some parts where the regular channels do not reach, and also to command all the yin and yang collaterals of the whole body.

The superficial collaterals are those collaterals running superficially and often appear in the surface. They are distributed widely without fixed region, playing roles of communication among the channels and transporting qi and blood onto the body surface. The minute collaterals are the tiniest and smallest collaterals distributed all over the body and numerous in the number. They are the sub-branches of the collaterals.

5. Twelve Muscle Regions　The twelve muscle regions are the system of tendons, muscles and joints where the qi of the twelve regular channels "concentrate, accumulate, distribute and connect". Their distribution is similar to the twelve regular channels. Muscles and tendons of the whole body can be divided into three yin and three yang of the hand and foot according to their distribution. In general, muscle regions originate at the extremities and converge at the bones and joints. Some of them enter the chest or abdominal cavity. However, they do not connect with *zang-fu* organs like the regular channels. The twelve muscle regions maintain the integrity of the body by connecting the limbs and the bones of the body, govern the movement of the joints and allow the movement of the body.

6. Twelve Cutaneous Regions　The twelve cutaneous regions are the segments of the skin that are under the influence of a particular channel. They reflect the functional activities of the twelve regular channels, and also are the locations where the channel qi distributes. The cutaneous regions protect the body against invasion of exterior pathogenic factors. They are also very important in diagnosis as they represent the areas on the skin where the qi of the internal organs and channels manifests outwardly.

II. Acupuncture Point

i. Concept of the Acupuncture Point

Acupuncture points, "*shù xué*,腧穴" in Chinese, refer to specific sites where qi and blood of *zang-fu* organs

一条络脉，加上躯干后的督脉络、躯干前的任脉络以及躯干侧的脾之大络，称为"十五络脉"。十五络脉的主要功能是加强相为表里的两条经脉之间在体表的联系，通达某些正经所没有到达的部位，可补正经之不足，还具有统领周身阴阳诸络的作用。

此外，从络脉分出、浮行于浅表的络脉称为"浮络"，其分布广泛，没有定位，起着沟通经脉，输达肌表的作用。最细小的络脉称为"孙络"，孙络分布全身，难计其数。

5. 十二经筋　十二经筋是十二经脉之气"结、聚、散、络"于筋肉、关节的体系，其分布范围与十二经脉大体一致，也分成手足三阴三阳。经筋均起于四肢末端，结聚于骨骼和关节部位，有的进入胸腹腔，但不像经脉那样络属脏腑。经筋有连缀四肢百骸、主司关节运动的作用。

6. 十二皮部　十二皮部是指与十二经脉相应的皮肤部分，是十二经脉在体表的功能活动部位，也是络脉之气血的散布所在。皮部具有抗御外邪、反映病证和协助诊断的作用。

二、腧穴

（一）腧穴的概念

腧，通"输"，意为转输、输注；穴，有孔、隙之意。腧穴是人体脏腑经络之气血输

as well as channels are transported to the surface of the body. "*Shù*" means to transport while "*xué*" means hole or valley.

Acupuncture points are not only sites where qi and blood are transported to the body surface, but they are also reflecting places of disorders, and sites to receive the stimulation by acupuncture, acupressure, cupping and moxibustion. Therefore, acupuncture of these points may help to promote flow of qi and blood in *zang-fu* organs, and regulate the balance between yin and yang so as to achieve the purpose of disease prevention and treatment.

ii. Classification of the Point

Points are generally classified into three groups, namely: channel points, extra points and *ashi* points.

1. Channel Point　Channel points, which are collectively known as "points of the fourteen channels", refer to the points that are distributed along the course of the twelve regular channels as well as *Ren Mai* and *Du Mai*. There are 361 of them in total. Each channel point has its definite name, fixed location and specific indications.

2. Extra Point　Extra points refer to the points that have definite name, fixed location and specific indications but are not recognized as points of the fourteen channels. They are also known as "extra points outside the channels". Extra points are very effective for treatment of some specific disorders.

3. *Ashi* point　*Ashi* points refer to the points that have neither the definite name nor fixed location, but are used for acupuncture and moxibustion by means of the tender spots or other reflecting spots. *Ashi* points are usually located near to the affected areas. Acupuncture of these points may serve to dredge the channel for treatment of diseases.

iii. Effect of the Point

Since they are sites where qi and blood are transported and stimulation spots for acupuncture and moxibustion used for prevention and treatment of diseases, points have the function of receiving stimulation, preventing and treating diseases. The stimulation of points by acupuncture and moxibustion may dredge the channel, regulate the flow of qi and blood, restore balance between yin and yang, and harmonize *zang-fu* organs so as to achieve the purpose of strengthening the healthy qi and eliminating the pathogenic qi.

1. Local Therapeutic Effect　This means that all points can treat the disorders of adjacent locations.

注于体表的特殊部位。

腧穴是气血输注的部位、疾病的反应部位，又是针刺、穴位按压、拔罐、艾灸等方法的施术部位，刺激腧穴可以促进脏腑气血运行，调和机体阴阳平衡，达到疾病预防和治疗作用。

（二）腧穴的分类

腧穴通常分为经穴、奇穴、阿是穴三大类。

1. **经穴**　经穴，指分布于十二经脉以及任、督二脉的腧穴，总称"十四经穴"，共计361个。经穴都有具体的穴名和固定的位置，分布在十四经循行路线上，有明确的针灸主治证。

2. **奇穴**　奇穴，指未归入十四经穴范围，但是既有明确位置、又有固定穴位名称和治疗作用的腧穴，又称"经外奇穴"。奇穴对某些病证有特殊的治疗作用，多为经验穴。如：四缝穴治小儿疳积等。

3. **阿是穴**　阿是穴，指没有固定位置和具体名称，只是以压痛点或其他反应点作为针灸施术的部位，又称不定穴。阿是穴大多位于病变附近，针刺后可疏通经气，达到治疗作用。

（三）腧穴的主治作用

腧穴是气血输注的部位、针灸防治疾病的刺激点，有接受刺激、预防治疗疾病的作用。针刺腧穴，可以通经络、调气血、平衡阴阳、调和脏腑，达到扶正祛邪的治疗目的。

1. **近治作用**　近治作用，指每一个腧穴都能治疗其所在部位及邻近部位的病证。近

Local therapeutic effect is a characteristic property shared by all three groups of points. For example, BL 1(*jīng míng*), ST 1(*chéng qì*) and ST 2(*sì bái*) located around the eyes can be used for treatment of ophthalmic diseases.

2. Remote Therapeutic Effect　This means that some points are effective not only for disorders of adjacent location, but also effective for disorders of remote locations on the course of their pertaining channels. The remote therapeutic effect is a property of the channel points and especially those points of the twelve regular channels located distally to the elbow and knee joints. For example, LI 4(*hé gǔ*) not only serves to treat diseases of the upper limbs, but also diseases of the neck, head and face.

3. Special Therapeutic Effect　In addition to the local and remote therapeutic effects, points are also of some other special effects, namely: bi-directional regulation, general regulation and other relatively specific effects.

(1) The bi-directional regulation effect means that some points have the bi-directional regulation function. For example, ST 25 (*tiān shū*) may be used to relieve constipation for treatment of constipation, and relieve diarrhea for treatment of diarrhea.

(2) The general regulation effect means that some points may serve to treat general disorders. These points are usually located along the course of yangming channels, and Ren and Du channels.

(3) The relatively specific effect means that some points may be specifically effective for treatment of certain diseases. For example, EX-LE7 (*lán wěi*) is effective in treating appendicitis.

iv. Method of Locating Point

The methods of locating points refer to the basic methods of determining the locations of points. Commonly used methods include the following three: measurement with anatomic landmarks, measurement with bone-length proportional units, and measurement with fingers.

1. Measurement with Anatomic Landmark This is a method for locating points by referring to the anatomic landmarks on the body surface. Anatomic landmarks may be divided into two types of fixed and moving ones.

(1) Fixed anatomic landmarks: Fixed anatomic landmarks include the five sensory organs, hair, nails, nipples, umbilicus, and prominences and depressions of bones and muscles. These obviously found landmarks can be used directly to locate points. For example, EX-HN

治作用又称为局部作用，是经穴、奇穴、阿是穴共同具有的特点。例如：眼区的睛明、承泣、四白各穴都能治疗眼病。

2. 远治作用　远治作用，指某些腧穴不仅能治局部病证，而且能治本经循行所到达的远隔部位的病证。远治作用又称为循经作用，是经穴尤其十二经脉在四肢肘、膝关节以下的腧穴的主治特点。例如：合谷穴，不仅能治疗上肢病证，而且还能治疗颈部和头面部病证。

3. 特殊作用　除近治作用、远治作用之外，腧穴还具有双向调整、整体调整和相对特异治疗的作用。

（1）双向调整作用：指针刺某些腧穴对机体的不同状态，可以起到双向的良性调整作用。例如：天枢穴，便秘时针刺可通便，泄泻时针刺可止泻。

（2）整体调整作用：指针刺某些腧穴可以起到调治全身性病证的作用，这些腧穴多见于手足阳明经穴和任督二脉经穴。

（3）相对特异治疗作用：指有些腧穴的治疗作用具有相对的特异性。例如：阑尾穴可治阑尾炎。

（四）腧穴的定位方法

腧穴的定位法，指确定腧穴位置的方法，又称为取穴法。常见的方法有解剖标志定位法、骨度分寸定位法、手指同身寸定位法三种。

1. 解剖标志定位法　解剖标志定位法，是以人体解剖标志作为依据来确定穴位位置的方法，又称为自然标志定位法。解剖标志可分为固定标志和活动标志两类。

（1）固定标志定位法：指利用五官、毛发、爪甲、乳头、脐窝、骨节凹凸、肌肉隆起等固定标志来取穴的方法。例如：两眉之间取穴印堂。

3 (*yìn táng*) is the point located in the center of the two eyebrows.

(2) Moving anatomic landmarks: Moving anatomic landmarks refer to the depressions and folds on the joints, muscles and skin with reference to specific body movements. For example, SI 19 (*tīng gōng*) and GB 2 (*tīng huì*) are located when the mouth opens.

2. Bone-length Proportional Measurement

This is a method by taking the bones and joints of the body as major markers to measure the length and size of certain body parts and then converting their length or size into proportional units based on the measuring criteria for locating points. The proportional measurements of different parts of the body are introduced in table 2-6.

（2）活动标志定位法：指利用关节、肌肉、皮肤随活动而出现的孔隙、凹陷、皱纹等活动标志来取穴的方法。例如：张口取穴听宫、听会。

2. 骨度分寸定位法　骨度分寸定位法，指以骨节为主要标志测量人体周身各部的大小、长短，并依据该尺寸按比例折算作为确定穴位标准的方法，又可称为骨度法。人体周身各部骨度分寸见表 2-6。

Table 2-6　Standards for Bone-Length Proportional Measurement

Portion of the body	Distance	Proportional measurement	Method	Notes
Head	Anterior hairline to posterior hairline	12 cun	Longitudinal measurement	If the anterior and posterior hairlines are indistinguishable, the distance from the glabella to *DU* 14 (*dà zhuī*) is measured as 18 cun. The distance from the glabella to the anterior hairline is taken as 3 cun, and the distance from *DU* 14 (*dà zhuī*) to the posterior hairline is 3 cun
	Between the two frontal angles along hairline	9 cun	Transverse measurement	For locating points on the head by transverse measurement
	Between the two mastoid processes	9 cun		
Chest and abdomen	*RN* 22 (*tiān tū*) to Xiphosternal symphysis	9 cun	Longitudinal measurement	The longitudinal measurement of the chest and hypochondriac region is generally based on the intercostals spaces. Each intercostals space is taken as 1.6 cun [the distance between *RN* 22 (*tiān tū*) and *RN* 21 (*xuán jī*) as 1 cun is an exception]
	Xiphosternal symphysis to center of umbilicus	8 cun		
	Between the center of the umbilicus and the upper border of the symphysis pubis	5 cun		
	Between the two nipples	8 cun	Transverse measurement	For females, the distance between two mid-clavicular lines can be taken as the substitute of the transverse measurement of the two nipples
Back	*DU* 14 (*dà zhuī*) to sacrum	21 vertebra	Longitudinal measurement	The longitudinal measurement of the back is based on the spinous processes of the vertebral column.
	Between the two medial borders of the scapula	6 cun	Transverse measurement	Usually, the lower angle of the scapula is about at the same level of the 7th thoracic spinous process, and the iliac spine is about at the same level as the 4th lumbar spinous process

continued

Portion of the body	Distance	Proportional measurement	Method	Notes
Lateral side of the trunk	Tip of the axillary fossa on the lateral side of the chest to tip of the 11th rib	12 cun	Longitudinal measurement	
	Tip of the 11th rib to prominence of the greater trochanter of femur	9 cun	Longitudinal measurement	
Upper limbs	End of the axillary anterior fold to transverse cubital crease	9 cun	Longitudinal measurement	For locating points of three yin and three yang channels of the hand
	Transverse cubital crease to transverse wrist crease	12 cun		
Lower limbs	Upper border of symphysis pubis to medial condyle of femur	18 cun	Longitudinal measurement	
	Lower border of medial condyle of the tibia to tip of medial malleolus	13 cun	Longitudinal measurement	
	Prominence of the greater trochanter of the femur to popliteal transverse crease	19 cun	Longitudinal measurement	The distance between the transverse creases of the hip to the middle of the patella is measured as 14 cun
	Popliteal transverse crease to tip of lateral malleolus	16 cun		
	Tip of lateral malleolus to sole	3 cun		

表 2-6　常用骨度表

部位	起止点	折量寸	度量法	说明
头部	前发际至后发际	12 寸	直	如前发际不明，从眉心至大椎穴作 18 寸，眉心至前发际 3 寸，大椎穴至后发际 3 寸
	前额两发角之间	9 寸	横	用于量头部的横寸
	耳后两完骨（乳突）之间	9 寸		
胸腹部	天突至歧骨（胸剑联合）	9 寸	直	胸部与胁肋部取穴直寸，一般根据肋骨计算，每一肋骨折作 1.6 寸（天突穴至璇玑穴可作 1 寸，璇玑穴至中庭穴，各穴间可作 1.6 寸计算）
	歧骨至脐中	8 寸		
	脐中至横骨上廉（耻骨联合上缘）	5 寸		
	两乳头之间	8 寸	横	胸腹部取穴横寸，可根据两乳头间的距离折量，女性可用锁骨中线代替

部位	起止点	折量寸	度量法	说明
背腰部	大椎以下至尾椎	21 椎	直	背腰部腧穴以脊椎棘突作为定位标志
	两肩胛骨脊柱缘之间	6 寸	横	一般两肩胛骨下角连线平第 7 胸椎棘突；两髂嵴连线平第 4 腰椎棘突身侧部
身侧部	腋以下至季胁	12 寸	直	季胁此指第 11 肋端下方
	季胁以下至髀枢	9 寸	直	髀枢指股骨大转子高点
上肢部	腋前纹头（腋前皱襞）至肘横纹	9 寸	直	用于手三阴、手三阳经的骨度分寸
	肘横纹至腕横纹	12 寸		
下肢部	横骨上廉至内辅骨上廉	18 寸	直	内辅骨上廉指股骨内侧踝上缘
	内辅骨下廉至内踝尖	13 寸	直	内辅骨下廉指胫骨内侧踝下缘
	髀枢至膝中	19 寸		
	膝中至外踝尖	16 寸	直	臀横纹至膝中，可作 14 寸折量
	外踝尖至足底	3 寸		

3. Finger Measurement　This is a measurement by using the length and width of the patient's finger(s) as a standard to locate points. There are usually three methods: middle finger measurement, thumb measurement and four-finger measurement.

(1) Middle finger measurement: This means that when the patient's middle finger is bent, the distance between the two medial ends of the creases of two interphalangeal joints is taken as one cun.

(2) Thumb finger measurement: This means that the width of the interphalangeal joint of the patient's thumb is taken as one cun.

(3) Four-finger measurement: This means that when the patient's four fingers (index, middle, ring and little fingers) extend and touch closely together, the width of the four fingers at the level of the crease of the proximal interphalangeal joint of the middle finger is taken as three cun.

v. Common-used Points

Each point is of its own relatively extensive indications. The locations, indications of the common-used points are listed in table 2-7.

3. 手指同身寸定位法　手指同身寸定位法，指以患者的手指为尺寸折量标准来量取穴位的方法，又可称为手指比量法和指寸法。常用的手指同身寸有以下三种：

（1）中指同身寸：以患者的中指中节屈曲时，内侧两端横纹间距离作为 1 寸量取穴位。

（2）拇指同身寸：以患者的拇指骨关节的横纹宽度作为 1 寸量取穴位。

（3）横指同身寸：令患者示指、中指、无名指、小指四指并拢，以中指中节近端横纹为标准，四指宽度为 3 寸量取穴位。

（五）常用穴位

每个腧穴都有较为广泛的主治范围。常用腧穴的定位、主治见表 2-7。

Table 2-7　Common-used Points

Channel	Point	Location	Indications
Hand *Taiyin* Lung Channel	LU 5 (*chǐ zé*)	On the cubital crease, at the lateral side of the tendon of biceps brachii	Spasmodic pain in the elbow and arm, cough, asthma, distending pain of the chest and rib-side, infantile convulsion
	LU 6 (*kǒng zuì*)	7 cun above the wrist crease, on the line joining LU 9 (*tài yuān*) and LU 5 (*chǐ zé*)	Cough, hemoptysis, hoarseness, sore-throat and pain in the elbow and arm
	LU 7 (*liè quē*)	1.5 cun above the transverse crease of the wrist, above the styloid process of the radius	Cough, shortness of breath, rigid neck and headache, toothache
	LU 9 (*tài yuān*)	At the radial end of the transverse crease of the wrist and in the depression on the radial side of the radial artery	Cough, asthma, distension of breast, sore-throat and pain of the wrist
	LU 10 (*yú jì*)	On the midpoint of the 1st metacarpal bone, at the junction of the white and red skin	Pain in the chest and back, headache, dizziness, sore-throat, fever and aversion to cold
	LU 11 (*shào shāng*)	On the radial side of the thumb, 0.1 cun posterior to the corner of the nail	Faint due to apoplexy, spasmodic pain in the fingers and infantile convulsion
Hand *Yangming* Large Intestine Channel	LI 4 (*hé gǔ*)	Between the 1st and 2nd metacarpal bones, on the midpoint of the 2nd metacarpal bone	Headache, toothache, fever, sore-throat, spasmodic pain of fingers; pain of arm and distorted face
	LI 10 (*shǒu sān lǐ*)	2 cun below LI 11 (*qū chí*)	Spasm of elbow, difficulty in stretching and bending the arm, numbness and aching pain of the arm
	LI 11 (*qū chí*)	In the depression lateral to the elbow crease when the elbow is bent	Fever, hypertension, swelling and pain of the arm and paralysis of the upper limbs
	LI 15 (*jiān yú*)	In the depression below the acromion when the arm is raised	Pain of the shoulder, dysfunction of the shoulder joints and paralysis
	LI 20 (*yíng xiāng*)	0.5 cun lateral to the nose and in the naso-labial groove	Rhinitis, nasal obstruction and distorted face
Foot *Yangming* Stomach Channel	ST 2 (*sì bái*)	Directly below the pupil and in the depression at the infraorbital foramen when looking straight forward	Distorted face, redness and itching of eyes
	ST 4 (*dì cāng*)	0.4 cun lateral to the corner of mouth	Drooling and distorted face
	ST 7 (*xià guān*)	In the depression between the zygomatic arch with mandibular notch which is visible when the mouth is open and invisible when the mouth is closed	Facial paralysis and toothache
	ST 8 (*tóu wéi*)	0.5 cun directly above the anterior hairline at the corner of the forehead	Headache
	ST 25 (*tiān shū*)	2 cun lateral to the navel	Diarrhea, constipation, abdominal pain, irregular menstruation
	ST 36 (*zú sān lǐ*)	3 cun below ST 35 (*dú bí*) and one finer-breadth lateral to the anterior border of the tibia	Abdominal pain, diarrhea, constipation, cold numbness of the lower limbs and hypertension
	ST 40 (*fēng lóng*)	On the middle of the line between the lateral part of the knee and the external ankle	Headache, cough, swollen limbs, constipation, mania and epilepsy, and paralysis of the lower limbs

continued

Channel	Point	Location	Indications
Foot *Taiyin* Spleen Channel	SP6 (*sān yīn jiāo*)	3 cun above the tip of the medial malleolus, posterior to the center of the tibial border	Insomnia, abdominal distension, anorexia, enuresis, unsmooth urination, women diseases
	SP 8 (*dì jī*)	3 cun below SP 9 (*yīn líng quán*)	Abdominal pain, diarrhea, edema, unsmooth urination, seminal emission
	SP 9 (*yīn líng quán*)	In the depression posterior and inferior to the medial condyle of the tibia	Aching pain of the knee joints, unsmooth urination
	SP 10 (*xuè hǎi*)	2 cun above the medio-superior border of the patella	Irregular menstruation, aching knees
	SP 15 (*dà héng*)	4 cun lateral to the navel	Diarrhea and dysentery due to deficiency-cold, constipation, lower abdominal pain
Hand *Shaoyin* Heart Channel	HT 1 (*jí quán*)	In the center of armpit	Chest oppression and hypochondriac pain, coldness and numbness of the arm and elbow
	HT 3 (*shào hǎi*)	In the depression at the ulnar side of the elbow crease when the elbow is bent	Pain of the elbow joint, tremor and spasm of elbow
	HT 5 (*tōng lǐ*)	1 cun above HT 7(*shén mén*)	Palpitation, severe palpitation, vertigo, sore-throat, sudden loss of voice, difficulty to speak due to stiffness of the tongue, pain of wrist and arm
	HT 7 (*shén mén*)	On the radial side of the tendon of the flexor carpi ulnaris and at the transverse crease of the wrist	Palpitation, insomnia and amnesia
Hand *Taiyang* Small Intestine Channel	SI 1 (*shào zé*)	At the lateral to the ulnar side of the small finger, about 0.1 cun posterior to the corner of the nail	Fever, unconsciousness in apoplexy, lack of lactation and sore-throat
	SI 3 (*hòu xī*)	In the depression proximal to the 5th metacarpophalangeal joint, on the junction of the red and white skin	Stiffness and pain in the head and neck, deafness, sore-throat, toothache, cataract and spasmodic pain in the arm and elbow
	SI 9 (*jiān zhēn*)	1 cun posterior to the crease of armpit	Aching pain in the shoulder joint, difficulty in movement, and paralysis of the upper limbs
	SI 11 (*tiān zōng*)	In the centre of the depression of the subscapular fossa	Aching pain of the shoulder and back, difficult movement of the shoulder joint, and stiffness of the neck
Foot *Taiyang* Bladder Channel	BL 1 (*jīng míng*)	0.1 cun lateral to the inner canthus	Eye disorders
	BL 2 (*cuán zhú*)	In the depression proximal to the eyebrow	Headache, insomnia, pain in the orbital bone, and redness of eyes
	BL 10 (*tiān zhù*)	1.3 cun lateral to the DU 15 (*yǎ mén*) and in the depression on the lateral side of the trapezius	Headache, stiff neck, stuffed nose, and pain in the shoulder and back
	BL 11 (*dà zhù*)	1.5 cun inferior to and lateral to the 1st thoracic vertebra	Fever, cough, stiff neck, aching pain in the scapula
	BL 12 (*fēng mén*)	1.5 cun lateral to the 2nd thoracic vertebra	Common cold, cough, stiff neck and pain in the waist and back

Channel	Point	Location	Indications
	BL 13 (fèi shù)	1.5 cun inferior to and lateral to the 3rd thoracic vertebra	Cough, panting, chest oppression, muscular overstrain it the back
	BL 15 (xīn shù)	1.5 cun interior to and lateral to the 5th thoracic vertebra	Insomnia, palpitation
	BL 17 (gé shù)	1.5 cun inferior to and lateral to the 7th thoracic vertebra	Vomiting, dysphagia, panting, cough and night sweating
	BL 18 (gān shù)	1.5 cun inferior to and lateral to the 9th thoracic vertebra	Hypochondriac pain, hepatitis and blurred vision
	BL 19 (dǎn shù)	1.5 cun inferior to and lateral to the 10th thoracic vertebra	Hypochondriac pain, bitter taste in the mouth and jaundice
	BL 20 (pí shù)	1.5 cun inferior to and lateral to the 11th thoracic vertebra	Distending pain in the stomach, dyspepsia and chronic infantile convulsion due to fright
	BL 21 (wèi shù)	1.5 cun inferior to and lateral to the 12th thoracic vertebra	Stomach disease, infantile vomiting of milk and indigestion
Foot *Taiyang* Bladder Channel	BL 22 (sān jiāo shù)	1.5 cun inferior to and lateral to the 1st lumbar vertebra	Borborygmus, abdominal distension, vomiting, and stiffness and pain in the waist and back
	BL 23 (shèn shù)	1.5 cun inferior to and lateral to the 2nd lumbar vertebra	Kidney asthenia, lumbago, seminal emission, irregular menstruation
	BL 24 (qì hǎi shù)	1.5 cun inferior to and lateral to the 3rd lumbar vertebra	Lumbago
	BL 25 (dà cháng shù)	1.5 cun inferior to and lateral to the 4th lumbar vertebra	Pain in the waist and leg, lumbar muscular sprain, intestinal inflammation
	BL 26 (guān yuán shù)	1.5 cun inferior to and lateral to the 5th lumbar vertebra	Lumbago and diarrhea
	BL 32 (cì liáo)	In the second sacral foramina	Pain in the waist and leg, disorders of the urinary and reproductive systems
	BL 54 (zhì biān)	3 cun lateral to and inferior to the 4th sacral foramina	Pain in the waist and thigh, flaccidity of the lower limbs, unsmooth urination, constipation
	BL 60 (kūn lún)	In the depression between internal malleolus and the tendo calcaneus	Headache, stiff neck, lumbago and sprain of ankle
	BL 62 (shēn mài)	In depression at the lower border of the lateral malleolus	Mania and epilepsy, aching pain in the waist and leg
Foot *Shaoyin* Kidney Channel	KI 1 (yǒng quán)	In the depression of the sole	Migraine, hypertension and infantile fever
	KI 3 (tài xī)	In the depression between internal malleolus and the tendo calcaneus	Sore-throat, toothache, insomnia, seminal emission, impotence and irregular menstruation
	KI 6 (zhào hǎi)	In the depression below the medial malleolus	Irregular menstruation

Channel	Point	Location	Indications
Hand *Jueyin* Pericardium Channel	PC 6 (*nèi guān*)	2 cun above the wrist crease and between tendon palmaris longus and tendon of flexor carpi radialis	Stomachache, vomiting, palpitation, mental derangement
	PC 7 (*dà líng*)	In the middle of the wrist crease and between tendon palmaris longus and tendon of flexor carpi radialis	Stomachache, palpitation, stomachache, vomiting, epilepsy and pain in the chest and hypochondrium
	PC 8 (*láo gōng*)	In the palmar crease and between the second and third metacarpal bone	Palpitation and tremor
Hand *Shaoyang* Sanjiao Channel	SJ 3 (*zhōng zhǔ*)	In the depression at the lower border of the fourth and fifth between the metacarpal bone	Migraine, inflexibility of the fingers, and pain of the elbow and arm
	SJ 4 (*yáng chí*)	On the transverse crease of the dorsum of wrist and on the ulnar side of the tendon of the extensor digitorum communis	Pain of the shoulder and wrist, malaria, consumptive disease and deafness
	SJ 5 (*wài guān*)	2 cun above the dorsal crease of the wrist and between the radius and ulna	Headache, pain and inflexibility of the elbow, arm and fingers
	SJ 14 (*jiān liáo*)	Inferior to the acromion and in the depression about 1 cun posterior to SJ 14 (*jiān liáo*)	Aching pain of the shoulder and arm, difficult movement of the shoulder joint
Foot *Shaoyang* Gall Bladder Channel	GB 20 (*fēng chí*)	Between musculi sternocleidomastoideus and trapezius muscle, parallel to DU 16 (*fēng fǔ*)	Migraine, headache, common cold and stiff neck
	GB 21 (*jiān jǐng*)	On the middle of the line between DU 14 (*dà zhuī*) and acromion	Stiff neck, pain of shoulder and back, difficulty to raise hands
	GB 30 (*huán tiào*)	On the point 1/3 lateral and 2/3 median of the line between the Greater trochanter of femur and sacral hiatus	Lumbago, leg pain and paralysis
	GB 31 (*fēng shì*)	On the middle point lateral to the high and 7 cun above the popliteal crease	Paralysis, aching pain of the knee joints
	GB 34 (*yáng líng quán*)	In the depression anterior and inferior to capitulum fibulae	Aching pain of the knee joints and hypochondriac pain
	GB 37 (*guāng míng*)	5 cun above the external ankle and on the posterior border of the fibula	Aching knees, pain of the lower limbs, pain of eyes, night blindness and breast distension
	GB 40 (*qiū xū*)	Anterior and inferior to the external ankle, in the depression lateral to the tendon of long extensor muscle of toe	Pain of the ankle joint, chest and hypochondrium
	GB 41 (*zú lín qì*)	On the dorsum of foot and 1.5 cun above the crease of the fourth and fifth toes	Scrofula, hypochondriac pain, foot swelling, pain and spasm
Foot *Jueyin* Liver Channel	LV 3 (*tài chōng*)	On the dorsum of foot, in the depression between the first and the second metatarsal bone	Headache, vertigo, hypertension and infantile convulsion
	LV 5 (*lí gōu*)	5 cun above the internal ankle and on middle of the median side of the tibia	Unsmooth urination, irregular menstruation, flaccidity of tibia
	LV 13 (*zhāng mén*)	At the end of the 11ᵗʰ rib	Pain of chest and hypochondrium, chest oppression
	LV 14 (*qī mén*)	Directly below the nipple and the sixth costal space	Chest and hypochondriac pain

continued

Channel	Point	Location	Indications
Ren Mai	RN 4 (*guān yuán*)	3 cun below the navel	Abdominal pain, dysmenorrheal and enuresis
	RN 6 (*qì hǎi*)	1.5 cun below the navel	Abdominal pain, irregular menstruation, enuresis
	RN 12 (*zhōng wǎn*)	4 cun above the navel	Stomachache, abdominal distension, vomiting, and indigestion
	RN 17 (*dàn zhōng*)	On the front midline and parallel to the 4th costal space	Cough, asthma, chest oppression and pain
Du Mai	DU 1 (*cháng qiáng*)	0.5 cun below the point of sacrum	Diarrhea, constipation and proctoptosis
	DU 4 (*mìng mén*)	Below the second lumbar vertebral spinous process	Pain of the waist and spine
	DU 14 (*dà zhuī*)	Below the 7th vertebral spinous process	Common cold, fever and stiff neck
	DU 16 (*fēng fǔ*)	1 cun directly above the middle of the posterior hairline	Headache and stiff neck
	DU 20 (*bǎi huì*)	7 cun directly above the middle of the posterior hairline	Headache, vertigo, coma, hypertension and prolapse of anus
	DU 26 (*shuǐ gōu*)	On the middle point 1/3 above and 2/3 below the nasolabial groove	Convulsion and distorted face
Extra Points	EX-HN 3 (*yìn táng*)	On the middle of the line between the brows	Headache, rhinitis and insomnia
	EX-HN 5 (*tài yáng*)	In the depression 1 cun posterior to the point between the brow and the outer canthus	Headache, common cold and eye problems
	EX-HN 4 (*yú yāo*)	Middle of the brows	Pain of the orbital bone, redness and pain of eyes, tremor of the eyelids
	EX-B 7 (*yāo yǎn*)	In the depression 3.5 cun lateral and below the fourth lumbar vertebral spinous process	Lumbar sprain and ache of the waist and back
	EX-B 2 (*jiā jǐ*)	0.5 cun below the first to the 5th thoracic and vertebral spinous process	Painful and stiff spine, visceral disease
	EX-UE 11 (*shí xuān*)	Tips of the ten fingers, 0.1 cun to the nails	Coma
	EX-LE 2 (*hè dǐng*)	In the depression on the middle of the upper border of patella	Swelling and pain of knee joint
	EX-LE 6 (*dǎn náng*)	1 cun directly below GB34 (*yáng líng quán*)	Colic of gallbladder
	EX-LE 7 (*lán wěi*)	2 cun below ST 36 (*zú sān lǐ*)	Appendicitis and abdominal pain

表 2-7　常用腧穴表

经络	穴名	位置	主治
手太阴肺经	尺泽	肘横纹中，肱二头肌腱桡侧	肘臂挛痛、咳喘、胸胁胀痛、小儿惊风
	孔最	在尺泽与太渊连线上，腕横纹上 7 寸	咳嗽、咯血、音哑、咽喉痛、肘臂痛
	列缺	桡骨茎突上方，腕横纹上 1.5 寸	咳嗽、气急、头项强痛、牙痛
	太渊	腕横纹桡侧端，桡动脉桡侧凹陷中	咳嗽、气喘、乳胀、咽喉痛、手腕痛
	鱼际	第一掌骨中点，赤白肉际	胸背痛、头痛、眩晕、喉痛、发热恶寒
	少商	拇指桡侧指甲角旁约 0.1 寸	中风昏仆、手指挛痛、小儿惊风
手阳明大肠经	合谷	手背，第一、二掌骨之间，约平第二掌骨中点处	头痛、牙痛、发热、喉痛、指挛、臂痛、口眼㖞斜
	手三里	曲池穴下 2 寸	肘挛、屈伸不利、手臂麻木酸痛
	曲池	屈肘，当肘横纹外端凹陷中	发热、高血压、手臂肿痛、肘痛、上肢瘫痪
	肩髃	肩峰前下方，举臂时呈凹陷处	肩膀痛、肩关节活动障碍、偏瘫
	迎香	鼻翼旁 0.5 寸，鼻唇沟中	鼻炎、鼻塞、口眼㖞斜
足阳明胃经	四白	目正视、瞳孔直下，当眶下孔凹陷中	口眼㖞斜、目赤痛痒
	地仓	口角旁 0.4 寸	流涎、口眼㖞斜
	下关	颧弓与下颌切迹之间的凹陷中，合口有孔，张口即闭	面瘫、牙痛
	头维	额角发际直上 0.5 寸	头痛
	天枢	脐旁 2 寸	腹泻、便秘、腹痛、月经不调
	足三里	犊鼻穴下 3 寸，胫骨前棘外一横指处	腹痛、腹泻、便秘、下肢冷麻、高血压
	丰隆	外膝眼与外侧踝尖连线中点	头痛、咳嗽、肢肿、便秘、狂病、下肢痿痹
足太阴脾经	三阴交	内踝上 3 寸，胫骨内侧面的中央	失眠、腹胀纳呆、遗尿、小便不利、妇科病
	地机	阴陵泉下 3 寸	腹痛、泄泻、水肿、小便不利、遗精
	阴陵泉	胫骨内侧髁下缘凹陷中	膝关节酸痛、小便不利
	血海	髌骨内上方 2 寸	月经不调、膝痛
	大横	脐中旁开 4 寸	虚寒泻痢、大便秘结、小腹痛
手少阴心经	极泉	腋窝正中	胸闷胁痛，臂肘冷麻
	少海	屈肘，当肘横纹尺侧端凹陷中	肘关节痛、手颤肘挛
	通里	神门穴上 1 寸	心悸、怔忡、头晕、咽痛、暴暗、舌强不语、腕臂痛
	神门	腕横纹尺侧端，尺侧腕屈肌腱的桡侧凹陷中	惊悸、怔忡、失眠、健忘
手太阳小肠经	少泽	小指尺侧指甲角一旁约 0.1 寸	发热、中风昏迷、乳少、咽喉肿痛
	后溪	第五掌指关节后尺侧、横纹头赤白肉	头项强痛、耳聋、咽痛、齿痛、目翳、肘臂挛痛
	肩贞	腋后纹头上 1 寸	肩关节酸痛、活动不便、上肢瘫痪
	天宗	肩胛骨冈下窝的中央	肩背酸痛、肩关节活动不便、项强

经络	穴名	位置	主治
	睛明	目内眦旁 0.1 寸	眼病
	攒竹	眉头凹陷中	头痛失眠、眉棱骨痛、目赤痛
	天柱	后发际正中直上 0.5 寸（哑门穴），旁开 1.3 寸，当斜方肌外缘凹陷中	头痛、项强、鼻塞、肩背痛
	大杼	第一胸椎棘突下，旁开 1.5 寸	发热，咳嗽、项强、肩脚酸痛
	风门	第二胸椎棘突下，旁开 1.5 寸	伤风、咳嗽、项强、腰背痛
	肺俞	第三胸椎棘突下，旁开 1.5 寸	咳嗽气喘、胸闷、背肌劳损
	心俞	第五胸椎棘突下，旁开 1.5 寸	失眠，心悸
	膈俞	第七胸椎棘突下，旁开 1.5 寸	呕吐、噎隔气喘、咳嗽、盗汗
	肝俞	第九胸椎棘突下，旁开 1.5 寸	胁肋痛、肝炎、目疾
	胆俞	第十胸椎棘突下，旁开 1.5 寸	胁肋痛、口苦、黄疸
足太阳膀胱经	脾俞	第十一胸椎棘突下，旁开 1.5 寸	胃脘胀痛、消化不良、小儿慢惊风证
	胃俞	第十二胸椎棘突下，旁开 1.5 寸	胃病、小儿吐乳、消化不良
	三焦俞	第一腰椎棘突下，旁开 1.5 寸	肠鸣、腹胀、呕吐、腰背强痛
	肾俞	第二腰椎棘突下，旁开 1.5 寸	肾虚、腰痛、遗精、月经不调
	气海俞	第三腰椎棘突下旁开 1.5 寸	腰痛
	大肠俞	第四腰椎棘突下，旁开 1.5 寸	腰腿痛、腰肌劳损、肠炎
	关元俞	第五腰椎棘突下，旁开 1.5 寸	腰痛、泄泻
	次髎	在第二骶后孔中	腰腿痛、泌尿生殖系疾患
	秩边	第 4 骶椎棘突下，旁开 3 寸	腰臀痛、下肢痿痹、小便不利、便秘
	昆仑	外踝与跟腱之间凹陷中	头痛、项强、腰痛、踝关节扭伤
	申脉	外踝下缘凹陷中	癫狂痫、腰腿酸痛
	涌泉	足底中、足趾跖屈时呈凹陷处	偏头痛、高血压、小儿发热
足少阴肾经	太溪	内踝与跟腱之间凹陷中	喉痛、齿痛、不寐、遗精、阳痿、月经不调
	照海	内踝下缘凹陷中	月经不调
	内关	腕横纹上 2 寸，掌长肌腱与桡侧腕屈肌腱之间	胃痛、呕吐、心悸、精神失常
手厥阴心包经	大陵	腕横纹中央，掌长肌腱与桡侧腕屈肌腱之间	心痛、心悸、胃痛、呕吐、癫痫、胸胁痛
	劳宫	手掌心横纹中，第二、三掌骨之间	心悸、颤抖
	中渚	握拳第四、五掌骨小头后缘之间凹陷中	偏头痛、掌指痛屈伸不利、肘臂痛
手少阳三焦经	阳池	腕背横纹中、指总伸肌腱尺侧缘凹陷中	肩臂痛、腕痛、疟疾、消渴、耳聋
	外关	腕背横纹上 2 寸，桡骨与尺骨之间	头痛、肘臂手指痛、屈伸不利
	肩髎	肩峰外下方，肩髃穴后寸许凹陷中	肩臂酸痛、肩关节活动不便

经络	穴名	位置	主治
足少阳胆经	风池	胸锁乳突肌与斜方肌之间，平风府穴（后发际正中直上1寸）	偏正头痛、感冒项强
	肩井	大椎穴与肩峰连线的中点	项强、肩背痛、手臂上举不便
	环跳	股骨大转子与骶裂孔连线的外1/3与内2/3交界处	腰腿痛、偏瘫
	风市	大腿外侧中间，腘横纹水平线上7寸	偏瘫、膝关节酸痛
	阳陵泉	腓骨小头前下方凹陷中	膝关节酸痛、胁肋痛
	光明	外踝上5寸，腓骨前缘	膝痛、下肢疾痹、目痛、夜盲、乳胀
	丘墟	外踝前下方，趾长伸肌腱外侧凹陷中	踝关节痛、胸胁痛
	足临泣	足背，第四、五趾间缝纹端上1.5寸	瘰疬、胁肋痛、足跗肿痛、足趾挛痛
足厥阴肝经	太冲	足背，第一、二跖骨底之间凹陷中	头痛、眩晕、高血压、小儿惊风
	蠡沟	内踝上5寸，胫骨内侧面的中央	小便不利、月经不调、足胫痿痹
	章门	第十一肋端	胸胁痛、胸闷
	期门	乳头直下、第六肋间隙	胸胁痛
任脉	关元	脐下3寸，前正中线上	腹痛、痛经、遗尿
	气海	脐下1.5寸	腹痛、月经不调、遗尿
	中脘	脐上4寸	胃痛、腹胀、呕吐、消化不良
	膻中	前正中线，平第四肋间隙处	咳喘、胸闷、胸痛
督脉	长强	尾骨尖下0.5寸	腹泻、便秘、脱肛
	命门	第二腰椎棘突下	腰脊疼痛
	大椎	第七颈椎棘突下	感冒、发热、落枕
	风府	后发际正中直上1寸	头痛、项强
	百会	后发际正中直上7寸	头痛、头晕、昏厥、高血压、脱肛
	水沟（人中）	人中沟正中线上1/3与下2/3交界处	惊风、口眼㖞斜
经外奇穴	印堂	两眉头连线的中点	头痛、鼻炎、失眠
	太阳	眉梢与目外眦之间向后约1寸处凹陷中	头痛、感冒、眼病
	鱼腰	眉毛的中点	眉棱骨痛、目赤肿痛、眼睑瞤动
	腰眼	第四腰椎棘突下，旁开3.5寸凹陷处	腰扭伤、腰背酸楚
	夹脊	第一胸椎至第五腰椎，各椎棘突下旁开0.5寸	脊柱疼痛强直、脏腑疾患及强壮作用
	十宣	十手指尖端，距指甲0.1寸	昏厥
	鹤顶	髌骨上缘正中凹陷处	膝关节肿痛
	阑尾	足三里穴下约2寸处	阑尾炎、腹痛
	胆囊	阳陵泉直下1寸	胆绞痛

(Ma Xue-ling)　　　　　　　　　　　（马雪玲）

Key Points

1. The theory of yin-yang studies the connotation, movement and change laws of yin-yang. It is the world outlook and methodology by which people understand and explain the occurrence, development and changes of things and phenomena in nature.

2. The concept of yin-yang is abstracted into a general division of any given thing (including living things, inanimate objects, feelings, actions, *etc.*) into two polar attributes that are related to each other.

3. The theory of yin-yang mainly includes four basic contents of opposition and restriction, interdependence and reciprocity, wane-wax and balance, and mutual transformation of yin and yang.

4. Five phases theory studies the connotation, feature and the laws of promotion, restriction, subjugation, and violation of the five phases: wood, fire, earth, metal and water. It is an ancient Chinese philosophy theory by which people understand and explain the occurrence, development and changes of things and phenomena in nature.

5. Five phases actually refer to the movement and transformation of these five phases as well as their relationships.

6. Wood is characterized by bending and straightening. Fire is the flaming upward. Earth is the sowing and reaping. Water is the moistening and descending. Metal is the working of change.

7. The theory of visceral manifestation is a theory covering the conception of viscera and manifestations, the morphological structure and physio-pathology of *zang-fu* organs, as well as the relationship among various *zang-fu* organs, or the relationship among *zang-fu* organs and the organism, Jing, qi, blood, body fluid, as well as the natural and social environment.

8. *Zang* is the intrinsic base of xiang and xiang is the external manifestations of *zang*. According to their characteristics of morphological structure and functions, the internal organs can be divided into *zang* organs, *fu* organs and extraordinary *fu* organs.

9. *Zang* organs include the heart, lung, spleen, liver and kidney, which collectively are called the five *zang* organs. Their common functions are to produce and store essence-qi, meanwhile store spirit, and their characteristics are that "they can be full of essence-qi instead of containing food".

10. *Fu* organs include the gallbladder, stomach, small intestine, large intestine, *sanjiao* and the urinary bladder, collectively called the six *fu* organs. Their common functions are to receive, digest and transmit the food, and their characteristics are that "they can be full of food

要点

1. 阴阳学说研究阴阳的内涵、运动和变化规律。它是人们认识和阐释自然界中事物和现象的发生、发展和变化的世界观和方法论。

2. 阴阳的概念被抽象为宇宙间相互关联的事物或现象（包括有生物、事物、情感、动作等）对立双方属性的概括。

3. 阴阳学说包括阴阳对立制约、互根互用、消长平衡和相互转化四个基本内容。

4. 五行学说研究的是木、火、土、金、水的内涵特征，以及相生、相克、相乘、相侮关系。它是人们认识和阐释自然界中事物和现象的发生、发展和变化的一种古代哲学理论。

5. 五行实际上研究的是五行的运动变化及其相互关系。

6. 木曰曲直，火曰炎上，土爰稼穑，水曰润下，金曰从革。

7. 藏象学说是研究藏象的概念，脏腑的形态结构与生理病理，脏腑之间，以及脏腑与形体官窍、精气血津液、自然社会之间的相互关系的理论。

8. "藏"是"象"的内在基础，"象"是"藏"的外在表现。根据其形态结构和功能特点，内脏可分为脏、腑和奇恒之腑。

9. 脏，即心、肺、脾、肝、肾，合称为五脏，其共同的功能是化生和贮藏精气，这一特点被概括为"藏精气而不泻"。

10. 腑，即胆、胃、小肠、大肠、三焦和膀胱，合称为六腑，其共同的功能是受盛、传化水谷，这一特点被概括为"传化物而不藏"。

instead of storing essence-qi".

11. The extraordinary *fu* organs are the brain, marrow, bone, vessel, gallbladder and uterus. Their physiological characteristics are to store the essence-qi, like the five *zang* organs, but their shapes are mostly hollow like the six fu organs. Their shapes and functions are distinctly different to five *zang* and six *fu*, thus being called as "extraordinary *fu* organs".

12. The essence, qi, blood and body fluid are the basic substances that constitute the human body and maintain its life activity. They are produced by the functional activities of the viscera, channels, tissues and organs.

13. Pathogenic factors refers to the cause of diseases, mainly including the externally-contracted six pathogenic factors, seven emotions, improper diet, overstrain and over ease, phlegm retention and blood stasis, of which the latter two are pathological outcome of disorder of *zang-fu* organs.

14. Pathomechanism refers to the fundamental mechanism of the onset, development and progress of the disease. TCM holds that diseases are complicated and changeable, but their pathological processes generally fall into several types of struggle between the healthy qi and the pathogenic qi, imbalance of yin and yang, disorder of qi and blood, disorder of metabolism of body fluid and so on.

15. The channel system connects internally with zang-fu organs and externally with the tendons, muscles and skin. Channels and collaterals together assume the responsibility of circulating qi and blood, communicating so as to connect all the viscera, organs, orifices, skin, muscles, tendons and bones to form an integral organic whole.

16. The methods of locating points refer to the basic methods of determining the locations of points. Commonly used methods include the following three: measurement with anatomic landmarks, measurement with bone-length proportional units, and measurement with fingers.

11. 奇恒之腑包括脑、髓、骨、脉、胆和女子胞。它们的生理特点是贮藏精气，与五脏相似，形态上中空有腔，与六腑相似，似脏非脏，似腑非腑，与五脏和六腑都有明显区别，故被称为"奇恒之腑"。

12. 精、气、血、津液是构成人体和维持生命活动的基本物质，是由脏腑、经络及组织器官功能活动所化生。

13. 病因，是指引起人体发生疾病的原因（又称致病因素），主要包括六淫、七情、饮食、劳逸、痰饮和瘀血等，其中痰饮和瘀血是脏腑病理产物形成的病因。

14. 发病机制即病机，是指疾病发生、发展与变化的机理。中医学认为尽管疾病种类繁多，表现错综复杂，但究其根本，都不外乎邪正盛衰、阴阳失调、气血失常、津液代谢障碍等方面。

15. 经络系统在内连属于脏腑，在外连属于筋肉、皮肤。经脉和络脉共同担负着运行气血，联络沟通等作用，把人体所有的脏腑、器官、孔窍以及皮肉筋骨等组织联结成一个统一的有机整体。

16. 腧穴的定位法，指确定腧穴位置的方法（又称为取穴法）。常见的取穴方法有解剖标志定位法、骨度分寸定位法、手指同身寸定位法三种。

Chapter 3 Basic Characteristic and Principle of TCM Nursing

第三章 中医护理的基本特点和原则

Learning Objectives

Mastery

1. To accurately summarize the basic contents of the "holistic concept", the concept and significance of "nursing determination based on pattern differentiation".

2. To correctly describe the concept of "treat heat with the heat" "treat cold with the cold" "treat the blocked by blocking" "treat the flowing by promoting its flow" "the same disease can be treated in many different ways" and "many different diseases can be treated in the same way".

3. To correctly describe the concept, contents and significance of "preventing disease before it arises".

4. To accurately summarize the basic principle of "nursing suitable for the season, locality and individual".

Comprehension

1. To use the examples to illustrate the relationship between human and nature, and human and society.

2. To distinguish the concept of disease, pattern and symptoms.

学习目标

识记

1. 能复述整体观念的基本内容、辨证施护的概念和意义。

2. 能复述热因热用、寒因寒用、塞因塞用、通因通用、异病同护和同病异护的概念。

3. 能复述治未病的概念、内容和基本原则。

4. 能复述三因制宜的基本原则。

理解

1. 能用实例说明人与自然界、社会相统一。

2. 能正确区分病、证和症的概念。

3. To use the examples to demonstrate the guiding principle of "paradoxical assistant".

Application

To use the knowledge that has been learned in this chapter to analyze and review the concept of holism and the significance of nursing determination based on pattern differentiation in clinical nursing practice.

3. 能用实例说明中医护理学反护法的指导原则。

运用

能运用本章所学的知识进行分析、评论整体观念和辨证施护在护理实践中的意义。

Case Study

Patient, female, 58 years old, makes a living by selling diner in the outdoors. She always has to work extra hours and tiredly go back home late. She saw a doctor because of the symptoms of fever and sore throat. Her axillary temperature was 38.0℃, and the fever got aggravated in the evening. She has the symptoms of aversion to cold, limbs cold and sweating-out. She complained of sore throat, poor appetite, restlessness, and sleep loss. And she always felt backache and fatigue. She urinates normally and her bowel movements are normal. She has the symptoms of red tongue with thin tongue fur and pulse rapid floating, hyperaemia and edema in the throat accompanied by the mild swelling in the local lymph nodes. Diagnosis: pharyngitis and laryngitis; yin deficiency with lack of moisture in the throat.

Question 1. According to the patient's condition, please give the TCM dialectical nursing.

Question 2. What nursing principle should be followed when caring the patient?

Question 3. What nursing measures should be given to the patient?

TCM nursing is based on the theory of TCM under the guidance of holistic concept, which is to take care of patients with the method of dialectical nursing, and to protect, maintain and restore human health with unique nursing technology. With the development of the society and the vigorous improvement of TCM, TCM nursing formed a unique theoretical system gradually.

导入案例与思考

患者，女，58 岁，一年四季经营户外快餐车，平素早出晚归。患者因发热、咽喉部疼痛而就诊。患者发热（腋温 38.0℃），晚间明显，稍有恶寒，肢冷，有汗出，自述咽干、喉部疼痛，饮食不佳，心烦少寐，平素腰痛，常常自感神疲乏力，二便尚可；查患者舌淡红，脉浮数；喉部水肿、充血，局部淋巴结轻度肿大。诊断：咽、喉炎，中医辨证：阴虚咽喉失濡证。

问题 1：根据患者的病情，请给出其中医护理辨证。

问题 2：针对患者的病情，应遵循什么护治原则？

问题 3：应为患者采取哪些护理措施？

中医护理学是以中医理论为基础，在整体观念指导下，运用辨证施护的方法，对患者加以照料，并施以独特的护理技术，以保护、维持、恢复人类健康。随着社会的进步，中医药事业的蓬勃发展，中医护理逐步形成了独具特色的护理理论体系。

Section 1　Basic Characteristic of TCM Nursing

TCM nursing faithfully adheres to theoretical system of TCM, inherits and develops the basic theory of TCM, namely "concept of holism" and "treatment based on pattern differentiation". TCM nursing formed the characteristics of "concept of holism" and "nursing determination based on pattern differentiation".

I. Concept of Holism

Concept of holism refers to the understanding

第一节　中医护理的基本特点

中医护理学秉承了中医学的整体观念和辨证论治，经中医护理人员的传承和发扬，形成了整体观念和辨证施护两个基本特点。

一、整体观念

整体观念是指对事物的完整性、统一性

of the integrity, unity, and the interconnectedness of all elements, which forms the item. TCM considers that "human" is an organic whole in which all-constituent parts are structurally inseparable, functionally coordinative and interactive, and pathologically inter-influencing. Meanwhile, the characteristics of human are closely related with the human's natural and social environments. TCM nursing not only manages to maintain and promote the health of the internal environment of human body, but also regulates the external environment to meet the needs of human health.

i. Human Body Being an Organic Whole

In the concept of TCM, human body is an integral unity, and is five *zang*-viscera-centered. The five *zang* organs, six *fu* organs, bones and tissues of the whole body are contacted and communicated through the channel system, performing the unifying and coordinative functions *via* the actions of essence, qi, blood and body fluid. So, during the examination, the internal pathological alterations of the viscera and qi and blood can be represented through the external changes of sense organs, orifices, body constituents, complexion and pulse conditions. The nurses grasp the abnormal information about the patient's body by careful observation so that they can make the right nursing diagnosis using proper nursing measures to promote patient's recovery early. For instance, the observation of tongue can be used to assess the hyperfunction or hypofunction of an internal viscus, the sufficiency or deficiency of qi and blood, and the exuberance or lack of the body fluid, as well as the severity or relief of a disease. The tongue of patient with heart heat is always crimson. Patients with stomach fire have the symptom of yellowish fur. For another example, the patient with qi and blood deficiency has the symptom of pale tongue and light-colored lips and nail beds. Meanwhile, TCM nursing prevents disease and cares clients from the perspective of holistic concept. For example, paraglossa under the tongue is related with the heat of heart or spleen. Clearing the heat of heart is used for treating the heart fire hyperactivity. Purging the pathogenic fire of spleen heat is appropriate for treating the splenic fever. Importantly, human's psychological activities are closely related to the physiological activity. Grief damages the lung, and the ecstatic joy restricts grief. Excessive joy damages the heart, and fear restricts joy. Fear damages the kidney, and thinking restricts fear. Excessive thinking damages the spleen. Anger restricts thinking (*Basic Questions·Yin Yang Ying Xiang Da Lun, Sù Wèn·Yīn Yáng Yìng Xiàng Dà Lùn*, 素问·阴阳应象大论). TCM nursing emphasizes coexistence, interdependence and interaction between the

和组成事物各个要素的联系性的认识。中医护理学的整体观念体现在人是一个有机的整体,构成人体的各组成部分在结构上完整统一,在生理上相互分工,在功能上相互协调,在病理上相互影响;同时,认为"人"是生理、心理及社会相统一的整体的人。中医护理活动既考虑维护和促进人的机体内部环境的健康,又要调节人体所处的外部环境。

(一)人是一个有机的整体

中医护理学认为人体的各组织器官在结构上不可分割,是以五脏为中心,通过经络系统的联络与沟通,将六腑、五体、官窍及筋肉、骨骼等全身组织紧密联系形成完整的有机整体。人体的生理功能互相协调、相互为用,各脏腑、组织和器官通过精、气、血、津液等作用维持、协调生理活动的平衡。脏腑功能的情况,也可以通过经络在体表和组织反映出来。各脏腑、组织和器官病理过程相互影响,如脾失运化,则水湿停滞,气血生化失源,而出现相应的水肿、气血不足等临床表现。所以在护理实践的过程中,从整体出发观察患者的外在变化,如官窍、形体和色脉等,可以了解机体脏腑的情况,从而做出正确的护理诊断,如通过对舌的观察可测知内在脏腑之虚实、气血之盛衰,舌尖赤红可见于心火旺者,舌中苔黄可见于胃火旺者,舌质淡白并唇甲色淡可见于气血亏者。在治疗护理方面,运用整体观作为指导,调节脏腑功能而治疗护理局部病变,促进患者的早日康复。如舌下肿者与心、脾热盛有关,心火盛者,选用清心治疗;脾火盛者,则泄脾热。人体的脏腑生理功能又与情志变化密切相关,如《素问·阴阳应象大论》中指出:"忧伤肺,喜胜忧""喜伤心,恐胜喜""恐伤肾,思胜恐""思伤脾,怒胜思"。从整体观出发,也应重视情志在治疗中的重要作用。

body and mind, and pays more attention to the important role of psychological factors in the interventions for patients.

ii. Close Relation of Human with the Surrounding

1. Unity of Human and Nature Human lives in the environment, which is a part of the material world. Human body can be accordingly affected by the changes of natural environment. During one year, physiological and pathological reactions of human body are regulated by the climatic changes to adapt to the different seasons. For example, in spring and summer, yang qi goes outward and flourishes. Qi and blood of the body has a trend to go and superficially circulates, which is shown by the relaxation of the skin, more sweating and less urine, and the pulse is usually superficial and large. However, in autumn and winter, yang qi goes inward and astringes. Qi and blood of the body tend to go internally. People manifest the compaction of skin, less sweating and more urine with deep and small pulse. The qi and blood and yin yang of the body also conduct an adaptable change according to the changes of the day and night. At noon, yang qi of human gets supreme, and its function has increased. In the evening, yang qi is internally astringed, which facilitates rest and promotes the energy recovery (*Basic Questions· Sheng Qi Tong Tian Lun, Sù Wèn·Shēng Qì Tōng Tiān Lùn*, 素问·生气通天论). Human's yang qi rises to drive the functional activities of tissues and organs with the changes of time during a day. Furthermore, the geographical difference in living environment is another important factor, which directly influences the physiological function of human body. For example, in the southeast of China, people struggle with poor soils, damp and hot. The striae of people who live in those places is porous. In contrast, in the northwest plateau of China, it is dry and cold. The striae of people who live in those places is compact. The people there are usually well-build. On the other hand, people's ability of adapting to the natural environment has a certain limit. Once the climate abruptly changes and the adaptability of people is beyond the demands caused by the change, then there will be disorder of regulating functions of the body, and people are prone to develop diseases.

2. Close Relation of Human and the Society Social environment is the sum of material and spiritual conditions in which human lives and moves. Society, including the whole system of social economy and culture, is the direct environment of human life. Human affects society through social activities, and different social environment and changes lead to different psychological

（二）人与环境的统一性

1. **人与自然环境的统一性** 人生活在环境中，是整个物质世界的一部分，自然环境发生变化时，人体就会受到相应的影响。如一年四季中，随着气候的变化，人体也以不同的生理变化来适应。春夏季节阳气升发，气血易浮于体表，人体的生理调适表现为皮肤松弛，腠理开泄，发汗散热，排尿偏少，脉象多浮大；秋冬季节阳气收敛内藏，气血趋向于内里，人体表现为皮肤致密，出汗减少而排尿较多，脉象多沉小。人体的气血阴阳不但随季节气候的变化而发生规律性的变化，而且随着昼夜的变化而出现规律性的波动。《素问·生气通天论》指出"日中而阳气隆，日西而阳气已虚"，人体的阳气朝始生、午最盛、夕始弱、夜半衰。同时，地域的不同，亦在一定程度上影响人的生理和心理活动。中国东南地势低，气候多湿热，人体腠理多疏松，人多表现为体格瘦削；西北地处于高原，气候多燥寒，人体腠理多致密，人体格多壮实。人类对自然环境的适应能力有一定的限度，如果气候剧变超过了机体的调节能力，或机体的调节功能障碍，无法对自然环境的变化做出相应生理调节，人体就可能发生疾病。

2. **人和社会环境关系密切** 社会环境是人类生存和活动范围内物质和精神条件的总和，是人类生活的直接环境，包括整个社会经济文化体系。人类通过社会活动影响社会，而对于社会环境的差异和变化，人们会相应地产生不同的心理反应，从而引起身心

reaction. Also, the psychological reactions may cause the different physical and mental changes. The harmonious social relationships, good interpersonal communication and harmonious family atmosphere are of benefit to the prevention and treatment of disease and rehabilitation. On the contrary, a bad social environment will give rise to the side effects on human's physiological and psychological health. TCM nursing emphasizes the unity of human and the society.

II. Nursing Determination Based on Pattern Differentiation

Disease is the overall process that the human body is in the pathological changes of the disharmony between yin and yang under certain pathogenic factors. Pattern is a pathological summary of a given stage of a disease, and the signs, symptoms and pathological information during the process of illness. Symptoms are the patients' subjective description about pain or discomfort, such as the complaints of headache, amaurosis, tinnitus, dizziness, thirst, sweat-out and *etc.*. Signs are the patients' abnormal conditions achieved through observation or test, such as yellow tongue fur, rapid-string pulse, swelling in lower extremity, erosion and bleeding in gums, and so on. Pattern differentiation is beneficial to correctly reveal the nature of the disease. For example, patients with the patterns of both liver fire invading the lung and lung yin deficiency have symptoms of cough, less sputum and viscous phlegm, or phlegm containing blood. However, patients with liver fire invading the lung show the signs of pain in the chest and rib-side, dizziness and bitter taste in the mouth, being edgy and irritable and the symptoms of red face and eyes, rough yellow tongue fur and *etc.*. In contrast, patients with lung yin deficiency often complain of dry throat accompanying the symptoms of emaciation, red tongue with scant liquid and hoarse voice.

"Nursing determination based on pattern differentiations" includes two elements, which are pattern differentiations and nursing determination. "Pattern differentiation" is to synthetically analyze the patients' history, signs and symptoms by inspection, auscultation-olfaction inquiry, pulse examination and palpation. The process of pattern differentiation is to differentiate and recognize the syndrome of the disease, identify the nature of the illness, the cause of the position and the relationship between healthy qi and pathogenic factor, so as to determine the patient's general condition. Nursing determination is to formulate the appropriate nursing method in accordance with the result of pattern differentiation.

健康的差异和变化。如和谐的社会关系、良好的人际沟通、和睦的家庭氛围对疾病的预防、治疗及康复起到积极的作用；相反，则会影响人类健康。中医学护理强调人与社会的统一。

二、辨证施护

疾病是机体在一定致病因素作用下所发生的阴阳失调的病理变化的总过程。证，又称证候或证型，是指在疾病的发展过程中，对某一阶段的病理概括，包括患者在患病过程中表现出的症状、体征和相关的病理信息；症状是患者对自身感到的痛苦或不适的主观描述，如自述头痛、黑矇、耳鸣、眩晕、口渴、汗出等。体征是指通过客观地观察、检测而得到的关于患者的异常征象，如舌苔黄、脉弦数、下肢水肿、齿龈糜烂出血等。通过以症为据，从症辨证，有利于正确地揭示疾病的本质，如肝火犯肺和肺阴虚的患者都有咳嗽、痰少黏稠或痰中带血的症状；不同的是肝火犯者常自述胸胁疼痛，急躁易怒，眩晕口苦，患者面红目赤，舌苔黄糙等；相比较，肺阴虚者则自述咽喉干燥，患者消瘦乏力、舌红少津、声音嘶哑等。

辨证施护由辨证和施护两个部分组成。辨证是指以中医的基本理论为指导，经望、闻、问、切四诊，收集患者的病情资料，并结合环境、正气的强弱和疾病的特点进行分析、综合，辨清患者患病的原因、疾病的性质、发生部位和正邪关系，从而判断患者的证。施护是护理人员根据辨证的结果，确定护理原则并制订相应的护理方案。

Pattern differentiation is the prerequisite and basis for nursing determination. Accordingly, nursing determination is the means and methods for caring patients. The effects of nursing measure demonstrate whether the conclusion derived from the analyzing of pattern differentiation is right. Generally, different nursing measures should be adopted for different symptoms of different disease. On the other hand, it occurs that several different syndromes can be summarized into one clinical disease. The same syndrome can be analyzed into different diseases. Thus "the same disease can be treated in many different ways" and "many different diseases can be treated in the same way" can be performed in clinic nursing.

"The same disease can be cared in many different ways" means that the nursing measures for the same disease are sometimes different because different patients may have different reactions due to geographic location, different stages of disease or at different time. For instance, for treating phlegm pattern, "heat phlegm pattern should be treated by clearing heat and transforming phlegm" while "damp phlegm pattern should be given the intervention of dispelling dampness". It is written in *Medical Faculty Marking Line* (*Yī Lín Shéng Mò*, 医林绳墨) that "patients that suffered from wind phlegm pattern may be managed by means of dissipating wind".

"Many different diseases can be cared in the same way" means that the same or similar nursing measures can be used for different diseases, which presents the same pathomechanism during the course of disease development. For example, though enuresis and prolapse of the uterus are different disease, they can be treated by the same nursing intervention of upraising center qi if both of these two diseases present middle qi collapse syndrome. TCM nursing pays more attention to pattern differentiation. Nursing method should be selected according to the pathomechanism and syndrome.

(Wang Chun-yan)

Section 2　Principle of TCM Nursing

The foundation of nursing principle is based on the therapeutic principle of TCM, guided by the concept of holism and pattern differentiation. It is regarded as a

辨证是施护的前提和遵循依据，施护是促进患者康复的手段和措施，通过施护的效果观察可以检验辨证结果的正确性。一般情况下，异病异证应采取不同的护理方法，而在临床上有时可以见到一种病包括几种不同的证，而不同的病在其发展过程中出现同一种证，在护理工作中需采用"同病异护"和"异病同护"的策略。

"同病异护"：同一种病，因发病时间、地区和患者的机体反应性的不同，或者处在疾病不同的发展阶段，所表现的证不同，施护的方法则应相应不同。例如痰证，"热痰则清之，湿痰则燥之，风痰则散之"（《医林绳墨》）。

"异病同护"：不同的病，在其发展的过程中，因出现了相同的病机，可以采用同一种护理方法。例如遗尿和子宫下垂，实为不同的病，但如果均有中气下陷证，则可以采用相同的升提中气的护理方法。因此，中医护理坚持辨证与辨病相结合，有针对性地护理。

（王春艳）

第二节　中医护理的原则

中医护理原则是在遵循中医学治疗的基本原则的基础上，在整体观念、辨证施护的

universal guiding principle for caring the patients with different diseases.

I. Reinforcing Healthy Qi and Dispelling Pathogen

The course of a disease is the process of struggle between two contradictory aspects, which are healthy qi and pathogenic factors. "Pathogenic factors can hardly attack the body if the anti-pathogenic qi is strong" (*Basic Questions·Discussion on Acupuncture Technique, Sù Wèn Yí Piān·Cì Fǎ Lùn*, 素问遗篇·刺法论). When the healthy qi gains the upper hand, the disease will subdue. "Where evils converge, the qi must be deficient" (*Basic Questions· Discussion on febrile disease, Sù Wèn·Píng Rè Bìng Lùn*, 素问·评热病论). When the pathogen gains the upper hand, the disease will progress. Thus strengthening the healthy qi and dispelling the pathogen should be carried out during the TCM nursing to change the ratio of these two sides in order to enable the patients to recover quickly.

"Reinforcing healthy qi" means to build up a good physique, raising the resistance of the body against pathogens by treating and caring. For example, for the patients with vacuity and lack of strength, nurse should advise them to take more rest, and give them appropriate nutraceuticals and nutrition therapies in addition to proper exercise. TCM nursing pays attention to the regulation of patients' mind and spirit and *etc.*. By enhancing physique, adjusting function, and putting disease-resistant positive factors of human body into full play, people achieve the goal of dispelling the pathogen. "Dispelling the pathogenic" means to eliminate pathogens of the disease by applying therapies of medicament, acupuncture and cupping to achieve the goal of resuming the healthy qi. It is suitable when there is an excess of pathogens with no deficiency of the healthy qi.

The application of principle of "reinforcing healthy qi and dispelling pathogen" in nursing practice should be done according to the exuberance and debilitation of pathogenic qi or healthy qi. Importantly, it should be distinguished when reinforcing healthy qi is suitable and when the method of dispelling the pathogen is proper, and under which circumstances, strengthening the healthy qi and dispelling the pathogen should be used simultaneously. We should follow the strategy of supporting the healthy qi without letting the evil remain and dispelling the pathogen without undermining the healthy qi.

指导下制订的，对临床病证的护理具有普遍指导意义。

一、扶正祛邪

扶正祛邪，即扶持正气，祛除邪气。疾病发生、发展的过程，是正、邪力量斗争的过程。《素问遗篇·刺法论》指出"正气存内，邪不可干"，正气充沛，人体的抗病能力则较强；"邪之所凑，其气必虚"（《素问·评热病论》），正气不足，邪气增长，疾病就会发生或向更坏的方面发展。中医护理目的是通过护理干预改变正、邪双方力量的对比，扶助正气，祛除邪气，使病情向康复的方向转变。

扶正即运用扶助正气的治疗和护理方法，如气虚乏力者，嘱多休息，适当给予滋补的药物，饮食调护加强营养，指导恰当的体育锻炼及调摄精神情志等；通过增强体质，调整功能，调动、发挥人体抗病的积极因素，以扶助正气，保持和促进健康。扶正适用于疾病的主要矛盾是正气虚弱的病证。祛邪即驱除病邪，以保存正气，如运用药物、艾灸、拔罐等方法恢复正气，适用于以邪实为主而正气未衰的病证。

在护理工作中，扶正祛邪原则的具体运用要注意分析正邪双方相互消长盛衰的情况，区分单纯正虚、单纯邪盛和正虚邪实的实际情况，针对性地运用单纯扶正法、单纯祛邪法、扶正祛邪法先后或同时进行的护理方法，并注意要做到扶正不留邪、祛邪不伤正，达到邪去正安的目的。

II. Nursing Aiming at the Root of a Disease

"Nursing aiming at the root of a disease" means that nurses must seek for the cause of disease, and treat the patient by addressing disease's root. "The root" is corresponding to the "the branch", and has multiple meanings. "It is necessary to seek the root when treating disease" (*Basic Questions·Yin Yang Ying Xiang Da Lun*). "The branch" is the phenomena of disease. "The root" is the essence of disease. For example, regarding the two sides of healthy qi and pathogen, healthy qi is the root and pathogenic qi is the branch. In terms of disease's cause and symptom, the cause is the root and the symptom is the branch. Considering the position of human body, the viscera are the root, and the periphery is the branch. In terms of the order of disease, old or primary disease is the root, while new or secondary one is the branch. It is the cardinal principle for nurses to care the patients based on pattern differentiation, aiming at the root of a disease. It is required that nurses should not only observe the symptoms and signs of patient, but also consider the external environmental factors of patients, such as life style, eating habits, emotional status, sleep patterns and so on. After dialectical analyses, nurses should determine the root of disease, find the nursing problem to be solved, make plans and take nursing measures. Generally, the external phenomena of diseases are consistent with the internal essence, but in some diseases the external phenomena and internal essence are not consistent. Therefore, a nurse must understand the essential information about the root and the branch, so that the appropriate nursing intervention can be properly used.

i. Orthodox Nursing

Orthodox nursing is used for a case that the signs and symptoms are consistent with its essence. The methods commonly used are "when there is cold, treat it with heat" "when there is heat, treat it with cold" "when there is deficiency, treat it with supplementation" and "when there is excess, treat it with drainage". Because the nursing intervention goes against the essence of a disease, it is also named "allopathic nursing". Take the example of vomiting and diarrhea: if the cause is the failure of movement and transformation, the intervention is to supplement the spleen, and to promote the movement and transformation. If it is difficult to discern the nature of the disease in a short time, the clinical interventions need to be cautious.

ii. Paradoxical Nursing

In some chronic diseases, obstinate diseases or critical illness, the inconsistence may possibly occur

二、护病求本

护病求本是指在护理患者的过程中，必须寻求疾病的根本原因，根据其本质采取针对性的护理措施。"本"是与"标"相对应的，有多种含义，本是本质，标是现象。《素问·阴阳应象大论》提出"治病必求于本"，例如，就正邪而论，正气为本，邪气为标；以病因和症状区分，则病因为本，症状为标；就病变的部位而言，内脏为本，体表为标；从疾病新旧划分，旧病为本，新病为标；从发病先后区分，先病为本，后病为标。护病求本要求护理人员充分了解患者的病情：不但观察患者症状、体征，还要考虑外界环境因素、患者的生活方式、饮食习惯、情志状态、睡眠模式等因素，进行辨证分析，判断疾病发生的根本原因，找出需要解决的护理问题，针对性地制订计划并采取护理措施。一般情况下，多数疾病的临床表现和其本质是一致的，但是也存在疾病的某些临床表现与本质相矛盾或相反的情况，因此，护理人员还要根据"本"与"标"的实质情况，恰当地采用正护法或反护法。

（一）正护法

正护法是指当疾病的临床表现和疾病的本质相一致时，针对疾病的本质，从正面进行护理，即逆病性而护的方法，因而又称之为逆护法。常用的有"寒者热之，热者寒之，虚则补之，实者泻之"。例如，吐泻症状，如果是由于运化功能低下、不能运化饮食而引起的，需采取补脾和增强运化作用的护理方法。在临床上很短时间内无法弄清病情、难以辨明疾病的性质时，需采用谨慎的态度。

（二）反护法

有些慢性病、疑难病和危重病可能出现证因不符、寒热真假和虚实真伪的情况，增

between syndrome and cause, between true or false, between cold and heat, or between deficiency and excess. Sometimes, manifestations of these cases are opposite of the nature of disease, which increases the difficulty of treating patients following pattern differentiation in clinic. Nurses are required to grasp the essence through the phenomena. Paradoxical nursing, also named "consistent nursing", can be used under these circumstances. Common methods are as follows.

1. Treat Heat with Heat　Warm and heat medicine and approaches may be applied to the patients suffering from the true cold with false heat. When the essence of disease is true cold, its external appearance is false heat, various warm and heat medicines should be selected to intervene the disease. The principle above is named "treat heat with heat". Take a patient who has a fever as an example: he has the symptoms of dry mouth, red tongue and rapid floating pulse. His symptoms above look like wind-heat common cold. But if the patient is also averse to the wind with the symptoms of nausea and vomiting, the patient's condition may be *taiyang* wind-invasion syndrome. Warm and hot medicines should be given to the patient to harmonize *ying-wei* levels.

2. Treat Cold with Cold　It is a method to treat the false-cold signs with various cold and cool medicines or measures in order to lower the temperature. It is suitable for patients in true heat syndrome but with false cold signs. For instance, patients sometimes have the cold signs in some acute febrile diseases under critical conditions, such as extreme cold limbs, greenish-blue facial complexion and fine rapid pulse. However, those symptoms are false-cold signs. In essence, the heat exuberance is true. Cold-cool medicine and other cold approaches for nursing should be used in this condition.

3. Treat the Blocked by Blocking　Sometimes, the patients in obstructive disease caused by viscera debilitation or insufficiency of qi and blood have the false obstruction signs. They should be treated by the method of "treat the blocked by blocking". The patient in spleen-stomach weakness displays abdominal fullness and distention, and obstruction because of the insufficiency of center qi and abnormal ascending and descending. Fortifying the spleen, boosting the qi and opening the obstruction by tonics can be used to solve the problem.

4. Treat the Flowing by Promoting Its Flow　It is a method to treat the syndrome with diarrhea sign by using various evacuant medicines or dredging methods. It is suitable for the patients with diarrhea or blood leakage because of the accumulation and stagnation in the interior or internal static blood obstruction. For example, flooding

加了临床辨证施治的难度，需要护理人员透过现象究其本质，采取反护法。反护法又称从护法，是指顺从疾病的现象而采取的护理方法，常用方法包括：

1. **热因热用**　用温热性药物或温热的方法护理具有假热征象的病证。意指疾病本质是寒，但是其外在表现为热，对其进行治疗和护理时，应针对寒的本质，避免被其热的假象所迷惑。如患者发热，自述口干，查舌偏红，脉浮数，似属风热感冒或温病征象，但问及患者有恶风，并有恶心、欲吐，故考虑为太阳中风证，因此，应给予其调和营卫的温热性药物。

2. **寒因寒用**　用寒凉药、寒凉法护理具有假寒征象的病证。如某些急性发热的疾病，在急危重症的情况下，常可表现为肢冷色青，脉细数之寒象，但分析病机，其寒象是假，体内热毒蕴郁太甚是其本质。因此，应该使用具有寒凉作用的方剂和方法，对患者进行治疗和护理。

3. **塞因塞用**　指用补益法护理具有闭塞不通症状的方法。塞因塞用在临床适用于脏腑衰弱、气血不足所致的滞塞不通的病证。如脾胃虚弱者，因中气不足，气机升降失常，证见脘腹胀满、阻滞不通，采用健脾益气法护理，促进脾胃升降功能的恢复，消除腹胀，达到开塞的目的。

4. **通因通用**　用通利的方法护理具有实性通泄症状的方法。通因通用适用于有积滞或者瘀血内结，而表现为腹泻或漏血症状的病证。如妇科由于瘀血所致崩漏，应正确使用通因通用，通过活血化瘀、使瘀血可祛、血循常

and spotting of female can be treated with the method of "treat the flowing by promoting its flow". By invigorating blood and dissolving stasis, blood stasis can be dispelled so that the blood circulation is recovered to normal, and menstrual cycle can be set right so that the effects of stanching bleeding and freeing stasis can be obtained.

5. Contrary Nursing in Medicine Taken Firstly, the contrary may be embedded in the prescription. For instance, if the pathogen is relatively light cold or heat syndrome, heat or cold medicines may be directly given to the patients. However, if the pathogen shows serious cold or heat syndrome, patients with great heat or cold syndrome may vomit due to the repellence between yin and yang when taking the medicine. It is unable to achieve therapeutic effects. So, it is necessary to use the medicines that can make disease and qi concomitant to avoid the repellence. For example, febrifuge is used for the true heat with false cold and cold-dispelling medicine is used for the true cold with false heat. Secondly, the contrary may be embedded in the temperature of medicine. It is necessary to take in a cold-cool natured decoction when it is hot, and to take in warm-hot natured decoction when it is cool.

III. Balancing Yin and Yang

The occurrence, development and deterioration of a disease are essentially the outcome of superiority or inferiority of yin and yang due to the destruction of their relative balance. "Carefully examine and adjust the yin and yang, aiming for the balance" (*Basic Questions. Zhi Zhen Yao Da Lun, Sù Wèn. Zhì Zhēn Yào Dà Lùn*, 素问·至真要大论) is the treatment principle of TCM. Therefore, coordinating yin and yang to restore their relative balance is one of the cardinal principles in clinical nursing. By eliminating the surplus and supplementing the deficiency, nurses help human body to calm yin and to sound yang so as to help patients to get life-long health promotion and disease prevention.

1. Eliminating the Surplus "Eliminating the surplus" is also named "reducing the superabundance". It is clinically followed in nursing course and is suitable for the cases with an excess of yin or yang. For example, patients with excess-heat syndrome due to the exuberance of yang-heat always have the signs of vigorous heat, less sweating, rough breathing, dry mouth and *etc.*. Nurses may clear away yang-heat with the nursing strategies of cold natured remedy, including room ventilation, avoiding over-excited emotion, taking in decoction when it is cool, and eating cold-cool natured food, such as watermelon

道、月讯有期，从而得止血通瘀的效果。

5. 药物护理的反佐法 药物的反佐一般指两个方面：一是处方上的寒热相佐，例如对于邪气较为轻浅的寒、热证候，可直接给予热药和寒药即可。但是，对于邪气较甚之寒、热重证，经投热药、寒药，可能发生阴阳格拒，出现呕吐不纳，难获其效。此时，常采用与病气相从的药物，如真热假寒证佐用热药，而真寒假热证佐用寒凉药，以求不发生格拒。二是服药时，药物温度的寒热相佐，寒凉药温服法或热药冷服法，诱病受药，以求更好地发挥药性。

三、调整阴阳

疾病的发生、发展和变化是由于阴阳的偏盛或偏衰，阴阳失调导致机体内环境稳定性的破坏。《素问·至真要大论》指出"谨察阴阳所在而调之，以平为期"，是中医治疗疾病的根本法则。临床具体护理工作应调整阴阳盛衰，恢复阴阳相对平衡的状态，损其有余、补其不足，达到阴平阳秘，从而促进健康和预防疾病。

1. 损其有余 损其有余又称损其偏盛，是指对于阴或阳的一方偏盛有余的病证所遵循的护理原则，适用于一方偏盛有余，而其相对的一方并无偏衰现象。如阳热亢盛的实热证，患者常表现为壮热、无汗、气粗、口干等，护理上采用治热以寒的方法，清泻热邪，如加强室内通风、避免情绪过激、药物冷服和饮食上辅以凉性的西瓜汁、梨汁、绿豆等清热生津之品。而对于阴寒内盛的实寒

juice, pear juice, mung bean and *etc.* to clear heat and promote fluid production. To treat patients with excess-cold syndrome due to exuberance of internal yin-cold, the nursing intervention should be focused on dispelling yin-cold with heat natured remedy. The nursing strategies include keeping proper room temperature, taking the decoction as it is hot and eating warm-hot natured food.

2. Supplementing the Deficiency Supplementing the deficiency is a nursing strategy for the cases with inferiority of yin or yang. Enriching yin, supplementing yang, or supplementing both yin and yang are respectively performed in view of the conditions of yin deficiency, yang vacuity or deficiency of both yin and yang. If yin fails to restrict yang due to its deficiency, such as vacuity heat pattern caused by yin vacuity with yang hyperactivity, the nursing measures to enrich yin so as to restrict yang should be taken. The nursing measures include keeping the room cool and ventilating, preventing patient from catching a cold because of his enjoying coolness, providing food with the action of nourishing yin, reducing heat and *etc.*. However, if yang fails to restrict yin due to its deficiency, such as vacuity cold pattern, the nursing measures to supplement yang so as to restrict yin should be taken. The nursing measures include keeping the room warm, providing food with the action of supplementing yang and restricting yin and *etc.*. Furthermore, health requires interdependence between yin and yang. The inferiority of either yin or yang may involve the other. For dual deficiency of yin and yang, supplementing both yin and yang is needed. Most importantly, in nursing an inferiority of either yin or yang, nurses should also pay attention to "seek yin from yang" or "seek yang from yin". When nursing the patients with yin detriment accompanied by affecting yang, the methods of nourishing yin and supplementing yang should be appropriately considered. When nursing the patients in yang detriment accompanied by affecting yin, supplementing yang and nourishing yin also should be appropriately considered.

IV. Emergency or Chronicity and Root or Branch

Disease is a complex process, and the development of disease is affected by various factors. Also, the condition of illness demonstrates different degrees of priority. The nursing plan should be formulated depending on the emergency or chronicity of the root and branch of disease. Nursing methods should be selected according to the principle of "in urgent conditions, caring the branch" "in

证，则用治寒以热的方法，用温散寒邪，如保持室内温度、药物热服和给予温热饮食等。

2. 补其不足　补其不足是指对于阴阳偏衰不足的病证所采取的护理策略。根据患者阴虚、阳虚或阴阳两虚的具体情况，针对性地给予滋阴、补阳或阴阳双补。例如阴虚不能制阳，可表现为阴虚阳亢的虚热证，应采用滋阴制阳的方法，可以保持病室内凉爽通风、调整湿度为40%~60%，防过燥，给予滋阴降火的饮食等。对于阳虚不能制阴的虚寒证，应采用补阳制阴的方法，可调整病室温度加强保暖，给予补阳制阴的饮食以温经散寒。同时，阴阳是互根的，阴损可及阳，而阳损亦可及阴，当阴阳都不同程度的不足时，须采取阴阳双补的原则，运用时必须分清主次。阴损及阳者，应在充分滋阴的基础上配合补阳之方；阳损及阴者，须在充分补阳的基础上配以滋阴之品。

四、标本缓急

疾病是一个复杂的过程，而且在疾病发展过程中的不同阶段，又受到多种不同因素的影响，使病情出现轻重缓急的不同表现。在护理过程中要针对标本缓急设计护理方案，采用"急则护其标，缓则护其本，标本俱急则标本同护"的灵活方法。

moderate conditions, caring the root" and "nursing the branch and the root simultaneously".

1. Nursing the Branch for Emergency　　When the branch aspect of the condition is very emergent and serious, and if it was not addressed promptly, it would endanger the life of the patient or affect the treatment and nursing of the root condition. At this time, the principle of "in urgent conditions, caring the branch" should be taken first, and the branch becomes the primary aspect of the disease. It should be taken first to handle the branch condition, and then deal with the root condition. For instance, for the patients with febrile convulsion, massive bleeding, asthmatic crisis, no matter what kind of disease it is, emergency measures should be taken first for the branch, then the root condition should to be cared.

2. Nursing the Root for Chronicity　　When the branch aspect of the condition is not emergent or serious, or has been properly disposed, TCM nursing should focus on the essence of the disease and grasp the root causes. Patients in chronic illness or in the recovery phase of the disease always face the condition. For example, in the case of cough caused by phlegm-damp obstructing the lung, cough is the branch and phlegm-damp obstruction is the root. When the symptom of cough is not serious, the nursing intervention should focus on transforming phlegm and dispelling dampness to deal with the root. When the root is solved, the symptom can be relieved.

3. Nursing the Branch and the Root Simultaneously　When both the branch and the root conditions are acute, the branch and the root should be cared at the same time so as to enhance the intervention effects and shorten the course. As for the patients in ulcerative colitis, spleen-kidney yang deficiency is the root. The condition involves external pathogenic factors invasion, excessive taxation, internal damage, enduring diarrhea and edema. The branch is the damp-heat and internal brewing. The patient's symptoms include mild fever, fatigued spirit and lack of strength, laziness to speak, tiredness in the body, glomus and oppression in the chest and stomach duct, nausea and torpid stomach intake, abdominal distention and loose stool. It is the syndrome of equal-stress in the branch and the root. When nursing, the root and the branch should be paid equal attention to. For the case above, measures include clearing the intestines and transforming dampness to care the branch, warming the kidney and fortifying the spleen to treat the root.

1. **急则护其标**　　如标病甚急，在疾病的发展过程中出现了严重的症状，不及时解决将危及患者的生命或影响其本病的总体治疗和护理，护理上应遵循急则护其标的原则，先护其标病，再护其本病。如病程中出现高热惊厥、大出血、哮喘危象、剧烈呕吐、昏迷等危重症状的患者，首先应采取积极措施护其标，待病情有所缓解再护其本病。

2. **缓则护其本**　　在标病不急或标病已得到妥善处理的情况下，护理的重点应根据疾病的病因而护本，多见于慢性病或恢复期的患者。如痰湿阻肺所致的咳嗽，咳嗽是标，痰湿阻滞是本，在症状不急时，在护理上采用化痰祛湿的方法以护其本，本病得愈，咳嗽的症状也随之减轻或消失。

3. **标本同护**　　在标病和本病俱急或并重的情况下，应标本同护，以提高效果，缩短病程。例如溃疡性结肠炎者，脾肾阳虚是本，外邪入里、劳倦内伤、久泻久痢、水邪久踞；湿热内蕴是标，患者表现为热势缠绵，神疲懒言，肢体困重，胸脘痞闷，恶心纳呆，腹胀便溏，属标本并重的证候，此时应标本同护，即清肠化湿以治标，温肾健脾以固本。

V. Three Considerations of Time, Person and Place in Nursing

The occurrence, development and transformation of disease can be affected by many factors, such as season, climate, geographic environment, especially the patient's physical constitution. So nurses should consider the factors above when caring patients, and suit the nursing measures according to the season, the locality and the individual.

1. Administer Nursing to the Season It is warm in the spring, hot in the summer, dry in the autumn and cold in the winter. Climatic changes of four seasons exert some certain impacts on physiological functions and pathological changes. Generally, in spring and summer yang qi rises. The striae of the skin and muscles get loose and open with more perspiration. In autumn and winter, yin prevails and yang declines. The striae of the skin and muscles are compact with less perspiration, and yang qi goes internally. Nurses should suit nursing for patients according to the season. Considering the warm breeze prevailing in spring, if a patient is suffering from contraction of wind-cold, the cool-cold natured herbs should be given to him. In summer, the weather is hot and the temperature is higher. It rains frequently and it is usually humid. Patients in the disease caused by summer-heat evil are always treated by means of resolving the summer heat and dispelling dampness. When a patient is in the condition of external contraction of autumn-dryness, the treatment should be cold-pungent and moistening dryness. Considering the cold-wind in winter, when a patient suffering from contraction of wind-cold, he should be given warm natured herbs to release the exterior with acrid-warm. Meanwhile, some chronic diseases, such as asthma and stroke, usually break out or get deteriorated when the climate changes. So, precautionary nursing measures should be taken ahead of time. Abnormal climatic change is a key factor of inducing diseases. For example, if it should be warm but it is abnormal cold in spring, the signs of patients in externally contracted disease are wind-cold exterior pattern. If it should be cold but it is abnormal warm in winter, the patients in externally contracted disease may show wind-heat exterior pattern. Furthermore, the changes of yin and yang during the day and night should be cared. In general, a disease is slight in daytime but serious at night because of the turning from excitation to inhibition of the body's function with the rising and declining of yin and yang, which easily results in the invasion of pathogens. Nurses should monitor the illness changes in the evening on the basis of principle of

五、三因制宜

疾病的发生、发展和转归受到多方面因素的影响，如时令气候、地理环境、个体差异等；因此，在护理中必须综合考虑影响疾病的各方面的因素，根据三因制宜的原则，即因人、因时、因地而制订恰当的护理措施。

1. **因时制宜** "时"指气候、季节等，一年四季有春温、夏暑、秋燥、冬寒之分；气候的变化对人体的生理、心理和病理变化有着一定的影响。一般情况下，春夏季节，气候逐渐由温转热，阳气升发，人体腠理疏松开泄；而秋冬季节，气候逐渐由凉转寒，阴盛阳衰，机体腠理致密，阳气内敛。护理必须因时制宜，春季风温，外感用药应辛凉解表；夏季常暑多兼湿，对暑邪致病者要注意解暑化湿；而外感秋燥，宜辛凉润燥；冬季风寒，外感用药宜辛温解表。同时，一些慢性疾病，例如哮喘、中风等，常在季节交替时发作或加重，护理时应注意在气候变化之前采取恰当的预防措施，以防疾病的发作或加重。另外，还需注意昼夜间阴阳盛衰的变化。一般情况下，患者的病情为昼轻夜重，原因可能与夜间机体阴盛阳衰、功能由兴奋转向抑制，病邪乘虚加甚有关。因此护理人员应加强观察，注意患者夜间病情的变化。

"suiting nursing to the season".

2. Administer Nursing to the Locality In different regions, geographic environments, climatic conditions and people's customs are different, so people are also different in physiological activities and pathological features. "The topography is different in height or low. Weather is cold in the higher terrain, and is hot in the lower terrain." The reference of *Wu Chang Zheng Da Lun* (*Wǔ Cháng Zhèng Dà Lùn*, 五常政大论) explains that with the changes of topography from height to low, weather changes from cold to hot. With the difference of natural geographical environment, yin and yang are also varied. Meanwhile, human's diet and behavior habit are closely related to the geographical environment that they live (*Basic Questions· Yi Fa Fang Yi Lun*, *Sù Wèn· Yì Fǎ Fāng Yì Lùn*, 素问·异法方宜论). In the eastern part of China, human like eating fish and salty food. The character of fish belongs to fire nature, which easily makes human accumulate heat toxin. Salt can get into the blood. Eating too much salt may injure the blood. So the skin of most people there are dark, and the interstices of their flesh are loose. The human's disease is also associated with the territory. In the eastern part of China, abscesses and ulcers are prone to be disseminated. In the western part of China, the diseases are usual developed from inside (*Basic Questions· Yi Fa Fang Yi Lun*). Thus nursing methods should differ according to the characteristics of geographical environment of patients and their life habits.

3. Administer Nursing to the Individual A principle in nursing determination based on the characteristics of patient's age, gender and physical constitution is known as "suiting nursing to the individual". The physiological states and pathological feature are different in people at their different age. Children are full of vitality, but their qi and blood are not abundant enough. They are likely to suffer from cold and heat evil. Therefore, the tonics should be carefully prescribed for children, and the dosage of herbs should be distinguished with the age, while the body weight should be considered. The vitality of aged people is gradually declining, and the qi and blood of old men are deficient. The old often suffer from syndromes of deficiency or healthy qi vacuity and evil repletion. For the old with excess pathogen, the drug used to dispel pathogen should be paid more attention to avoid damage healthy qi for the old. Among the young people, the constitution of yin-deficient, damp-heat and qi depression is common, which is probably related with their life style. For example, they like eating the fried food, and they are facing various

2. 因地制宜 不同的地区，由于地势、气候条件和生活习惯差异，人的生理活动和疾病的特征也不同。《五常政大论》指出"地有高下，气有温凉，高者气寒，下者气热"，解释了因地域高下之不同，气候亦有寒热温凉之差异。随着自然地理环境的不同，阴阳之气盛衰也各有差异；同时，人的饮食、行为习惯等方面都与其生活的地理环境密切相关。"东方之域，其民食鱼而嗜咸""鱼者使人热中，盐者胜血，故其民皆黑色疏理"（《素问·异法方宜论》），意指中国东部地区的人习惯吃鱼和咸的食物，因鱼性属火，易使人积热，而咸能走血，食用过多易伤血，因此该地区的人大多数皮肤色黑，肌腠松疏。人体的疾病也表现出地域的相关性。"东方之域，其病皆为痈疡""西方者，其病生于内"（《素问·异法方宜论》）。护理工作中，应根据不同地区的地理环境特点和其生活习惯确定相应护理措施。

3. 因人制宜 因人制宜指根据患者的年龄、性别和体质等不同特点而制订适宜的护理措施。不同年龄的人，其生理功能和病变特点也不相同；小儿生理功能旺盛，但气血未充，易寒易热，因此，对于小儿，当慎用补剂，用药剂量须根据年龄加以区分；老年人气血衰少，生理功能减退，患病多虚证或正虚邪实，虚证宜补，而对于邪实须攻者应注意用药的配方，避免损伤正气；在年轻人中，阴虚体质、湿热体质、气郁体质多见，可能与年轻人喜欢使用吃煎炸烧烤等食物及生活压力大有关，嘱其少食辛温燥烈之品、调节情志。女性有经、带、胎、产等生理情况，护理中须加以考虑，如在妇女妊娠期禁用活血破气、滑利攻下类的药物；对产后妇女则应考虑其恶露及气血亏虚等情况，禁用寒凉泄下和太过补益作用的药物。由于每个

life pressures and so on. Nurses should tell the young not to eat irritating food and appropriately regulate their emotion. Females have their special conditions such as pregnancy, delivery and menstruation. Nurses should consider those conditions when making the nursing measures. For example, the drugs for blood-activating, breaking qi, lubricating and offensively precipitating are forbidden to be used for females during the period of pregnancy. Considering the lochia and their qi and blood vacuity, the cold and cool herb, purgative formula and excessively supplementary prescription are limited to be used in postpartum women. Because of the differences in innate endowment and health care after birth, individuals have different types of physical constitution such as cold or heat. Generally, a person with a physical constitution of yang deficiency should keep warm and be given warm and hot natured food and tonics. A man with spleen-stomach weakness should avoid taking excessive rich and slimy medicine. The one that his physical constitution is yang exuberant should avoid being treated with hot tonics, and a person whose physical constitution is yin should be exuberated to use the cold.

In summary, the principles of suiting nursing to the season, locality and individual fully embody the concept of holism in the TCM nursing. During the nursing intervention, a nurse should not only pay attention to the features of the individual, but also consider the season and locality.

人的先天禀赋和后天调养的差异，个人体质亦有偏寒偏热的不同。例如：体质偏寒者应注意保暖、可辛温饮食；脾胃虚弱者须避免服用太过滋腻的药材；素体阳旺者慎用温热，素体阴盛者慎用寒凉。

综上所述，三因制宜的互利原则充分地体现了中医护理学的整体观，护理实践中注重强调人的体质、气候时令和地理环境等因素对人的健康的影响。

VI. Prevention

Modern health care has been changed from the illness-oriented to the health-centered. Health promotion and illness prevention have been increasingly attached importance by people, and are identified as the fundamental concepts for nursing practice, and are regarded as the core content of nursing work.

Prevention means taking measures in advance to stop the occurrence and development of diseases. Prevention is also named "nursing the undiseased" in TCM nursing. The concept of "nursing the undiseased" derives from the thought of "preventive treatment" (*The Yellow Emperor's Inner Classic*). "A wise man does some preventions before the disease occurs, and nips the chaos in the bud" (*Basic questions· Si Qi Tiao Shen Da Lun, Sù Wèn·Sì Qì Tiáo Shén Dà Lùn*, 素问·四气调神大论). There are some warning signs before the onset of febrile disease in the five viscera. For example, there may appear "redness" in different parts of the face, and it is

六、预防为主

现代护理由原来的"以疾病为中心"的模式转变为"以健康为中心"的模式，健康促进及疾病预防日益受到护理实践工作的重视，成为护理工作的核心内容。

预防即事先做好防备，是指采取一定的措施和手段防御疾病的发生和发展，中医称治未病。治未病的思想源自《黄帝内经》："是故圣人不治已病治未病，不治已乱治未乱"（《素问·四气调神大论》）；"病虽未发，见赤色者刺之，名曰治未病"（《素问·刺热》），意指五脏热病在发病前会有些先兆征象，可在面部的不同部位出现赤色，为热的表现，及时发现并给予早期干预可阻止发病或减轻

the expression of the heat. Disclosing in time and giving early intervention can prevent or alleviate the disease, which is also named "prevention before a disease" (*Basic questions· Ci Re, Sù Wèn·Cì Rè*, 素问·刺热). Zhu Zhen-heng (AD 1281-1358) in the Yuan Dynasty advocates the aftercare and prevention before disease occurrence rather than treatment when it comes to the disease (*Teachings of [Zhu] Dan-xi, Dān Xī Xīn Fǎ*, 丹溪心法). The prevention includes "preventing disease before it arises" "controlling the development of existing disease", and "preventing recurrence after healing".

1. Prevent Disease before It Arise　This implies that various measures should be taken to prevent the disease occurrence. Nursing prevention measures include regulating the physical fitness, mental condition, diet, life style and using medicinal prevention.

(1) Taking good care of the body: Human body is the essence and carrier of life. It is the material basis with which a person performs the life activities. A healthy body provides support for abundant vigor, and a healthy physique often results from unremitting physical exercises. Many famous Chinese doctors have created a series of classical exercises. For example, Hua Tuo of the Han Dynasty created the *five mimic-animal exercise* (*wǔ qín xì*, 五禽戏) according to the ancient method of physical and breathing exercise (*dǎo yǐn*, 导引). Eight-sectioned exercise (*bā duàn jǐn*, 八段锦) has been handed down from the Northern Song Dynasty (AD 1127-1279). The traditional Chinese fitness boxing *Tai Ji* (*tài jí quán*, 太极拳) of China closely combines the consciousness and breathing with movement.

(2) Cultivating mental health: TCM nursing not only pays special attention to take good care of the body, but also attaches importance to take good care of the people's emotion. Mental and emotional activities take essence, qi, blood and body fluid as their substantial foundation, and are closely related to visceral function and activity. Sadness and sorrow may influence the heart, and heart alteration may affect viscera (*Spiritual Pivot· natural life span, Líng Shū·Tiān Nián*, 灵枢·天年). Negative emotions may lead to qi stagnation and blood stasis, and do harm to the viscera, resulting in the disease. In contrast, pleasant feelings may make the qi and blood flow smoothly, and make the viscera work vigorously. "When a person is able to maintain mental mood calm and do not have too much desire and distractions, his qi will always maintain adequate status, and he is more resistant to illness" (*Basic Questions· Shang Gu Tian Zhen Lun, Sù Wèn· Shàng Gǔ Tiān Zhēn Lùn*, 素问·上古天真论). So, TCM nursing emphasizes the mental regulation for

病痛。元代朱震亨在《丹溪心法》中指出："与其求疗于有疾之后，不若摄养于无疾之先"，生动地指出了治未病的重要意义。治未病包括未病先防、既病防变和愈后防复三个方面。

1. **未病先防**　未病先防是在疾病发生之前采取各种措施以防止疾病的发生。护理工作的内容主要包括调养形体、调摄精神、调理饮食、调整起居及药物预防等。

（1）调养形体：形体是生命的本质和载体，是人进行生命活动的物质基础，健康的体魄为充沛的精力提供支持。体育锻炼是促进人健康的一项重要措施。我国古代医家发明了多种健身方法，如汉代著名医学家华佗根据古代导引法创造了五禽戏；北宋有八段锦，记载了运动健身的方法；传统的健身拳术太极拳，将意识、呼吸、动作密切结合。

（2）调摄精神：中医护理学不但重视形体的调养，而且注重调摄精神活动。人的精神情志活动以精、气、血、津液为基础，与脏腑的功能活动密切相关。"悲哀愁忧则动心，心动则五脏六腑摇"（《灵枢·天年》），消极的情绪使气滞血瘀，伤及五脏而致病；而愉快的情绪，可使人气血通畅，功能旺盛。"恬淡虚无，真气从之，精神内守，病安从来""气自安而不惧，形劳而不倦"（《素问·上古天真论》）。故中医护理强调精神调养，指导患者保持安静、平和、愉悦的情志状态，对内外环境的变化能做出积极的应对、调适，保持心理平衡。

patients, and tells the patients that it is important to keep a peaceful and happy mood with humility, and to make a positive response, adjust and maintain the psychological balance to the changes of outside.

(3) Having a proper diet: The essence coming from the five flavors balance of diet is the substantial foundation for maintaining normal physical functions, and is the necessary condition for assuring the survival and health. The imbalance diet can damage the organs and lead to the occurrence of disease. Eating too much will hurt the intestines and stomach (*Basic Questions· Bi Lun Pian, Sù Wèn·Bì Lùn Piān*, 素问·痹论篇). Having too much salty food will increase the risk of atherosclerosis and make the skin dark. Feeding too much bitters will lead to dry skin and hair loss. Having too much pungent food will result in the sinews tension and palm withered. Having too much acids will make muscle callus and lips crack. eating too much sweets will lead to bone pain and the hair loss (*Basic Questions· Development of Five-Viscera, Sù Wèn·Wǔ Zàng Shēng Chéng Piān*, 素问·五脏生成篇). TCM nursing emphasizes "proper diet", which means the diet should be appropriate and regular. One should cultivate a good dietetic habit, neither starvation nor satiety. One should pay attention to the regulations of the nature and flavor to make heat and cold harmonized, and the five flavors balanced. Cold food can easily damage yang qi of stomach, causing yang deficiency of stomach. Overheating diet can damage the stomach yin qi, leading to yin vacuity (*Supplement to 'Important Formulas Worth a Thousand Gold Pieces', Qiān Jīn Yì Fāng*). So, the temperature of food should be warm but not heating the lips, and cool without freezing the tooth. Furthermore, one should also pay attention to dietetic hygiene in order to avoid "disease entering by the mouth".

(4) Having a regular daily life: TCM nursing guides regimen according to environmental changes and the law of the biological clock. Working and resting with a regular daily life and having a good life habit can improve the body's ability to adapt to the natural environment, avoid and reduce the occurrences of the disease. For example, summer is suitable for nourishing yang. So, in order to promote the yang qi stretching, one should keep the habits such as going to bed late and getting up early, going out for a walk, increasing activities in appropriate and stretching form in summer. In winter, vegetation withers away, and worms are dormant. Just like the nature, the waxing and waning movement of human being gets slow in winter, and the metabolism of body is the same: essential qi is internally blocked and hidden. So one should gather yang, and save yin in winter. People should get up late and go to

（3）饮食有节：饮食五味和调所化生的精气，是维持人体生理功能，保证其生存和健康的必要条件。倘若饮食五味失调，可损伤脏腑，导致疾病的发生，"饮食自倍，肠胃乃伤"（《素问·痹论篇》），"多食咸，则脉凝泣而变色；多食苦，则皮槁而毛拔；多食辛，则筋急而爪枯；多食酸，则肉胝而唇揭；多食甘，则骨痛而发落"（《素问·五脏生成篇》）。中医护理强调饮食有节，是指饮食要适宜、规律，食量适中，不可过饱、过饥，要谨和五味；寒温适中，意指寒冷的饮食容易损伤胃的阳气，导致胃阳不足；过热饮食可损伤胃的阴气，引起胃阴虚耗。因此，《千金翼方》中指出要"热无灼唇，冷无冰齿"，不可偏食，并注意保持饮食卫生，防止病从口入。

（4）起居有常：中医护理应根据四季环境的变化，按生物钟的规律进行生活活动来指导养生。保持规律的起居作息及良好的生活习惯，能提高人体对自然环境的适应能力，避免和减少疾病的发生。如夏养阳，应晚睡早起，可适当出外散步，增加活动量，伸展形体，会促进阳气的生发；冬季草木凋零，蛰虫蛰伏，人与自然界一样，阴阳消长代谢缓慢，精气内闭潜藏，冬季则应敛阳护阴，宜早睡晚起，适当减少外出时间，避免受寒，便于阳气的潜藏，肾气的蓄积。

bed early, and go out less, avoiding catching cold in winter. These may facilitate the yang qi to be reserved in the body and the kidney qi to be accumulated.

(5) Medicinal prevention: TCM nursing holds the concept that drug prevention is an important means in preventing disease. Ancient doctors summarized some effective preventions and treatments through constantly exploration on drug prevention. The prescription of antiphlogistic tablet is recorded (*Basic Questions· Discussion on Acupuncture Technique*): "Take ten tablets have the effect of disease resistance." It is recorded by Sun Si-miao (AD 581—682) that Tusu Liquor (*tú sū jiǔ*, 屠苏酒) can resist the epidemic, and effectively prevent warm disease and typhoid (*Important Formulas Worth a Thousand Gold Pieces for Emergency*). Eating vulgaris may nourish yin and dispel dampness (*The Grand Compendium of Materia Medica*). Modern people use the fumigant of vulgaris for air disinfection. Study observed that the fumigant of vulgaris can inhibit adenovirus, herpes virus, influenza virus and the mumps virus. In the fight against the infectious atypical pneumonia in 2003, Chinese medicine played an important role in the early intervention, blocking the course of the disease, relieving symptoms, shortening the recovery time of the patients with fever, promoting inflammation absorption, reducing the complications and *etc.*. The significant values of Chinese herbal medicine in preventing diseases have been given attention.

2. Control the Development of Existing Disease
TCM nursing emphasizes the early diagnosis and treatment for the sick. Meanwhile, nurses should grasp the dynamic changes of illness so as to avoid further development and transmission of the disease. "One should get treatment or aftercare although there is only a little uncomfortable in the body. Do not regard it as nothing or neglect it in case that the illness gets aggravated. Do not struggle to stay afloat without treatment, which will make the condition worsen and result in greater harm" (*Treatise on the Origin and Development of Medicine, Yī Xué Yuán Liú Lùn*, 医学源流论). At the same time, during the process of caring the patient, the nurses should treat the affected area, master the regular pattern of disease development and alterations, correctly predict the trends of pathogenic changes, and take protective measures in advance so as to avoid the disease spreading to other areas of the body. For example, in clinical treatment for a liver disease, the method of strengthening the spleen is often taken as an auxiliary method, which means that not only treating and nursing the liver disease but also strengthening the spleen should be done to prevent the transmission of liver disease, although his spleen has not get affected yet (*The*

（5）药物预防：中医认为药物预防是在预防疫病中的重要手段。关于药物预防，历代医者通过不断地探索，总结出了一些有效的防治方法，如《素问遗篇·刺法论》记载小金丹方，"服十粒，无疫干也"；孙思邈的《备急千金要方》记载了屠苏酒方能"避疫气，令人不染温病及伤寒"；《本草纲目》记载艾叶"服之则走三阴，而逐一切寒湿"，现代人用艾叶烟熏剂进行空气消毒预防，研究发现艾叶烟熏剂对腺病毒、疱疹病毒、流感病毒和腮腺炎病毒等均有抑制作用。中草药预防疾病的效果愈来愈受到人们的认可。

2. 既病防变　对于已经生病者，中医注重疾病的早期诊断和及早治疗，同时要掌握疾病动态变化的规律，避免疾病的进一步发展、恶化。"凡人少有不适，必当即时调治，断不可忽为小病，以致渐深；更不可勉强支持，使病更增，以贻无穷之害"（《中国医学源流论》）。同时，在诊治、护理患者时，不但要对患者已发生病变的部位进行处理，还须掌握疾病发展传变的规律，正确地预测病邪传变的趋向，对可能被影响的部位，预先采取防护措施，以免疾病传至该处，如"见肝之病，知肝传脾，当先实脾气，无令得受肝之邪"（《难经·七十七难》），意指肝病常影响到脾，当肝病还尚未累及脾时，要治肝、护肝，又要治脾、护脾，防止肝病传变；中风的患者，在发病之初，其便秘、苔黄厚等腑实证象可能并不典型，但随着病情的发展，如风邪渐减而痰、瘀等征象渐显，此时其毒

Classic of Difficult Issues· the Classic on Seventy-seven Difficult Issues, Nàn Jīng. Qī Shí Qī Nán, 难经·七十七难). In the early process of stroke, the bowel repletion syndrome of patients such as constipation, tongue fur yellow and thick may not be typical. But with the progress of stroke, such as the wind-pathogen is weakened, whereas, the phlegm and stasis are increasing obviously, which indicates that their damage of brain is rising rapidly and may get deteriorated. Therefore, nurses should closely observe the patient's symptoms and signs, such as fever, hazy mind and *etc.*. Intervention should be given accurately and timely in advance so as to prevent the adverse prognosis early.

3. Prevent Recurrence after Healing Healing means the period from the early phase of recovery to the complete rehabilitation. In the recovery phase, the healthy qi of the patient is deficient, whereas the pathogenic qi is remnant. At this stage, improper care can easily lead to the recurrence of the disease, or cause some new problems. Therefore, appropriate protective measures should be made to prevent the recurrence of disease according to the condition of particular case. It is stated (*Treatise on Cold Damage, Shāng Hán Lùn,* 伤寒论) that during the early stage of healing, the spleen and stomach of patient are weak, and they cannot digest excessive food. At this time, porridge is suitable to nourish the stomach. During the period of healing, on the basis of consolidating treatment, TCM nursing focuses on strengthening dietary nursing, paying more attention to regulating emotion, guiding patients with moderate activity, promoting the recovery of their physical constitution in order to prevent the recurrence of the disease.

(Wang Chun-yan)

Key Points

1. TCM nursing inherits and carries forward essential characteristics of TCM, namely: concept of holism and nursing based on pattern differentiation.

2. In the concept of TCM nursing, human body is an organic whole. The life activities of human being are closely related with the environment of nature and society.

3. The principle of TCM nursing is "strengthening the healthy qi and dispelling the pathogen" "balancing yin and yang" "emergency or chronicity and root or branch" "the three considerations of time, person and place" and "preventing disease before it arises".

4. The application of "strengthening the healthy qi and dispelling the pathogen" principle in nursing practice

---

损脑络可能迅速加剧而导致病情的恶化。因此，要密切观察患者的症状和体征，如发热、神识昏蒙等，事先准确及时地给予干预，早期预防不良预后的发生。

3. **愈后防复** 愈后是指疾病初愈至完全康复的这一段时间。患者在疾病的恢复期，机体正气尚虚，而余邪未尽，此时若调理不当，容易导致疾病复发或引发某些新的疾患，因此，应根据疾病恢复期的具体情况采取恰当防护措施，防止疾病复发。在《伤寒论》中说明了病情初愈时脏腑的一般情况：脾胃尚弱，不能消化水谷，应稍给予糜粥以养胃气。中医护理注重在患者疾病初愈时在巩固治疗的基础上，加强饮食调养、关注情志的调摄、防御外邪的侵袭，指导患者适度的活动、促进体质的恢复以防止疾病的复发。

（王春艳）

要点

1. 中医护理继承和发扬中医的本质特征，即以整体观念为指导，采用辨证施护的方法对患者加以照料。

2. 中医护理学观念认为人是一个有机的整体，人类的生活活动与自然和社会环境密切相关。

3. 中医护理的原则：扶正祛邪，护病求本，调整阴阳，标本缓急，三因制宜，预防为主。

4. "扶正祛邪"原则要求护理人员在护理实

should be done according to the exuberance and debilitation of pathogenic qi or healthy qi. Importantly, it should be distinguished when strengthening the healthy qi is suitable, when the method of dispelling the pathogen is proper, and at what circumstances, strengthening the healthy qi and dispelling the pathogen should be used simultaneously.

5. "When nursing, it is necessary to seek the root" requires that nurses should not only observe the symptoms and signs of patient, but also consider the external environmental factors of patients. After dialectical analyzing, nurses should determine the root of the disease, find the nursing problem need to be solved, make plans and take nursing measures.

6. Orthodox nursing is used for a case that the signs and symptoms are consistent with its essence.

7. Paradoxical assistant can be used under the circumstances that the manifestations of the cases are opposite to the nature of disease.

8. The "paradoxical nursing" includes "treating heat with heat" "treating cold with cold" "treating the blocked by blocking" "treating the flowing by promoting its flow" and "contrary nursing in medicine taken".

9. "Balancing yin and yang" consists of "eliminating the surplus" and "supplementing the deficiency".

10. The nursing plan should be formulated depending on the emergency or chronicity of the root and the branch of the disease, and in accordance with the principle of "nursing the branch for emergency" "nursing the root for chronicity" and "nursing the branch and the root simultaneously".

11. The "prevention" includes "preventing disease before it arises" "controling the development of existing disease", and "preventing recurrence after healing".

践中注意分析正邪双方相互消长盛衰的状况。尤其应注意区分实际情况，针对性地运用单纯扶正法、单纯祛邪法、扶正祛邪法先后或同时进行的护理方法。

5. "护病求本" 原则要求护理人员在护理实践中不但要观察患者的症状和体征，而且要考虑患者的外部环境因素，经过辨证分析，判断疾病的根本原因，找出需要解决的护理问题，制订计划，采取护理措施。

6. 正护法用于疾病的临床表现和疾病的本质相一致的病例。

7. 反护法用于证因不符、寒热真假和虚实真伪的情况，需要护理人员透过现象究其本质。

8. 反护法常用的护理方法包括 "热因热用" "寒因寒用" "塞因塞用" "通因通用" 及 "药物护理的反佐法"。

9. "调整阴阳" 包括 "损其有余" "补其不足"。

10. 护理计划的制订要针对标本缓急的情况，遵循 "急则护其标，缓则护其本，标本俱急则标本同护" 的原则。

11. 治未病包括未病先防、既病防变和愈后防复三个方面。

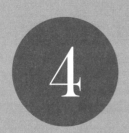

Chapter 4 General Nursing

第四章 一般调护

Learning Objectives

Mastery

1. To repeat the main contents of inspection of spirit, inspection of complexion, tongue inspection and inquiry.

2. To repeat the basic principles of seasonal health preservation and the detailed contents of daily life nursing in four seasons.

3. To repeat the principles of emotional nursing, the definition of nursing of inter-restriction among emotions, empathic therapy, method of persuasion and restraining.

4. To repeat the property of food, and the function and the basic principles of dietary nursing and restrictions.

5. To repeat the meaning of regulating of constitution in TCM exactly and to identify nine different kinds of TCM constitution exactly.

6. To repeat the meanings of nursing at the convalescent phase of disease and to describe five aspects of nursing at the convalescent phase of disease.

学习目标

识记

1. 能复述望神、望色、望舌和闻诊的主要内容。

2. 能复述四时养生必须遵循的基本原则和生活起居护理的具体内容。

3. 能复述情志护理的原则，以情胜情、移情易性法、说理开导法、节制法的概念。

4. 能复述食物的性能，饮食调护的作用、基本要求和饮食禁忌。

5. 能复述体质调护的含义，并能鉴别九种中医体质。

6. 能复述病证后期调护的含义及病证后期调护的五方面。

Comprehension

1. To give examples to explain significance of complying with the four seasons to keep yin-yang balance.
2. To give examples to explain the relationship between emotion and health.
3. To give examples to explain what is the performance of food and its function.
4. To understand the interventions applied to patients with various kinds of TCM constitution.
5. To give examples to explain the importance of nursing at the convalescent phase of disease

Application

1. To correctly take the pulse for a patient and to inquire a patient.
2. To correctly apply the methods of emotional nursing.
3. To give examples to describe the dietary restrictions and the TCM dietary formulas for specific patterns.
4. To choose the correct nursing method according to the different constitution.
5. To correctly educate the patient at the convalescent phase of disease according to individual's condition.

理解

1. 能用实例说明"顺应四时，平衡阴阳"的意义。
2. 能用实例说明情志与健康的关系。
3. 能用实例说明食物的性能和作用。
4. 能用实例说明各种体质的调护方法。
5. 能用实例说明病证后期调护的重要性。

运用

1. 能运用所学知识，对患者进行脉诊和问诊。
2. 能正确应用情志调护的方法。
3. 能用实例说明特殊病证的饮食禁忌及特殊病证的食疗方。
4. 能根据患者的体质，选择正确的调护方法。
5. 能根据患者的病情，正确指导患者进行病证后期调护。

Chapter 4

Case Study

Patient, male, 63 years old, has hypertension for 10 years. The patient has been suffered from angina for 4-6 minutes each time while feel fatigue, which is pointing radially to left shoulder, back and the inside of left hand, and also has the symptoms of chest oppression, diaphoresis and palpitation. These symptoms could be relieved after rest. The TCM symptoms include dark red tongue with white thin coating and petechias, wiry and tight pulse.

Question 1: What are the dietary restriction and recommendation for this patient?

Question 2: To give an example of TCM dietary formulas for this patient.

General nursing means recuperation and maintenance. In broad sense, it is to prevent diseases and enhance well-being based on theories and methods of TCM. In narrow sense, it refers to TCM nursing, which consists of daily life nursing, dietary nursing, emotional nursing, exercise nursing, *etc.*. Whether the nursing measures are implemented correctly or not will directly affect the recovery and prognosis of patients. So it is very important to conduct general nursing well.

Section 1 Observation of the State of Illness

Observation of the state of illness is a process by which nursing staff collect patient's information, sort, summarize, synthesize and analyze various clinical manifestations based on pattern differentiation, so as to understand the causes, pathomechanism, nature and location of the illness, and make judgements about the illness. Observation of the state of illness is a basic responsibility of nurses and also important contents for nursing work. Timely and accurate observation of the state of illness can help to detect disease's change as early as possible, get to know the therapeutic effects and provide basis for nursing planning and implementation.

I. Requirement for Observation

i. Comprehensive and Focus

Nurses should collect information about disease comprehensively, and with clear focus. "Comprehensive" means thorough observation of the patient, including his/

导入案例与思考

患者，男，63岁，既往高血压病史10年，近日来劳累后出现胸前区绞痛，向左肩背部及左手内侧放射，每次持续4~6min，发作时伴胸闷、出汗、心悸，休息后可逐渐缓解。舌质暗红，有瘀点瘀斑，舌苔薄白，脉弦紧。

问题1：请说出患者的饮食宜忌。

问题2：举例一项适宜的食疗方。

调护，即调理、养护。广义的调护，是指运用中医理论和方法来预防疾病，促进健康。狭义的调护，是指中医护理的具体方法。中医一般调护包括起居调护、饮食调护、情志调护、运动调护等。这些调护措施实施恰当与否，直接影响疾病的转归与预后。因此，做好一般调护具有十分重要的意义。

第一节 病情观察

病情观察是指护理人员运用四诊的方法收集患者的病情资料，对疾病的各种表现进行整理和归纳、综合和分析，以了解疾病的病因、病机、病性和病位，通过辨证对病情做出判断的过程。病情观察是护士的基本职责，也是护理工作的重要内容。及时、准确的病情观察可及早发现病情变化，了解治疗效果，为有效制订护理计划、实施护理措施提供依据。

一、病情观察的要求

（一）内容全面，重点明确

对病情的观察，要做到内容全面，重点明确。所谓的全面是指对患者全方面的观察，

her past history, current illness's status and treatment, *etc.*. At the same time, nurses should observe the patient with clear focus and purpose. For example, for patients with diarrhea, nurses need to know the onset of diarrhea, the frequency, characteristics, color, volume of stool and accompanying symptoms. If there is any treatment, nurses need to observe the treatment effects and side effects of medications, whether the illness is improving or worsening, *etc.*. The current focus is on whether there is diarrhea and whether there is deficiency of body fluid *etc.*. In this way, nurses can know fairly well about the patient and provide targeted nursing care. The observation's focus is different for different patients. For example, for patients with depression syndrome, the focus of observation is on the emotional change. For patients with pulmonary abscess, the focus is on cough and the change of color, quality and quantity of phlegm, *etc.*.

ii. Scientific and Accurate

Whether the method of observation is correct or not will have a direct influence on the illness' evaluation and the efficiency of nursing implementation. Nurses should be skilled at all kinds of observation methods, and analyze comprehensively based on four diagnostic methods. They should observe the illness carefully and accurately, using all opportunities to observe, ruling out all confounding factors, listening carefully, observing attentively and recognizing possible false appearances so as to detect the changes of illness timely and accurately. For example, pain has different characteristics such as dull pain, sudden pain, burning pain, cramps, *etc.*. Nurses should observe carefully and accurately so as to reflect the true condition.

iii. Summarize and Evaluate Accurately

Nurses should analyze the observation's results comprehensively to make correct judgements. They should not make arbitrary conclusions based on temporary, local or partial phenomenon or symptoms, particularly when there are contradictory results among each other. Nurses need to analyze comprehensively, summarize the findings, eliminate the false and retain the true, and make judgements comprehensively. For example, a patient with abdominal pain feels his/her pain relieved. He/she used to toss and turn while groaning, but now he/she becomes quiet and still. This generally indicates the condition has become better. However, if the patient is apathetic with cold limbs, blue in the face, cold sweat, weak pulse or no pulse at all, this might be shock and indicate a critical situation.

iv. Record Observation Truly and Objectively

Nurses should record the observation's results

包括既往史、现病状况及治疗等全过程。同时还应有重点、有目的地进行病情观察。如对腹泻患者，要掌握腹泻出现的时间，大便的次数、性状、颜色、量及其伴随症状等。如有治疗还应观察效果和用药反应，重点掌握是否还有腹泻及有无津亏等情况，从而了解目前病情是好转还是恶化等，做到心中有数，以进行针对性护理。不同患者，观察的重点也不同。如郁证患者应重点观察情绪变化，肺痈患者应重点观察咳嗽性质与痰液的色、质、量等变化。

（二）方法科学有效，细致准确

病情观察的方法正确与否，将直接影响病情判断以及护理措施落实的有效性，护士应熟练掌握各种病情观察方法，运用四诊合参，综合分析。要认真倾听，仔细观察，识别可能的假象，及时、准确地发现患者的病情变化。如疼痛有隐痛、阵痛、灼痛、绞痛等不同情况，应观察细致准确，才能真实反映病情。

（三）归纳总结，准确判断

对病情观察所得到的结果，必须全面分析，才能得出正确的判断，切忌根据一时或局部、片面的现象或症状，武断地下结论，尤其是观察结果之间互相矛盾时，更需全面分析、归纳总结、去伪存真、综合判断。如腹痛患者腹痛减轻或消失，患者由辗转呻吟变为静默不动，一般来讲表示病情好转，但如果患者神情淡漠，四肢厥冷，面色发青，出冷汗，脉象微弱甚至摸不到，则可能是休克，病情危重。

（四）记录结果，客观真实

对观察结果要及时、真实的记录，必要

timely and truly, with bedside handover if necessary. They should use numbers to describe the condition as much as possible, such as body's temperature, urinary volume, *etc.*. For those symptoms and signs that cannot be quantified, nurses should describe them objectively and truly. They should record not only the main symptoms, but also other accompanying symptoms and signs. For example, for patients with pain, they could use "talk and smile as usual" "curl up and remain still" "toss and turn" to express the severity of pain.

II. Basic Method of Illness Observation

Illness observation is a basic method for inspecting and analyzing disease and judging the development and progression of disease, and its basic parts are four diagnostic methods, namely inspection, listening and smelling, inquiry, pulse feeling and palpation. The four diagnostic methods are used to examine disease from different aspects and they have their own specific contents, scope of application, functions and cannot replace each other in diagnosis. So in clinical practice, they are usually used in combination for systematic understanding of a disease in order to ensure comprehensive analysis and correct diagnosis.

i. Inspection

Inspection means that the nurse use his or her eyes to examine the patient's whole body or local region for the purpose of understanding pathological conditions. Inspection should be done in the place with full light, especially natural light.

1. Inspection of the Whole Body　Inspection of the whole body, also known as general inspection, refers to purposeful examination of the spirit, color, shape and posture of the whole body so as to have a general understanding of the disease.

（1）Inspection of vitality (spirit): Vitality (spirit) refers to the general manifestations of life activities. The material base of vitality is essential qi, which comes from congenital essence and is being nourished continuously by the acquired essence developed from food as well as protected by the normal *zang-fu* organs' functions. That is why the vitality is said to be the external manifestations of the conditions of *zang-fu* organs and essential qi. By inspection of vitality, doctors or nurses can understand whether the essential qi is exuberant or deficient and whether the *zang-fu* organs' functions are strong or weak. Such an understanding is important for analyzing whether the pathological conditions are light or serious and whether the prognosis is benign or malignant.

时进行床头交接班。对能用计量表示的要记录具体数量，如体温、尿量等；对不能量化的症状和体征，描述要客观、真实。不仅记录主要症状，而且还应记录其伴发的症状与体征。如对疼痛患者以谈笑如常、蜷卧不动、转侧不安等表达疼痛的轻重程度。

二、病情观察的基本方法

病情观察是诊察分析病情，判断疾病发生发展的基本方法，其基本内容包括望诊、闻诊、问诊、切诊，简称"四诊"。四诊从不同侧面诊察病情，各有其特定的内容、适用范围和作用，彼此不能互相替代。因此，临床上应四诊合参，综合分析，才能全面系统地了解病情。

（一）望诊

望诊，是护理人员运用视觉观察患者全身和局部情况，以了解病情的一种诊察方法。望诊须在充足的光线下进行，尤以自然光线为佳。

1. **望全身情况**　望全身情况又称整体望诊，是对患者全身的神、色、形、态进行诊察，以对疾病有一个大概的了解。

（1）望神：神是指人体生命活动的综合外在表现。神的物质基础是精气，包括先天之精气和后天水谷精气的不断补充，还有赖于脏腑的正常生理功能。因此，神是脏腑精气盛衰的外部征象。通过望神，可以了解个体精气的盛衰、脏腑功能的强弱，对分析病情轻重和预后的良恶有重要意义。

The manifestations of vitality are multiple. The emphasis is on observing patients' consciousness, mental state, emotional expressions, complexion, eye expressions, speech, breath, posture, *etc.*. By examining the aspects mentioned above, man can differentiate whether the spirit is in existence, deficient, lost, false or in disorder.

1) Presence of vitality: also known as "vigorous vitality". The main manifestations are clear in consciousness, normal spirit, natural facial expressions, ruddy complexion, eyes with brightness and vitality, accurate verbal expression, normal breath, normal and natural movement of the limbs. These manifestations suggest the sufficiency of *zang-fu* essential qi, prosperity of healthy qi, and normality of life activities. Even if the person is sick, he/she has no impairment of healthy qi and the condition is mild with favorable prognosis.

2) Lack of vitality: It also known as "insufficiency of vitality". The main manifestations are clear in consciousness, but dispiritedness, pale complexion, dull expressions of eyes, short of breath, no desire to speak, low voice, and slow movement. These manifestations suggest weak *zang-fu* organs' functions and mild consumption of healthy qi. The manifestations are usually seen in patients with mild illness, at recovering stage or with weak constitution. It is slightly more serious than patients with presence of vitality, and has favorable prognosis.

3) Loss of vitality: It also known as "depletion of vitality". The main manifestations are dim in awareness, dispiritedness, pale complexion, dull eye expressions, faltering speech, slow response, difficulty in movement, even paraphasia, with delirium and floccillation, or sudden falling down with closed eyes, open mouth, loose hands, enuresis, *etc.*. These manifestations suggest extreme consumption of *zang-fu* essential qi, great impairment of healthy qi, severe state of illness, and unfavorable prognosis.

4) False vitality: False vitality refers to a false manifestation of spirit in disagreement with the nature of the disease. It is a misleading manifestation that occurs in a prolonged disease or serious disease. It's not a favorable sign and a sign of end of life. The main manifestations are that confused and slowly responsed patients suddenly change into excitation but with restlessness, or patients with no desire to speak, low and weak voice suddenly change into talkative and hope to see families alongside, or dull complexion suddenly changes into reddish cheeks, or poor appetite suddenly changes into good appetite *etc.*. These phenomena suggest the critical sign of separation of yin and yang, just like "the last light of a dying-out candle" and "the last radiance of setting sun". Clinicians should

神的表现是多方面的，望神的重点在于观察患者的神志精神、表情、面色、眼神、语言、呼吸和体态等。通过诊察上述各方面的情况，辨别得神、少神、失神、假神和神乱。

1）得神：又称为有神，主要表现为神志清楚，精神良好，表情自然，面色荣润，两目明亮有神，言语对答准确，呼吸平稳，肢体活动自如。它提示脏腑精气充足，正气强盛，生命活动正常；即使有病，也是正气未伤，属于轻病，预后良好。

2）少神：又称神气不足，主要表现为神志清楚，精神不佳，面色少华，目光乏神，少气懒言，语音低弱，动作迟缓。它提示脏腑功能虚弱，正气轻度亏损。常见于轻病或恢复期患者，也可见于体质虚弱者。病情比得神者稍重，预后良好。

3）失神：又称无神，主要表现为神志淡漠，精神萎靡，面色无华，目光晦滞，语言断续，反应迟钝，动作失灵；甚至语言错乱，循衣摸床，撮空理线或卒倒而目闭口开、手撒、尿遗等。它提示脏腑精气亏虚已极，正气大伤，病情严重，预后不良。

4）假神：是指久病、重病的患者精神突然好转，表现出与病情本质不符的假象，并非佳兆，而是临终前的先兆。其主要表现为原来意识模糊，反应迟钝，突然神情兴奋，烦躁不安；或原来默默不语，语声低微，突然言语不休，想见亲人；或原来面色晦暗，突见面赤如妆；或不欲饮食，突然食欲增加等。这是阴阳即将离绝的危候，犹如"残灯复明""回光返照"，临床应予特别注意。

pay special attention to that.

5) Mental disorder: It also known as mental confusion. It is usually seen in patients with epilepsy, mania and insanity. The usual manifestations are indifferent expression, taciturn and depression, laughing and then crying, which are usually due to stagnation of phlegm and confuse the mind. The manifestations, like dysphoria, running wildly, shouting, and fighting against people, are usually due to disturbance of the heart by phlegmatic fire. The manifestations like sudden coma, drooling, staring upwards, convulsion of limbs and groaning like a pig or goat, usually indicate epilepsy due to endogenous liver wind and phlegm confusing the mind, which can heal himself or herself.

(2) Inspection of the complexion: Inspection of the complexion is also known as "color inspection". It is a method for understanding pathological condition by observing the changes of the color and luster of the skin and face. The skin's color and luster are the signs of qi and blood of the *zang-fu* organs, so inspection of the complexion can enable one to understand the state of *zang-fu* organs' function, qi and blood. The facial skin is soft and thin. The luster is visible and easy to observe. Therefore, the inspection of the complexion mainly observes the color and luster of face, also including skin, eyes, fingernails *etc.*.

1) Normal complexion: The normal and healthy complexion is known as normal complexion. It is ruddy and lustrous, indicating exuberance of essential qi and normal functions of the *zang-fu* organs. Normal complexion is further divided into normal individual complexion and varied normal complexion. Normal individual complexion refers to the color of skin and face that never changes due to constitutional factors. Varied normal complexion refers to the changes of facial and skin's color in correspondence to the variations of the seasons and climates, emotions and exercises. The normal complexion of a healthy Chinese should be red with slight yellow, ruddy and lustrous.

2) Pathological (sick) complexion: Facial color during the course of a disease is called pathological (sick) complexion. It consists of blue, red, yellow, white and black, which correspond to different *zang-fu* organs and indicate different nature of diseases. Bright and moist color indicates mild illness, no insufficiency of qi and blood, while dull and dry color indicates serious illness, impairment of visceral essence.

3) Bluish complexion: Bluish complexion indicates cold syndrome, pain syndrome, stasis syndrome, convulsive syndrome and liver disease. Bluish color is usually a sign

5）神乱：即精神意识错乱，常见于癫、狂、痫的患者。如表现为表情淡漠，寡言少语，闷闷不乐，哭笑无常，多为痰气凝结，阻蔽心神的癫病；如烦躁不宁，登高而歌，弃衣而走，呼号怒骂，打人毁物，多属痰火扰心的狂病；如突然昏仆，口吐涎沫，双目上视，四肢抽动，口中如做猪羊叫声，一般能自行恢复，多属痰迷心窍，肝风内动的痫病。

（2）望色：又称色诊，是通过观察面部和全身皮肤色泽变化来诊察病情的方法。皮肤色泽是脏腑气血之外荣，望色能了解脏腑功能状态和气血盛衰情况。面部皮肤薄嫩，色泽变化易显露于外，便于诊察。因此，望色多以观察面部的颜色和光泽为主，兼望肤色、目睛、爪甲等部位。

1）常色：人体正常健康状态时的面色称为常色。常色的特征是鲜明润泽，含蓄不露，表示脏腑精气充足，功能正常。常色又分为主色和客色。主色是指因禀赋所致，终身不变的色泽。客色是指随季节气候、情绪运动等因素影响所致的面色、肤色变化。我国健康人的面色应是微黄透红，明润光泽。

2）病色：人体在疾病状态下的面色称为病色。病色大致可分为青、赤、黄、白、黑五种，分别提示不同脏腑和不同性质的疾病。若患者面部色泽鲜明、荣润，表明病情轻浅，气血未衰；若面色晦暗、枯槁，表明病情深重，精气已伤。

3）青色：主寒证、痛证、瘀证、惊风和肝病。青色是气血运行不畅，经脉瘀阻的

of inhibited flow of qi and blood and stagnation of vessels and meridians.

4) Red complexion: Red complexion indicates heat syndrome. It results from sufficient blood circulating in the meridians and skins. Flushed face is a sign of excess heat pattern due to hyperactivity of visceral yang and fever from external contraction. Flushed and delicate cheeks indicate deficiency heat syndrome due to endogenous heat resulting from yin deficiency.

5) Yellow complexion: Yellow complexion indicates dampness syndrome and deficiency syndrome. Yellow indicates malnutrition of muscles due to insufficiency of qi and blood resulting from failure of the spleen to transport, or due to internal accumulation of dampness.

6) White complexion: White complexion indicates syndrome of deficiency, cold, and loss of blood. White indicates yang deficiency, insufficiency or stagnant movement of qi and blood.

7) Black complexion: Black complexion indicates kidney deficiency syndrome, cold syndrome, blood stasis syndrome and fluid retention syndrome. Black complexion is the sign of kidney yang exhaustion, yin-cold predominance and exuberance of water or stagnation of qi and blood.

(3) Inspection of body: It is mainly to understand the function of *zang-fu* organs and the conditions of qi and blood by observing the shape and development of body. Strength refers to the strong physique, and the manifestations of which are lustrous skin, strong muscles, wide chest and thick bones. Weakness refers to decline of body's strength, and the manifestations of which are dry skin, lean muscles, thin chest and bones. Obesity is characterized by round head, short and thick neck, wide and flat shoulders, wide-short-round chest, big belly, smaller body, flabby muscles, pale and lusterless skin, usually suggesting insufficiency of yang qi. Emaciation is characterized by long head, thin and long neck, narrow shoulders, narrow and flat chest, small belly, higher body, thin muscles and dryness of skin which usually suggest insufficiency of yin blood. Deformity such as chicken chest and tortoise back are caused by insufficiency of congenital kidney essence or spleen and stomach failing to be nourished after birth.

(4) Inspection of postures: Inspection of postures mainly examines the patient's postures in quiescence and actions as well as abnormal movement. Yang governs action and yin quiescence. A tendency to be active, lying on a supine position with limbs stretching out, clothes and quilt removed, and face turning outwards, usually indicates yang syndrome, heat syndrome, and excess

征象。

4）赤色：主热证。赤色乃血液充盈皮肤脉络所致。满面通红，多为外感发热及脏腑阳盛所致的实热证；两颧潮红，多为阴虚内热的虚热证。

5）黄色：主湿证、虚证。黄色为脾虚失运，气血不充，肌肤失养或湿邪内蕴的表现。

6）白色：主虚证、寒证、失血证。白色为阳气虚弱，气血不足或运行不畅的表现。

7）黑色：主肾虚证、寒证、瘀血证、水饮证。黑色为肾阳衰微、阴寒水盛、气血凝滞的表现。

（3）望形体：主要是观察患者形体的胖瘦及发育情况，以了解脏腑功能的强弱和气血的盈亏。形体强指身体强壮，表现为皮肤润泽，肌肉结实，胸廓宽厚，骨骼粗大。形体弱指身体衰弱，表现为皮肤干燥，肌肉瘦削，胸廓狭窄，骨骼细小。形体胖表现为头圆形，颈短粗，肩宽平，胸廓宽短呈圆形，大腹便便，身材偏矮，肌肉松软，肤白无华，多为阳气不足。形体瘦表现为头长形，颈细长，肩狭窄，胸廓狭长平坦，腹部瘪瘪，身材偏高，肌肉瘦削，皮肤干燥，多为阴血不足。畸形如鸡胸龟背，多见先天肾气不足或后天脾胃失养。

（4）望姿态：主要观察患者的动静姿态及肢体的异常动作。"阳主动，阴主静"。患者喜动，卧时仰面伸足，揭去衣被，面常向外者，多属阳证、热证、实证；患者喜静，卧时蜷缩成团，喜加衣被，面常向里者，多属阴证、寒证、虚证。如头摇不能自主，四肢

syndrome. A tendency to be quiet, lying down huddling up with preference to put on more clothes and facing inward usually indicates yin syndrome, cold syndrome, and deficiency syndrome. Shaking head and trembling of limbs usually indicate internal disturbance of liver wind. Hemiplegia and distortion of commissure are usually caused by apoplexy. Pain, swelling and numbness in joints and difficulty in movement usually suggest obstructive syndrome. Sudden coma, foam around the mouth, convulsion and returning to normal after a seizure are signs of epilepsy. Flaccid limbs, motion difficulty or atrophy of muscles are usually signs of atrophy-flaccidity disease.

2. Inspection of the Local Region　The inspection of the local region, also known as regional inspection, is used to closely examine some regional areas to obtain necessary clinical data on the basis of general inspection according to the pathological conditions in question.

(1) Inspection of head and hair: Head is the region where all yang meridians converge and the house of spirit. Hair is the external manifestation of kidney and the extending part of blood. Thus, inspection of head and hair is helpful for understanding the condition of kidney, spleen and stomach as well as qi and blood.

1) Inspection of head: The inspection of head means to examine the external shape and movement of head. Bigger or smaller head with low intelligence in children is usually caused by inadequate innate endowment or insufficiency of kidney essence. Sunken fontanel in children usually indicates deficiency syndrome. Protrusion of fontanel usually indicates excess heat. Delayed closure of fontanel is frequently caused by congenital insufficiency of kidney essence or maldevelopment. Involuntary shaking head in both children and adults usually means internal disturbance of liver wind.

2) Inspection of hair: The inspection of hair mainly examines the luster, shape, growth and loss of hair. In the yellow race, black, dense and lustrous hair is a sign of sufficient kidney essence and exuberance of qi and blood. Yellow, sparse, dry hair and loss of hair is the sign of deficiency of kidney essence, qi and blood. Sudden patch loss of hair is called "alopecia areata", and usually due to blood deficiency and wind attack. Sparse hair and loss of hair in young people usually result from consumption of kidney essence or blood heat. Appearance of infantile hair like tassels with yellowish lusterless dryness is usually due to malnutrition.

(2) Inspection of five sense organs: The inspection of five sense organs includes inspection of eyes, ears, nose, mouth, lips, *etc.*. Each organ itself is closely related to several

时而颤动，多为肝风内动；半身不遂或口角歪斜，多为中风；关节肿痛或麻木不仁，行动不便，多为痹证；若卒然昏仆，口吐涎沫，四肢抽搐，醒后如常者，属痫证；如肢体软弱无力，行动不便，甚至肌肉萎缩者，多为痿证。

2. 望局部情况　望局部情况，又称分部望诊，是在整体望诊的基础上，根据病情及诊断需要，对患者的某些局部进行重点、细致的诊察，以进一步获取与疾病诊断有关的临床资料。

（1）望头与发：头为诸阳之会，精明之府；肾之华在发，发又为血之余。故望头与发可了解肾、脾胃和气血的盛衰。

1）望头：主要诊察头的外形和动态。小儿头形过大或过小，伴智力低下，多属先天禀赋不足或肾精亏损；小儿囟门下陷，多属虚证；囟门高突，多为实热；囟门迟闭，多为肾气不足，发育不良；无论大人或小儿，头摇不能自主者，多为肝风内动。

2）望发：主要诊察头发的色泽、形态和生长脱落情况。黄色人种头发色黑，浓密润泽，为肾精充足，气血旺盛之征象。发黄稀疏易落，或干枯不荣，为肾精不足，气血虚亏之征象；突然大片脱发，称斑秃，多属血虚受风；青壮年头发稀疏易落，多属肾虚或血热；小儿发结如穗，枯黄无泽，多为疳积。

（2）望五官：望五官包括望目、望耳、望鼻、望口唇等。五官与内脏有着密切的关系，

viscera. Therefore, the inspection of five sensory organs is not only helpful for the selection of treatment of sensory organs themselves based on pattern differentiation, but also helpful for understanding the pathological changes of the *zang-fu* organs.

1) Inspection of eyes: Eyes are the orifices related to the liver. All the visceral essence flows upward into the eyes. Inspection of eyes includes expression, color, shape and movement of the eyes. Redness of the white part largely attributes to wind-heat of lung meridian. Red and swollen eyes and pain in the eyes largely attributes to wind-heat of liver meridian. Yellowish change of the white part mostly attributes to jaundice. Sunken orbit is often due to loss of body fluid. Dropsy of the eyelids usually indicates edema. Staring straight upward and obliquely mostly indicates internal disturbance of liver wind. Immobile straight staring with perfect round eyeballs usually indicates exhaustion of *zang-fu* essential qi. Platycoria is usually a sign of essential qi exhaustion. Miosis usually indicates poisoning. Anisocoria usually suggests blood stasis in the brain.

2) Inspection of ears: Ears are the orifices related to the kidneys and the places where all meridians converge. Inspection of ears should concentrate on the color, shape and inner part of ears. Red and ruddy helix is favorable. Whitish color indicates cold syndrome. Bluish and blackish color is usually seen in pain syndrome. Thin and dry ears are usually a sign of insufficiency of kidney essence. Scorching dry and black color of ears usually signifies extreme loss of kidney essence. Cold in base of ears and red collaterals in the back of ears is mostly a sign of measles. Pus discharging from inner ear is called otorrhea, which is mostly attributes to damp-heat of the liver and gallbladder.

3) Inspection of nose: Nose is the orifice related to lung, corresponding to spleen channel and connecting with the stomach channel. The inspection of nose mainly concentrates on examining the excreta as well as the color and shape of nose. Reddish swelling with sore of nose is usually caused by exuberant heat in stomach or blood heat. The enlargement of nose tip with thickened skin, bulging surface like acne is called rosacea, which is mostly caused by accumulation of heat in the lung and stomach. Sinking of nose bridge with the loss of brows is usually a critical condition in leprosy. Wheezing, high fever, and nares flaring attribute to accumulation of phlegm-heat in lung. Chronic nares flaring and wheezing with profuse sweating like oils indicate decline and exhaustion of essential qi of lung and kidney. Watery nasal discharge mostly attributes to exogenous pathogenic wind-cold, while turbid nasal discharge mostly attributes to exogenous pathogenic

诊察五官的异常变化，不仅有助于对其本身病变的辨证施治，还可了解脏腑的病变。

1）望目：目为肝之窍，五脏六腑精气皆上注于目。望目，除诊察眼神外，还应注意目色、目形及动态异常。白睛红赤，多为肺经风热；目赤肿痛，多为肝经风热；白睛黄染，多属黄疸；目窝内陷，多为津液亏耗；眼睑浮肿如卧蚕，多为水肿；两目斜视、上视，多为肝风内动；两目直视，不能转动，目睛正圆，多为脏腑精气衰竭；瞳孔散大，多为精气衰竭；瞳孔缩小，多为中毒；两侧瞳孔不等大，多为颅内淤血。

2）望耳：耳为肾之窍，宗脉之所聚。望耳，应注意耳的色泽、形态和内耳的情况。耳轮以红润为佳，色白多属寒证，色青而黑多属痛证。耳肉薄而干枯，多为肾精不足；耳轮焦黑干枯多为肾精亏极。耳根发冷，耳背有红脉者，多为麻疹先兆；耳内流脓水，称为脓耳，多为肝胆湿热所致。

3）望鼻：鼻为肺之窍，脾经之所应，胃经之经过。望鼻，主要望鼻的色泽、外形及鼻内的分泌物。鼻红肿生疮，多为胃热炽盛或血热。鼻头增大，皮肤变厚，表面高低不平或生粉刺，称为酒糟鼻，多由肺胃蕴热所致。鼻柱崩塌，眉毛脱落，多为麻风恶候。喘促、高热、鼻翼煽动，为痰热壅肺；久病鼻煽，喘促汗出如油者，为肺肾精气衰绝危候；鼻流清涕，多为外感风寒；鼻流浊涕，多为外感风热；久流黄稠浊涕而腥臭者为鼻渊。

wind-heat. A long duration of discharging yellow, thick and fishy nasal snivel is called nasosinusitis.

4) Inspection of mouth and lips: The spleen opens to mouth, flourishes on lips and is internally and externally related with stomach. Inspection of mouth and lips is helpful for understanding the functions of spleen and stomach as well as the pathological changes of qi and blood in the whole body. Inspection of mouth and lips mainly focuses on inspecting the color, luster, dryness, moisture and shape. The normal color of lips is reddish, fresh and moist. Pale lips mostly attribute to qi and blood deficiency. Blue and purplish lips usually indicate cold obstruction and blood stasis. Deep red and dry lips indicate consumption of fluid by exuberant heat. Purplish and brownish dry lips indicate extreme exuberance of stagnant heat. Bright red lips indicate yin deficiency and exuberant fire. Lips as red as cherry usually indicates poisoning of CO. Dry and fissuring lips is often caused by exogenous dryness pathogen or injured fluid due to pathogenic heat. Red and swelling lips with ulceration are often caused by heat accumulation of spleen and stomach. Distortion of commissure is often caused by apoplexy. Closed mouth or trembling lips usually attributes to internal disturbance of liver wind.

5) Inspection of tooth and gums: Tooth and gums are connected with the collaterals of *yangming* channel. So inspection of tooth and gums is helpful for understanding the pathological changes of the stomach. Inspection of gums mainly concentrates on examining the color of gums. Normally, gums are light red and moist. Pale gums indicate blood deficiency. Reddish swelling and painful gums indicate exuberance of gastric fire. Dry teeth are usually caused by stomach heat injuring body fluid. Teeth being as dry as dried bone are usually caused by exhaustion of kidney yin. Loose and sparse teeth with exposure of root are mostly attributes to kidney deficiency or exuberance of deficiency-fire.

6) Inspection of throat: Throat is the door to lung and stomach, the pathway for breathing and eating and the region over which kidney channel circulates. So inspection of throat is helpful for examining the pathological changes of lung, stomach and kidney. Inspection of throat mainly concentrates on the color and shape of throat. Red and swollen throat with soreness is commonly caused by accumulated heat of lung and stomach. Red, swollen and ulcerous throat with yellowish and white pyogenic spots is induced by accumulation and hyperactivity of heat-toxin of lung and stomach. Bright and tender color with slight pain mostly attributes to fire hyperactivity from yin deficiency. Light red throat without swollen which can't be healed over long time is usually due to flaming up of deficiency-

4）望口唇：脾开窍于口，其华在唇，与胃互为表里。诊察口唇，可了解脾胃功能及全身气血变化。望口唇主要诊察口唇的色泽、润燥和形态。正常唇色红而鲜润。口唇淡白，多属气血两虚；唇色青紫，多为寒凝血瘀；唇色深红而干，为热盛伤津；唇色绛紫而干焦，为淤热盛极；唇色鲜红，为阴虚火旺；唇色如樱桃色，多为一氧化碳中毒。唇干裂、皲裂，多为外感燥邪或邪热伤津；唇红肿糜烂，多为脾胃蕴热；口角歪斜，多为中风；口噤或抽搐不止，多为肝风内动。

5）望齿龈：齿龈为阳明脉络所系，诊察齿龈异常变化，可了解胃的一些病变。望齿龈，主要诊察齿龈的色泽变化。正常齿龈色泽红而润泽。龈色淡白，为血虚不荣；齿龈红肿疼痛，为胃火上炎；牙齿干燥，多为胃热伤津；齿干如枯骨，为肾阴枯涸；牙齿松动稀疏，齿根外露者，多属肾虚或虚火上炎。

6）望咽喉：咽喉为肺、胃之门户，呼吸、饮食之通路，肾经循行之处。望咽喉可了解肺、胃、肾的病变。望咽喉主要诊察咽喉色泽、形态的变化。咽喉红肿而痛，多属肺胃积热；红肿溃烂，有黄白腐点，为肺胃热毒壅盛；若色鲜娇嫩，疼痛不甚，多为阴虚火旺；色淡红不肿，久久不愈，多为虚火上浮。若咽喉部出现灰白色假膜，擦之不去，重擦出血，随即复生，为白喉，急需隔离治疗。

fire. False whitish membrane on the throat that is not erasable, bleeding when rubbed heavily and reappearing is diphtheria. It must be treated immediately by isolation.

3. Inspection of Skin　Skin is distributed over the surface of body and is the defending barrier of body and nourished by qi, blood and body fluid through meridians. Inspection of skin is not only helpful for diagnosing skin disorders, but also helpful for understanding the nature of the disease, the condition of the *zang-fu* organs and the state of qi and blood. Inspection of skin mainly concentrates on the color, shape, rash *etc.*. The normal skin color of the yellow race is reddish and yellowish, moist and lustrous, and elastic. Yellow skin accompanied by yellow eyes and urine is jaundice, in which bright yellow is yang jaundice and dark yellow is yin jaundice. Dropsy of skin is often due to spreading of dampness. Dry skin is often due to consumption of body fluid. Dry and rough skin is often due to malnutrition of the muscles and skin. Macules refer to reddish or purplish uneven patches on skin. It cannot be felt by hands and does not fade when pressed. Red macula on skin is caused by warm and heat pathogen invading the blood system, in which red and moist macula indicates favorable prognosis and dark red or purple means unfavorable prognosis. Rash refers to reddish points like millet that can be felt by hands and fade when pressed. Measles which is red and moist and appears in proper order, abatement of fever after eruption is favorable. Red, purple and dark measles is indicative of excessive heat and toxin in the interior. Measles being light but not red and suddenly vanishing is indicative of pathogenic factors dominating over healthy qi and the prognosis is unfavorable, which man should pay attention to. White miliaria-like crystal blister indicates dampness retention and excessive heat. The inspection of skin should also include boils, furuncle, phlegmon, carbuncle, *etc.*.

4. Inspection of Tongue　The inspection of tongue also known as tongue diagnosis, is an important part of inspection diagnosis in TCM. Changes of the tongue can objectively reflect the growth and decline of healthy *qi*, location of pathogen, nature of pathogenic qi and prognosis of a disease, helping nurses to estimate changes and prognosis of a disease, and to provide important basis for nursing implementation based on pattern differentiation.

(1) Relationship between tongue and *zang-fu* organs: Tongue is generally divided into four portions, as the tip of tongue, the center of tongue, the root of tongue and the margin of tongue, which correspond to organs (Fig. 4-1). The tip of tongue corresponds to heart and lung. The center of tongue corresponds to spleen and

3. 望皮肤　皮肤居一身之表，是机体的屏障，气血津液通过经络外荣皮肤。望皮肤，不仅有助于皮肤病证的诊断，还可了解疾病性质、脏腑虚实和气血的盛衰。望皮肤主要诊察患者皮肤的色泽、形态和皮疹等。正常黄种人肤色红黄隐隐，荣润光泽，富有弹性。皮肤色黄伴目黄、尿黄属黄疸，色鲜明为阳黄，色暗晦为阴黄。皮肤虚浮肿胀，多属水湿泛溢；皮肤干瘪枯燥，多为津液耗伤；皮肤干燥粗糙，多为肌肤失养。皮肤出现色红或紫，大小不一，不高出皮肤者，压之不褪色者，称为斑。皮肤发斑，斑色红为温热之邪入营血，红润为顺，暗红或紫赤则为逆；皮肤出现色红，点小如粟，高出皮肤者，压之褪色者，称为疹。麻疹色红润，依次出疹，疹出热退为顺，若疹点赤紫暗滞则为热毒内盛，淡而不红或突然蛰伏不见是正虚邪气内陷，多属逆象，应提高警惕。皮肤上出现白色小颗粒，晶莹透亮，属湿郁热盛；观察皮肤形态还应观察有无疔、疖、疽、痈等。

4. 望舌　望舌又称舌诊，是中医观察病情的重要内容。舌象的变化，能客观地反映"正气盛衰，病邪深浅，邪气性质，病情进退"，可以帮助护理人员判断患者的疾病转归和预后，为辨证施护提供重要依据。

（1）舌与脏腑的关系：舌体分为舌尖、舌中、舌根、舌边四个大致区域，分别与内脏相对应（图4-1）。其中舌尖对应心肺，舌中对应脾胃，舌根对应肾膀胱，舌边对应肝胆。

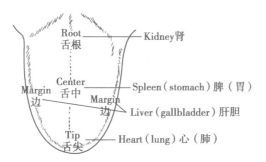

Fig. 4-1　Correspondence of Tongue to Viscera

图 4-1　舌诊脏腑部位分属图

stomach. The root of tongue corresponds to kidney and bladder. The margin of tongue corresponds to liver and gallbladder.

(2) Methods and precautions for tongue inspection: The patient is asked to sit down or lie in supine, facing the light source. Tongue is protruded naturally with a reasonable time period. Mouth is opened wide to make tongue be exposed fully. Attention should be paid to stained coating, also known as "dyed tongue coating", which caused by some medicine or food. For example, olive discolors the coating black and *huáng lián* discolors the coating yellow. Being protruded too long, sticking out too much, being rolled up, after eating or eating colored food will cause a false tongue appearance.

(3) Content of tongue inspection: Inspection of tongue mainly includes the examination of tongue body and tongue coating. Tongue body refers to the condition of muscle tissues of tongue and coating relates to fur on the surface of tongue that is also known as lingual papillae. The sequence of inspection of tongue begins from the tip of tongue, then the center and margin of tongue, and finally the root of tongue. Inspection begins with tongue body first and then moves to tongue coating. The normal tongue is soft, flexible, light red, moist, and the coating of tongue is evenly scattered, white and thin, neither wet nor dry. It is often described as "light red tongue and thin and white coating", suggesting normal functions of *zang-fu* organs, sufficiency of qi, blood and body fluid as well as superabundance of gastric qi.

1) Inspection of tongue body: It mainly includes tongue spirit, color, shape and movement of tongue.

Inspection of tongue spirit: It also known as luster and lusterlessness of tongue. Luster means tongue is moist, red and lustrous, with flexible movement. It is called existence of spirit. Even the person is ill, there will be good prognosis. Lusterlessness is dry, dark and wizened, with inflexible movement, also called depletion of spirit. There

（2）望舌的方法和注意事项：望舌时应让患者取坐位或仰卧位，面向光源，自然张口伸舌于口外，充分暴露舌体，时间不宜过长。还应注意某些药物、食物造成的"染苔"，即舌面着色。如橄榄可使舌苔染黑，黄连可使舌苔染黄等。伸舌过久、过分用力、蜷曲、进餐后或着色食物会造成舌象变化的假象。

（3）望舌的内容：主要包括望舌质和望舌苔两方面。舌质指舌的肌肉脉络组织，舌苔为舌表面的苔，也称舌乳头。望舌的顺序，一般先看舌尖，再看舌中、舌边，最后看舌根。先看舌质，后看舌苔。正常舌象为舌体柔软，活动自如，颜色淡红、润泽，舌苔均匀、薄白而干湿适中，常简述为"淡红舌、薄白苔"，提示脏腑功能正常，气血津液充盈，胃气旺盛。

1）望舌质：包括主要舌神、舌色、舌形和舌态。

望舌神：指舌的荣枯。"荣"为容润红活，有生气，有光彩，活动灵敏自如，谓之有神，虽病也有善候；"枯"为干枯死板，暗滞，运动失灵，谓之无神，乃是恶候。

will be a poor prognosis of that.

Inspection of tongue color: A pale tongue indicates syndromes of deficiency and cold often caused by insufficiency of yang qi and blood. A reddened tongue indicates a heat syndrome caused by exuberant heat and stasis of qi and blood. A bright red tongue with scanty fur indicates excessive fire and yin deficiency. A deep red tongue is a sign of exuberant heat, which indicates exogenous heat invading the nutrient and blood systems, fire excess from yin deficiency and blood stasis. A purple tongue indicates extreme heat, excessive cold, blood stasis, and alcohol intoxication. A cyanotic tongue indicates syndromes of yin-cold and blood stasis, and is the manifestation of qi stagnation and blood stasis.

Inspection of tongue shape: Rough tongue is marked by rough texture, dry surface and dull color. Rough tongue usually indicates excess syndrome and heat syndrome. Tender tongue is characterized by fine texture, moistened and lustrous surface, light color and bulgy appearance. Tender tongue usually indicates deficiency syndrome and cold syndrome. An enlarged tongue with light color indicates internal retention of dampness and phlegm. A swollen tongue means the tongue is swollen and the mouth cannot be closed, and the tongue even can't retract in severe cases, indicating heat stagnation and intoxication. A thin tongue is thinner than usual, indicating deficiency of yin blood. Various fissures on the tongue is called "fissured tongue", indicating the deficiency of yin fluid. A prickly tongue shaped by hyperplasic lingual papillae with prickly feeling when touched indicates interior heat accumulation. The margins of tongue printed with tooth marks are called teeth-marked tongue, indicating qi deficiency or yang deficiency and internal retention of dampness.

Inspection of tongue motility: A stiff and inflexible tongue is called stiff tongue, which indicates invasion of the pericardium by heat, consumption of fluid due to high fever and collateral obstruction due to wind and phlegm. A flaccid and soft tongue that is too weak to protrude and withdraw is called flaccid tongue, indicating consumption of yin fluid and insufficiency of qi and blood. A trembling tongue means tongue is involuntarily tremoring, indicating endogenous liver wind. A deviated tongue is a tongue deviated to one side, suggesting liver wind complicated by phlegm, liver wind complicated by stagnation in the collaterals of tongue or wind stirring from yin deficiency. Tongue protrudes out but is unable to retreat is called protruding tongue. Tongue that frequently protrudes out but immediately draws back or licks the lips or corners of the mouth is called wagging tongue. Both conditions suggest heat in heart and spleen. A shortened tongue is a

望舌色：淡白舌为虚证、寒证，多为阳气虚弱、气血不足；红舌为热证，为热盛气血壅滞；鲜红少苔，为阴虚火旺；绛舌（深红色）主热盛，为邪热深入营血，阴虚火旺及瘀血；紫舌主热极、寒盛、瘀血或酒毒；青舌主阴寒证、血瘀证，为气血瘀滞之象。

望舌形：舌体纹理粗糙，舌面干燥，舌色较暗，形质坚敛苍老，称为苍老舌，多主实证，热证；舌体纹理细腻，舌面湿润，舌色浅淡，形质浮胖娇嫩，称为娇嫩舌，多主虚证、寒证；舌体胖大，舌色偏淡，主水湿痰饮证；舌体肿大，甚则不能闭口，不能缩回者，称肿胀舌，主热郁、中毒；舌体瘦小而薄，称瘦薄舌，为阴血亏虚；舌面有明显裂沟，称裂纹舌，多为阴液亏耗之征；舌面乳头增生、肥大，高起如刺，抚之棘手，称为芒刺舌，多为里热炽盛，邪热内结之象；舌体边缘有牙齿压迫的痕迹，称为齿痕舌，多为气虚或阳虚，水湿内停。

望舌态：舌体强硬，不能活动，称为强硬舌，主热陷心包、高热伤津或风痰阻络；舌体软弱，伸缩无力，称为萎软舌，主阴液亏损或气血俱虚；舌体不自主颤动，称颤动舌，主肝风内动；舌体不正，伸舌时舌体歪向一侧，称为歪斜舌，多见于肝风挟痰，痰瘀阻络或阴虚风动；舌伸出口外，不能缩回者，称为吐舌；舌不时伸出口外，立即缩回或反复转弄者，称为弄舌。吐弄舌，多为心脾有热；舌体卷缩，不能伸出口外，称为短缩舌，多属危重证候。

tongue contracted and cannot protrude, or cannot even reach the teeth, usually indicating critical condition.

2) Inspection of tongue coating: Including inspection of texture and colors of tongue coating.

Inspection of tongue coating texture: Inspection of tongue coating texture includes the examination of its thickness, moistness, greasiness, exfoliation, *etc.*.

Thickness: If tongue body is "bottom visible", it is thin coating. If tongue body is "bottom invisible", it is thick coating. Thin tongue coating is seen in normal people or at the primary stage of illness, suggesting that the pathogenic factors are superficial and the disease is mild or insufficiency of healthy qi. Thick coating indicates development of pathogenic factors from the exterior to the interior, superiority of the pathogenic factors or pathogenic retention in the interior.

Moistness and dryness of tongue coating: The tongue coating that is moist with moderate dampness is called moist coating. The tongue coating is with excessive dampness and the saliva is ready to drop when the tongue protrudes, which called a glossy coating. The tongue coating that is dry, without fluid or even fissured is called dry coating. The tongue coating that is dry, rough and sandy is called a rough coating. A moist or glossy tongue coating suggests normality of fluid or retention of fluid. A dry tongue coating suggests consumption of fluid and dysfunction of fluid transportation.

Greasy and curd tongue coating: Tongue coating compact and difficult to exfoliate which is thick on the center and thin on the margins is called greasy coating. It's often due to dampness, phlegm, retention of indigestive food. A thick, loose and spare tongue coating with large granules that resemble the crushed bean curd is called curd-like coating. It's often caused by retention of indigestive food or retention of turbid phlegm.

Exfoliating tongue coating: Exfoliating tongue coating means that the coating on tongue has exfoliated partially or completely during the course of a disease. Partial exfoliation of tongue coating is divided into anterior exfoliated tongue coating, medium exfoliated tongue coating and patched exfoliated tongue coating. If the tongue coating is completely exfoliated as smooth as a mirror, it is called mirror-like tongue. It is a sign of exhaustion of stomach yin and deficiency of stomach qi.

Inspection of colors of tongue coating: Examining color of tongue coating, so as to analyze the state of disease. Colors of tongue coating are commonly seen in white, yellow and grayish black, which may appear seperately or simultaneously.

2）望舌苔：包括苔质和苔色。

望苔质：苔质，即舌苔的形质。望苔质主要诊察舌苔的厚薄、润燥、腻腐、剥落等变化。

厚薄：以能见底者为薄苔，不能见底者为厚苔。苔薄者，可见于正常人或疾病初起，提示病邪在表、病轻或正气不足；厚苔，病邪已由表入里，病邪较盛或里有积滞。

润燥：舌苔干湿适中为润苔；若舌面过滑，伸舌欲滴，为滑苔；舌苔干燥，扪之无津，甚则干裂，为燥苔；舌苔毫无水分，苔质粗糙如砂石，称为糙苔。舌苔润滑者说明津液未伤或津液内停，舌苔干燥者说明津液亏损或津液输布障碍。

腻腐：若苔质颗粒细腻而致密，边薄中厚，紧贴舌面，刮之不易脱落，称为腻苔，为湿浊、痰饮、食积所致；若苔质颗粒较大，疏松而厚，形如豆腐渣堆积舌面，刮之即去，称为腐苔，为食积、痰浊久积不化所致。

剥落：舌面的舌苔在病程中部分或全部剥落，称为剥落苔。部分舌苔剥落，根据舌苔剥落部位，可分为前剥苔、中剥苔和花剥苔。舌苔全部脱落，舌面光洁如镜，称为光剥苔，又称镜面舌。剥落苔为胃气匮乏，胃阴枯竭所致。

望苔色：诊察苔色变化，分析病情。常见的苔色有白苔、黄苔、灰黑苔，可单独出现，也可结合出现。

White tongue coating: White tongue coating is usually seen in external syndrome and cold syndrome. A thin, white and moist tongue coating usually indicates wind-cold external syndrome. A thin, white and dry tongue coating usually indicates wind-heat external syndrome. A white, thick, sticky and greasy tongue coating is mostly due to dampness and phlegm. A powder-like thick and white tongue coating is usually seen in pestilence and internal abscess.

Yellow tongue coating: Yellow tongue coating usually indicates internal syndrome or heat syndrome. Light-yellow tongue coating indicates mild heat, deep-yellow tongue coating signifies severe heat and sallow tongue coating suggests extreme heat. A thin and light yellow tongue coating is often a sign of heat transformed from wind-cold or exogenous wind-heat. A yellow, thick and sticky tongue coating often indicates damp heat of the stomach and intestine and retention of phlegm and indigestive food. A yellow and dry tongue coating is a sign of consumption of fluid due to exuberant heat.

Grayish black tongue coating: Grayish black tongue coating suggests severity of internal syndrome or severe internal cold syndrome. A moist, grayish black tongue coating indicates yang deficiency and cold exuberance, accumulation of cold-dampness or retention of phlegm and fluid. A dry grayish black tongue coating indicates consumption of fluid due to extreme heat.

5. Inspection of Excreta　The inspection of excreta mainly includes examination of its form, color, quality, volume, *etc.*, so as to assess the condition of a disease. Generally speaking, whitish or light-colored and thin excreta often indicate cold syndrome and deficiency syndrome. Yellowish or deep-colored and thick excreta often indicate heat syndrome and excess syndrome.

(1) Inspection of sputum and saliva: including inspection of sputum and inspection of saliva.

1) Inspection of sputum: Sputum is a kind of sticky fluid excreted from lung and trachea. Thin, white, and profuse sputum, or with grayish black is considered as cold sputum. Thick and yellow sputum is considered as heat sputum. If sputum is white and in large amount, slippery and easily expectorated, it is regarded as damp sputum. Scanty, sticky sputum difficult to expectorate, or with unproductive cough, is dry sputum. Bloody sputum or hemoptysis is often due to invasion of heat into lung collaterals. If sputum appears like purulent blood or with foul smell, it is usually seen in pulmonary abscess.

2) Inspection of saliva: Frequent salivation from the corners of mouth in children is usually due to failure to control fluid caused by spleen deficiency or stomach

白苔：苔见白色，称为白苔，多见于表证、寒证。苔薄白而润，多为风寒表证；薄白而干，多为风热表证；苔白厚而滑腻，多为湿浊、痰饮内停；苔白厚如积粉，多为瘟疫或内痈。

黄苔：苔见黄色，称为黄苔，多见于里证、热证。淡黄热轻，深黄热重，焦黄热极。苔薄微黄，多为风寒化热或外感风热；苔黄而厚腻，多为胃肠湿热，痰食阻滞；苔黄而燥，为热盛伤津。

灰黑苔：苔见灰黑，称为灰黑苔，主里证或里寒证的重证。苔灰黑而滑润，为阳虚寒盛，寒湿、痰饮内停；苔灰黑而干燥，为热极津伤。

5. **望排出物**　指观察患者排出物（排泄物、分泌物）的形、色、质、量等方面的变化，以诊察疾病的方法。一般来说，凡排出物色白、清稀者，多属虚证、寒证；色黄、稠浊者，多属实证、热证。

（1）望痰涎：包括望痰和望涎。

1）望痰：痰是由肺和气道排出的黏液。痰稀、色白、量多，或有灰黑点，为寒痰；痰稠色黄，坚而成块，为热痰；痰色白量多，滑而易咯出，为湿痰。痰少而黏，难以咯出，甚则干咳无痰，为燥痰；痰中带血，或咯血，多为热伤肺络。咯吐脓血腥臭痰，多为肺痈。

2）望涎：小儿口角流涎，多属脾虚不能摄津，亦可见于胃热、虫积或消化不良；成

heat, intestinal parasitosis and indigestion. Spontaneous drooling in adults is usually seen in sequela of apoplexy.

(2) Inspection of vomitus: Vomiting is caused by upward adverse flow of gastric qi. Thin vomitus without foul smell usually indicates cold vomit. Turbid and sour vomitus often indicates heat vomit. Sour and fetid vomitus with indigested food is usually caused by retention of food. Vomiting of indigested food without sour and fetid smell is usually caused by deficiency-cold in spleen and stomach. Vomiting of clear fluid, sputum and saliva is usually due to dysfunction of spleen in transportation or retention of fluid in stomach. Vomiting of yellowish and greenish bitter fluid is often due to accumulation of damp heat or heat accumulation in liver and gallbladder. Vomiting of fresh blood or purplish blood with clot or with food dregs is often due to stomach heat or liver heat invading stomach, impairing the collaterals of stomach causing blood fail to circulate in vessels.

(3) Inspection of feces: Loose stool like porridge is often indicative of deficiency cold. Dry and hard stool is often indicative of excess heat. Deep yellow and sticky stool with foul smell is often indicative of damp-heat in stomach and intestines. Watery stool mixed with indigested food is often indicative of cold-dampness. Sticky stool mixed with pus and blood indicates dysentery. Brown-black blood being seen after defecation indicates that bleeding occurs in distant part, whereas bright red blood being seen before defecation indicates that bleeding occurs in the proximal part.

(4) Inspection of urine: Urine being clean and in large amount mostly indicates deficiency cold. Urine being yellow and red and in small amount often indicates heat syndrome. Turbid urine indicates downward flow of turbid dampness. Hematuria is often a result of blood and collateral injury due to heat. Urine with sand and stone is called urolithiasis. Urine with cream and fat is called unctuous strangury.

6. Inspection of Infantile Index Finger Vein

Inspection of infantile index finger veins means to examine the length, color, shape, *etc.* of the veins along the palmar margin to detect pathological changes. This method is applicable for the diagnosis of infants under the age of three.

Infantile index finger vein is divided into wind pass, qi pass, and life pass. Between the first and the second stems of the index finger is wind pass. Between the second and the third stems of the index finger is qi pass. Between the third stem and the top of the index finger is life pass (Fig. 4-2). Appearance of the index finger vein on the wind pass indicates that the disease is mild. If it extends to the

人口角流涎不止，可见于中风后遗症。

（2）望呕吐物：呕吐是由胃气上逆所致。呕吐物清稀无臭，多为寒呕；呕吐物秽浊酸臭，多为热呕；吐出酸腐夹杂不消化食物，多属食积；吐出不消化食物而无酸腐气，多属脾胃虚寒；呕吐清水痰涎，多因脾失健运，胃有停饮所致；呕吐黄绿苦水，多为肝胆湿热或郁热；呕吐鲜血或紫暗有块，夹杂食物残渣，多属胃有积热或肝火犯胃，热伤胃络而血不归经。

（3）望大便：大便溏薄属虚寒，大便燥硬属实热；便黄如糜，溏黏恶臭多属肠胃湿热；便稀如水样，夹有不消化食物，多属寒湿；便如黏冻，夹有脓血，是为痢疾；先便后血，其色褐黑者是远血，先血后便，其色鲜红者是近血。

（4）望小便：小便清澈而量多者，多属虚寒；小便黄赤而量少者，多属热证；小便混浊不清，多为湿浊下注；尿血者，多是热伤血络；尿有砂石者为石淋；尿如膏脂者为膏淋。

6. 望小儿示指脉络 望小儿示指脉络是诊察患儿示指掌面前缘脉络的长短、色泽和形态等，以了解病情，适用于 3 岁以内的小儿。

小儿示指脉络分为风、气、命三关。示指的第一节至第二节横纹之间，为风关；第二节至第三节横纹之间，为气关；第三节横纹至示指末端，为命关（图 4-2）。示指脉络显于风关者，病情较轻；脉络至气关者，病情较重；脉络直达指端者，病情凶险，预后

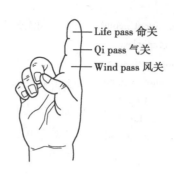

Fig. 4-2　Three Passes of Infantile Index Finger Vein
图 4-2　小儿示指脉络三关图

qi pass, it means that the disease is relatively serious. If it stretches directly to the tip of the finger, it indicates critical condition and unfavorable prognosis.

Light-colored and whitish vein indicates insufficiency of qi and blood. Reddish vein often indicates exogenous wind and cold. Red or purplish vein often indicates internal exuberance of heat. Bluish vein often indicates pain syndrome. Visible and floating vein indicates that the pathogenic factors are superficial, and it is often seen in exterior syndrome caused by exogenous factors. Deep and indistinct vein means that the pathogenic factors are in the interior, and it is often seen in the case of interior syndrome caused by internal injury.

ii. Listening and Smelling

Listening and smelling means listening to various sounds and noises made by the patient and smelling the odor and excreta from body of the patient so as to understand the pathological conditions of the patient.

1. Listening to Sound　Listening to sounds means listen to speech, respiration, cough, vomit and hiccup of a patient so as to assess the condition of the disease.

（1）Speech: In listening to speech, attention should be paid to detect whether the voice is strong or weak, whether the words are coherent and whether the expression is clear and fluent. The speech of normal person is natural in pronunciation, smooth in tone, clear and fluent in expression and consistent in words. Since the *zang-fu* organ, constitution and physical building are different from person to person, the voice is also different. For example, male voice is often low and full, while female voice is often high and clear. Children's voice is sharp and melodious, while voice of the aged is low and deep. Generally speaking, high and sonorous voice in healthy people is a manifestation of sufficiency of original qi and lung qi. There is a close relation between speech and emotions. For example, the voice in joy is lively and cheerful, and the voice in rage is stern and quick.

不良。

脉络色淡白，多为气血不足；色鲜红，多为外感风寒；色紫红，多为内热炽盛；色青，多为痛证。脉络浮现易见者，病位较浅，多见于外感表证；脉络沉隐模糊者，主病在里，多见于内伤里证。

（二）闻诊

闻诊是通过听患者发出的各种声音和嗅患者身体及其排出物散发出的气味，以了解病情的诊察方法。

1. 听声音　听声音是指通过听患者的语言、呼吸、咳嗽、呕吐、呃逆等各种声响，来判断疾病的寒热虚实。

（1）听语言：应注意语音的强弱，语言内容是否言与意符，语言是否清晰流利。正常人的语言发音自然，音调和畅，言语清楚流利，言与意符。由于个体脏腑、形质、禀赋差异，正常的声音也有所不同。如男性多声低而浊，女性多声高而清，儿童则声尖清脆，老人则声浑厚低沉。一般认为，正常人声音高亢洪亮，是元气和肺气充沛的表现。语言与情志的变化也有密切的关系。如喜时发声欢快而和畅，怒时发声忿厉而急疾。

Loud and sonorous voice and talkativeness usually indicate excess syndrome and heat syndrome. Low, weak voice and oligologia often indicate deficiency syndrome and cold syndrome. Hoarseness in a new disease is called "sudden hoarseness", indicating excess syndrome related to impaired lung qi caused by exogenous pathogenic factors attacking lung. Hoarseness or aphonia in a chronic disease often indicates deficiency syndrome due to internal injury, deficiency of lung and kidney yin, and body fluid unable to reach the glottis.

Words are the voice of the mind. Paraphasia often belongs to diseases of heart and mind. Delirious speech means raving with high and sonorous voice in a confused state of mind. Such a morbid condition pertains to excess syndrome due to heat disturbing the mind. Fading murmuring is marked by unconsciousness, repeated and incoherent murmuring in a low voice. It is often caused by excessive consumption of heart qi and is a deficiency syndrome of mental derangement. Soliloquy is marked by mental depression, talking to oneself, incoherent speech and stop talking when seeing people, and usually caused by coagulation of phlegm confusing the mind or by severe impairment of heart qi. Paraphasia means that the patient speaks nonsense in consciousness and is aware of it afterwards. Such a morbid is often due to insufficiency of heart qi and malnutrition of spirit. Slurred speech is marked by unclear and slow expression without fluency, and usually seen in apoplexy.

(2) Respiration: Lung governs qi and controls breathing, while kidney governs the reception of qi. The patient's nomal breath indicates body being injured and qi not being injured. The patient's abnormal breath indicates both body and qi being injured. Acute onset disease with rapid breath and high voice often pertains to excess syndrome and heat syndrome. The disease with long duration, weak breath and shortness of breath in movement often pertains to deficiency syndrome and cold syndrome. Panting refers to difficulty in breath, shortness and rapidity in breath, or even difficulty in opening the mouth, raising the shoulders and flapping the nose wings in breathing as well as inability to lie down flat. Wheezing is marked by rapid breath, stridor in the throat, and repeated relapse. It is usually caused by internal retention of phlegm complicated by exogenous pathogenic factors' attacks. Simultaneous appearance of panting and wheezing is called wheezing and panting. Shortness of breath means that the breath is not continuous like dyspnea and that the patient raises shoulders when breathing. Usually there is no sputum. Such a morbid condition is usually seen in various diseases of excess or deficiency nature. The

语音高亢有力，多言者属实证、热证；低微无力，少言者多属虚证、寒证。新病音哑者，为暴哑，多为外邪袭肺，肺气不宣，属实证；久病音哑或失音，多为内伤，肺肾阴虚，津液不能上承声门所致，属虚证。

言为心声，语言错乱多为心神病变。神志不清，胡言乱语，声高有力，称为谵语，多属热扰心神之实证。神志不清，语言重复，时断时续，声低无力，称为郑声，多属心气大伤，精神散乱之虚证。情志抑郁，自言自语，语无伦次，见人则止，称为独语，多属痰气凝结，蒙蔽心神或心气大伤所致。神智清醒而语言错乱，言后自知说错，称为错语，多因心气不足，神失所养而致。说话不流利，含糊不清，缓慢涩滞，多见于中风。

（2）听呼吸：肺主气，司呼吸，肾主纳气。患者呼吸如常，是形病而气未病；呼吸异常，是形气俱病。发病急，呼吸气粗而快，多属实证、热证。病程长，呼吸气微，动则气短，多属虚证、寒证。呼吸困难，短促急迫，甚或张口抬肩，鼻翼煽动，难以平卧者为喘。呼吸急促而喉间有哮鸣音，常反复发作为哮，多因内有素痰伏肺，复感外邪引动而发，喘与哮常同时发生，故常合称为哮喘。呼吸短促而不相连接，气短不足以息，似喘而不抬肩，气急而无痰声为短气，可见于多种疾病，有虚实之分。虚证以气短声低息微为特征，实证以气短声粗为特征。呼吸微弱，短而声低，气少不足以息，为少气，主诸虚劳损，身体虚弱。

deficiency syndrome is marked by shortness of breath, low voice and weak breath. The excess syndrome is marked by shortness of breath and hoarseness of voice. Weak breathing is marked by feeble and short breath and low voice. It is often due to deficiency and over strain of body and frailty.

(3) Cough: Cough is due to lung failing to diffuse and govern descent and ascending counterflow of lung qi. Deep cough usually indicates excess syndrome. Low cough usually indicates deficiency syndrome. Whitish thin sputum is usually due to exogenous wind-cold. Yellowish thick sputum is often due to invasion of pathogenic heat into lung. Profuse thin sputum easy to expectorate is often due to cold dampness or phlegm retention in lung. Dry cough refers to cough without sputum. Infantile paroxysmal and continuous cough like the crying of an egret in the end and shortness of breath while coughing is called whooping cough. Cough like barking of a dog accompanied by hoarseness and dyspnea indicates diphtheria.

(4) Vomiting, hiccup and belching: Vomiting slowly with weak sound often indicates the cold pattern and deficiency pattern. Vomiting acutely with loud voice means excessive-heat syndrome. Vomiting in the evening of food eaten in the morning or vomiting in the morning of food eaten in the evening, with indigestive food in the vomitus is called regurgitation. It is often caused by stomach cold, spleen deficiency and indigestion of food. Sudden projectile vomiting is often caused by pathogenic heat disturbing mind. If vomiting and diarrhea occur simultaneously after eating, food poisoning should be considered.

1) Hiccup: Hiccup also known as "burp", is caused by upward rise of stomach qi and involuntary short and frequent gurgling noise in the throat. Repeated hiccup with sonorous voice often indicates heat syndrome. Deep long and weak hiccup occurring intermittently is often due to deficiency-cold. Hiccup in a new disease with sonorous voice is usually caused by cold pathogen or heat pathogen attaching stomach. Hiccup in chronic diseases or severe diseases with low voice indicates decline of gastric qi.

2) Belching refers to deep, long and slow noise made in throat due to upward rise of qi from stomach. Belching with acid and putrid odor is due to retention of food in stomach. Repeated sonorous belching is due to emotional upset often caused by invasion of liver qi into stomach. Intermittent belching with deep voice accompanied by poor appetite is often due to weakness of spleen and stomach.

2. Smelling Smelling means to smell various

（3）听咳嗽：咳嗽是肺失宣降，肺气上逆的表现。咳声重浊，多属实证；咳声低微无力，多属虚证。痰白而清稀多为外感风寒；痰稠色黄，多为肺热；咳即痰出，痰多而稀，多为寒湿或痰饮犯肺；干咳无痰，多为燥咳。咳嗽阵发，连声不绝，咳而气急，终止时常有鸡鸣样回声者，称为顿咳，多见于小儿。咳声如犬吠，伴声音嘶哑，吸气困难，见于白喉。

（4）听呕吐、呃逆与嗳气：呕吐徐缓，声音微弱者，多属寒证、虚证；呕吐急剧，声音洪亮者，为实热证。朝食暮吐或暮食朝吐，吐出不消化食物，称反胃，多因胃寒脾虚，不消水谷所致。呕吐来势急，呈喷射状，多为热扰神明。食后吐泻并作，应注意是否为食物中毒等病证。

1）呃逆，俗称打呃，是胃气上逆，从咽喉部冲出，声短而频，呃呃作响的一种不能自主的声音。呃声频作，连续有力，高亢而短，多属实热；呃声低沉而长，气弱无力，良久一作，多属虚寒；新病呃逆，其声有力，多属寒邪或热邪客于胃；久病、重病出现呃逆，声低无力，多为胃气衰败。

2）嗳气是气从胃中上逆，致咽喉部发出沉长而缓的声音。嗳气有酸腐气味，为宿食内停；嗳气频作，其声响亮，发作与情志不舒有关，多为肝胃不和；嗳气声低断续，伴食欲缺乏，多为脾胃虚弱。

2. 嗅气味 嗅气味是指嗅患者体内发出

odors of the body, secretions, and excretions and smells in the wards so as to understand the pathological changes.

(1) Odor of the patient: Foul breath is seen in caries or due to stomach heat. Sour odor from mouth indicates retention of food in stomach and intestine. Putrid odor from mouth suggests ulcerative gingivitis or internal abscess. The sour and putrid secretion and excrement of a patient often indicates excess syndrome and heat syndrome. Offensive smell of fish or no smell often indicates deficiency syndrome and cold syndrome. For instance, sour, putrid and foul odor of stool or with pus and blood often indicate retention of food or heat accumulation in stomach and intestine. Foul and stinking urine indicates damp-heat pouring downward. Stinking and foul sputum with pus and blood is due to lung abscess.

(2) Odor of ward: Ammonia in a ward is often found in edematous patients at the advanced stage. A smell of rotten apple is usually attributable to diabetic patients at the late stage. Both indicate critical pathological conditions.

iii. Inquiry

Inquiry means purposeful investigating on the basis of initial impressions from inspection as well as listening and smelling so as to understand more about the state of the disease. The subjects of inquiry include patients, family members, accompany person, *etc.*. The contents of inquiry include general information and the "ten questions of TCM".

The general information includes name, age, marital states, occupation, *etc.* of the patient, chief complaints, the onset, development, treatment of the disease, related past medical history, family history, personal life history, *etc.*. The ten questions include: the first, inquiring about fever and cold; the second, inquiring about sweating; the third, inquiring about head and face; the fourth, inquiring about excrement; the fifth, inquiring about diet; the sixth, inquiring about symptoms of chest; the seventh, inquiring about hearing; the eighth, inquiring about water taking; the ninth, inquiring about past medical history; the tenth, inquiring about pathomechanism. Meanwhile it is necessary to observe the change of disease while giving medicine. Women patients should be inquired about menstrual cycle, advanced or delayed menstruation, amenorrhea, and uterine burst of bleeding. For children, measles and smallpox should be inquired.

1. Inquiry of Fever and Cold   Inquiry of fever and cold means asking the patient whether he or she has the sensation of fever and aversion to cold, their severity, time of onset, how long it lasts and associated symptoms.

的各种气味及排出物和病室的气味，以了解疾病情况。

（1）嗅气味：若患者口气臭秽，多属胃热或有龋齿；口气酸馊，是食积肠胃；口气腐臭，多为牙疳或内痈。患者的分泌物及排泄物凡气味酸腐臭秽者，多属实证、热证；略带腥味或无臭者，多属虚证、寒证。如大便酸腐臭秽或兼脓血者，多为宿食或肠胃积热；小便臊臭混浊者，为湿热下注；咳吐脓血，腥臭味异常者，为肺痈。

（2）嗅病室气味：若病室内闻及尿臊味，多见于水肿病晚期；烂苹果味多见于消渴病患者，均属危重证候。

（三）问诊

问诊是在望诊、闻诊所获得的初步印象的基础上，通过有目的地询问以了解更多病情的一种方法。问诊的对象包括患者、患者家属、陪诊者等。问诊的内容包括一般情况和"中医十问"。

一般情况包括患者姓名、年龄、婚姻、职业等资料，疾病的主要症状、起始、发展、诊治经过及其与疾病有关的患者体质、既往病史、家族史和个人生活史等。"中医十问"即"一问寒热二问汗，三问头身四问便，五问饮食六问胸，七聋八渴俱当辨，九问旧病十问因，再兼服药参机变，妇女尤必问经期，迟速闭崩皆可见，再添片语告儿科，天花麻疹全占验。"

1. **问寒热**   问寒热是询问患者有无怕冷、发热的感觉及寒热出现的时间，寒热的轻重、持续的时间、有关的兼症等。

(1) Aversion to cold with fever: If aversion to cold with fever is seen at the initial stage of a disease, it often indicates external syndrome due to exogenous factors. Serious aversion to cold with mild fever indicate external syndrome due to wind-cold. Serious fever with mild aversion to cold indicates external syndrome due to wind-heat. Mild fever with aversion to wind indicates external syndrome due to wind attack.

(2) Fever without chills: Fever without chills means that the patient only has fever and does not feel chilly, usually accompanied by thirst and constipation. Such a problem usually pertains to internal heat syndrome. High persistent body temperature (above 39℃) without aversion to cold is known as high fever, indicating interior syndrome of excess heat. Tidal fever refers to the condition that the patient's fever recurs daily like the regular rise and fall of the tide, indicating excess syndrome of *yangming*, damp-warm disease or yin deficiency syndrome. Low fever between 37℃ and 38℃ is known as mild fever, which is often found in diseases of endogenous injury and late stage of warm-febrile diseases.

(3) Chills without fever: Chills without fever means that the patient only feels chilly but there is no fever, which indicates interior-cold syndrome. Aversion to cold in a new disease is usually caused by serious invasion of cold that stagnates yang qi and deprives the warmth of body. Fear of cold in chronic disease is usually caused by decline of yang qi and lack of the warmth of body.

(4) Alternating chills and fever: Alternating chills and fever means that aversion to cold and fever occur alternately. It is seen in *shaoyang* disease or malaria.

2. Inquiry of Sweating　Sweating is transformed from body fluid by yang qi and excretes from the sweat pores. Sweating becomes abnormal due to the invasion of pathogenic factors and imbalance between *yin* and *yang* inside the body. Inquiry of sweating includes whether there is sweating, time, quantity and location of sweating, its accompanying symptoms, *etc.*.

Absence of sweating associated with aversion to cold and fever often indicates exterior excess syndrome. Sweating accompanied by a fever and aversion to wind indicates exterior deficiency syndrome. Spontaneous sweating means that the patient sweats in daytime and gets worse after exercises, accompanied by aversion to cold, fatigue, lassitude, *etc.*. It often indicates qi deficiency or *yang* deficiency. Night sweating refers to sweating during sleep and ceasing of sweating while one awakes. It often indicates yin deficiency. Shiver sweating refers to a condition in which a patient is first attacked by severe chills, and then perspiration follows. It indicates a confrontation between

（1）恶寒发热：疾病初起，恶寒与发热同时并见，多为外感表证；恶寒重、发热轻为风寒表证；发热重、恶寒轻为风热表证；发热轻而恶风为伤风表证。

（2）但热不寒：患者只发热不寒冷，兼口渴便秘，多为里热证。患者高热不退（体温超过 39℃），不恶寒，称为壮热，属里实热证；定时发热或定时热甚，如潮汐之有定时，谓之潮热，属阳明实证、湿温病或阴虚证；轻度发热，热势较低，体温多在 37~38℃，称为微热，常见于某些内伤和温热病后期。

（3）但寒不热：患者只怕冷，不发热，多为里寒证；新病恶寒，多因寒邪较重，阳气被遏，机体失于温煦所致；久病畏寒，多因阳气虚衰，形体失于温煦所致。

（4）寒热往来：恶寒与发热交替发作，称寒热往来，属少阳病或疟疾。

2. **问汗**　阳气蒸化津液从玄府出于体表而成为汗。病邪的侵扰和机体的阴阳失调使患者汗出异常。主要询问患者有无出汗，出汗时间、多少及部位，主要兼症等。

无汗发热恶寒，多为表实证；有汗发热恶风，多为表虚证。经常汗出不止，活动后更甚，兼见畏寒神疲乏力等症，谓之自汗，多为气虚、阳虚；睡时汗出，醒后即止，谓之盗汗，多属阴虚；恶寒战栗之后，继之出汗，称为战汗，为正邪相争剧烈之时，是疾病发展的转折点。若汗出热退，脉静身凉，为邪去正安，若汗出仍烦躁不安，脉来疾急，为邪盛正衰。汗出量多，津液大泄为大汗，临床有虚实之分，兼高热、烦渴、脉洪大，

pathogenic factors and healthy qi. It is regarded as the turning point of an illness. If fever abates, pulse calms down and the body turns cool after sweating, it is a sign that pathogenic factors are being expelled. If there are restlessness and rapid pulse after sweating, it is a sign of domination of pathogenic factors and decline of healthy qi. Profuse sweating refers to excessive perspiration and profuse evaporation of the body fluid in various conditions. Clinically, it is divided into deficiency and excess types of sweating. An excessive heat syndrome is often marked by profuse sweating and a high fever, extreme thirst, and a full pulse. When a patient has profuse cold perspiration, accompanied by lassitude, feeble breathing, cold limbs and a faint pulse, it is a *yang* exhaustion syndrome due to *yang* deficiency and depletion of qi.

3. Inquiry of Pain　Inquiry of pain includes pain's location, nature, degree, time, *etc.*.

Distending pain means pain accompanied by a distending sensation, indicating qi stagnation. Stabbing pain means a sharp pain as if caused by a stab, indicating blood stasis. Scurrying pain means that the pain is not fixed and is migratory. Wandering pain of joints is usually seen in obstructive diseases due to wind and dampness attack. Wandering pain over the chest, hypochondrium, epigastrium and abdomen are often caused by qi stagnation. Burning pain refers to pain with scorching sensation, and a preference for cold, indicating fire-heat. Colicky pain means sharp pain like a knife stabbing, often caused by substantial pathogenic factors obstructing the activity of qi. Dull pain means that the pain is not sharp or tolerable, but constant. It is usually due to deficiency syndrome. It often occurs in the head, stomach, abdomen and low back. It is often caused by insufficiency of qi and blood, leading to inner production of *yin*-cold. Cold pain means that the pain is accompanied by cold sensation and a preference for warmth, aggravated by cold and alleviated by warmth. It is usually seen in the head, low back and the abdomen, mostly caused by an attack of meridians by cold or insufficiency of yang qi, which fails to warm up the *zang-fu* organs and meridians.

4. Inquiry of Diet and Taste　Inquiry of diet and taste include thirst, drinking water, intake of food, taste, *etc.*.

(1) Thirst and drinking water: Thirst means a desire for water. Drinking water means the quantity of water being drunk. In clinic, nurses should inquire the characteristics of thirst and the amount of water being drunk. It is a reflection of the condition of the body fluid and its distribution. Generally speaking, one has no thirst but desires to drink water which indicates the body fluid is

多为里实热证；冷汗淋漓，神疲气弱，肢冷脉微，是阳虚气脱的亡阳危证。

3. **问痛**　主要询问疼痛的部位、性质、程度、时间等。

胀痛指疼痛伴有胀满的感觉，主气滞；刺痛指疼痛如针刺之状，主瘀血；窜痛指痛处游走不定，或走窜攻痛，肢体关节疼痛而游走不定，多见于风湿痹证。胸胁脘腹走窜攻痛，多因气滞所致；灼痛指疼痛伴有灼热感而喜凉，主火热；绞痛指疼痛剧烈如刀绞，多因有形实邪阻闭气机所致；隐痛指疼痛较轻微，但绵绵不休，多属虚证；多见于头、脘、腹、腰部，多因气血不足，阴寒内盛。冷痛指疼痛且有冷感而喜暖，遇寒则甚，得温痛减，常见于头、腰、脘腹部，多因寒邪阻络或阳气不足，脏腑、经络失于温煦而致。

4. **问饮食口味**　包括对口渴、饮水、进食、口味等情况的询问。

（1）口渴与饮水：口渴指口干渴的感觉。饮水指饮水量的多少。临床应注意询问口渴特点及饮水量的多少，是体内津液盛衰和输布状况的反映。一般地说，口不渴为津液未伤，多见于寒证。口渴多饮是津液损伤的表现，多见于热证。其中渴喜冷饮，面赤壮热

not consumed, usually seen in cold syndrome. Thirst and polydipsia suggest impairment of body fluid. It is often seen in heat syndrome. Thirst with preference for cold drinks, accompanied by reddened complexion and high fever, indicates excess heat syndrome. Thirst with much drinking of water, accompanied by profuse urination, polyphagia and gradual emaciation is consumptive disease. When one feels thirsty but has no desire to drink, it's a sign of mild consumption or maldistribution of body fluid. It is due to yin deficiency, dampness-heat, phlegm-retained fluid, blood stasis, *etc.*.

(2) Appetite and food intake: Appetite refers to the demand for food and enjoyable sensation of taking food. Food intake refers to the actual amount of food being taken. Inquiry of appetite and food intake is helpful in understanding the conditions of spleen and stomach as well as the prognosis of the disease. One has reduced appetite or no desire to eat and indigestion mostly indicates dysfunction of spleen and stomach. A gradual reduced appetite in the course of a disease usually indicates weakness of spleen and stomach. Regaining appetite usually indicates recovery of stomach qi. Polyphagia and frequent eating are caused by exuberance of stomach fire. Polyphagia and frequent eating with emaciation are often seen in consumptive disease. One has hunger without desire for food, but burning sensation in the stomach often indicates stomach *yin* deficiency. One dislikes greasy or rich food is often due to the retention of food in stomach, as well as accumulation of damp heat in the liver, gallbladder spleen and stomach. Anorexia in the gravida is due to upward adverse flow of qi in the thoroughfare vessel which prevents the stomach qi from descending. A preference for eating raw rice or earth *etc.* is frequently seen in children with parasitic infestation.

(3) Taste: Taste refers to the sense in mouth. Abnormal taste in mouth may reflect the disorders of spleen and stomach as well as other *zang-fu* organs. A bland taste in mouth is often seen in deficiency of gastrosplenic qi. Bitter taste in mouth often indicates exuberance of liver and gallbladder fire, and upward adverse flow of gallbladder qi. A sweet and sticky sensation in mouth is usually caused by the damp-heat in spleen and stomach. Sour taste in mouth or acid regurgitation often indicates accumulated heat in liver and stomach. A sour and putrid taste in mouth mostly indicates retention of undigested food. Salty taste in mouth is usually due to deficiency of kidney and cold syndrome.

5. Inquiry of Sleep　Sleep is in close relation with the circulation of wei qi and the conditions of yin and yang. To a certain degree, it is in relation with the condition of qi and blood as well as the functions of heart and kidney.

者，属实热证；大渴喜饮，小便量多，能食而瘦者，为消渴病。渴不多饮是轻度伤津或津液输布障碍的表现，可见于阴虚、湿热、痰饮、瘀血等。

（2）食欲与食量：食欲指进食的欲望和对进食的欣快感觉。食量指实际的进食量。询问患者的食欲与食量，有助于判断脾胃功能的强弱及疾病预后转归。食欲减退或不欲食，胃纳呆滞，多为脾胃功能失常。若病程中食量渐减，多为脾胃虚弱；食量渐增，多为胃气渐复；消谷善饥，为胃火炽盛；若消谷善饥，形体反见消瘦，多见于消渴病。饥不欲食，胃中灼热、嘈杂者，多为胃阴不足；厌食油腻厚味，多为食积内停，或肝胆、脾胃湿热内蕴；孕妇厌食，多因妊娠后冲脉之气上逆，影响胃之和降。嗜食生米、泥土等，多见于小儿虫积。

（3）口味：口味指口中的味觉。口味异常可反映脾胃及其他脏腑的病变。口淡乏味，多为脾胃气虚；口苦，多为肝胆火旺，胆气上逆；口甜而黏腻，多为脾胃湿热；口中泛酸，多为肝胃蕴热；口中酸馊，多为伤食；口中味咸，多为肾虚及寒证。

5. 问睡眠　睡眠与人体卫气循行、阴阳盛衰密切相关，与气血的盛衰及心、肾功能也有一定关系。主要询问睡眠时间的长短、

Inquiry of sleep mainly includes whether sleep time is long or short, whether it is easy or difficult to fall asleep, whether there is dream or not, *etc.*. Clinically disturbed sleep includes insomnia and somnolence.

(1) Insomnia: Insomnia is also called sleepless. It is characterized by difficulty in falling asleep, or easiness to wake up and difficulty in falling asleep again, or shallow sleep or easiness to be disturbed in sleep, or even inability to fall asleep all night, usually accompanied by profuse dreaming. Insomnia accompanied by palpitation, amnesia, lusterless complexion, poor appetite and lassitude mostly results from worrying too much, deficiency of both heart and spleen. Insomnia with tidal fever, night sweating, soreness and weakness of low back and knees often results from imbalance between heart and kidney. Difficulty to fall asleep or easily waking up during sleep, with vertigo, chest distress, vexation and bitter taste in mouth usually results from stagnation of gallbladder qi and attack of phlegmatic heat. Insomnia accompanied by chest distress, belching, and abdominal distention, often indicates food stagnation in stomach caused by dysfunction of stomach qi.

(2) Somnolence: Somnolence is also called drowsiness. It refers to sleepiness in both daytime and at night, spontaneously falling asleep, waking up after being called and wanting to sleep again after waking up. It is usually due to yang deficiency and yin abundance. Drowsiness and hypersomnia, accompanied by dizziness, heavy body and abdominal stuffiness, which mostly indicates phlegm-dampness. Postcibal somnolence accompanied by spiritual lassitude, reduced appetite and indigestion is often due to insufficiency of center qi (*zhōng qì,* 中气) and failure of the spleen to transport. Somnolence found in recovery period after serious illness indicates that healthy qi has not been regained.

6. Inquiry of Urination and Defecation   The inquiry of urination and defecation is a way to understand the digestive function of body and metabolism of fluid. It's also an important evidence to determine whether the disease is cold or heat and excess or deficiency. Inquiring about defecation and urination should focus on frequency, quality, color, odor, amount, time and feeling of defecation and urination, other accompanying symptoms, *etc.*.

(1) Defecation: Normally a person defecates once a day and the stool is marked by normal shape, with no dryness, but proper dampness, smooth discharge, mostly yellow color without pus, mucus, indigested food, *etc.*. Constipation means difficulty in defecation or prolonged or even no defecation in several days due to dry feces. Constipation accompanied by fever, thirst, abdominal distention and pain often indicates excess heat.

入睡难易、有无多梦等情况。临床上常见失眠与嗜睡两种表现。

（1）失眠：又称不寐，以经常不易入睡，或睡而易醒不能再睡，或睡而不酣，时易惊醒，甚至彻夜不眠为特点，且常见多梦。失眠，兼见心悸健忘、面色无华、食少无力，多为思虑过度，心脾两虚；不易入睡，兼潮热盗汗，腰膝酸软者，多为心肾不交；若失眠而时时惊醒，兼眩晕胸闷、心烦口苦者，多为胆气不宁，痰热内扰；若失眠而兼胸闷嗳气、脘腹胀满，多为食滞内停，胃气不和。

（2）嗜睡：又称多寐，指患者睡意浓深，不分昼夜，时时欲睡，呼之即醒，醒之欲寐。嗜睡的病机是阳虚阴盛。困倦多眠，兼头昏、身重、脘闷者，多为痰湿；饭后嗜睡，兼神疲倦怠、食少纳呆，多为中气不足，脾失健运所致。大病之后精神疲乏而嗜睡，为正气未复的表现。

6. 问二便　询问大小便状况，可了解机体消化功能，水液代谢情况，也是判断疾病寒热虚实的重要依据。主要询问排便的次数，大小便的性状、颜色、气味、便量、时间及排便的感觉和伴随症状等。

（1）大便：正常人一般每天大便一次，成形不燥，干湿适中，排便通畅，多呈黄色，便内无脓血、黏液及未消化的食物等。便秘指大便燥结难解，排便间隔时间延长，甚至多日不排便。便秘兼发热口渴、腹满胀痛，多属实热；久病、老人、孕妇或产后便秘，

Constipation in the elderly, in patients who suffer from a prolonged illness and in pregnant women or women who have just given birth, often denotes deficiency of body fluid and blood or deficiency of both qi and yin. Diarrhea accompanied by burning pain in anus and scanty dark urine indicates diarrhea due to heat attack. Diarrhea accompanied by abdominal dull pain, poor appetite and cold abdomen, indicates diarrhea due to cold attack. Long-term diarrhea following abdominal pain before dawn is called morning diarrhea. It indicates kidney yang deficiency. Diarrhea accompanied by sour stool and abdominal pain alleviated after defecation often indicates accumulation of indigestive food. Diarrhea accompanied by tenesmus, mucous stools mixed with pus and blood indicates dysentery from dampness-heat. Bleeding preceding stool with fresh blood is usually due to damp heat injurying collateral or hemorrhoid bleeding. Bleeding following stool with purplish black blood indicates spleen failing to control blood or blood stasis. Prolapse of anus during defecation refers to the syndrome of qi deficiency.

(2) Urination: Normally a person urinates 3-5 times in the daytime and 0-1 time in the night, while the volume of urine discharged in a day and a night is 1 200-2 000ml. Clear and profuse urine is usually due to deficiency cold syndrome. Dark scanty urine often suggests heat syndrome. If it is accompanied by difficulty and pain in urination and turbid urine, it is usually due to dampness-heat in the urinary bladder and blood stasis. Frequent and profuse urination or spontaneous urination or urinary incontinence mostly result from deficiency of kidney or qi deficiency.

7. Inquiry of Head and Face　Inquiry of head and face includes vertigo, tinnitus, deafness, hearing impairment, dizzy vision, itching eye, eye pain, blurred vision, night blindness, pain, numbness of tongue, *etc.*.

(1) Vertigo: Vertigo means that the patient subjectively feels swirling over head. In severe cases, the patient feels his or her body or the things in sight are swirling, and he or she cannot stand still. Vertigo may be caused by up-flaming of liver fire, hyperactivity of liver yang, encumbrance and stagnation of phlegmatic dampness, insufficiency of qi and blood as well as deficiency of kidney essence.

(2) Tinnitus, deafness, and hearing impairment: Tinnitus refers to noise in the ears like chirping of a cicada or tidal sound. Fulminant tinnitus like the noise made by a frog or tide, which cannot be reduced by pressure, is of excess syndrome due to exuberant liver and gallbladder fire to disturb the upper orifices. Low and gradual tinnitus like chirping of a cicada, which can be reduced or stopped by pressure, is of deficiency syndrome due to deficiency

多为津亏血少或气阴两虚。腹泻、肛门灼热，小便短赤者为热泻；腹泻、腹痛绵绵，不思饮食，腹部冷者为寒泻；长期黎明前腹痛泄泻为"五更泻"，属肾阳虚衰；腹痛泄泻，泻下酸腐，泻后痛减者，多为伤食积滞；便下脓血，里急后重，为湿热下痢；便前下血，血色鲜红，为湿热伤络或痔疮下血；先便后血，血色紫黑，为脾不统血或瘀血内阻；便时脱肛，为气虚下陷。

（2）小便：健康成人一般日间排尿 3~5 次，夜间 0~1 次，每昼夜尿量约 1 200~2 000ml。小便清长而量多，多属虚寒；小便短赤，多为热证；若兼尿痛，排尿不畅而混浊，多为膀胱湿热和瘀血；小便频数，甚至自遗或失禁，多为肾虚或气虚。

7. **问头面**　包括头晕、耳鸣、耳聋、重听、目眩、目痒、目痛、目昏、雀盲、舌痛、舌麻等。

（1）头晕：头晕是指自觉头部有晕眩感，病重者感觉自身或视物旋转，站立不稳。肝火上炎、肝阳上亢、痰湿困滞、气血不足、肾精亏虚等，均可导致头晕。

（2）耳鸣、耳聋、重听：耳鸣是指自觉耳内鸣响，如闻蝉声，或如潮声。突发耳鸣，声大如蛙聒，或如潮声，按之鸣声不减，属实证，多因肝胆火盛，上扰清窍所致；耳鸣渐起，声音细小，如闻蝉鸣，按之鸣声减轻或暂止，属虚证，多因肝肾阴虚，肝阳上亢

of liver and kidney yin and hyperactivity of liver yang, or deficiency of kidney essence and insufficiency of brain which fails to nourish ears. Deafness means hypoacusis or even anakusis. The condition of hypoacusis, unclear hearing and hearing of repeated voice is called hearing impairment. Sudden deafness and hearing impairment are often in excess pattern. Deafness and hearing impairment in prolonged disease are usually of deficiency pattern.

(3) Dizzy vision, itchy eye, and eye pain: Dizzy vision means swirling of things like sailing on a boat. It often appears together with vertigo. It is caused by pathogenic wind and fire attacking the upper orifices or phlegmatic dampness confusing the upper orifices, and it is of excess syndrome. It can also due to deficiency of essence and blood as well as malnutrition of eyes and it is of deficiency syndrome. Itchy eye means itching sensation in eyelid, canthus or pupil of eyes. Itchy eye in severe cases is usually of excess syndrome. Mild itching and dryness of eyes are often due to malnutrition of eyes caused by insufficiency of liver blood or deficiency of liver and kidney yin. Eye pain refers to pain of one or two eyes which is usually of excess pattern.

(4) Blurred vision, night blindness: Blurred vision refers to a dim vision and man cannot see things clearly. Night blindness refers to normal vision during the daytime but man cannot see things clearly at night. It is often seen in patients with chronic diseases or the aged and weak people. They are usually caused by the deficiency of liver and kidney, insufficiency of essence and blood and malnutrition of eyes.

8. Inquiry of Chest and Abdomen　Inquiry of chest and abdomen mainly includes chest oppression, palpitation, hypochondriac distention, stomach cavity pǐ, abdominal distension, borborygmus, *etc.*.

(1) Chest oppression, palpitation: Chest oppression is a subjective sensation of discomfort and fullness in the chest, usually due to inhibited circulation of qi in heart, lung and liver. Palpitation refers to subjective feeling of quick heart beating and throbbing, which usually is a sign of the disorder of heart or heart spirit.

(2) Hypochondriac distention, stomach cavity pǐ: Hypochondriac distention refers to distension and discomfort over one side or both sides of hypochondrium, usually seen in disorders of liver and gallbladder. stomach cavity pǐ refers to subjective feeling of oppression and discomfort in epigastrium, usually seen in disorders of spleen and stomach.

(3) Abdominal distension and borborygmus: Abdominal distension refers to subjective sensation of distension and discomfort in abdomen, usually due

所致，或肾虚精亏，髓海不充，耳失所养而致。耳聋是指听力减退，甚至听觉丧失，亦称耳闭。重听是指听力减退，听音不清，声音重复。耳聋、重听突发，多属实证，久病逐渐出现耳聋、重听、多属虚证。

（3）目眩、目痒、目痛：目眩是指视物旋转动荡，如乘舟车，常与头晕相兼而作，称为眩晕。常因风火上扰清窍或痰湿上蒙清窍所致的实证，也可见于精血亏虚，目窍失养所致的虚证。目痒指眼睑、眦内或目珠有痒感，目痒甚者，多属实证。两目微痒而干涩，多是肝血不足或肝肾阴虚，目失所养所致。目痛是指单目或双目疼痛，所属实证。

（4）目昏、雀盲：目昏是指视物昏暗不明，模糊不清。雀盲是指白昼视力正常，每至黄昏视物不清。常见于久病或年老体弱者。多因肝肾亏虚，精血不足，目失濡养所致。

8. 问胸腹　主要包括胸闷、心悸、胁胀、脘痞、腹胀及肠鸣等。

（1）胸闷、心悸：胸闷是指自觉胸中痞闷不舒，多因心、肺、肝气机不畅所致。心悸是指经常自觉心跳、心慌，甚至不能自主，多是心神或心脏病变的反映。

（2）胁胀、脘痞：胁胀是指自觉胁恶一侧或两侧胀满不舒，多见于肝胆病变。脘痞是指自觉胃脘部痞闷不舒，多见于脾胃病变。

（3）腹胀、肠鸣：腹胀是指自觉腹部胀闷不舒，多因脾胃虚弱，食积胃肠，实热内结，

to weakness of spleen and stomach, food retention, internal retention of excess heat, mingling of qi, blood and fluid. Palpable abdominal distension is of deficiency syndrome due to weakness of spleen and stomach that fail to perform the normal functions of transportation and transformation. Unpalpable abdominal distension is of excess syndrome due to retention of food in the stomach and intestines or internal retention of excess heat that obstructs the circulation of qi. Borborygmus may be caused by deficiency of splenic qi, deficiency of splenic yang, internal exuberance of cold dampness, disharmony of liver and spleen, internal retention of fluid and disharmony of qi activity in intestines.

9. Inquiry of the Symptom about Loin, Back and Four Limbs Inquiry of the symptom over loins, back and four limbs includes cold sensation in back, aching loins, heaviness of body, numbness of four limbs, *etc.*. Cold sensation in back is often caused by exogenous wind and cold or predomination of yin due to yang deficiency or internal retention of phlegm and fluid. Aching loins refers to continuous discomfort and aching sensation in waist, usually caused by kidney deficiency, or by obstruction of wind and cold, or by sprain due to overstrain. Heaviness of body refers to the heavy, aching and lethargic sensation of body. If heaviness of body is accompanied by dropsy, it is often caused by failure of lung to disperse and descend, or failure of spleen to transport and transform, or failure of kidney to govern water. Heaviness of body, with spiritual lassitude and dyspnea is usually caused by failure of spleen to transform due to deficiency, and obstruction of yang qi. Numbness of four limbs refers to hypoesthesia or disappearance of the sense of muscles and skin on four limbs, usually caused by deficiency of qi and blood, or by internal disturbance of liver wind, or by damp phlegm and obstruction of the meridians and vessels by blood stagnation.

10. Inquiry of Symptom about Andropathy Inquiry of symptom in andropathy mainly includes impotence, seminal emission, and immature ejaculation. Impotence refers to inability to erect penis or weak erection of penis, usually due to insufficiency of kidney yang, deficiency of kidney essence, deficiency of both heart and spleen, spreading of damp heat as well as liver depression and qi stagnation. Seminal emission refers to frequent loss of sperm not caused by coitus. It is usually caused by yin deficiency and exuberant fire, by hyperactivity of kidney fire, by weakness of kidney qi, or by invasion of damp heat. Immature ejaculation refers to premature ejaculation of seminal fluid during the course of sexual life, leading to incapable of normal sexual life. It

气、血、水互积所致。腹胀喜按属虚，多因脾胃虚弱，失于健运所致。腹胀拒按属实，多因食积胃肠，或实热内结，阻塞气机所致。肠鸣可因脾气虚、脾阳虚、寒湿内盛、肝脾不调、水饮内停，肠腑气机不和所致。

9. **问腰背四肢** 包括背冷、腰酸、身重、四肢麻木等。背冷是指自觉背部冷凉，多因外感风寒、阳虚阴盛或痰饮内伏所致。腰酸是指腰部酸楚不适，绵绵不已，多因肾虚、风寒痹阻或劳损所致。身重是指身体有沉重酸困的感觉，身重伴水肿，多因肺失宣降、脾失健运或肾不主水所致；身重困倦，神疲气短，多因脾虚失运，阳气被遏所致。四肢麻木是指四肢肌肤感觉减退，甚至消失，多因气血亏虚，或肝风内动，或湿痰、瘀血阻络所致。

10. **问男科** 主要包括阳痿、遗精和早泄。阳痿是指阴茎痿软不举，或举而不坚，多因肾阳不足，肾精亏虚，心脾两虚，湿热浸淫，肝郁气滞所致。遗精是指不因性生活而精液频繁遗泄，多属阴虚火旺，相火妄动，肾气不固，或湿热浸淫所致。早泄是指在性生活过程中，精液过早泄出，以致不能进行正常的性生活。多因肾阳虚弱，肾气不固，或阴虚火旺，或肝郁气滞所致。

is usually caused by deficiency of kidney yang, weakness of kidney qi, or vigorous fire due to yin deficiency or stagnancy of liver qi.

11. Inquiry of Symptom about Gynecology
Physiologically, women are characterized by menstruation, leukorrhea, pregnancy and delivery of baby. Therefore, attention should be paid to whether she has married or not, menstruation, leukorrhea, pregnancy and delivery of baby in diagnosing diseases in women.

（1）Inquiry of menstruation: Menstruation refers to regular uterine bleeding in women of childbearing age. Menstruation normally occurs once a month. Inquiry of menstruation includes the cycle, duration, quantity, color, nature and accompanied symptoms of menstruation. If necessary, inquiry of menstruation should also include the date of the last menstruation, menarche or age of menopause. Normally menstruation occurs once every 28 days and lasts for 3-5 days. The menstrual blood discharged in a healthy woman is 50-100ml. The color of menstrual blood is marked by red color, proper in density and no mixture of blood clot. If menstruation occurs 8-9 days in advance, it is called early menstruation. The preceded menstrual cycle, accompanied by bright red blood, scanty menstruation, and pressure relieved abdominal pain, often indicates syndrome of qi and blood deficiency. If menstruation occurs 8-9 days later than usual is called delayed menstruation. Delayed menstruation accompanied by dark purple blood with clots, and abdominal pain before menstruation, mostly indicates blood stasis or cold syndrome. Menstruation occurring at irregular intervals, accompanied by unpalpable abdominal pain and breast distention before menstruation, is mostly due to liver qi stagnation. Amenorrhea refers to stoppage of menstruation for over three months without pregnancy at the age of menstruation or not during lactation in women. Amenorrhea accompanied by light red blood, fatigue, pale complexion and poor appetite mostly results from blood deficiency. Amenorrhea accompanied by depression, pain in the lower abdomen, dark purple tongue mostly results from qi stagnation and blood stasis. Profuse uterine bleeding is marked by sudden massive uterine bleeding, profuse in amount and long in duration. Vaginal dripping is marked by slight but persistent leakage of blood from the uterus. Menstruation accompanied by light red and thin blood, abdominal pain and fatigue, mostly indicates deficiency cold. Menstruation accompanied by profuse blood with bright red in color, heat in the palms and soles, vexation and poor sleep, often refers to heat of deficiency type. The purple menses clots with stabbing pain in lower abdomen are mostly due to blood stasis.

11. **问妇科** 经、带、胎、产是妇女特有的生理现象。对女性患者除常规问诊内容外，还须询问婚否、月经、带下、妊娠、产育等情况。

（1）月经：主要询问月经周期、行经天数，月经的量、色、质及伴随症状。必要时询问末次月经日期，初潮或停经年龄。正常月经约28d行经一次，行经期一般3~5d，每次排出血量一般50~100ml，经血正红，不稀不稠，不夹杂血块。若月经周期经常提前八九天以上，称为月经先期。月经先期，色鲜红而量少，腹痛喜按，多为气血两虚；月经周期经常错后八九天以上，称为月经后期。月经后期，色紫暗有块，经前腹痛，多为血瘀或寒证。经行无定期，腹痛拒按或经前乳胀，多为肝郁气滞。在行经年龄，若停经超过3个月而又未受孕，或不在哺乳期月经不来，称为闭经。闭经，兼见色淡，神疲气短，面色无华，食少，多为血虚；如兼精神抑郁，少腹拘急疼痛，舌质紫暗，多为气滞血瘀。经血突然大下，且量多不止，称为血崩；经血淋漓，日久不断，称为经漏；若经血色淡腹痛，体倦乏力，多为虚寒；经血色鲜红量多，手足心热，心烦少眠，多为虚热；经血色紫有块，少腹刺痛，多为血瘀。

(2) Inquiry of leukorrhea: Leukorrhea is a kind of milky, odorless and scanty vaginal excreta that can lubricate vagina. Inquiry of leukorrhea includes the quantity, color, texture and odor of leukorrhea. A large amount of whitish, watery vaginal discharge often indicates deficiency and cold in spleen and kidney. A yellowish and viscous vaginal discharge with offensive odor mostly refers to exuberance of damp-heat. A vaginal discharge with blood with offensive odor often suggests pouring down of damp-heat.

12. Inquiry of Symptom about Pediatric

Apart from the usual aspects included in inquiry, the inquiry of symptom in pediatrics should be done according to the infantile physiological and pathological features. Since diseases in the newborn (from the date of birth to one month after birth) are usually due to congenital factors or delivery conditions, inquiry should be emphasized on such aspects like the health condition of the mother during pregnancy and delivery periods, the contraction of diseases, his/her mother's condition before and after giving birth. Inquiry in pediatrics should emphasize the feeding, sitting, crawling, standing, walking, closed time of fontanel, eruption of tooth and learning to speak so as to understand the postnatal nutrition and development of infants. Infants at 6 months to 5 years of age are susceptible to acute infectious diseases. Nurses should inquire whether the infant is being infected by measles and varicella, whether the infant has received preventive inoculation before, whether the infant has the history of close contact with patients suffering from epidemic diseases, *etc.*. Infants' immune system is weak in resisting against diseases and regulating functions, and they are easy to be attacked by six exogenous pathogenic factors. So the infants and children should be inquired about whether he or she has the history of being frightened, catching cold, improper dietary disorders, *etc.*.

iv. Pulse-taking and Palpation

Pulse-taking means that the doctor use his or her hand to palpate, feel and press certain part of the patient's body to diagnose disease, including taking pulse and palpation.

1. Pulse-Taking Since the formation of the pulse condition is closely bound up with the condition of *zang-fu* organs, qi and blood, and body fluid, pathological changes may impede smooth flow of qi and blood, resulting in a change of the pulse condition. Then, through pulse-taking one may predict the location of a disease and its prognosis.

(1) Regions for taking pulse: *Cùn kǒu* (寸口) is the usual region selected to take pulse, which refers to pulsation of radial artery on the wrist. Pulse over *cùn kǒu* is

（2）带下：指妇女阴道内的一种少量乳白色、无臭的分泌物，具有濡润前阴的作用。主要询问带下的量、色、质和气味等情况。带下量多稀白，多为脾肾虚寒；带下量多色黄，质稠臭秽，多为湿热内盛；赤白带下，稠黏臭秽，多为湿毒下注。

12. 问小儿 小儿除一般问诊内容外，还需结合小儿的生理病理特点。新生儿的疾病多与先天因素或分娩情况有关，所以要询问其母妊娠期及产育期的营养健康状况、有无遗传疾病及分娩情况。婴幼儿应重点询问喂养方法及坐、爬、立、走、囟门闭合时间、出牙、学语的情况，从而了解小儿后天营养及生长发育情况。小儿6个月至5岁之间，易患急性传染病，应询问是否患过麻疹、水痘，是否预防接种，有无与传染病患者接触史等。小儿抗病力弱，调节功能低下，易感受六淫之邪，应询问有无受惊、着凉、伤食等情况。

（四）切诊

切诊是医者用手在患者体表的一定部位进行触、摸、按、压，以了解病情的一种诊察方法。包括脉诊和按诊两部分。

1. 脉诊 脏腑、气血、津液发生病变，血脉运行受到影响，脉象就会产生变化，故通过触按患者一定部位的脉搏，可以体察脉象，判断疾病的病位与推断疾病的预后。

（1）诊脉的部位：目前通行的是诊寸口，即手腕后桡动脉搏动处。寸口诊法把寸口脉

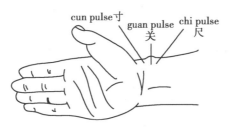

Fig. 4-3   Division of pulse over *cùn kǒu*
图 4-3   寸口脉寸关尺部位图

divided into three parts: *cùn, guān, and chǐ* (寸、关、尺). The part slightly below the styloid process of radius is *guān* pulse, the part anterior *guān* pulse is *cùn* pulse, and the part posterior *guān* pulse is *chǐ* pulse (Fig. 4-3). Both hands have three divisions of pulse, namely, *cùn* pulse, *guān* pulse and *chǐ* pulse. So altogether there are six divisions of pulse.

(2) The methods for taking pulse: The patient should rest for a while before pulse-taking. The patient sits erect or lies in supine and the forearms stretches out naturally to the level of the heart. At the time of taking pulse, the three fingers of the doctors are put at the same level and slightly arched to press the pulse with the belly of fingers. The middle finger of the doctor presses on the *guān* pulse, the index finger presses on *cùn* pulse, and the ring finger presses on *chǐ* pulse. The doctor keeps his or her own breath normal and calm to examine the pulse of the patient. The pulse should be taken at least for one minute each time in order to correctly examine the conditions of the pulse.

A normal pulse refers to the pulse conditions of a healthy person, with pulse presenting at three divisions over *cùn kǒu*, neither floating nor sunken, neither fast nor slow, gentle in sensation, moderate in size, soft, powerful, and regular in beating. It varies with factors such as age, gender, climate, diet, laboring, emotion *etc.*.

The pulse condition reflecting various pathological changes of a disease is known as the pathological pulse. Floating pulse is characterized by sensible under light pressure, while weak and constant beating under heavy pressure. Floating pulse often indicates external syndrome. Sunken pulse is characterized by sensible only under heavy pressure, which often indicates internal syndrome. Slow pulse is characterized by no more than 60 beats *per* minute, which indicates cold syndrome. Rapid pulse is characterized by beating over 100 times *per* minute, which indicates heat syndrome. Surging pulse is marked by wide size and full content, beating like roaring waves under light pressure as well as sudden flowing and ebbing, which indicates excess heat syndrome. Thready pulse is as thin

分为寸、关、尺三部。以掌后高骨稍内下方的部位为"关",关前为"寸",关后为"尺"(图 4-3)。左右两手各有寸、关、尺三部,共六部脉。

(2)切脉的方法:诊脉前请患者先休息片刻。取坐位或仰卧位,前臂自然伸展,与心脏同一水平。诊脉时医者中指定关,示指定寸,无名指定尺,三指平齐,手指略呈弓形,以指腹切按脉体。调匀自己的呼吸,静心凝神,体察脉象,每次诊脉时间至少在 1min以上。

正常脉象又称为平脉,表现为三部有脉,不浮不沉,不快不慢,从容和缓,不大不小,柔和有力,节律一致。平脉常受年龄、性别、气候、饮食、劳动、情绪等不同因素影响而产生相应的生理变化。

疾病反应于脉象的变化,即为病脉。轻取即得,按之稍弱而不空为浮脉,多主表证。轻取不应,重按始得为沉脉,多主里证。脉来迟缓,每分钟脉动不足 60 次为迟脉,主寒证。脉来快数,超过 100 次 /min 为数脉,主热证。脉体宽大,充实有力,滔滔满指,状如波涛,来盛去衰为洪脉,主里实热证。脉体细小如线,软弱无力,应指明显为细脉,多主气血两虚。往来流利,应指圆润,如珠走盘为滑脉,多主痰饮、食滞、实热。往来艰涩不畅,如轻刀刮竹为涩脉,主气滞、血

as a thread, weak and quite sensible under pressure, which often indicates deficiency of both qi and blood. Slippery pulse is beating freely and smoothly like the movement of beads of an abacus, which often indicates retention of phlegm and fluid, dyspepsia and excess heat. Choppy pulse is beating in an inhibited way like scraping a piece of bamboo, which indicates qi stagnation, blood stasis, essence injury and insufficiency of blood. Deficient pulse is marked by weak beating of the pulse at all the *cùn, guān, and chǐ* regions, which indicates deficiency syndrome. Excess pulse is marked by powerful sensation of pulse beating at *cùn, guān, and chǐ* regions under superficial, moderate and heavy pressure, which indicates excess syndrome. Pulse beats slowly with occasional and irregular intermittence is called knotted pulse, which indicates predominance of yin, qi stagnation and declination of qi and blood. Pulse beats slowly with regular and longer intermittence is called intermittent pulse, which indicates declination of visceral qi and deficiency of original qi. Hasty pulse beats fast with occasional and irregular intermittence, which often indicates exuberant yang and excessive heat, qi stagnation, blood stasis and retention of phlegm and food. Tight pulse appears like the pulling of a rope and flicks the finger when being pressed, which indicates cold syndrome, pain syndrome and retention of food. Wiry pulse appears straight, like the feeling of pressing the string of a violin, which indicates disorders of the liver and gallbladder, retention of phlegm and fluid, and pain syndrome. Soggy pulse is superficial and thin, which indicates deficiency syndrome and dampness syndrome. Weak pulse is deep and thin, sensible under heavy pressure, and insensible under light pressure, which indicates declination of both qi and blood. Faint pulse is very thin, soft, and almost insensible under pressure, which indicates declination of yang qi. The pulse beats over 140 times *per* minute is called racing pulse, which indicates near depletion of original qi.

2. Palpation   Palpation means to use fingers or palms to feel or press a patient's skin, hands and feet, chest and abdomen, and other regions to understand whether the local regions are cold or warm, soft or hard as well as whether there are tenderness, lump or other abnormal changes. Palpation can help to understand the location and nature of diseases.

(1) Palpation of skin: For a fever patient, when his or her skin is palpated, the fever gets higher at the first palpation, but lower after a long touch that indicates an exterior heat pattern. A lower fever has been felt at the first palpation, but higher after a long touch, which indicates an interior heat syndrome. Cold skin is indicative of yang

瘀、精伤、血少。三部脉举之无力，按之空虚为虚脉，主虚证。三部脉举按皆有力，浮沉皆得为实脉，主实证。脉来缓慢，时有中止，止无定数为结脉，主阴盛气结，气血虚衰。脉来缓弱，时有中止，止有定数，良久方来为代脉，主脏气衰微，元气虚损。脉来急促，时有中止，止无定数为促脉，多主阳盛实热，气血痰饮宿食停滞。脉来紧张，如牵绳转索，按之弹指为紧脉，主寒证、痛证、食积。端直以长，如按琴弦为弦脉，主肝胆病、痰饮、痛证。脉浮而细软为濡脉，主虚证、湿证。脉极软而沉细，重取始得，轻取不得为弱脉，主气血俱衰。脉极细极软，按之欲绝，若有若无，为微脉，主阳气衰微。脉来急疾，140 次 /min 以上为疾脉，主元气将脱。

2. **按诊**   按诊是用手指或手掌对患者的肌肤、手足、脘腹及病变部位施行触摸按压，以测知局部冷热、软硬、压痛、痞块或其他异常变化，从而推断疾病的部位和性质的一种诊病方法。

（1）按肌表：凡身热患者，按其皮肤，初按热甚，久按热反转轻者，为表热证；久按热更甚，热自内向外蒸发者，为里热证。皮肤凉，多为阳虚；皮肤干燥，为津液不足。肌肤肿胀，按之有凹陷，松手不能即起者为

deficiency. Dry skin is indicative of insufficiency of body fluid. When the swollen and distending skin is pressed and the depression on the skin fails to rebound, it is indicative of edema. If the depression on the skin disappears immediately after the touch, it is flatulence.

A swelling has been felt hard but without a hot sensation often indicates yin syndrome. A swelling with a burning sensation often refers to a yang syndrome. A stone-hard swelling without a hot sensation often indicates absence of pus. A swelling with a soft top, hard edge, hot skin and pain upon heavy pressure often indicates pus formation.

(2) Palpation of hands and feet: Cold hands and feet indicate deficiency of yang and abundance of cold. Hot hands and feet indicate abundance of yang and heat. A feverish sensation of the palms and soles indicates a fever due to interior injury. Hot sensation on the back of the hands and feet indicates a fever due to exogenous pathogenic factors. Both lower limbs feeling cold often indicates abundance of yin and cold. Both soles feeling feverish often indicates yin deficiency.

(3) Pressing epigastrium and abdomen: Epigastric and abdominal pain with preference for pressure and pain relieved after being pressed often indicate deficiency syndrome. Epigastric and abdominal pain with aversion to pressure often indicates excess syndrome. It's regarded as flatulence if the patient's abdomen sounds hollow like the sound of a drum on percussion and has no difficulty in urination. When the patient has difficulty in urination and the sound of water movement in abdomen can be heard on percussion, it's regarded as ascites. An abdominal mass is marked by a fixed pain, visible shape and it is not movable on percussion, which suggests problems of the blood system. It is named concretions or accumulations. If the mass is marked by a wondering pain and invisible shape, it indicates qi stagnation. It is named conglomerations or gatherings.

(4) Palpation of acupoints: Acupoints, the places where qi of *zang-fu* organs and channel converges and transmits, are the points that reflect visceral disorders on the surface of the body. In pressing acupoints, cares should be taken to see if there are tenderness, nodules and other sensitive responses. For example, nodules over BL 13 (*fèi shù*) and tenderness over LU 1 (*zhōng fǔ*) usually indicate lung diseases. Tenderness over BL 18 (*gān shù*) and LV 14 (*qì mén*) often indicate liver diseases.

(Zhou Yun-xian)

水肿，松手即起者为气肿。

疮疡按之肿硬不热多为阴证；肿处灼热，多为阳证；按之坚而不热，多尚未成脓；边硬顶软，患处灼热，重按跳痛更甚者，多为有脓。

（2）按手足：患者手足俱冷，多为阳虚寒盛；手足俱热，为阳热炽盛；手心热，多为内伤；手背热，多为外感；两足皆凉，多为阴寒内盛；两足心热，多为阴虚。

（3）按脘腹：腹痛喜按，按之痛减者多为虚证；腹痛拒按者多为实证；腹满叩之如鼓，小便自利者为气胀；小便不利，推之漉漉有声，为水臌；腹内有肿块，按之坚而不移，痛有定处者，为癥为积，多属血瘀；肿块时聚时散，按之无形，痛无定处者，为瘕为聚，多因气滞所致。

（4）按腧穴：腧穴是脏腑经络之气汇聚转输之处，是内脏病变反映于体表的反应点。按腧穴，应注意穴位处有无压痛、结节，以及其他敏感反应。如肺腧穴有结节或中府穴有压痛，多为肺病；肝腧穴或期门穴有压痛，多为肝病。

（周云仙）

Section 2　Daily Life Nursing

As for daily life, it refers to the basic activities in people's daily life including life style, habits, customs, work style, *etc.*. Daily life nursing means that people should comply with the changes in nature and live regularly. Daily life is closely related to health. People should follow the changes in nature, adapt to the seasonal changes, keep normal dietary and regular daily life in order to maintain health and prolong life. Conversely, people will fall to diseases if they eat improperly or live irregularly.

I. Complying with Four Seasons to Keep Yin-Yang Balance

i. Significance and Basic Principle of Complying with Four Seasons to Keep Yin-Yang Balance

The changes of yin and yang in the four seasons dictate the alterations in the world. In terms of changes in four seasons, yang qi works as the commander to generate and cultivate things in spring and summer, because yang qi is in charge of generation while yin qi is for nourishing. In autumn and winter all things are under the control of yin qi, when yang qi tends to wither up all things and yin qi to store them. And then, all things are sheltered for storage. In *Basic Questions·Yin Yang Ying Xiang Da Lun*, it is said that the function of the human body is corresponded to *Tian qi* (qi of nature), which means human can communicate with natural rules based on the changes of yin-yang in nature. Basically, health preservation in four seasons is to adjust yin-yang in human body according to the rise and fall of yin-yang in nature, thereafter the vital activities within body can correspond to the changes of nature.

It is recorded in the *Basic Questions· Si Qi Tiao Shen Da Lun*, that people should "nourish yang in spring and summer while nourish yin in autumn and winter", which is put forward according to the time, characteristics, states of the waxing and waning of yin and yang, qi's ascent and descent, viscera function's rise and fall. In spring and

第二节　生活起居调护

起居是指人们在日常生活中的基本生存活动，包括生活方式、生活习惯、劳作风格等。起居调护是指顺应自然变化的规律，合理安排日常生活、作息时间等。生活起居与健康有着密切的关系，《素问·上古天真论》曰："上古之人，其知道者，法于阴阳，和于术数，食饮有节，起居有常，不妄作劳，故能形与神俱，而尽享其天年，度百步乃去。"反之，若"以酒为浆，以妄为常……起居无节，故半百而衰也。"说明要保持身体健康，延年益寿，应懂得顺应自然变化的规律，适应四时气候变化，做到饮食有节，起居有常，生活规律；若饮食不节，起居无常，就会多病早衰。

一、顺应四时，平衡阴阳

（一）"顺应四时，平衡阴阳"的意义和基本原则

世间万物变化的根本原因，是四时阴阳的变化。《素问·阴阳应象大论》："阳生阴长，阳杀阴藏。"春夏为阳气当令，阳主生发，阴主长养，万物应以生、长；秋冬为阴气所主，阳主肃杀，阴主闭藏，万物趋于收、藏。人体的生命功能与天地自然之气相通应，生命本于自然阴阳变化。四时调养从根本上说，就是根据自然界阴阳的盛衰，来调节人体阴阳的盈虚，使人体的阴阳变化适应自然界阴阳变化的规律。

《素问·四气调神大论》曰："春夏养阳，秋冬养阴"，这是根据自然界和人体阴阳消长、气机升降、五脏盛衰的不同时间、特点、状态而提出的调摄原则。春夏时节，万物从冬藏中复苏、生发，以至于繁荣茂盛，这种

summer, everything recovers from dormant winter, and grows to prosperity. The growing of vitality from weak to strong is a symbol of yang qi of the natural world in spring and summer. Likewise, the function of yang qi prevails in human vital activities at that time. Therefore, people should adapt their vital activities to the natural changes for preserving yang. From autumn to winter, everything goes from fruition to hiding and storing, because the natural world is dominated by yin qi at that time, as well as human body. Therefore, it is time to store yang qi and nourish yin essence to adapt to natural changes. This is the basic principle of yin-yang changes in four seasons. If this basic principle is gone against within human body and yin-yang balance is broken, many diseases will occur. Therefore, people should follow the basic principle of "nourishing yang in spring and summer while nourishing yin in autumn and winter" in seasonal health preservation.

ii. Daily Life Nursing in Four Seasons

1. Daily Life Nursing in Spring In spring, yang qi gradually gets more and more prosperous and works predominantly in nature after being stored in winter. It governs the growth, and everything is about to boom. There is a vigorous picture in nature. People should comply with the healthy qi and adjust daily life.

(1) The principle of daily life nursing in spring: The principle of daily life nursing in spring is to follow the upward trend of yang qi in nature; be consistent with growing trend and the vitality of everything in nature, support yang qi within the human body; regulate the functions of the liver and gallbladder, keep away from pathogenic qi in nature in order to maintain exuberance of qi of the *shaoyang* meridian in the body and lay a solid foundation for health preservation in summer.

(2) Maintenance of daily activities: All the daily activities should be stretched, smooth, dispersing and unobstructed state in spring. In spring, people should go to sleep a little later at night; get up as early as possible in the morning; do some outdoor exercises; wear loose and comfortable clothes; leave one's hair loose and relax the body as comfortable as possible. If unrestrained, yang qi will be generated and enriched. Doing exercises in the daytime can relieve fatigue and having entertainment after a hard day at work in the evening would be helpful to relieve physical and mental stress. But, people should follow certain basic rules, which is, people should choose different exercises according to the individual constitutions and inclinations. Activities or exercises should not be too intense in case of physical over-exertion, so that the human body can be kept in a stretched and relaxed condition.

生机的由弱而强，是天地间春夏阳气的象征。人类在这一阶段的生命活动须适应自然界阴阳的变化以养阳。秋冬之令，万物渐趋结实、肃杀而至闭藏，是阴气主政，人体也以阴气为主导，宜适应自然变化以潜藏阳气，滋养阴精。背离这一阴阳变化的至理，就有可能影响人体整个阴阳的平衡，导致各种疾病的出现。所以，四时养生必须遵循"春夏养阳，秋冬养阴"的基本原则。

（二）四时起居调护

1. **春季起居调护** 春季，经过隆冬的秘藏，阳气已由弱而旺，自然界阳气当令，主万物的生发，自然界呈现蓬勃向上、生机盎然的景象。人们应顺应春时生发之气，调摄作息。

（1）春季生活起居的调护原则：应顺应自然界阳气生发的积极趋势，与天地万物蓬勃向上的趋势一致，扶助机体阳气，调畅肝胆气机，规避春季各种致病因素，保持人体少阳之气的旺盛，并为夏季的养"长"打下充实的基础。

（2）日常活动调养：春季各种起居活动均要考虑到舒展、宣泄通达。《素问·四气调神大论》曰："春三月……夜卧早起，广步于庭，披发缓行……此春气之应，养生之道也。"春季应稍迟些睡觉，在保证基本睡眠的前提下尽可能早起，进行一些室外活动，衣服保持宽松舒适，披散头发，尽量舒缓身体，在没有任何压抑束缚的情况下，促进阳气的生发。白天尽可能抽时间进行活动以舒缓机体的疲惫，晚上适当进行有益身心的娱乐活动以缓解一天的劳累。基本要求是根据个人不同体质及个人喜好，选择不同的活动，以舒缓、畅达为要。尽量进行强度不大而舒缓的活动，

Sitting, watching and sleeping for a long continuous time will be disadvantageous to relaxation of muscles and tendons and will block qi and blood circulation in the channels and collaterals, causing dysfunction of the liver and gallbladder. Man should stay less sedentary indoors and choose an outdoor venue, such as outdoor activities in the park or grass field to communicate with nature and breathe the fresh air. Thus yang qi in the human body will rise gradually in spring by doing these sports.

(3) "*Chun Wu*" (keeping warm in spring) fosters yang qi: "Keeping warm in spring" means that people should take off the winter clothing as late as possible, and keep warm energy in the body to foster inner condition for the generation of yang qi. In spring, yang qi begins to rise but is not strong enough and cold qi fades away gradually. It is cold in one minute, whereas, it could become hot in the next minute in the early spring. It is very difficult for the body to adapt to the changeable weather. Therefore, if people take off winter clothing too early, the cold pathogen will attack the human body easily and cause diseases ultimately, which because yang qi is still insufficient to resist the spring cold at this time. If the principle of "keeping warm in spring" is followed properly, yang qi will be prosperous. This also means that the healthy qi is strong enough so that deficiency-type pathogen and abnormal weather will have no opportunities to attack the body. Clothes in spring should be loose, soft and warm. Adding or taking off clothes should accord to the climatic changes. One should not take off winter clothing too early. Cold usually comes in from the foot, so traditional health preservation suggests dressing in spring should be thicker in feet and thinner in trunk, and young women should not wear skirt too early.

(4) "Deficiency-type pathogen and abnormal weather must be prevented in time": It refers that people must know how to recognize the pathogenic factors and keep away from them timely. In spring, it may be pleasant when it is warm with sunlight, but sometimes it may be cold when it rains continuously. Changeable weather in spring often cause infectious diseases of respiratory system such as flu and mumps, skin diseases such as neurodermitis and urticaria, as well as gastrointestinal diseases. Therefore, man must pay much attention to the changes of climate, and especially their influences on human body, to avoid attack of deficiency-type pathogen and abnormal weather.

2. Daily Life Nursing in Summer Yang qi is exuberant in summer. The heaven yang qi goes down from above, and yin qi of the earth goes up from below, leading to the integration of yin and yang qi, and the prosperity

使机体尽可能处于调达舒畅的状态。但不可过于疲惫，亦不宜久坐不动、久视不移、久睡不起，以免阻碍肌肉筋骨的舒缓，使经络气血淤积，有碍于肝胆之气的调畅。尽量少守舍，可选择空气清新的户外适宜场所，如公园、草地等地进行户外活动，多接触大自然，以呼吸自然界的新鲜空气，舒缓筋骨，使春天阳气生发。

（3）"春捂"以养阳气："春捂"指春季尽可能迟地卸减冬装，"捂"住身体的热气，以保证阳气生发的体内环境。春季阳气刚升而未盛，寒气将去而未衰，乍暖乍寒，机体很难适应这种变幻莫测的气候。寒温冷热不时，过早地脱去棉衣，寒气则趁虚而入，初生的阳气尚不足以与春寒抗衡，抵御能力减弱，极易感受各种疾病。"春捂"得宜，阳气旺则正气盛，虚邪贼风便无缘侵袭人体。春季着装既要宽松、柔软保暖，还应注意随气候变化而增减，切忌减衣太快。此外，由于寒多自下而上，传统养生主张春时衣着宜下厚上薄，青年女性尤为注意，不可过早换裙装。

（4）虚邪贼风，避之有时：认识各种致病因素以适时趋避。春季，晴时阳光普照、温暖宜人，阴时阴雨绵绵、寒气袭人，乍寒乍暖的气候易引起疾病，如流行性感冒、腮腺炎等呼吸道传染病，神经性皮炎、荨麻疹等皮肤病及胃肠道疾病等。因此，春季应尤其注意天气变化对人体的影响，在瞬息转变的时候，避开虚邪贼风的侵袭。

2. 夏季起居调护 夏季阳气旺盛，天阳下济，地热上蒸，天地阴阳之气上下交合，万物繁华茂盛。

and flourishing of all living things.

(1) The principle of daily life nursing in summer: With extremely exuberant characteristics of yang qi in summer, people should keep consistent with the growing tendency of all living things, comply with the strong yang qi in nature to nourish yang qi for raising the body, and nourish heart qi to assist yang qi. People should not only protect themselves from summer-heat pathogen in summer and dampness pathogen in long-summer, but also need to pay attention to protect yang qi in the human body. All the aspects of health preservation should follow the general rule of "nourishing yang qi in spring and summer" to lay a foundation for health promotion in autumn.

(2) Maintenance of daily activities: In summer, people should adapt to early sunrise and late sunset. It is good for people to go to bed later in the evening and get up earlier in the morning. As the daytime lasts longer, man should have a nap at noon to restore energy. People are likely to be attacked by wind-cold-dampness in summer, because the striae and interstices are loose and the sweating pores are open. People should not prefer coolness too much or have too much cold drink, which will result in the deficiency of center qi. Meanwhile, the summer-heat pathogen accompanied by wind-cold pathogen will take the chance to invade the human body. So in summer, people should not dress too few, and should pay more attention to keep the abdomen and the back warm since *du mai* is on the back, which governs yang qi of the whole body. The circulation of yang qi in the body will be blocked if the back gets cold. The point of the bellybutton belongs to the *ren mai*, the major function of which is to adjust qi and blood of yin channel. Catching cold on bellybutton and the back will not only affect the spleen and stomach, causing abdominal pain, diarrhea, *etc.*, but also result in the dysmenorrhea and menstrual disorder. In the meantime, it is inadvisable for people to sleep outside or sleep in air conditioned rooms with air conditioner blowing too hard. People should not stay in the passageway or under the eave, and should keep away from the slit of windows and doors in case of the invasion of wind pathogen. People should neither take a cold shower, swim in cold water to relieve heat nor walk in rain in order to avoid the invasion of cold-damp pathogen while the sweating pores are open. When it is too hot, taking a warm bath or toweling off sweat softly by warm and wet towel is strongly advised in order to avoid the striae and interstices shutting down immediately in cold circumstance, and consequently to avoid smooth-flowing of qi and leaving the pathogenic factors in the human body. The sunshine is sufficient in summer for its longer sunlight time. One should get out

（1）夏季生活起居的调护原则：应根据自然界阳气极度旺盛的特点，与天地间万物生长的趋势一致，顺盛阳以养阳，护阳气以养"长"，养心气以辅阳，既要盛夏防暑邪，长夏防湿邪，同时又要注意保护人体阳气，不离"春夏养阳"的总规律，为秋季的养"收"打下基础。

（2）日常活动调养。《素问·四气调神大论》曰："夏三月……夜卧早起，无厌于日……此夏气之应，养长之道也。"夏季人们应顺应自然界养长之势，宜入夜晚睡，清晨早起，以适应日出早而落日晚的规律。白天时间长，夜卧早起，午间适当小眠，以恢复体力。夏日炎热，腠理开泄，易受风寒湿邪侵袭，不可过于避热趋凉，或饮冷无度，致使中气内虚，暑热与风寒之邪趁虚而入。因此夏季穿衣不可太薄，尤其腹、背部更要注意保暖。因为人的背部是督脉所在，主管着人体一身的阳气，背部受寒易阻碍全身阳气的运行，而脐部属于任脉，调节阴经的气血。脐部和背部受寒不仅会影响到脾胃，使人体出现腹痛、腹泻等症状，更可引起痛经、月经紊乱等疾病。同时夏季睡眠时不宜夜晚露宿，空调房间不宜室内外温差过大。纳凉时勿在房檐下、过道里，应远离门窗缝隙，以防贼风入内。汗孔张开，不宜立即用冷水冲凉，或入冷水游泳，或冒雨贪凉，以防寒湿入侵。过热时，提倡温水浴，或用温湿毛巾擦抹，使机体腠理毛孔不致骤然闭拒，气不得泄，而致邪闭于内。夏季日照时间长，阳光充足，人体养护也要尽可能地进行户外活动，多接触阳光，使汗液排泄，排出体内毒素。夏季活动要注意：最好选择清晨或傍晚较凉爽时进行，场地宜选择公园、庭院等空气清新处，以散步、慢跑等强度较低的项目为宜，活动量要适度。

in the sun as often as possible to promote yang qi in the human body. One should carry on some outdoor exercises as possible as one can, and it can promote sweat excretion which regulates the human body fluid and takes away the waste from the body. When doing exercises in summer, it is better to do exercises in the morning or in the evening and in a place such as park or garden where there is abundant of fresh air. Moderate physical exercises such as taking a walk, jogging *etc.* should be chosen.

(3) Avoiding pathogenic factors to prevent diseases: The excessive summer-heat will lead to dizziness, chest oppression, nausea, thirst, and even coma. Hence, doing labor work or physical exercise should avoid burning sunshine, and necessary protection should be taken. In summer, one should protect himself from pathogenic dampness which prevails in the long summer. If pathogenic dampness and pathogenic heat work together, yang qi of the spleen and stomach is easily get hurt so that fluid in the body cannot normally metabolize. The diseases caused by summer-heat pathogen and pathogenic dampness are not easy to be cured. So one should avoid living in wet environment and do not sleep in the humid place for a long time. Simultaneously, people should be cautious about common summer illness such as "common cold in summer", heatstroke, bacillary dysentery, acute gastroenteritis, solar dermatitis, food poisoning and so on.

3. Daily Life Nursing in Autumn　In autumn, yang qi falls gradually and yin qi gets rising little by little in nature. Autumn is the transition from the abundant yang qi to the profuse yin qi. The rising and falling of yin-yang in body also corresponds with waxing and waning of yin-yang in nature. The qi movement transfers from the opening in strong state of yang qi into the accumulation in the abundant state of yin qi. It is also called that the "the rising in summer" is transferred to "gathering in autumn".

(1) The principle of daily life nursing in autumn: The principle of daily life nursing in autumn should follow the basic rule of "nourishing yin in autumn and winter" to foster the yin qi, gather the mature, care the lung and prevent the troubles from the autumn dryness. People should follow natural rules that yin qi grows gradually from weak to prosperous and then take cultivating yin qi of body as the most important task to build a good foundation for the winter storage.

(2) Maintenance of daily activities: In autumn, people should adapt to the dry weather and restraining characteristic in nature to work and rest, sleep early to comply with the collection of the yin essence and get up early to adapt the extension of yang qi. In the daily

（3）防病避邪：暑热过度可使人头昏、胸闷、恶心、口渴、甚至昏迷。因此，安排劳动或体育锻炼时，要避开烈日炽热之时，并注意加强防护。夏季还要防湿邪侵袭。长夏是湿邪最盛之时，湿邪与热邪相缠绕，极易损伤人体脾胃之阳气，使体内的水液不能正常代谢。暑湿伤人后引起的疾病，病程很长，不易恢复，所以在居住环境上要切忌潮湿，更不要久卧湿地。同时应注意预防一些常见病证，如夏季感冒（也称热伤风）、中暑（俗称发痧）、细菌性痢疾、急性胃肠炎（也称六月泻）、日光性皮炎、食物中毒等。

3. 秋季起居调护　秋季，自然界阳气渐降，阴气渐长，是由阳盛转变为阴盛的过渡时期。人体的阴阳盛衰也与天地阳消阴长相应，由阳盛的气机开泄，转为阴长的气机收敛，随"夏长"到"秋收"而相应改变。

（1）秋季生活起居的调护原则：应遵循秋冬养阴的基本规律，养阴、养收、养肺、防秋燥；应当适应自然界阴气渐生而旺的规律，把保养体内的阴气作为首要任务，为冬藏打基础。

（2）日常活动调养：《素问·四气调神大论》曰："秋三月，早卧早起……此秋气之应，养收之道也。"秋季的起居作息要适应秋燥之气和收敛之性，应早睡以顺应阴精的收藏，

activities, people should avoid overtiredness and excessive perspiration to protect yang qi from injuring and yin fluid from consuming. Exercise for health preservation in autumn should be classified into the following three levels. Firstly, the static-oriented exercises like *qigong* which involves rhythmic breathing coordinated with slow stylized repetition of fluid movement, a calm mindful state, and visualization of guiding qi through the body. Secondly, the moderate exercise aiming at relaxing the bones and muscles without sweating profusely and labor-consuming, such as the *taijiquan*, the *taiji* sword, and walking. Thirdly is the vigorous exercise with large amount of motion, which is suitable for the obese people to lose weight.

(3)"Enduring cold in autumn" to defend yang qi: The old saying of "keeping warm in spring and enduring cold in autumn" is a principle for health preservation in four seasons. The "keeping warm in spring" is helpful to raise yang qi, while "enduring cold in autumn" contributes to defend it. "Enduring the cold in autumn" is effective for cultivating health in the autumn, which has been paid much attention in both the ancient and modern times. Because the weather in autumn is cool but not yet too cold to endure at this time, people should follow the principle of storing up yin essence and defending yang qi in the autumn, do some cold-resistant exercise intentionally to strengthen their physique and gradually avoid over-dressing-induced perspiration which will lead to the consumption of yin fluid and leaks of yang qi. Of course, "enduring cold in autumn" should be carried on according to different people and weather. For instance, the old and the young children whose resistance are weak should pay attention to keep warm and add clothing in time in the deep autumn.

(4) Evading the deficiency-type pathogen and abnormal weather to prevent diseases: The weather changes greatly and all the heat pathogen, dryness pathogen and cold pathogen exist in the autumn. So people should be cautious in daily life to prevent the pathogenic factors from invading the body before getting sick. In autumn, people should mainly pay attention to the prevention of the following illnesses. The bronchial asthma often relapses suddenly when the autumn weather turns from hot to cool. The constipation caused by autumn dryness could consume the human body fluid, resulting in intestinal dryness. The autumn diarrhea is a typical seasonal sickness, which is the reason why much attention should be paid to maintain abdominal warm for the babies and infants, since the weather in autumn becomes cooler and cooler, and the children are likely to catch cold in the abdomen.

早起以顺应阳气的舒张。日常活动不可过度劳累，不可泄汗过多，以防阳气和阴液受损伤。秋季养生锻炼分为三个层次：一是以静养为主的气功锻炼法，强调呼吸内守、形神内敛；二是轻度运动养生法，如太极拳、太极剑、散步等，以舒展肌肉筋骨为目的，不要求大汗淋漓、消耗体力；三是对形体肥胖而需要减肥者，可以考虑运动量大一点的项目。

（3）"秋冻"以辅阳气：四季养生的一个原则是"春捂秋冻"，春捂以助阳气的升发；秋冻则是辅佐阳气的敛藏。秋冻含有积极意义，是古今养生都十分强调的秋天养生方法。秋虽凉还不至于寒，人们还能耐受，有意识地进行防寒锻炼，逐渐增强体质和避免因穿衣过多产生身热汗出而致阴津伤耗、阳气外泄，以顺应秋天阴精内蓄、阳气内守的需要。当然秋冻还要因人、因天气变化而异，如老人、小孩，由于抵抗力弱，在进入深秋时就要注意保暖，适时增加衣服。

（4）避虚邪贼风以防病：秋季气候变化较大，热、燥、寒气皆有，起居若不慎，便容易患病。故应慎起居，避虚邪，防秋病于未发之前。主要应注意以下病证的预防：支气管哮喘，多半在秋季气候由热转凉时发作；便秘，因秋天气候干燥，燥伤津液，肠道干涩而引起；秋季腹泻，是典型的季节病，要注意婴幼儿腹部保暖，因秋季气候渐凉，婴幼儿腹部容易受寒。

4. Daily Life Nursing in Winter　In winter, yang qi in nature is hidden and the yin qi works as a commander to control the accumulation and storage of everything. Yang qi is also accumulated in body complying with the changing rule of natural yin-yang.

(1) Principle of daily life nursing in winter: The principle of health preservation should comply with the characteristics of hiding and storing in winter, keep up with the tendency of storing energy in nature to nourish yin essence of the human body, gather the vitality and maintain yang qi, and keep warm against cold. Furthermore, people should protect the kidney qi to establish the foundation for the generating and rising in the next spring.

(2) Maintenance of daily activity: The cold pathogen in winter is very likely to damage yang qi in body. The basic principle of daily activity is to keep away from the cold and protect yang qi. People, especially the old, should go to sleep early and not get up before sunrise in cold winter, which is because in winter, the night becomes longer and the coldness is heavier. Going to sleep early may keep yang qi in body to prevent the coldness from invading, and getting up late may ward off the cold of the night. It's the basic measure to keep warm in the cold and the yang qi in body should follow the yang qi in nature. In winter, people, especially the old and the weak, should pay more attention to keep head, neck, back and feet warm. The wind-cold pathogen tends to invade human body from the back where is the yang within yang, and may cause respiratory and cardiovascular diseases. In addition, "cold invades from the feet", so people should pay attention to keep feet warm, which can protect people from catching cold in winter. Otherwise, the viscera may be affected by the encroaching cold pathogen, resulting in abdominal pain, diarrhea and so on.

(3) Disease prevention and health preservation in winter: The coldness is the strongest predisposing factor of lots of diseases in the severely cold winter. When human body gets over-stimulation of coldness, hypertension, heart diseases, cranial vascular disease and other diseases related to the circulatory system can be induced. Coldness may cause the coarseness and rahagades of exposed skin, the frostbite on the ear, nose, finger and so on. The facial paralysis can be induced in winter if the head is suddenly attacked by the cold air or cold wind. Keeping warm in winter is the key to prevent all above diseases.

4. 冬季起居调护　冬季，自然界阳气潜藏于内，阴气当令，主万物闭藏。人体阳气也顺应天地阴阳升降的规律而秘藏于内。

（1）冬季生活起居的调护原则：应顺应自然界冬气闭藏的特点，与天地间万物潜藏能量的趋势一致，滋养人体阴精，蓄养机体生机，保养阳气，防寒保暖，以保护肾气为根本，为春天的生发奠定基础。

（2）日常活动调养：冬令时节，由于风寒气冷，寒邪最易伤人体之阳气，故日常活动的重要原则就是防寒护阳。《素问·四气调神大论》曰："冬三月，早卧晚起，必待日光……养藏之道也。"人们在寒冷的冬天应早睡、晚起，起床的时间最好在日出之后。因为冬令夜愈深则寒气愈重，早睡可以使人体阳气免受阴寒的侵扰；待日出再起床，则能避开夜间的寒气。以自然界的阳气主张机体的阳气，是人们防寒保暖的基本措施。冬季要特别注意头部、颈部、背部和两足的保暖，年老体弱者尤应注意。背部是人体的阳中之阳，风寒等邪气极易通过背部侵入而引发呼吸系统疾病和心脑血管疾病。寒从脚起，冬季要注重两足的保暖，两足温暖者不易受寒感冒，而足部受寒，势必影响内脏，可引致腹痛、腹泻等疾病。

（3）冬季防病保健：严寒季节，寒气最易伤人，可诱发多种疾病。当过度的寒冷刺激时，对高血压、心脏病、脑血管病和其他循环系统疾病都有诱发作用；寒冷可使人体裸露部位的皮肤粗糙或皲裂、老化，耳、手指等常发生冻疮；冬天若让头部突然遭受冷空气，或长时间受到冷风的侵袭，易发生面神经麻痹。这些疾病的预防主要是防寒保暖。

II. Suitable Ward Environment to Avoid External Pathogen

The six pathogenic factors are closely related to seasonal climate and living environment. Nursing staff should be initiative to master the rules of climate change in the four seasons to prevent from wind pathogen in spring, to avoid the summer heat pathogen in summer, to restrain dampness in late summer, to hold back dryness pathogen in autumn, to retard coldness pathogen in winter, and then provide patients good environment for recuperation.

i. Arrangement of the Ward Based on the Syndrome

The ward should be arranged according to the character of the diseases. The patients with cold syndrome and yang deficiency syndrome should be arranged in the warm ward toward the sun to make them comfortable because they fear cold and wind. The patients with heat syndrome and yin deficient syndrome should be arranged in the cool ward backward the sun to make them cool and easeful because they hate heat and prefer cold.

ii. Quiet Ward

Quiet environment helps the patient to rest and rehabilitate. The noise can make people feel distracted. For example, patients with heart qi deficiency often catch palpitation because of the sudden sound. So they should be arranged in a quiet environment in which the noise should not surpass 40-60 decibels.

iii. Suitable Temperature and Humidity in the Ward

Temperature and humidity in the ward should be suitable. Generally, 18-22℃ are appropriate. If the temperature is too high, people are easy to feel dry and hot. Otherwise, if the temperature is excessively low, people are easy to feel cold and uncomfortable. The suitable range of the relative humidity indoors is from 50% to 60%. Excessively high humidity suppresses the human body to vaporize and exhale, and then makes the human body feel uncomfortable. Excessively low humidity is easy to make people feel dry and painful in the pharynx and larynx. Therefore, the temperature and humidity should be adjusted according to the climate and the different diseases. The temperature between 16℃ and 20℃ is suitable for the patients with yin deficiency syndrome and heat syndrome, and the temperature between 20℃ and 26℃ is suitable for the elderly, the infant, and the patients with yang deficiency syndrome and cold syndrome. The low humidity is appropriate for the patients with excessive dampness syndrome. The high humidity is appropriate for the patients with the dryness syndrome. The patients with

二、调摄环境，慎避外邪

六淫致病多与季节气候、居室环境密切相关。护理人员应主动掌握四时气候变化的规律，做到春防风，夏防暑，长夏防湿，秋防燥，冬防寒，为患者创造良好的休养环境。

（一）病室安置辨证而定

病室安排应根据病证性质的不同而定。如寒证、阳虚证者，多畏寒怕风，宜安置在向阳、温暖的病室内，使患者感到舒适；热证、阴虚证者，多恶热喜凉，可安置在背阴、凉爽的病室内，使患者感到凉爽、舒适、心静，以利于养病。

（二）病室安静

安静的环境有助于患者休息和调养。噪声的刺激会使人感到心烦意乱，尤其是心气虚的患者，常因突然的声响而心悸不已。故应创造一个安静的居住环境，噪声以不超过40~60分贝为宜。

（三）病室温湿度适宜

室内温、湿度应适宜。一般以18~22℃为宜，温度过高，易使人感到燥热；温度过低，易使人感到寒冷不适。室内相对湿度以50%~60%为宜，湿度过高，抑制人体蒸发散热，使人体感到不舒服；湿度过低，易使人感到口舌干燥、咽喉干痛。同时，应根据气候和不同病证调整室内温湿度。阴虚证、热证患者以16~20℃为宜；老年人、婴幼儿、阳虚证、寒证患者以20~26℃为宜；湿盛患者，湿度宜低；燥证患者，湿度宜高；阴虚者多热而偏燥，湿度宜高；阳虚者多寒而偏湿，湿度宜低。

yin deficiency feel hot and dry, so the humidity should be higher. The patients with yang deficiency feel cold and wet, so the humidity should be lower.

iv. Suitable Light in the Ward

Abundant light in the ward is required, which makes the patients feel comfortable and delighted. But the light should not be directly irradiated to the face of the patients. Patients with different syndromes require different kinds of light. For example, the patients with heat syndrome, excessive yang syndrome or neurasthenia, require caliginous light, but the patients with spasmodic syndrome or epilepsy require dark curtain to make room dullish because the strong light may induce convulsion.

III. Living Regularly, Working and Resting Moderately

i. Living Regularly

"Living regularly" contains the following meanings: working and resting on time, avoiding oversleep, doing exercises moderately to strengthen tendons and bones, eating three meals every day at fixed time and in fixed amount, taking meat with vegetables, combining exertion and rest, and keeping still and active alternatively. When this has been achieved, people can live out their lives according to *Basic Questions*. "Living regularly" is the important rule of adjusting spirit and qi. People can maintain spirit and qi, possess full of energy and exuberant vitality if they have regular living and reasonable work and rest. Otherwise, people will be lack of energy and their vitality will decline if they live irregularly.

ii. Working and Resting Moderately

Overstrain in TCM includes mental overstrain, labor overstrain and sexual overstrain. Excessive desires is one kind of mental strains, and it is caused by over preference which is nerve-racking. For this reason, the measures should be taken to conserve the spirit for health cultivation by cutting the origin of excessive desires and reduce desires. With regard to labor overstrain, "No overwork and over-rest" is the principle according to *Peng Zu health cultivation theory* (*Péng Zǔ Shè Shēng Yǎng Xìng Lùn*, 彭祖摄生养性论). It refers that people should neither be overtired, but increase activity gradually in their daily life, nor take too much rest, because it will make qi and blood stagnate, causing dysfunction of the tendons and bones. If people keep still without enough movement or even without movement, it will induce the stagnation of essence, flaccidities of tendons and even the decrease of longevity. Longtime lying injuries qi, while longtime

（四）病室光线适宜

一般病室内要求阳光充足，使患者感到舒适愉快。但不宜让日光直射患者面部。不同病证的患者对光线要求亦不同。如热证、阳亢患者、神经衰弱者等的病室光线宜偏暗；痉证、癫狂证者，强光可诱发痉挛，应用暗窗帘遮挡。

三、起居有常，劳逸适度

（一）起居有常

起居有常要求人们做到按时作息，力戒贪睡；适当锻炼，筋骨强健；一日三餐，定时定量；荤素粗细，搭配合理；劳逸结合，动静有度。《素问·上古天真论》曰："食饮有节，起居有常，不妄作劳，故能形与神俱，而尽终其天年，度百岁乃去。"起居有常是调养神气的重要法则。人们若能起居有常，合理作息，就能保养神气，使人体精力充沛，生命力旺盛；反之，若起居无常，天长日久则神气衰败，就会出现精神萎靡，生命力衰退。

（二）劳逸适度

劳包括神劳、形（体）劳和房劳。神劳很重要的一个方面是嗜欲，嗜欲是因为喜好太过而致偏爱成癖，欲望太过，必伤心神。关于体劳，《彭祖摄生养性论》云："不欲甚劳，不欲甚逸。"人体日常的运动，不宜过于劳累，要循序渐进，过劳于人不利；也不宜过于清闲安逸，静而少动甚至不动易导致精气郁滞，筋伤肉痿，从而缩短寿命。过多睡卧伤人元气，过多地坐着不动伤人肌力；性欲虽为人之天性，不可放纵而应有所节制。古人云："房中之事，能生人，能煞人，譬如水火，知用之者，可以养生，不能用之者，立可死矣。"

sitting hurts flesh. Although sexual desire is human's nature, it should be under control. As the old saying goes, sexual activities brought both benefits and harm to people. If people can take it reasonably, it will bring health benefits, otherwise it will harm people.

IV. Sleeping Abstemiously to Prolong Life

Sleeping abstemiously means that sleep in proper ways according to the rules of nature and the changes of yin-yang, so as to keep the quality of sleeping, get rid of tiredness, and restore energy. The ultimate purpose is to help people to strengthen constitution, prevent diseases and increase longevity. TCM attaches more importance to the rationality of sleep and holds that sleep and diet are important for health preservation. One third of the lifetime is spent on sleeping which is not only the physiological need, but also the essential way to assure health and regain energy.

TCM considers that the movement of celestial bodies and the change of yin and yang contribute to the alternation of day and night which is regard as yang and yin respectively. The body should comply with the law of the alternation of day and night. It is better to go to sleep when yin qi gets much more than yang qi, and it is better to get up in the opposite case.

i. Do and Don't for Sleeping

1. Do and Don't before Sleeping

(1) Calm down before sleep: Exultancy and rage may give rise to spiritual unpeace. Excessive reading and consideration induce qi disorder and stop yang transforming into yin. People should not take vigorous activity before sleep in case of affecting sleep's quality. People should slow down the breathing rate before sleep. People can guide themselves into relaxation and meditation by means of sitting still, taking a walk, watching slow rhythmic TV programs, listening to low and slow music, and so on, which is helpful to produce yin. And prosperous yin can bring sleep.

(2) Warm the feet: Firstly, washing feet with hot water before sleep to make the blood circulate downward to feet, relieving the brain congestion to promote sleep. Secondly is massaging KI1 (*yǒng quán*) point in the sole, which is an important point of the kidney meridian. Modern medical studies have proved that massaging the feet frequently can regulate the functions of automatic nerves and endocrine system, and promote the blood circulation, ultimately, help to relieve fatigue, improve sleep

四、睡眠有节，益寿延年

睡眠有节，是指根据自然界与人体阴阳变化的规律，采用合理的睡眠方法和调护措施，以保证睡眠质量，消除疲劳，恢复精力和体力，从而达到防病强身，益寿延年的目的。祖国医学历来重视睡眠科学，认为"眠食二者为养生之要务"。人的一生中有三分之一的时间在睡眠中度过，这既是生理的需要，也是健康的保证和恢复精神的必要途径。

中医学认为天体的运行、阴阳的变化促成了昼夜的交替，昼为阳，夜为阴。人体应与昼夜阴阳消长的规律相适应。当阳气衰、阴气盛的时候就该闭目安眠，而当阴气尽、阳气盛时就该起床。

（一）睡眠宜忌

1. 睡前宜忌

（1）睡前神宜定：忌七情过极，读书思虑，大喜大怒则神不守舍，读书思虑则神动而躁，致气机紊乱，阳不入阴。睡前亦不可剧烈运动，以免影响入睡。睡前应减慢呼吸节奏，可以适当静坐、散步、看慢节奏的电视、听低缓的音乐等，使身体逐渐入静，静则生阴，阴盛则寐。

（2）睡前宜暖足：一是睡前用温热水浸足，使血液下行，改善脑部充血状态，以利入眠；二是按摩足涌泉穴，该穴是足少阴肾经要穴，长期按摩以利睡眠。现代医学研究证明，经常按摩刺激脚部，能调节自主神经和内分泌功能，促进血液循环，有助于消除疲劳，改善睡眠，防治心脑血管疾病。

quality, and prevent and treat the cardio-cerebral-vascular diseases.

(3) Eat several small meals, neither too much nor too little: It is stated in the ancient book that "going to bed immediately after eating too much will impair qi". Eating too much before sleep may result in dysfunction of the spleen and stomach. It is difficult to fall into sleep when people feel hungry before sleep. Drinking tea or coffee can excite the central nerves and make it difficult for people to fall into sleep. In addition, drinking too much water before sleep causes frequent urination at night, which will affect people's sleep, especially for the old ones. People with poor sleep can drink milk or yogurt, or eat food with the effects of cultivating heart yin, such as a thick soup cooked with sugar candy, lily and lotus, which has a good effect of improving sleep. People should take a rest after eating for about 30 minutes before sleep.

2. Do and Don't during Sleep

(1) Avoid wind and fire: The wind pathogen can invade the brain easily, leading to face paralysis and hemiplegia if the head faces towards the door and windows, or the door and windows are open when people are sleeping. The fire pathogen is easy to attack the upper *jiao*, causing dry pharynx, red eyes, nose bleeding and even headache if the head faces towards the fire or heating facilities when people are sleeping.

(2) Avoid speaking and singing at sleep onset:The ancients said that "The lung like the bell is the marquee of the five organs. It should be constringed when people lie down to rest." If people speak and sing before they go to bed, the lung may shake, then the five organs can't be calm. As a result, the quality of sleep will be influenced.

ii. Sleeping Time and Posture

1. Sleeping Time "Sleeping at noon (11am-1pm) and at midnight (11pm-1am)" is one of the traditional sleeping regimens in China. TCM considers that yin and yang in the world connect each other at noon and midnight, when the qi and blood in body are very unbalanced, so people had better go to bed at that time. According to the changes of yin and yang in a day, it's the time of the most prosperous yin qi and the weakest yang qi from 11pm to 1am, so it is better to go to sleep to foster yin in body. Moreover, it's also a good time to nourish the liver for the qi and blood which just arrive in liver and gallbladder in the meridian. Modern study shows that the function of every organ in the human body is the weakest from 0-4 o'clock in the morning and the sympathetic nerve in the human body is the weariest from 11am to 1pm. So sleeping at noon and midnight is more accordant with physical rules,

（3）睡前饮食宜少食多餐，不宜过饱，也不宜过少。《彭祖摄生养性论》曰："饱食偃卧则气伤。"饱食即卧，则脾胃不运，食滞胸脘，化湿成痰，大伤阳气。饥饿状态入睡则饥肠辘辘，难以入眠。浓茶、咖啡能兴奋中枢神经，使人难以入睡，不宜多饮。睡前不宜大量饮水，饮水过多则排尿次数增多，特别是老年人，夜尿增多则起夜多，影响夜间休息。睡眠不佳者，就寝前可饮用牛奶或酸奶，也可食用养心阴的食物，如冰糖百合莲子羹、百合莲子汤等，将有良好的催眠效果。进食后宜休息半小时左右再就寝。

2. 睡中禁忌

（1）寝卧忌当风，对炉火：睡眠时头对门窗或大开门窗，风易入脑户引起面瘫、偏瘫。卧时头对炉火、暖气，易使火攻上焦，造成咽干目赤鼻衄，甚则头痛。

（2）卧忌言语哼唱。古人云："肺为五脏华盖，好似钟磬，凡人卧下肺即收敛"，如果卧下言语，则肺震动而使五脏俱不得宁，影响睡眠质量。

（二）睡眠时间和姿势

1. 睡眠时间 子午觉是古人睡眠养生法之一，即每天于子时（23~1点）、午时（11~13点）入睡。中医认为，子午之时，阴阳交接，极盛极衰，体内气血阴阳极不平衡，必欲静卧，以候气复。根据天地阴阳之气在一天中消长变化的规律，每天晚上的子时是阴气最盛、阳气最弱、阴阳之气交接之时，故此时是睡眠的最佳时期，此时最能养阴，而子时也是经脉运行到肝、胆的时间，养肝的时间应该熟睡。现代研究也发现，夜间0点至4点，机体各器官功能降至最低；中午11点至13点，是人体交感神经最疲劳的时间，因此睡子午觉更符合人的生理规律，可以起到事

and can achieve double results with half effort. However, a too long nap at noon is not good for the body, and half an hour to an hour is enough. The sleeping time may vary with age, gender, constitution, environment, *etc.*, while the recommend sleeping time is 8 hours. And the younger they are, the longer sleeping time and the more times they need.

2. Sleeping Posture   There are three kinds of sleeping position: lateral position, prone position and supine position. The one who sleeps in lateral position resembles a lying dragon, with *ren mai* and *du mai* connected, yin and yang harmonized. TCM health experts consider that lateral position is the most appropriate sleep position. When people lie in prone position with back upward and belly down, though limbs keep forceful and qi circulates smoothly, five *zang* organs are under stress, leading to disharmony of yin and yang and causing difficulty in sleeping peacefully. When people sleep with supine position, limbs are stretched and relaxed, while yin and yang conversed. Yin channel is upward and yang channel is downward, while *du mai* are under stress. As a result, though yin channel gets smooth, yang qi can't be stimulated. When falling asleep, yang qi will be trapped by turbid yin, and qi can't reach distal extremities.

3. Sleeping Direction   The sleeping direction is closely interrelated with health. The ancient doctors have already given some opinions on it. Some advocate the sleeping direction should be decided on the yin-yang characters of the four seasons. They argue that people should sleep towards the east in spring and summer since spring and summer pertain to yang, while people should sleep towards the west in autumn and winter because autumn and winter pertain to yin, which are in accordance with the principle of "nourishing yang in spring and summer while nourishing yin in autumn and winter". Some believe that people should sleep towards the east in all the four seasons. They consider that the head, on the top of the body, controls all the yang of the body, and should towards where qi and blood circulate. The east pertains to spring and helps to raise qi of everything in nature. So people sleep towards the east in order to elevate the clear and lower the turbid to make the head clear. Most of them hold that people should avoid sleeping towards the north. They claim that the north pertains to water, and is in charge of winter and cold. Cold qi may directly hurt the essential yang and original spirit of the body if people sleep towards the north.

(Su Chun-xiang)

半功倍的作用。午休时间不宜过长，以 30min 至 1h 为佳。每人每天睡眠时间因不同年龄、性别、体质、性格、环境因素等而不同，通常应为 8h，而年龄越小，睡眠时间越长，次数也越多。

2. 睡眠姿势   睡眠姿势有侧卧、俯卧、仰卧三种。侧卧者似卧龙，任督相通，阴阳和顺，中医养生专家认为侧卧是首选的睡姿。俯卧位，伏床而卧，背朝上腹朝下，虽有利四肢经气畅达，但五脏受压，阴阳不和，难于安眠。仰卧位，虽四肢舒展放松，但阴阳倒逆，阴脉在上、阳脉在下，督脉被压，尽管阴脉畅达，但阳气无法激荡，一觉睡熟，阳气尽为阴浊所陷，经气未能畅达四肢末梢。

3. 睡眠方位   睡眠的方位与健康紧密相关，中国古代养生家根据天人相应、五行相生理论，对寝卧方向提出过几种不同的主张。有的主张按四时阴阳定东西，认为春夏属阳，头宜朝东卧；秋冬属阴，头宜朝西卧，以符合"春夏养阳，秋冬养阴"的原则。有的主张一年四季都应寝卧东向，认为头为诸阳之会，人体之最上方，气血升发所向，而东方震位主春，能够升发万物之气，故头向东卧，可保证升清降浊，头脑清楚。而大多数养生家认为要避免北首而卧，认为北方属水，阴中之阴位，主冬主寒，恐北首而卧阴寒之气直伤人体元阳，损害元神之府。

（苏春香）

Section 3　Emotional Nursing

The so-called seven emotions refer to joy, anger, grief, thought, sorrow, fear and fright. The seven emotions are mental activities of people which are closely related to physiological activities and function of *zang-fu* organs. The seven emotions are not pathogenic when they are kept properly and normally. Only when the emotional stimuli are too abrupt, strong or continual to go beyond the normal range of human physiological activities, can they disturb the qi movement, disharmonize *zang-fu* organs, yin and yang, qi and blood, and consequently cause diseases. The seven emotions may not only cause various diseases, but also deeply affect the development of diseases. Therefore, nurses should try their best to help patients to eliminate their adverse emotional stimuli such as tension, fear, anger, and worry while help the patients to regulate emotions, maintain good spirit and promote health.

I. Relationship between Emotion and Health

i. Normal Emotion Lead to Harmony of *Zang-fu* Organ and Qi

The normal emotions reflect harmony of *zang-fu* organs, qi and blood, yin and yang. Furthermore, normal emotions can regular *zang-fu* organs and qi, enhance the body's resistance to disease, and play a positive role in maintaining the health of the human body. For example, joy is considered to be positive emotion. Proper joy can relieve the nervousness and help to regulate qi and blood. Joy is also beneficial to people's physical and mental health. Anger is considered to be negative emotion. However, as one of the people's basic emotions, anger is also beneficial to people's health. Liver is associated with anger in emotion. Proper anger helps the liver qi to flow. Therefore, if emotions are normal, *zang-fu* organs and qi will be harmony, and consequently strengthen the function of *zang-fu* organs.

ii. Abnormal Emotion Internally Damage *Zang-fu* Organ

1. Damage *Zang-fu* Organ Directly　If people's emotion is affected by adverse external stimuli, *zang-fu* organs, qi and blood will disharmonize, and consequently cause diseases. Because emotion is closely related to the five *zang* organs, excessive seven emotions often directly damage the related *zang-fu* organs. Generally, excessive joy damages the heart; anger damages the liver; excessive

第三节　情志调护

所谓情志，指人的七种情绪，即喜、怒、忧、思、悲、恐、惊，简称七情。七情属于人的精神情志活动，与人体脏腑功能活动有密切的关系。在正常情况下，七情不会使人致病，只有突然强烈或长期持久的情志刺激，超过人体的正常生理活动范围，使人体气机紊乱，脏腑、阴阳、气血失调，导致疾病的发生。七情不仅可以引起多种疾病的发生，而且对疾病发展也有重要影响。因此，作为护理工作者，应设法消除患者的紧张、恐惧、愤怒、忧虑等不良情志的刺激，帮助患者调节情志以保持良好精神状态，促进健康。

一、情志与健康的关系

（一）情志正常，脏气调和

正常的情志活动是体内脏腑、气血、阴阳调和的反映，同时又能反作用于人体，调达脏气，增强人体的抗病能力，对维护人体的健康起着积极的促进作用。如喜是一种积极、肯定的情志，适当喜的心情，可以缓和紧张情绪，有助于气血调畅。喜的心境有益于人的身心健康。一般情况下，怒被认为是一种消极、否定的情绪。但怒作为人的基本情感之一，对人体的健康也有着其积极的一面。怒为肝之志，正常情况下有助于肝气的疏泄条达。可见，情志正常，则脏气舒达调畅，从而使脏腑功能活动得到加强。

（二）情志异常，内伤脏腑

1. 直接伤及内脏　人的精神情志受到外界不良刺激，使脏腑气血失调，就会产生疾病。由于生理上情志与五脏有着密切的关系，因此，七情过激往往直接损伤相应的内脏。一般认为，喜伤心，怒伤肝，思伤脾，悲、忧伤肺，恐伤肾。从临床上看，七情致病以

thinking damages the spleen; grief damages the lung; fear damages the kidney. Clinically, seven emotions mainly cause disease from heart, liver and spleen. Because the heart governs the blood and then stores the spirit, the liver stores the blood and then governs the free flow of qi, the spleen governs transportation and transformation and then the spleen and stomach are the source of qi and blood production. Heart plays a leading role in the pathomechanism of seven emotions. Heart is the governor of the five *zang* organs, the abode of essence and spirit, and the adobe of seven emotions. Therefore, excessive seven emotions firstly damage the heart spirit, and then affect other *zang-fu* organs, and consequently cause diseases.

2. Affect Qi Movement of *Zang-fu* Organ　All diseases result from qi disorder. TCM considers that the disease is caused by ascending and descending disorder of qi movement. Abnormal change of emotion results in disorder of qi movement of *zang-fu* organs, dysfunction of ascending, descending, exiting and entering, as well as disharmony of *zang-fu* organs.

(1) Anger causes qi to rise: Excessive anger causes liver qi to rise, and then blood rises along with qi counterflow. This manifests red face and red eyes, hematemesis, and even fainting and cataplexy.

(2) Excessive joy causes qi to slacken: Excessive joy causes heart qi to dissipate, and leads to the failure of the spirit to keep to its abode. This manifests lack of concentration of essence and spirit, loss of vitality, mania, *etc.*.

(3) Sorrow consumes qi: Excessive sorrow consumes lung qi. This manifests depression, weak breathing, lack of strength, *etc.*.

(4) Fear causes qi to sink: Excessive fear causes kidney qi insecurity and qi leakage. This manifests aching and weak legs, incontinence of stool and urine, spontaneous seminal emission, *etc.*.

(5) Fright causes qi to be chaotic: Sudden fright causes the disorder of heart qi, disharmony of qi and blood, and abnormal heart spirit. This manifests palpitations, insomnia, profuse dreaming, night crying, *etc.*.

(6) Excessive thinking causes qi to knot: Excessive thinking causes binding constraint of spleen qi, disordered transportation and transformation. This manifests poor appetite and digestion, distention and fullness of stomach and abdomen, thin, unformed stool, diarrhea, *etc.*.

3. Affect the Change of Disease　In the course of the disease, abnormal changes of emotion can often influence the development and the change of disease. Patients are easy to have negative mood, then leading to

心、肝、脾三脏为多见，因为心主血而藏神，肝藏血而主疏泄，脾主运化，为气血生化之源。其中，心在七情发病中起主导作用，心为五脏六腑之大主，精神之所舍，七情发生之处。故七情太过首先伤及心神，然后影响到其他脏腑，而引起疾病。

2. 影响脏腑气机　"百病生于气也"。中医学认为，疾病之所以发生是由于体内气机升降异常所致。异常情志变化，导致脏腑气机紊乱，升降出入运动失常，脏腑功能活动失调。

（1）怒则气上：是指过度愤怒使肝气上冲，血随气逆，并走于上。临床可见面红目赤，或呕血，甚则昏厥猝倒。

（2）喜则气缓：是指过度喜乐，使心气涣散，神不守舍，出现精神不集中，甚则失神狂乱等症。

（3）悲（忧）则气消：是指过度悲忧，可耗伤肺气。临床常见意志消沉、精神萎顿、少气乏力等症状。

（4）恐则气下：是指过度恐惧，可使肾气不固，气泄于下。临床可见下肢酸软无力，二便失禁、滑精等症。

（5）惊则气乱：是指突然受惊，导致心气紊乱，气血失和，心神失常。临床可见心悸、失眠多梦，小儿夜啼等症。

（6）思则气结：是指思虑过度，导致脾气郁结、运化失常。出现纳呆，脘腹胀满，便溏泄泻等症。

3. 影响病情变化　在疾病过程中，情志的异常变化往往能影响病势的发展与变化。患者因自身脏腑气血功能失调，容易产生不

abnormal fluctuations of emotion due to dysfunction of *zang-fu* organs, qi and blood. Greater emotional fluctuations can aggravate the dysfunction of *zang-fu* organs, qi and blood, which exacerbate the disease, and even lead to rapid deterioration.

II. Principle of Emotional Nursing

i. Being Sincere and Considerate

The patient's emotion and behavior are different from those of the healthy people. Patients are easy to feel anxious, depressed and worried. Nurses should take care of the patients and be considerate of the patients' mood with scrupulousness, love, patience and responsibility.

ii. Nursing Based on the People

It is stated in the *The Yellow Emperor's Inner Classic The Spiritual Pivot (Huáng Dì Nèi Jīng Líng Shū,* 黄帝内经·灵枢) that "People's constitutions are different, some are firm and some are feeble, some are weak and some are strong, some are long and some are short, some are yang type and some are yin type". Patients' psychological states are different because of the difference of the gender, age, constitution, educational degree, economic condition, life experience, character, interests, ability, character and course of the disease. Therefore, nurses must clearly know the individual difference, and then adopt different emotional nursing for different patients.

1. Difference in Constitution　Chinese medicine considers that constitution will pathologically change when yin-yang in the human body is out of balance. Classification of constitution is based on individual characteristics in syndrome, pulse condition and the tongue. There are eight types of constitution in TCM: constitution of qi deficiency, constitution of yang deficiency, constitution of yin deficiency, constitution of phlegm-damp, constitution of damp-heat, constitution of blood stasis, constitution of qi stagnation and constitution of special intrinsic quality. Different constitution should be taken care of by different emotional nursing.

2. Difference in Age　Children can easily contract diseases by fright and fear because their *zang-fu* organs are delicate, qi and blood are not full, and their central nervous system has not developed consummately. Adults can easily contract diseases by anger or thoughtfulness because their qi and blood are just full, and they are in all kinds of complicated environments. Elderly people frequently feel lonely and they are easily to contract diseases by

良心境，引起情志的异常波动。而较大的情志波动，反过来又能加剧脏腑气血功能的失调，促使疾病加重，甚至导致病情迅速恶化。

二、情志调护的原则

（一）诚挚体贴

患者的情绪状态和行为不同于健康人，常常会产生焦虑、抑郁、烦躁、忧愁等不良情绪。《素问·汤液醪醴论》曰："精坏神去，荣卫不可复也"。故护理工作者应"见彼苦恼，若己有之"，以细心、爱心、耐心、责任心去关心、照顾患者，体谅患者的心情。

（二）因人施护

《黄帝内经·灵枢》曰："人之生也，有刚有柔，有弱有强，有长有短，有阴有阳"。由于患者的性别、年龄、体质、文化程度、经济条件、生活经历、性格、兴趣、能力以及疾病的性质和病程长短的不同，他们的心理状态也会有所不同。因此，护理工作者必须清楚了解患者的个体差异，因人施护，有的放矢，对不同的患者采用不同的情志护理方法。

1. 体质差异　中医认为，当人体的阴阳失去平衡时，体质也会发生病理变化。根据临床上的证候、脉象、舌苔，可以把人分为八种病理体质：气虚体质、阳虚体质、阴虚体质、痰湿体质、湿热体质、血瘀体质、气郁体质、特禀体质。体质不同，情志护理方法也应不同。

2. 年龄差异　儿童脏腑娇嫩，气血未充，中枢神经系统发育不完善，多易为惊、恐致病；成年人气血方刚，又处于各种复杂的环境中，多易为怒、思致病；老年人常有孤独感，多易为忧郁、悲伤、思虑致病。

depression, sadness and thoughtfulness.

3. Difference in Gender Man is ascribed to yang and mainly controls qi, thus man is bold and unconstrained, and is easily diseased by excessive joy and violent rage. Woman is ascribed to yin and mainly controls blood, thus woman is exquisite and fragile, and is more easily diseased by depression and sorrow.

iii. Avoiding Stimuli

It is stated in *Su Wen* that one should "be quiet then spirit is hidden, and be uneasy then spirit disappears". Quiet environment makes the patients comfortable and have enough sleep to promote health rehabilitation. Therefore, nurses ought to create a quiet and comfortable environment to help the patients avoid getting unnecessary bad stimuli. Four principles should be obeyed: walking lightly, closing the door lightly, speaking lightly, doing nursing job lightly. Visiting rules should be strictly carried out. Nurses should try their best to reduce the visitors in the ward and keep the ward quiet in the condition of insuring the patients acquiring the adequate emotional support.

III. Method of Emotional Nursing

Emotional changes can directly affect physiological function of the human body. It is stated in the *Basic Questions* that "diseases cannot be cured if people are lack of spirit and volition". Famous experts in the ancient times advocate again and again that "a good doctor surely cures physical disease on the premise of curing mental troubles". So strengthening emotional nursing is of great importance to improve disease rehabilitation and maintain health. There are following methods of emotional nursing which can be chosen based on individual actual condition in order to achieve the best effect.

i. Nursing of Inter-restriction among Emotion

The nursing of inter-restriction among emotions here also known as mutual restriction between seven emotions, is to use one emotion to restrict another emotion in order to relieve or eliminate bad mood, and to keep good mental state. It is stated in *Basic Questions* that "anger damages the liver, and sorrow overcomes anger; excessive joy damages the heart, fear overcomes joy; excessive thinking damages the spleen, anger overcomes thought, grief damages the lung, joy overcomes grief; excessive fear damages the kidney, thought overcomes fear." This kind of nursing method is formed on the basis of inter-restriction and inter-promotion relationship

3. **性别差异** 男性属阳，以气为主，感情粗犷，刚强豪放，易因狂喜、大怒而致病；女性属阴，以血为先，感情细腻而脆弱，一般比男性更易因情志为患，多因忧郁、悲哀而致病。

（三）避免刺激

《素问·痹论》曰："静则神藏，躁则消亡"。安静的环境不仅能使患者身体舒适，还能使其睡眠充足，有利于恢复健康。因此护理工作者应给患者创造一个安静舒适的环境，避免其受到不必要的恶性刺激。在工作中应做到四轻：走路轻、关门轻、说话轻、操作轻。严格探视制度，在保证患者得到亲人情感支持的情况下尽量减少病房内探视人员，保持病房安静。

三、情志调护的方法

情志变化可以直接影响人体的生理功能。《素问·汤液醪醴论》曰："精神不进，志意不治，故病不愈"。历代名医一再提倡："善医者，必先医其心，而后医其身"。因此，加强情志护理，对疾病的康复及维持健康都有重要的意义。情志护理的方法有多种，可根据个体的实际情况选择合适的方法，以便取得最佳效果。

（一）以情胜情法

以情胜情法又叫情志制约法，指以一种情志抑制另一种情志，以淡化或消除不良情绪，保持良好精神状态的一种方法。《素问·阴阳应象大论》指出："怒伤肝，悲胜怒""喜伤心，恐胜喜""思伤脾，怒胜思""忧伤肺，喜胜忧""恐伤肾，思胜恐"。以情胜情法是根据情志及五脏间存在的阴阳五行生克原理，用相互制约、相互克制的情志来转移和干扰原来对机体有害的情志，借以达到协调情志

among the seven emotions, yin-yang and the five *zang-fu* organs. One emotion that is able to restrict the other one can be used to transfer and disturb the other emotion if it becomes excessive enough to damage people's health. Nursing of inter-restriction among emotions can be used to harmonize the emotions. It is a special method of psychological nursing and rehabilitation in TCM.

The nursing of inter-restriction among emotions should be applied when the patients have a premonition about their emotional alterations. The nurses shouldn't abruptly use the method without any preparation. In addition, the nurses should master the patients' sensitivity to emotional stimuli in order to choose a proper stimulation, neither too strong nor too weak.

1. Using Joy to Overcome Grief　Using joy to overcome grief in accordance with the methods that use fire to restrict metal means to cheer the patient up by using humorous and amusing words or exciting words in order to restrict his excessive sad emotion and cure the related diseases. The nursing method can be applied in the diseases manifesting depression caused by excessive sadness.

Here is a case recorded in the ancient book, *The Fun Allusion of Medicine (Yī Yuàn Diǎn Gù Qù Shí*, 医苑典故趣拾)*. In the Qing Dynasty (AD 1616—1911), a milord always felt depressed and wore a long face with knitted eyebrows, so his family specially invited a famous doctor to make a diagnosis and give treatment for him. After asking about his disease history and feeling his pulse, the doctor determined that the milord had menstrual irregularities. After hearing this diagnosis, the milord laughed and said: "I am a man, and it is impossible for me to have menstrual irregularities, which is so ludicrous." Hence, he would laugh when recalling the case.

Zhu Dan-xi (AD 1281—1358), a famous doctor, once met a young man who cried and felt sad all the time for his wife's unexpected death shortly after their marriage, and he finally fell ill. Though he had seen many famous doctors and used all valuable medicines, but all his efforts were in vain. After feeling his pulse, Zhu Dan-xi said: "The pulse shows you are pregnant, and you have been pregnant for several months." The young man laughed and said: "Confounding man with women, you are such an empiricist." Hence, he would laugh and tell the jape to others. Then he got good appetite and good mood, and his disease was cured. The two stories above are typical cases of applying joy to overcome grief.

的目的。此为祖国医学独特的心理治疗与康复方法。著名医家张子和指出："悲可以制怒，以怆恻苦楚之言感之；喜可以治悲，以谑浪戏狎之言娱之；恐可以治喜，以恐惧死亡之言怖之；怒可以制思，以污辱欺罔之事触之；思可以治恐，以虑彼志此之言夺之。凡此五者，必诡诈谲怪，无所不至，然后可以动人耳目，易人听视"。

在使用以情胜情法时，要在患者有所预感时再进行正式的情志治疗，不要在患者毫无思想准备之时突然地进行，并且还要掌握患者对情志刺激的敏感程度，以便选择适当方法，避免太过或不及。

1. 喜胜悲法　喜胜悲法指火制约金法，即用各种幽默、逗人的语言，或使人兴奋的语言，让患者尽快高兴起来，以克制其原有悲忧过度所致情绪障碍及相关的躯体疾病。对于由于神伤而表现得抑郁、低沉的种种病证，皆可使用。

在《医苑典故趣拾》中有一病例：清代有位巡按大人，郁郁寡欢，成天愁眉苦脸。家人特请名医诊治，当名医问完其病由后，按脉许久，竟诊断为"月经不调"。巡按大人听罢，嗤之以鼻，大笑不止，连连说道："我堂堂男子焉能'月经不调'，真是荒唐到了极点"，从此，每回忆及此事，就大笑一番，乐而不止。

名医朱丹溪曾遇一青年秀才，婚后不久突然亡妻，故终日哭泣悲伤，终成疾病。求尽名医，用尽名药，久治无效。朱丹溪为其诊脉后说："你有喜脉，看样子恐怕已有数月了"。秀才捧腹大笑，并说："什么名医，男女都不分，庸医也"，此后，每想起此事，就会自然发笑，亦常将此事作为奇谈笑料告诉别人，与众人同乐。此后秀才食欲增加，心情开朗，病态消除。以上两例为运用喜胜悲法的典型例证。

There are two common ways to practice. Firstly, to make the patient happy and eliminate the diseases caused by excessive sadness and worry by joking with the patient or using unserious words. Secondly, if the patient feels unhappy for his unfulfilled demand, his demand should be satisfied to relieve his bad mood for his rehabilitation.

2. Using Grief to Overcome Anger　Using grief to overcome anger according to the rule of metal restricting wood means to make the patient sad by words or other methods in order to restrict his excessive anger and eliminate related diseases. In clinical practice, nurses can set different situation or make the patient sad with grievous and touching words to arouse his grief emotion. Threatening words can also be used to make the patient fearful and then grieved. Grief makes qi consumed so that the depressed qi in the chest can be dispersed.

3. Using Anger to Overcome Thought　Using anger to overcome thought according to the concept of wood restricting earth means making the patient angry with different methods in order to overcome his excessive thinking and eliminate related diseases.

It is recorded in the *Supplement to "Classified Case Records of Famous Physicians"* (*Xù Míng Yī Lèi Àn*, 续名医类案) that "a rich woman has bad sleep for two years because of over thinking. Zhang Zi-he (AD 1156—1228) said: 'Your pulse is slow because the spleen is affected, which is associated with thinking in emotion.' So he takes her money and drinks for several days with her husband in order to make her angry. Then the woman gets angry and perspires, then feels sleepy that night. After she has slept for nine days, she eats food and her pulse goes back to normal".

Another case is also recorded. "A young man who lives in the green-dragon bridge area caught a strange disease that he likes staying in a dark room alone and is afraid of the light. His disease would get aggravated once he is exposed to the light for a while. One day, Li Jian-ang, a famous doctor passes by the young man's house, and is invited to examine him. The doctor does not give prescription after examining, but he takes the young man's writing and reads it incorrectly. The young man asks angrily: 'Who is reading it?' Then Li Jian-ang reads more loudly. The young man is angry very much, so he runs out and takes the writing from the doctor and sits down beside the light, condemning him: 'You don't understand the sentences, how can you read it so loudly?' He recovers after his anger which gives full vent to her pensiveness

喜胜悲法常用的策略有两种：其一，可以以玩笑或不庄重的语言刺激患者，使患者兴奋起来，以消除因过度悲伤忧愁所致疾病；其二，若患者是因意念未遂、所求不得、郁郁寡欢，积久成疾者，则应顺其意，使患者情志舒畅而促使病愈。

2. 悲胜怒法　悲胜怒法即金制约木法，即用各种语言或方法使患者产生悲哀的情绪，以克制其原有愤怒过度所致情绪障碍及相关的躯体疾病。护理人员可创设不同情境，或以悲伤凄苦的动情语言感化患者，唤起他悲痛的情感；或用威吓的语言震慑患者，使其恐惧，继而转悲，悲则气消，胸中郁怒之气得以排解。

3. 怒胜思法　怒胜思法指木制约土法，即用各种方法使患者发怒，以克制其原有思虑过度所致情绪障碍及相关的躯体疾病。适用于长期思虑不解、气结成疾或情绪异常低沉的病证。

《续名医类案》记载："一富家妇人，因思虑过甚，二年余不寐。张子和看后曰：'两手脉俱缓，此脾受之也，脾主思故也。'乃与其丈夫怒而激之也，多取其财，饮酒数日，不处一法而去，其人大怒，汗出，是夜困眠，如此者，八九日不寐，自是而食进，脉得其平。"

《四川医林人物》里亦记载一例郁病怒激之病例：青龙桥有位姓王的儒生，得了一种怪病，喜欢独居暗室，不能接近灯光，偶尔出来则病情加重，遍寻名医而屡治不验。一天名医李健昂经过此地，家人忙请他来诊视。李氏诊毕，并不处方，却索取王生昔日之文，乱其句读，高声朗诵。王叱问："读者谁人"，李则声音更高。王气愤至极，忘记了畏明的习惯，跑出来夺过文章，就灯而坐，并指责李氏："你不解句读，为何在此高声嘶闹？"。儒生一怒之后，郁闷得泄，病也就好了。

emotion."

The two cases have shown that over thinking could affect the adjustment of human behavior and activity, then qi can't move but stagnates instead, or yin and yang disharmonize. Because excessive yang can't harmonize with yin, people have bad sleep. When people get angry, the upward flowing qi may break the qi blockage, while the excited yang may be released with perspiration, then yin and yang become balanced and disease is cured.

4. Using Thinking to Overcome Fear　Using thinking to overcome fear according to the principle that earth can restrict water means to overcome the patient's excessive fear and eliminating those related diseases by making him think.

It is recorded (*Jìn Shū · Yuè Guǎng zhuàn*, 晋书·乐广传) that "a familiar customer has not come for a long time. Yue Guang asks him the reason, the man says: 'Last time I came here, you gave me alcohol, when I just wanted to drink. I saw a snake in the glass, and I felt nausea and suffered from disease after drinking.' Guang hears that there is a bow on the wall, the reflection of which in water looks like a snake, so he takes the drink and puts it on the same place and says to the man: 'What do you see in the drink?' The man says: 'The same.' Guang tells him the reason. He understands." The case of "self-created suspicion" shows that the diseases suffered from fear can be treated by thinking to release fear and tension, then to eliminate disease and recover health.

5. Using Fear to Overcome Joy　Using fear to overcome joy according to the principle that the water can restrict the fire means to overcome the patient's excessive joy in order to eliminate the related diseases by using different methods to terrify him. The nursing method can be used to treat the diseases manifesting excitation and manic.

One story is recorded in the ancient book (*Huí Xī Yī Àn*, 洄溪医案). A man who newly became the Number One Scholar suddenly fell ill on his way back home to announce this good news. A doctor was invited. After examining, he told the man: "Your disease cannot be cured, and you will die in seven days. You should hurry on with your journey and go home as soon as possible." The man lost his spirits and hurried on with his journey day and night. Seven days had passed, but he was still alive. His servant said to him: "Here's a letter the doctor asked me to give you when you arrived home." The letter said: "After you have become the Number One Scholar, you were over-joy, which injured your heart. No drugs was suitable for you, so I frightened you by saying that you were dying to treat the disease. You are safe now."

以上二例，说明思之甚可以使人的行为和活动调节发生障碍，致正气不行而气结，或阴阳不调，阳亢不与阴交而不寐。当怒而激之时，逆上之气冲开了结聚之气，兴奋之阳因汗而泄，致阴阳平调而愈。

4. 思胜恐法　思胜恐法指土制约水法，即采用让患者思考问题的方法，以克制其原有惊恐过度所致情绪障碍及相关的躯体疾病。

《晋书·乐广传》记载："尝有亲客，久阔不复来，广（乐广）问其故。答曰：'前在坐，蒙赐酒。方欲酒，见杯中有蛇，意甚恶之，既饮而疾'。于时河南听事壁上有角弓，漆画作蛇，广意杯中蛇即角影也。复置酒于前处，谓客曰：'酒中复有所见不'，答曰：'所见如初'，广乃告其所以，客豁然意解，沉疴顿愈"。"杯弓蛇影"这一成语所讲的历史事实，说明由恐惧引起的疾病，可以用深思的方法来解除其恐惧紧张的心理状态，从而使疾病消除，恢复健康。

5. 恐胜喜法　恐胜喜法指水制约火法，即用各种方法使患者产生惊恐，以克制其原有的因喜乐过极所致情绪障碍及相关躯体疾病。适用于神情兴奋、狂躁的病证。

《洄溪医案》里亦记载一例喜病恐胜之病例：某人新考上状元，告假返乡，途中突然病倒，请来一位医生诊视。医生看后说："你的病治不好了，七天内就要死，快赶路吧，抓紧点时间可以回到家中"。新状元垂头丧气，日夜兼程赶回家中，七天后安然无恙。其仆人进来说："那位医生有一封信，要我到家后交给您"。只见信中讲到："公自及第后，大喜伤心，非药力所能愈，故假以死恐之，所以治病也，今无妨矣"。

ii. Empathic Therapy

Empathic Therapy means a series of methods to transfer or change one's emotion and attention with certain measures to dispel bad emotion. After suffering from a certain disease, some people tend to focus on the disease, worring about the de terioration of the condition, the poor prognosis, the influences of the disease on work, labor, study and life, thinking all day long, and setting him/her in depression, worry and fear. To those people, nurses may divert their attention from their disease to other things, or change the surrounding environment to protect them from harmful stimulation. There are many specific methods about empathic therapy, which should be employed flexibly based on the different psychological states and characteristics of different people. The main methods are as follows:

1. Empathic Therapy with Music, Chess, Book, Painting and Calligraphy   It is said in the ancient book *Bei Shi* (*Běi Shǐ*, 北史) that "listening to the music and reading books can cultivate spirit." It is also stated in *Rhymed Discourse on External Remedies* (*Lǐ Yuè Pián Wén*, 理瀹骈文) that "reading books and listening to the music are more effective on curing diseases caused by the seven emotions than taking medicine." So one could do such activities according to one's interests as calligraphy, painting, music, *etc.* to get rid of gloomy mood, smooth the flow of qi and foster the mind. Ou Yang-xiu (AD 1007—1072) recorded in his book *Song Yang Zhi Xu* (*Sòng Yáng Zhì Xù*, 送杨置序) that he once suffered from the disease caused by anxiety and his focus on music gradually helped him to dissipate his disease as if it had never occurred.

2. Empathic Therapy with Physical Exercise   When a person is hysterical or quarrelling with others, it is better to divert his attention to physical exercises like playing ball game, walking, *taijiquan* and so on, because mental tension can be eased by physical tension. Traveling can help to dissipate worry and improve rehabilitation of the patient. When people are under excessive anxiety and unhappiness, they should take a walk in the suburban area and enjoy natural scenery which can help to regulate his passive emotion and ease his tension by enchanting blue sky with interspersed cloud and intoxicating fragrance of flower mingled with bird chirping.

iii. Method of persuasion

The method of persuasion means to persuade patients by using correct and wise words to correct his viewpoint, let them realize the harm brought by their behavior, relieve their unnecessary worry, boost their

（二）移情易性法

以情胜情法又称转移法，即通过一定的方法和措施转移或改变人的情绪和注意力，以解脱不良情绪的方法。有些人患某种疾病后，往往将注意力集中在疾病上，担心病情恶化，担心预后不佳，担心因病影响工作、劳动、学习和生活，整天胡思乱想，陷入苦闷、烦恼和忧愁之中，甚至紧张、恐惧。在这种情况下，应分散患者对疾病的注意力，使其思想焦点从疾病转移于他处；或改变周围环境，使患者避免与不良刺激接触。移情易性的具体方法很多，应根据不同人的心理特点、环境等，采取不同的措施，灵活运用。主要方法如下：

1. **琴棋书画移情法**　《北史·崔光传》曰："取乐琴书，颐养神性"。《理瀹骈文》曰："七情致病者，看书解闷，听曲消愁，有胜于服药者矣。"故在烦闷不安、情绪不佳时可根据各自的兴趣爱好，从事自己喜欢的活动，如书法、绘画、音乐等，用这些方法排解愁绪、寄托情怀、舒畅气机、怡养心神。欧阳修《送杨置序》中记载了他"尝有幽忧之疾"，后来"受宫音数引，久而久之，不知疾之在体也"。

2. **运动移情法**　在情绪激动时或与别人争吵时，最好的方法是转移一下注意力，参加适当的活动，如打球、散步、打太极拳等；或参加适当的体力劳动，用形体的紧张去消除精神上的紧张。旅游亦可以驱除烦恼，有利于身心恢复健康。当思虑过度，心情不快时，应到郊外游玩，领略大自然的风光，让山清水秀的环境调节消极情绪。

（三）说理开导法

说理开导法是指通过运用正确、巧妙的语言，对人进行劝说开导，端正人对事物的看法，认识自己的行为所造成的危害，解除

confidence in fighting against the disease, follow doctors and nurses' advice to achieve early recovery.

If the method is used properly and skillfully, enlightening patients with reason, examples or emotionally moving, being targeted, people's mental burden will be relieved, their confidence will be boosted, and their mental and physical condition will be improved.

It has been pointed out in *The Yellow Emperor's Inner Classic* that doctor should inform the patient about the harm of a disease, impart the curability to the patient, guide the patient with the principles of treatment and relieve mental burden of the patient. This is the origin of the persuasion method. That means a few aspects. Firstly, "informing the patient of the harm of a disease" refers to tell the patient the character, causes, harm, severity of the disease in order to arise his attention, to make him treat his disease correctly, neither neglecting nor fearing. Secondly, "imparting the curability to the patient" refers to telling the patient that he will recover as long as he cooperates with the doctors and nurses and follow their advices, which can enhance his confidence in conquering the disease. Thirdly, "guiding the patient with the principles of treatment" refers to tell the patient the concrete measures about taking care and treatment. Fourthly, relieving mental burden of the patient refers to help him to relieve negative mental state and overcome bad mood.In the history of TCM, many famous doctors recorded their experience of curing diseases with the method of persuasion. It has been recorded in *Si You Zhai Cong Shuo* (*Sì Yǒu Zhāi Cóng Shuō*, 四友斋丛说) that Kuang Zi-yuan felt depressed and caught a disease because he failed to be an official in the government. An old monk diagnosed him and pointed out that he had too much desire. He had to give up his excessive desire if he wanted to recover from the disease. He took the monk's advice and recovered after sitting quietly for months.

iv. Method of Restraining

Restraining is a method to prevent drastic emotions through regulating feelings and controlling sentiments to achieve psychological balance. TCM regimen believes that internal injury caused by excess of seven emotions is the main reason for attack of diseases. Extreme emotion is harmful to the body, so people should lay stress on spiritual cultivation and emotional regulation to maintain psychological balance. *The Yellow Emperor's Inner Classic* points out that intelligent people should keep moderate joy and anger to preserve health. *Medical Revelations* (*Yī Xué Xīn Wù*, 医学心悟) concludes four important points

不必要的忧愁顾虑，提高战胜疾病的信心，积极配合治疗，使机体早日康复。

运用时要针对不同人的精神状态和个性特征，做到有的放矢、动之以情、晓之以理、喻之以例、明之以法，解除患者的思想负担，提高其自信心，以逐渐改善患者的精神状态和躯体状况。

《黄帝内经》曰："告之以其败，语之以其善，导之以其所便，开之以其所苦。"此为说理开导法的起源。其含义：第一，"告之以其败"，是向患者指出疾病的性质、原因、危害、病情的轻重，引起患者对疾病的注意，使患者认真对待疾病，既不轻视忽略，也不畏惧恐慌。第二，"语之以其善"，指告知患者只要与医务人员配合，及时治疗，是可以恢复健康的，以增强患者战胜疾病的信心。第三，"导之以其所便"，告诉患者调养和治疗的具体措施。第四，"开之以其所苦"，指帮助患者解除消极的心理状态，克服内心不良情绪。历代著名医家在临床诊疗中，善于运用疏导的方法治疗疾病。《四友斋丛说》载：邝子元求官不顺，郁闷积病，一老僧分析其疾病的原因是妄想太多，要想病好，就要消除妄想，按老僧建议"静坐月余，心疾如矢"。

（四）节制法

节制法指调节情绪，节制感情，防止七情过激，从而达到心理平衡的方法。中医养生学认为七情内伤是造成发病的重要原因，七情过用必成灾，人必须注意精神修养，节制自己的感情，维持心理平衡。《黄帝内经》指出"智者养生"，要"和喜怒"。《医学心悟》归纳了"保生四要"，其中"戒嗔怒"即为一要。

of regimen, one of which is to avoid anger.

Delighted mood is helpful to the human body. But suddenly excessive joy causes qi to slacken, which is heart qi dispelling. The heart governs the blood and vessels. Heart qi deficiency will cause failure of qi to circulate the blood. Disability of blood circulation results in blood stasis in vessels of the heart and then induces palpitations, angina, stroke and even death.

It is recorded in *Yu Yi Cao* (*Yù Yì Cǎo*, 寓意草) written by Yu Chang (AD 1585—1664), a famous doctor in the Qing Dynasty, that a man got a new position and was jaunty, but he died because of excessive joy before he went home. It is recorded in *Yue Shu Zhuan* (*Yuè Shū Zhuán*, 岳书传) that Niu Gao (AD 1087—1147) was too excited because he had beaten Wan Yan (AD ?—1148), then he laughed three times and died. It is recorded in *Ru Lin Wai Shi* (*Rú Lín Wài Shǐ*, 儒林外史) that Fan Jin took part in the test several times when he was young, but he failed every time. When he was more than fifty years old, he finally succeeded. He suddenly turned manic because of excessive joy. Those are the cases to show that excessive joy damages the heart.

Moderate anger helps regulate qi and calms the emotions. But excessive anger damages the liver and then the liver qi cannot flow smoothly. If liver qi invades the head, people will feel headache, marked by redness in the face and eyes, feeling pain in liver region. Or people are quiet, and don't say anything. In the most serious case, people's limbs may be twitch and asphyxia and even resulted in death.

When people meet annoying things, it is normal that they feel moderately worried. But if they are excessive worried, depressed, always sorrowful sullen, low-spirited, even strained with bad sleep, and irritable the function of *zang-fu* organs will be maladjusted due to disorder of qi movement, and people will have palpitations, stomachache, poor appetite, insomnia and so on.

When people get problems, they will think about it but excessive thought would result in many diseases. TCM holds that pensiveness leads to qi stagnation. The spleen is associated with thinking of seven emotions. So, pensiveness is most likely to impair spleen qi, which will lead to dysfunction of the spleen and stomach, manifesting poor appetite, distention in stomach, abdominal pain and so on.

It can be known from the above that extreme emotions do great harm to body, so people should consciously pay attention to controll their own emotions.

愉悦的心情在一定程度上来说对人体是有益的，但如果是突然的狂喜，就会喜则气缓，即心气涣散。心主血脉，心气虚则不能行血，血运无力导致血液瘀滞于心脉，出现心悸、心痛、中风甚至死亡。

清代医学家喻昌《寓意草》里记载："昔有新贵人，马上扬扬得意，未及回寓，一笑而逝。"《岳书传》中的牛皋因打败了完颜兀术，兴奋过度，大笑三声，气不得续，当即倒地身亡。《儒林外史》里记载范进少时多次进京赶考，屡考屡败，到五十多岁终于中举，由于过度高兴，突然癫狂。这些均是喜伤心的病例。

适度的生气有利于气机的宣泄和情志的调畅。但若暴怒，怒则气上，暴怒伤肝，则会导致肝气不疏，上犯头目，出现头胀头痛，面红目赤，肝区疼痛；或者气极反静，不言不语，重者会因气厥而四肢抽搐，甚至昏厥死亡。

人在遇到烦心事的时候适当地忧愁担心无可厚非，但是忧虑太过，终日愁眉苦脸、闷闷不乐、意志消沉，甚至紧张、烦躁难以入眠，就会因气机紊乱而导致脏腑功能失调，出现心悸、胃痛、食欲减退、失眠等种种不适。

每个人在遇到问题时都要思考，但若思虑过度也会导致多种病证。中医认为思则气结，脾在志为思，故过度思虑最易伤脾气，脾胃运化失职，就会造成食欲减低、胃脘胀满、腹胀、腹痛等。

基于七情过激对身体的伤害，故需要注意有意识地控制自己的情绪，做到大喜临门，

Don't be over-excited when encountering with good things and don't be too sad when encountering with bad ones. Immunity of the human body can be improved greatly by avoiding the unpleasant negative mood such as anger, depression and sadness, and keeping in an optimistic state. If the function of the brain and the entire nervous system can be improved and the function of all the organs are consistently harmonized, the mild psychological disorders or diseases such as anxiety, insomnia, headache, neurasthenic, can be avoided, and even the chance of catching severe psychological diseases such as schizophrenia can be also prevented.

(Su Chun-xiang)

Section 4　Dietary Nursing

Dietary nursing is a vital part in health promotion and disease treatment, guided by the principle of pattern differentiation, the essence of which is to provide strategies for nursing care on nutrition and dietary, thus to supplement the *zang-fu* organs, dispel pathogen and balance yin and yang.

I. Property and Function of Food

Based on the TCM theory of "the homogeneousness between medicine and food", food is similar to medicine, whose nature, flavor and channel entry are the key to the specific categorization and property. The natures of food include coldness, hotness, warmness, and coolness, which generally called the four natures. The flavors of food include acrid, sweet, sour, bitter and salty, which called the five flavors. The channel entry of food is defined as the obvious function on the *zang-fu* organs, channels and collaterals. Therefore, keeping balance of dietary ingredients based on the principle of pattern differentiation and the property of food is beneficial to health protection and disease treatment.

i.Food with the Function of Heat-clearing

Bitter-cold and sweet-cold food has the function of hear-clearing, fire-draining and toxin-resolving. This kind of food is beneficial to the patient with excess heat

不过分激动；悲伤时，适可而止。只要善于避免嗔怒、忧郁、悲伤等不愉快的消极情绪，使心理处于怡然自得的乐观状态，可大大地提高机体免疫能力。如能提高大脑及整个神经系统的功能，使各个器官系统的功能协调一致，不仅可避免焦虑、失眠、头痛、神经衰弱等轻度的心理疾病，也会减少精神分裂症等严重心理疾病的发生。

（苏春香）

第四节　饮食调护

饮食调护是指在治疗疾病的过程中，根据辨证施护的原则，利用食物自身的特性，对患者进行营养和膳食方面的指导和护理，以补益脏腑，祛邪扶正，调整阴阳，从而防病治病，促进健康。

一、食物的分类和性能

中医认为"药食同源"，故食物亦有偏性，为其性、味、归经之偏，各种偏性均有其相应的功能，称食物的性能。食物的性，即作用性质，具有寒、热、温、凉之四性（古称四气）；其味有辛、甘、酸、苦、咸之五味；食物的归经，为食物对人体脏腑及经络产生的明显作用。在选择食物时，必须根据患者的体质、疾病的性质不同，选择不同性能的食物进行配膳，做到寒热相宜，五味调和。

（一）清热类食物

苦寒、甘寒性质的食物，具有清热、泻火、解毒的功效。如苦瓜、冬瓜、丝瓜、西

syndrome, including balsam pear, wax gourd, loofa, watermelon, radish, cucurbit, tea, mung bean, coix seed, cholecyst of some animals, *etc.*. However, cold food might do damage to yang qi. Therefore, great caution should be paid by the patient with the syndromes of yang qi insufficiency and spleen-stomach weakness.

ii. Food with the Function of Clearing and Supplementing

Some salty-cold or sweet-cold food has the function of nourishing yin fluid, clearing deficiency-heat or draining deficiency-fire. This kind of food is beneficial to the patient with heat deficiency syndrome, including duck, geese, soft-shelled turtle, tofu, mung bean, bean sprout, pear, sugarcane, lotus seed, seaweed, spinach, Chinese cabbage, tremella, rocky candy, *etc.*. However, patient with yang deficiency should take them with caution.

iii. Food with the Function of Warming and Supplementing

Food with warm property has the function of center-warming, yang-assisting and cold-dissipating. This kind of food is beneficial to the patient with cold syndrome, including mutton, chicken, pigeon, walnut, longan, litchi, brown sugar, *etc.*. However, patient with heat syndrome or vigorous fire due to yin deficiency should use them with caution.

iv. Food with the Function of Neutral Supplementation

Neutral, in dietary nursing, is defined as the food with no obvious bias in the four natures, having the specific function of supplementing and boosting as well as center harmonizing. This kind of food is beneficial to all kinds of patients especially to those at the convalescent phase of disease, including beef, pork, egg, cuttlefish, silkworm chrysalis, broad bean, lentil, yam, lotus, black fungus, peanut, carrot, day lily, *etc.*.

v. Food with the Function of Acrid-Dispersing

Acrid-warm or acrid-hot food with the function of dispersing and qi moving is beneficial to the patient with yin-cold syndrome. This kind of food includes ginger, garlic bulb, prickly ash peel, fermented soybean, fennel, sweet basil, cassia twig and wine, *etc.*.

vi. Food with the Function of Dispersing

Food with the function of dispersing might be the trigger of recurrence of some diseases, especially skin diseases, and could aggravate some acute diseases. This kind of food includes the head of pig and chicken, as well as some vegetables such as mushroom, coriander, toona sinensis and some seafood such as shrimp and crab.

瓜、萝卜、葫芦、莴笋、茶叶、绿豆、薏米及各种动物的胆等，常用于实热证的调护。但寒性食物易损伤阳气，故阳气不足、脾胃虚弱患者应慎用。

（二）清补类食物

部分咸寒或甘寒的食物，具有养阴液、清虚热、泻虚火的功效。如鸭、甲鱼、豆腐、绿豆、豆芽、梨、甘蔗、莲子、海带、菠菜、白菜、银耳、冰糖等，常用于虚热证的调护，素体阳虚者应慎用。

（三）温补类食物

温热性质的食物，具有温中、助阳、散寒的功效。如羊肉、鸡、鸽子、核桃、桂圆、荔枝、红糖等，常用于寒性病证的调护，热证和阴虚火旺者慎用或禁用。

（四）平补类食物

所谓"平"，是指此类食物没有明显的寒、凉、温、热之偏性，其性较平和，具有补益、和中的功效。如牛肉、猪肉、鸡蛋、墨鱼、鹅、蚕蛹、蚕豆、扁豆、山药、莲肉、黑木耳、花生、胡萝卜、黄花菜等，适用于各类患者，尤其是疾病恢复期的患者。

（五）辛散类食物

辛温或辛热性质的食物，具有发散、行气的功效。如生姜、大蒜、花椒、淡豆豉、茴香、苏叶、桂枝、白酒等，常用于各种阴寒之证。

（六）发散类食物

发散类食物易于诱发旧病，尤其是诱发皮肤疾病，或加重新病的食物称为发散类食物。如禽畜类中的猪头、鸡头、牛肉，蔬菜类的蘑菇、芫荽、香椿，水产品类的虾、蟹等。

II. Function of Dietary Nursing

i. Reinforcing Healthy Qi and Supplementing Deficiency

The main cause of disease is the hypofunction of the whole body, including its tissues and organs. This mechanism is called healthy qi deficiency in TCM. The corresponding pattern named deficiency, including yin deficiency, yang deficiency, qi deficiency and blood deficiency. It is manifested as mental fatigue, weakness, shortness of breath, palpitations, inappetence, lumbus aching, legs limping, thin and weak pulse or thin and deep pulse.

In TCM, all the food with the function of supplementing the essentials or enhancing immunity or boosting energy are perceived as having the function of supplementing and boosting the *zang-fu* organ and reinforcing healthy qi. This kind of food includes animal product, milk, egg and grain products. The following examples are some foods with the specific function of reinforcing healthy qi and supplementing deficiency.

1. Food with the function of supplementing yang, e.g., walnut, leek, sword bean, mutton, sparrow, shrimp, *etc.*.

2. Food with the function of supplementing qi, e.g., japonica, glutinous rice, millet, soybean, tofu, *etc.*.

3. Food with the function of supplementing blood, e.g., pork liver, mutton liver, cow liver, *etc.*.

4. Food with the function of supplementing yin, e.g., duck egg, soft-shelled turtle, cuttlefish, pigskin, duck, fructus lycii, black fungus, tremella, *etc.*.

ii. Expelling Excess to Dispel Pathogen

Generally, the illness is caused by external pathogenic factors or *zang-fu* organ malfunction. If pathogenic qi is in excess, the excess pattern will occur. As a consequence, channel or *zang-fu* organs blocked by pathogenic factor, alternatively, qi stagnation or blood stasis, phlegm-damp or stagnation will happen. The common symptoms include gruff breathing, dysphoria, abdominal distension, intense pain, constipation, urinary stoppage, yellow greasy tongue coating and strong pulse.

Food with the function of expelling excess could remove pathogen and protect *Zang* organ, which could be devided into many categories. Those food will be introduced as followed:

1. Exterior-releasing food, especially for influenza, e.g. ginger, Chinese onion, fermented soybean.

二、饮食调护的作用

（一）扶正补虚

人体各种组织、器官和整体的功能低下，是导致疾病的重要原因，中医学把这种病理状态称为"正气虚"，其所引起的病证称为"虚证"。虚证的临床表现有阴虚、阳虚、气虚、血虚，各具证候特点，但总体上表现为精神萎靡、身倦乏力、心悸气短、食欲缺乏、腰疼腿软、脉象细弱或沉细。

凡是能够补充人体物质、增强人体正常功能，提高抗病能力，改善或消除虚弱证候的食物，都具有补益脏腑、扶助正气的作用。这类食物大多为动物类、乳蛋类或粮食类。

1. **补阳类** 核桃仁、韭菜、刀豆、羊肉、雀肉、虾等。

2. **补气类** 粳米、糯米、小米、黄豆、豆腐等。

3. **补血类** 猪肝、羊肝、牛肝等。

4. **滋阴类** 鸭蛋、甲鱼、乌贼、猪皮、鸭肉、枸杞子、黑木耳、银耳等。

（二）泻实祛邪

外界致病因素侵袭人体，或脏腑功能活动失调，皆可使人发生疾病。如果病邪较盛，中医称为"邪气实"，其证候则称为"实证"。实证的范围很广，如邪闭经络或脏腑，或气滞、血瘀、痰湿、积滞等。一般常见实证的症状有呼吸气粗、精神烦躁、脘腹胀满、疼痛难忍、大便秘结、小便不通或淋沥涩痛、舌苔黄腻、脉实有力等。

用于实证的食物，大都具有除病邪的作用，邪去则脏安，身体康复。泻实类食物的种类较多，分别介绍如下。

1. **解表类** 生姜、大葱、豆豉等，用于感冒。

2. Heat-clearing and fire-draining food for excess heat syndrome, e.g., balsam pear, lotus seed, watermelon.

3. Heat-clearing and dampness-drying food for damp-heat syndrome, e.g., eggplant, buckwheat, purslane.

4. Heat-clearing and toxins-resolving food for heat-toxin syndrome, e.g., mung bean, adzuki bean, balsam pear, tofu, pea.

5. Heat-clearing and summer heat-resolving food for summer heat syndrome, e.g., watermelon, mung bean, green tea.

6. Heat-clearing and sore throat relieving food for interior heat induced swelling and pain in throat, e.g., waternut, Chinese white olive, fig.

7. Heat-clearing and blood-cooling food for blood heat syndrome, e.g., eggplant, lotus rhizome node, luffa, black fungus.

8. Stagnation removing food for constipation, e.g., banana, spinach, bamboo shoot, honey, black sesame.

9. Wind-dampness expelling food for rheumatism, e.g., coix seed, chaenomeles fruit, cherry, eel.

10. Aromatic food for removing dampness, e.g., lentil, broad bean.

11. Urination promoting food for urinary stoppage, edema, gonorrhea or phlegm-rheum, e.g., corn, corn silk, black soybean, mung bean, adzuki bean, Chinese wax gourd, Chinese wax gourd peel, Chinese cabbage, carp.

12. Interior warming food for interior cold syndrome, e.g., dried ginger rhizome, cinnamon bark, prickly ash peel, fennel, pepper, mutton.

13. Qi moving food for qi stagnation, e.g., sword bean, rose flower.

14. Blood moving food for blood stasis, e.g., Chinese hawthorn fruit, alcohol, vinegar.

15. Phlegm-transforming food for phlegm stasis, e.g., alga, seaweed, laver, radish, almond.

16. Cough and panting relieving food for cough and panting syndrome, e.g., almond, pear, ginkgo nut, eriobotrya, lily bulb.

17. Spirit-calming food for neurasthenia and insomnia, e.g., lotus seed, wheat, lily bulb, longan, spiney date seed.

18. Astringency inducing food for diarrhea or frequency of urination, e.g., smoked plum, lotus seed.

iii. Preventing Disease and Prolonging Life

The diet as the essential to health must be properly arranged to guarantee sufficient qi and blood and the

2. 清热泻火类　苦瓜、莲子、西瓜等，用于实热证。

3. 清热燥湿类　茄子、荞麦、马齿苋等，用于湿热病证。

4. 清热解毒类　绿豆、赤小豆、苦瓜、豆腐、豌豆等，用于热毒证。

5. 清热解暑类　西瓜、绿豆、绿茶等，用于暑热证。

6. 清热利咽类　荸荠、青果、无花果等，用于内热咽喉肿痛证。

7. 清热凉血类　茄子、藕节、丝瓜、黑木耳等，用于血热证。

8. 通便类　香蕉、菠菜、竹笋、蜂蜜、黑芝麻等，用于便秘。

9. 祛风湿类　薏苡仁、木瓜、樱桃、鳝鱼等，用于风湿证。

10. 芳香化湿类　扁豆、蚕豆等，用于湿温、暑湿、脾虚湿盛证。

11. 利水类　玉米、玉米须、黑豆、绿豆、赤小豆、冬瓜、冬瓜皮、白菜、鲤鱼等，用于小便不利、水肿、淋病、痰饮等证。

12. 温里类　干姜、肉桂、花椒、茴香、胡椒、羊肉等，用于里寒证。

13. 行气类　刀豆、玫瑰花等，用于气滞证。

14. 活血类　山楂、酒、醋等，用于血瘀证。

15. 化痰类　海藻、海带、紫菜、萝卜、杏仁等，用于痰证。

16. 止咳平喘类　杏仁、梨、白果、枇杷、百合等，用于咳喘。

17. 安神类　莲子、小麦、百合、龙眼肉、酸枣仁等，用于神经衰弱和失眠。

18. 收涩类　乌梅、莲子等，用于泄泻、尿频等滑脱不禁之证。

（三）防病益寿

食物对人体的滋养作用是身体健康的重

normal function of *zang-fu* organ, which is interpreted as the interior healthy qi protecting the body from pathogenic factors.

Diet is also the key to keep a harmonious and balanced state of yin and yang. Guided by the principle of pattern differentiation and the properties of food, reasonable diet is defined as an important intervention to regulate yin and yang by reinforcing the deficient and reducing the surplus so as to restore the relative balance between yin and yang, which was recorded in the *Basic Questions. Yin Yang Ying Xiang Da Lun* (*Sù Wèn. Yīn Yáng Yìng Xiàng Dà Lùn*, 素问·阴阳应象大论).

In addition, some specific function of food can also directly prevent disease, e.g. garlic for preventing diarrhea, mung bean decoction for preventing heatstroke, scallion and ginger for preventing wind-cold induced influenza.

Diet also plays as a main role for slowing the aging process, especially for the aged. The ancient Chinese medical book named *How to Support Older Parents* (*Yǎng Lǎo Fèng Qīn Shū*, 养老奉亲书), had recorded the reason and method for diet in slowing the aging process.

III. Basic Principle of Dietary Nursing

Basic principle should be followed by dietary nursing in order to achieve the aim of health maintenance and disease treatment.

i. Adhering to an Abstemious and Regular Diet

1. Adhering to a Regular Diet　According to medical record from *Lv's Spring and Autumn* (*Lǚ Shì Chūn Qiū*, 吕氏春秋), regular diet with fixed time could prevent disease, which could be explained as irregular diet and overeating or excessive hungry might cause the dysfunction of spleen and stomach, and eventually do damage to health.

Nowadays, three-daily-meal as the worldwide dietary habits is scientific and practicable to fit the daily activity requirement. The following contents will introduce the principles of daily meals.

(1) Having a filling breakfast: A good night sleep with sufficient digestion and absorption could boost energy. However, because of the emptiness of gastrointestinal tract, keeping a nutritious and adequate diet in the morning is also necessary for energy supplies. The optimal food for breakfast includes carbohydrate foods (e.g. rice, flour) and

要保证。合理安排饮食，保证机体充足的营养供给，可以使气血充足，五脏六腑功能旺盛。正气存内，邪不可干。

饮食还可以调整人体的阴阳平衡，即《素问·阴阳应象大论》所说："形不足者，温之以气，精不足者，补之以味。"根据食物的气、味特点，及人体阴阳盛衰的情况，予以适宜的饮食，或以养精，或以补形，既是补充营养，又可调整阴阳平衡，不但保证机体健康，也是预防疾病的重要措施。

此外，发挥某些食物的特异作用，可预防某些疾病。例如：用大蒜预防腹泻；用绿豆汤预防中暑；用葱白生姜预防风寒感冒等，都是民间的宝贵经验。

对于老年人，饮食在延缓衰老方面起着十分重要的作用。如《养老奉亲书》说："高年之人真气耗竭，五脏衰弱，全仰饮食以资气血。"

三、饮食护理的基本要求

饮食护理并非无限度地补充营养，须遵循一定的原则和法度，以达到恢复元气，改善机体功能，治疗疾病的目的。

（一）饮食有节，定时定量

1. **进食有规律**　进食宜有较为固定的时间，《吕氏春秋》中说："食能以时，身必无灾。"如果食无定时，或零食不离口，或忍饥不食，打乱胃肠消化的正常规律，都会使脾胃失调，消化能力减弱，食欲逐渐减退，有损健康。

现在世界上大多数国家采用的是每日三餐制。它符合日常生活、工作与学习的安排，能使摄入的各种营养满足机体的需要。

（1）早饭宜饱：经过一夜睡眠，人体得到了充分休息，精神振奋，但胃肠经一夜时间，已经空虚，此时若能进食，则营养得以补充，精力充沛。所谓"饱"是指要保证一定的饮食量，提供充足的能量。除米面食品外，还

any soft food containing high protein, such as milk, soya-bean milk and egg.

(2) Having a rich lunch: Lunch As the intermediate link between breakfast and supper, must provide sufficient energy for working or learning activities in the afternoon. Rich lunch defined as a properly designed balanced meal, including reasonable ingredients combination and cooking methods.

(3) Having a light supper: Comparing to the reduction of food intake, food choices are also important at supper to reduce the burden of digestive system and ensure a good sleep. Eating before bedtime is not recommended. However, if this occurs, gentle activities will be encouraged. The recommending energy distribution ratio of three meals is 3∶4∶3.

2. Adhering to an Abstemious Diet In TCM, all the major tasks of digestion, absorption, transportation and distribution of nutrients are performed by spleen and stomach. Therefore, the normal function of two organs is the prerequisite and foundation for body's normal physiological functions. Without appropriate eating habits, either overeating or excessive hungry, will do damage to spleen and stomach, even the overall health, which could result in premature ageing.

In addition, chronic hunger is one of the common cause of malnutrition. On the other hand, overeating can lead to some gastrointestinal symptoms such as tight feeling in the stomach and unusual odor of feces. Overweight or even obesity is also resulted from the accumulative effects of overeating. The rule of diet and its significant meaning in healthy had been recorded in the ancient Book named *Guǎn Zī* (*Guǎn Zī*, 管子).

ii. Balancing the Property of Food

1. Balancing the Flavors of Food The five flavors of food have relative tropism to different organs. The sour flavor enters the liver. The bitter enters the heart. The sweet enters the spleen. The pungent enters the lung and the salty enters the kidney. They play different roles in the body and may have much to do with the function of five *zang* organs. As recorded by the *Yellow Emperor's Inner Classic: Basic Questions*, the diet with well-balanced flavors could supplement and boost *zang* qi, and enrich and nourish the five *zang* organs, thus, resulting in strengthening the body health and healthy life time.

If the five flavors cannot meet the needs of the internal organs, the correlated *zang* qi would be ups and downs. As a result, normal functions of the five *zang* organs would decline accordingly. For example, the acrid food has the effects of dispersing and promoting

可以食牛奶、豆浆、鸡蛋等优质蛋白。

（2）午饭宜好：午饭起着承上启下的作用。上午的活动告一段落，下午仍需继续进行。白天能量消耗较大，应当及时补充。所以，午饭要吃好，应荤素搭配、干稀搭配、粗细搭配，且佐以合适的烹饪方法。

（3）晚饭宜少：晚上接近睡眠，活动量小，不宜多食。如进食过饱，易使饮食停滞，增加胃肠负担，会引起消化不良，影响睡眠。也不可食后再睡，宜小有活动之后入寝。一般早、中、晚餐的能量分别占总能量的 30%、40%、30% 为宜。

2. 进食有节制 人体对饮食的消化、吸收、输布，主要靠脾胃来完成，进食定量，饥饱适中，恰到好处，则脾胃能够承受。饮食的消化吸收正常，人体就能及时地得到营养供应，以保证各种生理活动的进行。如果饮食不节，暴饮暴食，或饥一顿，饱一顿，则容易损伤健康，造成早衰。

长期过饥，可以导致营养不良；过饱，可能出现胃肠道症状，胃腹部胀满不舒，大便有异味，天长日久，有可能体重增加，日渐肥胖。正如《管子》所说："饮食节……则身利而寿命益。"

（二）搭配相宜，饮食随和

1. 谨和五味 中医将食物的味道归纳为酸、苦、甘、辛、咸五种，统称"五味"。五味与五脏的生理功能有着密切的关系，对人体的作用各不相同。酸味入肝，苦味入心，甘味入脾，辛味入肺，咸味入肾。五味调和能滋养五脏，补益五脏之气，强壮身体。正如《素问·生气通天论》所说："谨和五味，骨正筋柔，气血以流，腠理以密，如是则骨气以精。谨道如法，长有天命。"

如果五味偏嗜太过，久之会引起相应脏气的偏盛、偏衰，导致五脏的功能活动失调。比如，辛味食物可发散、行气、活血，因其能刺激胃肠蠕动，增加消化液的分泌，食之

the circulation of the qi and blood, therefore, it could stimulate peristalsis to promote the gastric acid secretion. Patient with hemorrhoids, anal fissure, peptic ulcer, constipation or panasthenia should avoid this kind of food. The sweet food has the effects of supplementing qi and blood, relieving pain and resolving toxins. However, eating excessive sweet food will result in catching phlegm, damage spleen and stomach, and even cause diabetic mellitus. The sour food has the effects of promoting appetite. However, excessive eating can stimulate gastric acid secretion. Therefore, people with spleen and stomach disease should take this kind of food in caution. The bitter food has the effects of clearing heat. However, excessive eating will lead to stomachache, diarrhea and dyspepsia. The salty food has the effects of softening hardness and relieving constipation by purgation. As an important trace element, sodium could regulate osmotic pressure and water-sodium metabolism. Moderate drinking salty water especially after vomiting, diarrhea and profuse sweating could supplement the drained sodium. However, excessive intake of sodium, generally more than 5g per day, will result in edema, hypertension and atherosclerosis.

2. Balancing the Nature of Food　Balancing the natures of food not only means the diet should be harmonious in four natures, but also should be in proper digestible temperature, or be eaten as the raw or the cooked according to the food characteristics. As recorded in *Yellow Emperor's Inner Classic* and indicated by Sun Si-miao, in order to prevent pathogenic factor damaging health, food should be taken in proper temperature, neither too hot nor too cold, which might burn the lip or freeze the teeth. This instruction could be explained by the theory from TCM theory that food with higher temperature could damage the yin fluids of spleen and stomach, while food with lower temperature could damage the yang qi of spleen and stomach, resulting to the unbalancing of yin and yang, which might cause some symptoms or diseases such as thirst, halitosis, constipation, hemorrhoids or body coldness, abdominal pain, diarrhea. In modern medicine, the pathphysiological mechanism could be explained that temperature could affect the function of digestive enzyme, which will eventually influence the normal process of digestion and absorption.

3. Guaranteeing Comprehensive Nutrition　*Yellow Emperor's Inner Classic* stated that "the five kinds of grains are basic foods; five kinds of fruits are supplementary foods; five domestic animals are beneficial foods; and five kinds of vegetables are nourishing foods." The above statement has generalized the structure and compositions of an optimal diet, which includes a variety

过量会刺激胃黏膜，故患有痔疮、肛裂、消化道溃疡、便秘以及神经衰弱的患者不宜食辛味食物。甘味具有补养气血、调和脾胃、缓解疼痛、解毒等作用，但过食甜腻之品，则会壅塞滞气、助湿生痰，甚至诱发消渴病。酸味可健脾开胃，促进食欲，但过量服食可引起胃酸增多，影响消化功能，故脾胃有病者宜少食。苦味具有清热燥湿、清热解毒、清热泻火等作用，多食则会引起胃疼、腹泻、消化不良等症。咸味能软坚润下，有调节人体细胞和血液渗透压平衡以及正常水钠代谢的作用，在呕吐、腹泻及大汗后，适量饮用淡盐水，可防止体内微量元素的缺乏。成人每天食 5g 左右盐已足够，过食可诱发水肿、高血压、动脉硬化等病证。

2. 寒热适宜　寒热适宜，一方面指食物属性的阴阳寒热应互相调和，另一方面指饮食入腹时的生熟情况或温度要适宜。《黄帝内经》指出："食饮者，热无灼灼，寒无沧沧。寒温适中，故气将持，乃不致邪僻也。"养生家孙思邈也指出："热无灼唇，冷无冰齿。"意即进热食时，口唇不能有灼热感；吃寒食时，也不能使牙齿感觉冰凉。这是因为过食温热之品，容易损伤脾胃之阴液；过食寒凉之物，容易损伤脾胃之阳气，从而使人体阴阳失调，出现口干口臭、便秘、痔疮或形寒肢冷、腹痛腹泻等病证。现代医学认为，人体中各种消化酶要充分发挥作用，其中一个重要的条件就是温度。只有当消化道内食物和人体的温度大致相同时，各种消化酶的作用才发挥得最充分，而温度过高或过低，均不利于食物营养成分的消化和吸收。

3. 营养全面　《黄帝内经》提出全面的营养供给应"五谷为养，五果为助，五畜为益，五菜为充"，概述了膳食的结构与内容，即以谷类、动物类食物补益人体，以蔬菜、水果类食物辅助补充，如此食物多样，荤素搭配，

of sources: grains, meat, vegetables and fruits. Diet arranged like this is rich in diversity, and well-balanced in meat and vegetables, which may prevent indulgence in any flavor so as to be well-proportioned in various nutritions. Referred to the "Five Grains", the refined grains taste better while lose a lot of dietary fiber and vitamin B compared with coarse grains. One of the basic dietary principles is the balancing intake of coarse and refined grains. Furthermore, the scope of grain is rather large in TCM, and always contains some kind of plant seed such as soybean which provides lysine while none of the other kind of grain contains. "Five Animals" is defined as the meat products including egg and milk, which provide a good resource of protein with high quality, lipid, fat-soluble vitamins and trace elements, having the function of enriching and nourishing human body. However, excessive consumption will result in dampness, phlegm and heat. It could be explained as that this kind of food contains large amount of saturated fatty acid and cholesterol, excessive consumption of which could result in hyperlipidemia, increasing the risk of disease such as cholelithiasis and obesity atherosclerosis. In addition, vegetable and fruit have the function of soothing, stimulating appetite and digestion. Reasonable proportion of vegetables and fruits consumption could supplement essential vitamins, trace elements and dietary fibers, providing a comprehensive nutrition.

iii. Guaranteeing the Dietary Sanitation

The food prepared for consuming should be fresh with normal appearance and odor. Anything suspicious of bacterial or toxic contamination should be avoided. In addition, dietetic hygiene should concern the dining environment, tableware and the catering. Unhygienic diet as one of the main factors could cause gastric intestinal disease with the symptoms such as stomachache, vomiting and diarrhea, or parasitic disease (e.g. ascaris lumbricoides, pinworm, cestode), the typical symptoms of which are abdominal pain, parorexia and malnutrition. Eating spoiled food contaminated by bacteria might produce toxins, cause poisoning, and even lead to coma or death. One of easy methods to sterilize food is cooking thoroughly. Generally, most of the food should be cooked, especially meat, which has been recorded in *Important Formulas Worth a Thousand Gold Pieces for Emergency* (*Bèi Jí Qiān Jīn Yào Fāng*,备急千金要方). Furthermore, well cooked food can promote the absorption of the nutrition, particularly for the elderly. This is the important principle in dietary sanitation.

iv. Keeping Delicate Diet

Excessive consumption of greasy, spicy food and alcohol could damage spleen and stomach. Food contains

粗细得当，促进全面营养。"五谷"指五谷杂粮及其精加工产物，包括豆制品，主张混合进食。豆类可弥补谷类赖氨酸之不足，杂食促进蛋白质互补。谷物经精加工后，口感较好，但丢失较多膳食纤维和 B 族维生素，宜粗细结合。"五畜"指猪、马、牛、羊等肉食，亦包括蛋类、乳类等，属滋养强壮之品，宜适量选食，补益机体。"五畜"富含优质蛋白、脂肪、脂溶性维生素和微量元素，美味可口。但偏嗜膏粱厚味，易助湿、生痰、化热，导致某些疾病的发生。现代医学认为动物性食物含大量饱和脂肪酸和胆固醇，过食会导致高脂血症、肥胖症、动脉粥样硬化等病证。"五菜为充，五果为助"是指除上述食物外，尚需补充适量菜果类。蔬菜、水果多具有疏利、开胃消食、疏通胃肠等作用，富含维生素、微量元素及膳食纤维，可补充人体所需的多种营养素，以达到全面营养。

（三）饮食卫生，新鲜洁净

食物应新鲜，无杂质、变色、变味，避免食用被细菌或毒素污染的食物，严防病从口入；进餐需注意卫生条件，包括进餐环境、餐具和供餐者的健康卫生状况。饮食不洁，可引发多种肠胃道疾病，出现腹痛、吐泻等症状，或引起寄生虫病，如蛔虫、蛲虫、绦虫等，临床可见腹痛、嗜食异物、面黄肌瘦等症。若进食腐败变质有毒食物，则可出现剧烈腹痛、吐泻等中毒症状，重者可出现昏迷或死亡。食物的烹调加热，在一定程度上可起到清洁消毒作用，且大部分食物不宜生食，肉类尤须煮熟。《备急千金要方·养性序》说："勿食生肉，伤胃，一切肉惟须煮烂。"这对老年人尤为重要。故饮食以熟食为主是饮食卫生的重要内容之一。

（四）饮食清淡，免伤脾胃

中医一贯主张饮食清淡，即避免进食过

substantial amounts of fat may promote dampness and phlegm, causing the symptoms of ascendant hyperactivity of liver yang and internal stirring of liver wind. The cause of furuncle and carbuncle especially on the head and face is also related to the overeating of greasy food. Salty food should be avoided as well, which could cause hypertension. Delicate diet with low fat and salt is the essential principle for life cultivation and health preservation, which had been recorded in many ancient medical books such as *Important Formulas Worth a Thousand Gold Pieces for Emergency*. There is a saying that goes, "meat generates fire, fat produces phlegm, vegetables and tofu keeps body healthy".

v. Reasonable Processing

Food processing includes the procedures about cleaning, cooking and preservation. Reasonable processing could facilitate individual's appetite, digestion and absorption. For example, the time of rice-rinsing should be reduced, for the reason that 2 or 3 times rinsing procedure will lead to 29%-60% loss of vitamin B_1, and 23%-25% of vitamin B_2 and nicotinic acid, as well 70% of the trace elements. In order to reduce nutrient loss, some food preparation tips such as keeping rice soup while cooking and washing vegetable before cutting are recommended. Quick stir-fry with appropriate amount of farina and simmering dishes with pot cover could prevent the loss of vitamins C. In short, reasonable food processing should balance the flavors, sensory and nutritional content of foods.

vi. Pattern Differentiation for Diet

1. Individuality-concerned Diet　Dietary nursing should consider the differences among individuals. The factors influencing the selection of foods include age, constitution, personality of individuals, *etc.*.

(1) People with overweight or obesity: People with overweight or obesity generally have a symptom of phlegm-damp, which might be aggravated by the intake of greasy food. Therefore, delicate food with low calorie is recommended, such as vegetable and fruit. Compared with other kinds of food, the calories contained in the seafood are lower than the most of meat and poultry, while wild fowl is lower than the domestics. Refers to meat, beef and mutton are lower than pork. Moreover, skim milk is lower than whole milk. Similar to edible animal product, vegetable also differs when compared by the different

多油腻或辛辣食物及大量饮酒，以免损伤脾胃、诱发疾病。肥厚油腻食物可助湿生痰，造成肝阳上亢，肝风内动。再如各种疮疡肿毒的发生，也多与进食油腻食物有关，尤其是头面部、颈部的痈、疖、疡与饮食有关。临床上常见到疖痈初发患者，如果继续进食油腻及煎炸食物，则病情发展较快。古代医家还特别强调饮食不宜过咸，应少食盐。《备急千金要方》指出："咸则伤筋，酢则伤骨，故每宜淡食"。在实践中，中医十分强调饮食清淡，这样可确保健康，预防疾病，延年益寿。俗语说"肉生火、油生痰，青菜豆腐保平安"就含此理，饮食清淡可有利于健康长寿。

（五）合理加工，提高营养

食物的加工包括清洗、烹调与保存。科学合理的食物加工可增强食欲、促进消化，有利于胃肠道的吸收。为减少食物营养成分流失，做米饭时，应尽量减少淘米次数.因大米淘洗 2~3 次后，维生素 B_1 可损失 29%~60%、维生素 B_2 和烟酸可损失 23%~25%、无机盐可损失 70%；另外，煮饭时不要丢弃米汤；蔬菜最好先洗后切；烹调可急火快炒，同时可加适量淀粉，以保护维生素 C；煮菜时间不要太久，煮菜时加锅盖，以防止维生素流失。总之，菜肴烹调方法既要讲究食品的风味和感官性状，又要注意营养成分的保存。

（六）辨证施食，三因制宜

1. 因人制宜　饮食调护应根据不同的年龄、体质、个性等方面的差异，分别予以不同的调摄。

（1）体胖者：体胖多痰湿，饮食宜清淡、化痰之品，如青菜、水果等，忌食肥甘厚腻，以免助湿生痰；体胖者热量过剩宜食用热量低的食物，如鱼虾热量低于其他肉类、禽类食物，飞禽类的热量低于家禽类的热量；畜肉中，牛羊肉的热量低于猪肉的热量；脱脂牛奶比全脂牛奶的热量低；同样是绿叶蔬菜，瓜类蔬菜的热量比根茎类蔬菜低。体瘦者多阴虚内热，宜食滋阴生津、养血补血的食物，

types. For instance, melon vegetable is lower than root vegetable. People with low body weight generally have a pattern of yin deficiency with internal heat. The diet should nourish yin, promote fluid production and supplement the blood. However, spicy food should be avoided.

(2) Pregnant woman: During the gestation period, because of the growth of fetus, pregnant woman generally has the pattern of yin blood deficiency. Therefore, the yang qi will be exuberant. For this special crowd, diet should be sweet, cool and even supplement, even supplementing with sweet or coolness, such as fish, milk, vegetable and fruit, while avoiding hot and spicy or warm and dry food, which could affect the fetus by assisting yang and generating fire. This is a diet principle called cool diet during the gestation period. In the period of lactation, woman will have a pattern of qi and blood deficiency and stasis. The diet should be nourishing, digestible, delicate and supplement, e.g. millet congee, jujube, bone broth and egg. Cold, cool, acrid, sour and dry food should be avoided. This is the diet principle called warm diet during the lactation period.

(3) Teenager: Teenager is a special group with tender yin and tender yang. The diet for them should be neutral supplement, digestible, fortifying spleen and promoting appetite. Food should be diversity and balanced in grains, meat and vegetables. Monophagia or consume fatty and drastic supplementing food should be avoided in order to prevent overweight or low weight.

(4) Old and those who recovered from serious illness: The old and those who recovered from serious illness usually have dysfunctional digestion, named spleen-stomach weakness, transportation and transformation weakness. The diet for them should be delicate, warm and soft, avoiding raw, cold, thick and hard food. When considering the supplementation, instead of drastic supplementing, which could result in pathogens stasis, frequent and small amounts of intake is recommended. Furthermore, the old generally have constipation, so plant seed or root vegetable containing dietary fiber is more beneficial.

2. Time-concerned Diet Climate as the important influencing factor on the process of physiology and pathology should be considered in diet to promote health.

(1) Spring: In spring, yang qi ascents and disperses. The diet in this period should be delicate and warm, e.g. wheat, jujube, pork, peanut. The consumption of sesame, raw, cold and greasy food should be well controlled.

(2) Summer: During this hot season, delicate, thirst-

忌食辛辣动火之品，以免伤阴。

（2）孕产妇：孕产妇在妊娠期，由于胎儿生长发育的需要，机体的阴血相对不足，而阳气偏盛，宜食性味甘平、甘凉的补益之品，如鱼肉、乳类、蔬菜、水果等，忌食辛热、温燥之物，以免助阳生火动胎气，即所谓"产前宜凉"；哺乳期由于胎儿的娩出，气血受到不同程度的损伤，机体多虚多瘀，此时宜食有营养、易消化、补而不腻之物，如小米粥、大枣、骨头汤、鸡汤、蛋类等，忌食寒凉、辛燥、酸性食物，即所谓"产后宜热"。

（3）儿童：儿童身体娇嫩，为稚阴稚阳之体，宜食性味平和，易于消化，又能健脾开胃的食物，而且食物的品种宜多样化，粗细结合、荤素搭配，不可偏嗜，以免过胖或过瘦，忌食滋腻、峻补之品。

（4）老年或大病初愈之人：老年或大病初愈之人脾胃功能虚弱，运化无力，宜食清淡、温热、熟软之品，忌食生冷、黏硬、不易消化之物，且因其体质虚弱，不宜大剂量强补，而应少量多次进补，防止偏补太过或因补滞邪。肠燥便秘者，宜多食含油脂的植物种仁或多纤维的菜根之品。

2. 因时制宜 由于春、夏、秋、冬四时气候的变化对人体的生理、病理有很大影响，因此应当在不同的季节合理选择调配不同的饮食，帮助患者增强体质，恢复健康。

（1）春季：春季三月，风和日暖，阳气升发，宜食清温平淡之物，如麦、枣、猪肉、花生、芝麻等，少食生冷、黏腻之物。

（2）夏季：夏季三月，酷热难耐，应进食

quenching and heat relieving food should be concerned, e.g. watermelon, Chinese wax gourd, mung bean soup, smoked plum and adzuki bean soup, agastache tea and rock candy water. However, physiological characteristic of human body in summer is external yang and internal yin; hence, cold or greasy food should be avoided. Furthermore, the dose of some Chinese medicine such as rén shēn, lù róng and fù zǐ should be well controlled for people with yang deficiency.

(3) Autumn: Due to the arid climate in autumn, diet should have the function of enriching yin to moisten lung. Mild food with the function of boosting the stomach and promoting fluid production, such as sesame, honey, pineapple, milk, sugarcane and glutinous rice are recommended. Acrid food such as green onion, ginger or chili should be taken as less as possible. When considering supplementation, food should also have the function of promoting fluid's production.

(4) Winter: Due to the cold climate in winter, protecting yang qi, as well as nourishing and storing essence to reinforce and consolidate healthy qi is the basic principle in dietary nursing, whih could strengthen immunity and protect the body from the warm disease in the spring. High-calorie food with the function of enriching yin and subduing yang could be considered. This kind of food includes grain, mutton, testudinate and wood ear. In addition, all meals in winter should be served warm.

3. Local Condition-Concerned Diet　China has a vast territory, and the climate is very different between the south and north. The climatic characteristics in south-east China are high temperature and high humidity, therefore the corresponding diet feature should be delicate and with the function of removing dampness. The climatic characteristics in north-west China are low temperature and dryness, therefore the corresponding diet feature should be warm and with the function of promoting fluid's production and moistening dryness. Refers to the altitude, high altitude hypoxia might cause low appetite or anorexia. In this circumstance, individuality-concerned cooking methods should be paid more attention to. Furthermore, multiple meal with small amount for each one, and sour fruit or drink are recommended. No matter in any circumstance, delicate diet with low greasy, low gas production and proper fiber contained should be taken.

vii. Keeping Good Eating Habit

1. Proceeding Slowly　A good habit to build is to eat slowly and chew well, which could stimulate appetite by increasing the flow of saliva and digestive juices. Furthermore, as the main link in the digestive

清淡、解渴、生津、消暑之品，如西瓜、冬瓜、绿豆汤、乌梅小豆汤、藿香茶，冰糖煎水代茶饮等。但夏季人体又有阳外阴内的生理特点，故切忌过食寒凉、厚味之品；平素阳虚体质，常服用参茸、附子之品者，也应注意节制。

（3）秋季：秋季三月，炎暑渐消，气候干燥，饮食应以滋阴润肺为主，可适当食用一些柔润食物，如芝麻、蜂蜜、菠萝、乳品、甘蔗、糯米等，以益胃生津，尽可能少食葱、姜、辣椒等辛辣之品；进补时也应注意在平补的基础上再合以生津养液之品。

（4）冬季：冬季三月，万物凋谢，朔风凛冽，宜食用具有滋阴潜阳作用且热量较高的食物，如谷类、羊肉、龟鳖、木耳等，而且宜热饮热食，以保护阳气。由于冬季以养精、藏精为主，此时进补可扶正固本，有助于体内阳气生发，增强抵抗力，可有效地预防开春的时行瘟病，为来年身体健康打下较好的基础。

3. 因地制宜　东南地区气温偏高，湿气重，宜食清淡、渗湿食物；西北地区气温偏低，燥气盛，宜食温热、生津、润燥食物；高原地区易缺氧可引起食欲下降或厌食，应注意烹调方法，少食多餐，餐间增加酸性水果和酸甜饮料。膳食应多清淡少油腻，避免摄入产气和含纤维素过多的食品。

（七）保持良好的进食习惯

1. **进食宜缓**　进食时应该从容和缓，细嚼慢咽，这样既有利于各种消化液的分泌，又能稳定情绪，也是促进消化吸收的重要环

and absorption processes, it also could stabilize mood. Overeating or rushing meals could increase the burden of gastrointestinal system. In addition, it is also the main cause for choke and bucking.

2. Focusing on Eating　Focusing on eating is beneficial to people to taste the real flavors of food, as well as beneficial to digestion and absorption. Conversely, having meals while watching TV or reading books as a heath hazard should be avoided, which will influence the digestion and absorption.

3. Creating a Pleasant Atmosphere　The flow of qi is governed by liver, the free activity of which could promote the function of spleen and stomach. Hence, being in a bad mood could influence the normal function of liver, which could lead to dysfunction of spleen and stomach. Therefore, tranquil, neat and pleasant dining environment with relaxed music is beneficial to appetite and digestion.

4. Paying Attention to Oral Hygiene　Food particles between teeth and the gum line is the main factor for bad breath even the tooth decay and periodontitis. Hence, oral hygiene and good oral care should be paid attention to. Postprandial rinsing to remove food residue could reduce the dental caries and oral secondary infection. In the Han Dynasty, the ancient physicians had already recorded the mouthwash behavior to protect tooth and avoid bad breath in the ancient medical book named *Essentials from the Golden Cabinet* (*Jīn Guì Yào Lüè*, 金匮要略).

5. Taking a Walk after Meal　Running or laying down after dinner should be avoided, while the former behavior could damage the *zang-fu* organ and the later behavior could affect the normal function of spleen and stomach. Taking a walk after meal is recommended, which is beneficial to digestion, and in a word, is good to health. The ancient medical book named *Formulas of Health Cultivation at Beside* (*Shè Yǎng Zhěn Zhōng Fāng*, 摄养枕中方) also recorded the healthy behavior, just as the old saying: after dinner sitting a while and after supper walking a mile.

6. Massaging Abdominal Area　Massaging abdominal area to stimulate the gastrointestinal peristalsis is beneficial to digestion and absorption. This method had already been recorded in the ancient medical book named *Supplement to 'Important Formulas Worth a Thousand Gold Pieces'*. The procedure of massaging abdominal area is clockwise massaging the abdomen along the colon for 20

节以保护肠胃。急食暴食，则会骤然加重肠胃负担，还容易发生噎、呛、咳等意外。

2. 进食宜专　进食时，应尽量将头脑中的各种琐事抛开，把注意力集中到饮食上来，做到专心致志，这样既可品尝食物的味道，又有利于消化吸收；反之，若边吃饭边看电视或书报，则纳食不香，影响消化吸收，从而影响人体健康。

3. 进食宜乐　进食时应保持环境宁静和整洁、气氛轻松和愉快，同时可适当配以轻松舒缓的音乐。安静愉快的情绪有利于胃的消化，乐观的情绪和高兴的心情都可使食欲大增，这就是所说的肝疏泄畅达则脾胃健旺；反之，情绪不好，则肝失条达，抑郁不舒，致使脾胃受其制约，影响食欲，妨碍消化功能。

4. 食后漱口　食后还要注意口腔卫生。早在汉代，《金匮要略》中即有"食毕当漱口数过，令牙齿不败口香"之说。进食后，口腔内容易残留一些食物残渣，若不及时清除，往往引起口臭，甚至发生龋齿、牙周病。经常漱口可使口腔保持清洁，牙齿坚固，并能防止口臭和口腔疾病。

5. 食后散步　一般饭后切忌饱后急行，也不宜食后即卧。食后即卧可导致宿食停滞，影响脾胃健运。如饱后急行，则会损伤脏腑。饭后一般宜缓行散步，有利于消化吸收，也有益于健康。《摄养枕中方》中说："食止、行数百步，大益人。"俗话说："饭后百步走，能活九十九。"进食后，活动身体，有利于胃肠蠕动，促进消化吸收，而散步是最好的活动方式。

6. 食后摩腹　摩腹对于促进食物的消化吸收也有重要的作用。《千金翼方》说："平旦点心饭讫，即自以热手摩腹。"又说："中食后，还以热手摩腹。"食后摩腹的具体方法是：进食以后，自左而右，可连续做 20~30 次不等。这种方法有利于腹腔血液循环，可促

to 30 times. Massaging while walking is recommended as the combined effect.

IV. Dietary Restriction

Food selection should consider individual's health status, specific function of foods and their combinations. Otherwise it might lead to malnutrition or disease. Although all the eatables could provide certain nutrition, therapeutic effects of them are limited. Misuse of a certain food could result in some adverse reactions or side effects. The similar principle on dietary restrictions had been recorded in the ancient medical book named *Essentials from the Golden Cabinet Birds, Animals, Fish and Worms prohibition and Treatment* (*Jīn Guì Yào Lüè Niǎo Shòu Chóng Yú Jìn Jì Bīng Zhì Piān*, 鸟兽鱼虫禁忌兵治篇).

i. Incompatibility of Food in Diet Prescription

Generally, foods are more effective in combination than alone, either for taste-masking or improving specific effect. When taking the urination promotion into consideration, the corresponding diet could be adzuki bean combined with cyprinoid. Similarly, huáng qí is combined with coix seed for urinating promotion and dampness percolation. Fish or crab is combined with zǐ sū yè for toxin-resolving and fishiness removing. Inversely, some foods could not be used together, because some ingredients might interact with each other to produce toxin, which is so-called incompatibility. Some typical incompatible foods include persimmon combined with crab, scallion combined with honey, turtle combined with amaranth. Although many Chinese materia medica or dietary book have recorded amount of incompatibility of food in diet prescription, generally they are empirical evidences. Therefore, these records should be discriminated carefully, and even some scientific technologies could be used if necessary.

ii. Dietary Restriction for Pattern

1. Avoiding Raw and Cold Food　Patients with cold pattern, deficiency pattern, deficiency-cold of spleen and stomach, deficiency-cold constitution, yang deficiency or being susceptible to wind-cold should avoid raw or cold foods. For those with chronic colonitis or gastritis should be particularly pay attention to. This category of food includes some kinds of fruits such as pear, banana, lotus rhizome, peach, waternut, and some salads made from cucumber, lettuce, *etc.*.

进胃肠消化功能，经常进行食后摩腹，不仅有益于消化，对全身健康也有促进作用。如果在饭后，边散步，边摩腹，则效果更佳。

四、饮食宜忌

在某种情况下，某些食物不能食用，否则会导致身体出现偏差，甚至引起病变。不同食物性能有差异，尽管都有可食性和营养功能，但在防治疾病时是有一定范围的。如果滥用即可产生不良反应和副作用。《金匮要略·禽兽鱼虫禁忌兵治篇》曾指出"所食之味，有与病相宜，有与身为害。若得宜则益体，害则成疾，以此致危。例皆难疗。"

（一）配伍禁忌

一般情况下食物都可以单独食用，有时为了矫味或提高某些方面的作用，常常将不同食物搭配起来食用，即协同作用。如赤小豆配鲤鱼可增强利水作用，黄芪加薏米可加强渗湿利水的作用，鱼及蟹加苏叶可解毒去腥等。其中有些食物不宜在一起配合应用，也就是所谓配伍禁忌，即相悖相克作用。如柿子忌螃蟹，葱忌蜂蜜，鳖忌苋菜等。关于食物配伍禁忌，历代本草中都有不少记载，但古人的这些食物禁忌因经验成分比较多，应灵活分析看待，也有必要运用现代科学技术作进一步研究。

（二）不同病证类型的食物禁忌

1. **忌生冷**　寒证、虚证、脾胃虚寒或体质虚寒者，阳虚者、平时易感风寒者及胃肠消化功能差者（如慢性结肠炎、胃炎等），均应忌食生冷食物，包括某些瓜果，如梨、香蕉、鲜藕、桃、荸荠等，及凉拌菜，如凉拌黄瓜、凉拌莴笋等。

2. Avoiding Fried Food Patients with heat pattern, dyspepsia, damp-heat accumulation syndrome, jaundice, phlegm-damp should avoid fried food, so as for some infectious disease such as pneumonia or hyperthermia, and gastroduodenal ulcer, hypertension. This category of food includes fried meat or fried shrimp *etc.*.

3. Avoiding Greasy Food Patients with dyspepsia, hyperlipidemia, coronary heart disease, hypertension, cholecystitis, cholelithiasis or pancreatitis should avoid greasy food. This category of food includes pig's trotters, fat meat, animal organs, *etc.*.

4. Avoiding Spicy Food Patients with high fever should avoid spicy food, including ginger, scallion, garlic bulb, prickly ash peel, cinnamon, alcohol, chili, *etc.*.

5. Avoiding Dispersing Food Patients with acute infectious diseases such as acute abdominal disease, hepatitis or furuncle and carbuncle should avoid dispersing food, which could exacerbate disease, including fish, crab, shrimp, cock, bamboo shoot, shepherd's purse, brassica juncea, fragrant-flowered garlic, cockscomb, *etc.*.

iii. Dietary Restrictions for Five *Zang* Disorder

1. Heart Disorder The heart disorder signs include palpitation, chest bì (*xiōng bì*, 胸痹), insomnia, *etc.*. Patients with heart disorder generally have hyperlipidemia, therefore, diet should be delicate and particularly low fat. Lean meat and fish are recommended; however, adipose, animal organs, alcohol, tobacco, strong tea or coffee should be avoided.

2. Lung Disorder The lung disorder signs include cough, panting, lung abscess, lung consumption, pleural rheum, silicosis, *etc.*. Delicate diet especially containing vegetable and fruit is recommended to the patients with the above signs. Spicy, greasy, sweet or gooey food, tobacco, alcohol should be avoided. Foods with the function of heat clearing and phlegm dissolving, such as turnip, orange, pear and loquat are recommended to the patients with severe lung heat, particularly to the patients with the symptoms of cough and yellow sputum. Foods with the function of heat clearing and lung moistening, such as waternut, lotus rhizome juice, watermelon, are recommended to the patients with the symptom of bloody sputum. Cold fruit should be avoided to the patients with lung cold. Food with the function of yin enriching and lung supplementing, such as lily bulb, tremella, turtle are recommended to the patients with lung yin deficiency. The patients with coughing and panting should avoid dispersing food such as sea-fish, shrimp, and coriander.

2. 忌煎炸 热证、食滞、湿热积、黄疸、痰湿甚者、感染性疾病（如肺炎、高热、胃及十二指肠溃疡、高血压病等）均应忌煎炸食物，如油炸肉类、油炸虾等。

3. 忌油腻 对消化不良、高脂血症、冠心病、高血压病、胆囊炎、胆石症、胰腺炎等疾病均应忌油腻及含脂肪多的食物，如蹄膀、肥肉、动物内脏等。

4. 忌辛辣 对热性病均忌辛辣食物，如生姜、葱、大蒜、花椒、桂皮、酒、辣椒等。

5. 忌发物 有些病要忌发物，如各种急证、疖痈等感染性疾病、急腹症、肝炎等。发物中包括鱼、虾、蟹、公鸡、芋艿、竹笋、荠菜、芥菜、韭菜、鸡头等。如不忌发物，往往会加重病情。

（三）五脏病证的饮食宜忌

1. **心系病证的饮食宜忌** 包括心悸、胸痹、失眠等病证。血脂正常者，一般营养食物均适宜；血脂增高者，以清淡素食为主，少进瘦肉、鱼类之品，忌食动物脂肪、内脏等肥腻之品以及烟酒、浓茶、咖啡等刺激品。

2. **肺系病证的饮食宜忌** 包括咳嗽、哮喘、肺痈、肺痨、悬饮、硅沉着病等病证。宜食清淡素食、水果。忌食辛辣、烟酒、油腻、甜黏之品。咳嗽痰黄，肺热盛者，宜食萝卜、橘子、梨、枇杷等清热化痰之品；痰中带血者，宜食荸荠、藕汁、西瓜等清热润肺、止血之品；痰白清稀、肺寒者，忌食生冷瓜果；肺阴虚者，宜食百合、银耳、甲鱼等滋阴补肺之品；哮喘患者忌食海鱼、虾、香菜、羊肉等发物。

3. The Spleen and Stomach Disorder　The signs and symptoms of spleen and stomach disorder include epigastric pain, vomiting, diarrhea, constipation. The diet should be nutritious, soft, warm and digestible for patients with the above signs. Raw, cold, fried, and hard food should be avoided. For the patients with deficiency-cold of spleen and stomach, ginger and green pepper are recommended. For the patients with stomach heat, cold fruit is recommended. Food containing alkali such as noodle could be recommended to the patients with hyperchlorhydria. Inversely, patients with achlorhydria could take some vinegar or Chinese hawthorn fruit after meal. For the patients with diarrhea, semi-liquid food or soft meal with controlled cooking oil should be recommended. However, cold and moistening food, such as amaranth, garland chrysanthemum, eggplant, cold fruit should be avoided.

4. Liver and Gallbladder Disorder　The signs and symptoms of liver and gallbladder disorder include jaundice, tympanites, dizziness, stroke, epilepsy and constraint syndrome. The diet should be nutritious with low saturated fat and sodium, such as fresh vegetable and lean meat, chicken, fish, *etc.*. Spicy food, alcohol or cigarette should be avoided. Furthermore, the diet for the patients with hepatic disease should consider the different disease stages. Vegetarian diet is recommended for the patients in the acute stage of hepatic disease, while during the remission or convalescence, diet with controlled intake of meat is recommended. Diet with low or no sodium should be followed for the patient with cirrhotic ascites, and a stricter diet on the meat intake is necessary for the patients with hepatic coma.

5. Kidney Disorder　The kidney disorder signs and symptoms include edema, strangury, wasting-thirst (*xiāo kě*, 消渴), urinary retention, flaccidity syndrome, and seminal emission. The diet should be delicate and nutritious. Therefore, foods or spices containing large amount of sodium, alkali, or sour and spicy food should be avoided. Foods with the functions of promoting urination and detumescence, such as Chinese wax gourd, bottle gourd, adzuki bean, shepherd's purse, coix seed and crucian are recommended to the patient with edema. Supplementing and nourishing foods such as pork, beef, mutton, chicken and egg are beneficial to the patient with kidney deficiency. Diet with low or no sodium is necessary for the patient with nephritis. Fat or protein should be avoided by the patient with the symptom of chyluria.

3. **脾胃系病证的饮食宜忌**　包括胃脘痛、泄泻、便秘等病证。宜食营养丰富、软、烂、热、易于消化的食物，忌食生冷、煎炸、硬固之品。脾胃虚寒者，宜食姜、椒类；胃热者，宜食凉性水果；胃酸过多者，宜食含碱食物，如热干面；胃酸缺乏者，饭后宜食适量的醋或山楂片；腹泻者，宜食少油、半流质食物或软饭，忌食苋菜、茼蒿、茄子、生冷瓜果等寒凉滑润之品。

4. **肝胆系病证的饮食宜忌**　包括黄疸、臌胀、眩晕、中风、癫痫、郁证等病证。宜食新鲜蔬菜及营养丰富的瘦肉、鸡、鱼类，忌食辛辣、烟酒等刺激品，少进动物脂肪。肝胆疾病急性期以素食为主，缓解期或恢复期可进荤食；肝硬化腹水，宜食低盐或无盐饮食；肝昏迷时期，应控制动物蛋白类食物。

5. **肾系病证的饮食宜忌**　包括水肿、淋证、消渴、癃闭、萎证、遗精等病证。宜食清淡、营养丰富的食物以及多种动物性补养类食物，忌食盐、碱过多和酸辣太过的刺激之品。水肿者，宜食冬瓜、葫芦、赤豆、荠菜、薏苡仁、鲫鱼等利尿消肿之品；肾虚者，宜食猪、牛、羊、鸡、蛋类等补养品；肾炎宜食低盐或无盐饮食；乳糜尿应忌食脂肪、蛋白类食物。

V. TCM Dietary Formulae

Dietary therapy plays an important role in health promotion and disease prevention. It establishes a more effective food-based and Chinese medicinal supplemented formulas system to enhance the therapeutic effect and taste.

i. Five-Shen Soup (*Wǔ Shēn Tāng*, 五神汤)

In the *Empirical Formula from Huizhi Tang (Huì Zhí Táng Jīng Yàn Fāng*, 惠直堂经验方).

[Ingredient] *Jīng jiè* 10g, *zǐ sū yè* 10g, tea 6g, ginger 10g, brown sugar 30g.

[Processing] First put the *jīng jiè, zǐ sū yè*, tea and ginger in the casserole, then place one bowl of water, boils in gentle fire, and stir in brown sugar.

[Administration] Drink while warm.

[Function] Inducing sweating to release the exterior.

[Indication] Wind-cold pattern with exterior symptoms of cold, body aches, absence of sweating.

ii. Hongyan Wine (*Hóng Yán Jiǔ*, 红颜酒)

In the *Restoration of Health from the Myriad Diseases (Wàn Bìng Huí Chūn*, 万病回春).

[Ingredient] Walnut 100g, sweet almond 30g, jujube 50g, honey, ghee, white wine 1 000ml.

[Processing] Mash the walnuts and jujubes; blanch the sweet almonds by soaking off the skin in the boiled water, add water repeatedly and let it boil 4-5 times , then dry and mash them; put the above mashed food into the white wine, sealed immersion for a week.

[Administration] Twice a day; 10 to 20ml for each time.

[Function] Enriching and nourishing the lung and kidney, supplementing and boosting the spleen and stomach, moisturizing the skin.

[Indication] Rough skin, pale complexion.

iii. Glutinous Rice and Colla Corii Asini Porridge (*Nuò Mǐ Ē Jiāo Zhōu*, 糯米阿胶粥)

In the *Reflections on Dietotherapy (Shí Yī Xīn Jiàn*, 食医心鉴).

[Ingredient] *ē jiāo* 30g, glutinous rice 50g, brown sugar.

[Processing] Cook porridge from cleaned glutinous rice, stir in the mashed *ē jiāo*, cook for 2 to 3 minutes while boiling, then stir in the brown sugar.

五、常用食养食疗方

食疗通过药食相配，以食物为主，药物为辅，达到保健强身，防治疾病的作用。食物与药物的性能相通，二者配合应用，可以更好地发挥作用。食疗无苦药之弊，寓养生于美味食品之中，因而受到人们的欢迎。

（一）五神汤（《惠直堂经验方》）

【组成】荆芥、苏叶各 10g，茶叶 6g，生姜 10g，红糖 30g。

【制作】荆芥、苏叶、茶叶、生姜入锅加水小火煎沸，倒入红糖溶解搅匀即成。

【用法】趁热饮。

【功效】发汗解表。

【应用】适用于风寒感冒初起见恶寒、身痛、无汗等。

（二）红颜酒（《万病回春》）

【组成】核桃肉 100g，甜杏仁 30g，红枣 50g，蜂蜜、酥油适量，白酒 1 000ml。

【制作】先将核桃肉、红枣捣碎；甜杏仁泡去皮，煮 4~5 沸，捞出晒干捣碎，备用。白蜜、酥油溶化后，与上三味食物倒入白酒中，密封，浸泡 7d 即可饮用。

【用法】每次 10~20ml，每日 2 次。

【功效】滋补肺肾，补益脾胃，润肤美容。

【应用】适用于皮肤粗糙、面色苍白者。

（三）糯米阿胶粥（《食医心鉴》）

【组成】阿胶 30g，糯米 50g，红糖适量。

【制作】将糯米淘洗净，入锅加清水煮至粥将熟时，放入捣碎的阿胶，边煮边搅拌。稍微煮至 2~3 成沸，加入红糖搅拌均匀。

[Administration] Twice a day with warm on an empty stomach. Three days is one course of treatment.

[Function] Enriching yin and supplementing the blood.

[Indication] Yin blood deficiency, cough due to deficiency-consumption, hematemesis, epistaxis, bloody stool, menstrual irregularities, vaginal bleeding (painless spotting) during pregnancy.

iv. Radix et Rhizoma Glycyrrhizae, Wheat, Jujube Soup (*Gān Mài Dà Zǎo Tāng*, 甘麦大枣汤)

In the *Essentials from the Golden Cabinet.*

[Ingredient] *Gān cǎo* 20g, wheat 100g, ten jujubes.

[Processing] Put the *gān cǎo* and 500ml water into the casserole, boiled on high heat then switch to low heat to 200ml, and keep the juice. Cook the cleaned jujubes, wheat and water in the casserole on low heat until the wheat cooked thoroughly, then add the *gān cǎo* juice, and heat it till boiling.

[Administration] Take warm on an empty stomach.

[Function] Nourishing the heart and calming the spirit.

[Indication] Heart deficiency, mind restlessness due to liver constraint, mental trance, insomnia.

v. Adzuki Bean Carp Soup (*Chì Xiǎo Dòu Lǐ Yú Tāng*, 赤小豆鲤鱼汤)

In the *Arcane Essentials from the Imperial Library* (*Wài Tái Mì Yào*, 外台秘要).

[Ingredient] Adzuki bean 100g, one carp (about 125g), one piece of ginger, salt, aginomoto, Chinese rice wine, plant oil.

[Processing] Soak the cleaned adzuki bean for half an hour; clean the ginger and carp, remove the gill and organs while keeping the scales; fry the carp with plant oil, then add water, adzuki bean, ginger and Chinese rice wine, boiled on high heat then switch to low heat till the adzuki bean well cooked; add in salt and aginomoto.

[Administration] Eat together with rice or eat as you wish.

[Function] Promoting urination and detumescence.

[Indication] Water-dampness or people with dysuria.

vi. Duck Cooked with Cordyceps (*Dōng Chóng Xià Cǎo Yā*, 冬虫夏草鸭)

In the *Supplement to 'The Grand Compendium of Materia Medica'* (*Běn Cǎo Gāng Mù Shí Yí*, 本草纲目拾遗).

[Ingredient] One male duck, 5-10 Cordyceps, salt,

【用法】每日分 2 次趁热空腹服食，3d 为一疗程。

【功效】滋阴补血。

【应用】适用于阴血不足、虚劳咳嗽、吐血、衄血、便血、妇女月经不调、胎漏等。

（四）甘麦大枣汤（《金匮要略》）

【组成】甘草 20g，小麦 100g，大枣 10 枚。

【制作】将甘草放入砂锅内，加入清水 500ml，大火烧开，小火煎至 200ml，去渣，取汁，备用。将大枣洗净，去杂质，同小麦一起放入锅内，加水适量，用小火煮至麦熟时，加入甘草汁，煮沸后即可食用。

【用法】空腹温热服。

【功效】养心安神。

【应用】适用于心虚、肝郁引起的心神不宁、精神恍惚、失眠等。

（五）赤小豆鲤鱼汤（《外台秘要》）

【组成】赤小豆 100g，鲤鱼 1 条（250g），生姜 1 片，盐、味精、黄酒、食用植物油适量。

【制作】将赤小豆洗净，加水浸泡半小时；生姜洗净；鲤鱼去鳞去鳃、肠脏，洗净。起植物油锅，煎鲤鱼，加清水中量，放入赤小豆、生姜、黄酒少许。先大火煮沸，改小火焖至赤小豆熟，调上盐、味精即可。

【用法】随量食用或佐餐。

【功效】利尿消肿。

【应用】适用于水湿泛溢，症见小便不利等。

（六）冬虫夏草鸭（《本草纲目拾遗》）

【组成】雄鸭 1 只，冬虫夏草 5~10 枚，食

scallion, ginger.

[Processing] Remove the feather and organs of the male duck. Put the duck, Cordyceps, salt, scallion, ginger and water in the casserole, simmered until thoroughly cooked.

[Administration] Regular consumption.

[Function] Supplementing deficiency and assisting yang.

[Indication] Weakness, spontaneous sweating, limbs coldness, impotence, seminal emission.

vii. Steamed Stuffed Yam and Poria Bun (*Shān Yào Fú Líng Bāo Zi*, 山药茯苓包子)

In the *Confucians' Duties to Their Parents* (*Rú Mén Shì Qīn*, 儒门事亲).

[Ingredient] Flour of common yam rhizome 100g, flour of poria 100g, wheat flour 200g, white granulated sugar 300g, plant oil, red and green dyed tangerine pericarp.

[Processing] Stir the flour of common yam rhizome and poria in water and steamed for half an hour; add in the wheat flour and ferment it, then neutralize the acidic scent with alkali. Make steamed buns with red and green dyed tangerine pericarp and plant oil and steam them.

[Administration] Regular and continuing consumption.

[Function] Tonifying qi and strengthening the spleen, supplementing yin and consolidating essence.

[Indication] Unhealthy spleen and stomach, frequency of urination, seminal emission, enuresis.

viii. Stew Hen with Dāng Guī and Dǎng Shēn (*Guī Shēn Dùn Mǔ Jī*, 归参炖母鸡)

In the *Life in Heaven and Earth* (*Qián Kūn Shēng Yì*, 乾坤生意).

[Ingredient] One hen, *dāng guī* 15g, *dǎng shēn* 15g, scallion, ginger, Chinese rice wine, salt.

[Processing] Remove the feather and organs of the hen. Put the *dāng guī*, *dǎng shēn*, scallion, ginger and Chinese rice wine and salt into the abdominal cavity of the hen. Simmer the hen on low heat in a casserole till thoroughly cooked.

[Administration] Regular consumption.

[Function] Tonifying qi and supplementing blood, warming the center and supplementing deficiency.

[Indication] Weakness due to the chronic illness, regurgitation and poor appetite.

ix. Lotus Leaf and Waxgourd Soup (*Hē Yè Dōng Guā Tāng*, 荷叶冬瓜汤)

In the *Chinese Dietotherapy Encyclopedia* (*Zhōng Guó Yào Shàn*, 中国药膳大全).

盐、葱、姜等调料各适量。

【制作】雄鸭去毛及内脏，洗净放入锅内，加冬虫夏草、食盐、葱、姜等调料，加水以小火煨炖至熟烂即可。

【用法】经常食用。

【功效】补虚助阳。

【应用】适用于久病体弱、肢冷自汗、阳痿、遗精等。

（七）山药茯苓包子（《儒门事亲》）

【组成】山药粉 100g，茯苓粉 100g，面粉 200g，白砂糖 300g，食用植物油、青丝、红丝适量。

【制作】山药粉、茯苓粉放在大碗中，加水适量，搅拌成糊，上蒸笼蒸半小时，加入面粉后发酵、加碱；用植物油、青丝、红丝等为馅，包成包子，蒸熟即可。

【用法】连续随量食用。

【功效】益气健脾，补阴涩精。

【应用】适用于脾胃不健、尿频、遗精、遗尿等。

（八）归参炖母鸡（《乾坤生意》）

【组成】母鸡 1 只，当归 15g，党参 15g，葱、姜、黄酒、食盐适量。

【制作】母鸡去毛及内脏，洗净，腹腔内装当归、党参、葱、姜、黄酒、食盐各适量，把鸡放在砂锅内，加水以小火煨炖，熟烂即可。

【用法】经常食用。

【功效】益气补血，温中补虚。

【应用】适用于久病体衰，反胃食少等。

（九）荷叶冬瓜汤（《中国药膳大全》）

[Ingredient] Fresh lotus leaf 50g, fresh waxgourd 250g.

[Processing] Put the cleaned lotus leaf and waxgourd in the casserole, boil it and season with salt.

[Administration] Take the waxgourd and soup, twice a day, one to three-day-course.

[Function] Dispel summer heat and remove dampness.

[Indication] Summer heat-warmth and summer heat-damp disease with the symptoms such as fever, boredom, headache, thirty, dark urine or dysuria.

x. Turnip and Chinese Waxgourd Peel Soup (*Luó Bo Dōng Guā Pí Tāng,* 萝卜冬瓜皮汤)

In the *Chinese Dietotherapy* (*Zhōng Guó Yào Shàn,* 中国药膳).

[Ingredient] Turnip 60g, Chinese waxgourd peel 10g, lettuce peel 15g.

[Processing] Decoct the turnip, Chinese wax gourd peel and lettuce peel.

[Administration] One or two a day, 150ml each time.

[Function] Strengthening the spleen, dispelling phlegm and dampness.

[Indication] Hyperlipidemia (the pattern of internal obstruction of phlegm-damp).

(Shan Ya-wei)

【组成】鲜荷叶 50g，鲜冬瓜 250g。

【制作】二者洗净置锅内，加水适量，熬汤至熟，加食盐调味即可。

【用法】食冬瓜，饮汤，每日 2 次，1~3d 为 1 疗程。

【功效】祛暑利湿。

【应用】暑温、暑湿病所致的发热烦闷、头痛口渴，尿赤或小便不利等。

（十）萝卜冬瓜皮汤（《中国药膳》）

【组成】白萝卜 60g，冬瓜皮 10g，莴笋皮 15g。

【制作】白萝卜、冬瓜皮、莴笋皮一起水煎。

【用法】直接饮用，每日 1~2 次，每次 150ml。

【功效】健脾，祛痰化湿。

【应用】适用于痰湿内阻型高脂血症。

（单亚维）

Section 5　Regulating of Constitution in TCM

I. Definition

Constitution is an important manifestation of human life activities, and refers to the inherent characteristics formed in the process of human life, obtained in the congenital and acquired base on morphological structure, physiological function and psychological state. As a human characteristic which is adapted to the natural and social environment in the process of growth and development, it is comprehensive and relatively stable. Based on individual life, theory of Constitution in TCM is to study

第五节　体质调护

一、中医体质的概念

体质是人类生命活动的一种重要表现形式，是指人体生命过程中，在先天禀赋和后天获得的基础上所形成的个体形态结构、生理功能和心理状态方面综合、相对稳定的固有特质；是人类在生长、发育过程中所形成的与自然、社会环境相适应的个体特征。中医体质学以生命个体的人为研究出发点，旨

the characteristics, evolution rules, influencing factors and classification criteria of different constitution, so as to apply to the prevention, diagnosis, treatment, rehabilitation and health preservation of diseases. Regulating of constitution in TCM emphasizes on individualized nursing applied for people with different constitution determined by TCM constitution classification and judgment.

II. Classification and Characteristic of Constitution in TCM

According to *Classification and Determination of TCM Constitution (Zhōng Yī Tǐ Zhì Fēn Lèi Yǔ Pàn Dìng*, 中医体质分类与判定)*, constitution can be divided into nine types, including gentle quality, qi deficiency, yang deficiency, yin deficiency, phlegm-damp, damp heat, blood stasis, qi stagnation and special intrinsic quality. Details are as follows:

i. Constitution of Gentle Quality

1. Characteristics of Body　The people with the constitution of gentle quality are fit and strong.

2. Psychological Features　Their personalities are amiable and optimistic.

3. Signs and Symptoms　They present as moist skin, thick shiny hair, lustrous eyes, having an acute sense of smell, red lips, fullness of energy, good tolerance to heat and cold, good sleep, good appetite, smooth urination and normal elimination of feces, pink tongue with thin white fur, and moderate to strong pulse.

4. General Characteristics　This kind of people maintains balance between yin and yang, qi and blood, with vigorous fitness body, and ruddy complexion.

5. IncidenceTendency　They rarely get sick.

6. Ability to Adapt to External Environment This kind of people has strong ability to adapt to the natural and social environment.

ii. Constitution of Qi Deficiency

1. Characteristics of Body　Muscle weakness is the main characteristic for the people with the constitution of qi deficiency.

2. Psychological Features　They have introverted personality and dislike taking adventure.

3. Signs and Symptoms　They present as lassitude, fatigue, soft weak voice, shortness of breath, easy sweating, pale tongue with teeth marks of tongue edge, deep and weak pulse.

4. General Characteristics　Qi deficiency means insufficiency of the primordial qi, so the main manifestations

在研究不同体质的构成特点、演变规律、影响因素、分类标准，从而应用于疾病的预防、诊治、康复与养生。

二、体质的分类及特征

根据王琦的《中医体质分类与判定》，人的体质可分为平和质、气虚质、阳虚质、阴虚质、痰湿质、湿热质、血瘀质、气郁质、特禀质九个类型，具体介绍如下：

（一）平和质

1. **形体特征**　体形匀称健壮。

2. **心理特征**　性格随和开朗。

3. **常见表现**　面色、肤色润泽，头发稠密有光泽，目光有神，鼻色明润，嗅觉通利，唇色红润，不易疲劳，精力充沛，耐受寒热，睡眠良好，胃纳佳，二便正常，舌色淡红，苔薄白，脉和缓有力。

4. **总体特征**　该类人群阴阳气血调和，以体态适中、面色红润、精力充沛等为主要特征。

5. **发病倾向**　平素患病较少。

6. **对外界环境适应能力**　对自然环境和社会环境适应能力较强。

（二）气虚质

1. **形体特征**　肌肉松软不实。

2. **心理特征**　性格内向，不喜冒险。

3. **常见表现**　平素精神不佳，容易疲乏，语音低弱，气短懒言，动则气喘，易出汗，舌淡红，舌边有齿痕，脉沉重、按无力。

4. **总体特征**　该类人群元气不足，以经常感觉身倦乏力、气短、动则汗出等气虚表

are fatigue, shortness of breath, and easy sweating.

5. Incidence Tendency   They are susceptible to catch a cold, gastroptosis, nephroptosis, and prolapse of the anus, having poor self-healing ability and slow recovery after disease. Women are more likely to suffer from uterine prolapse.

6. Ability to Adapt to External Environment   They cannot tolerant to pathogenic factors of wind, cold, summer heat and dampness.

iii. Constitution of Yang Deficiency

1. Characteristics of Body   The people with the constitution of yang deficiency are more likely have muscle weakness.

2. Psychological Features   Their personalities are quiet and introverted.

3. Signs and Symptoms   This kind of people often present as aversion to cold, cold extremities, preference to hot nature diet, low spirit, tender pale tongue, and deep weak pulse.

4. General Characteristics   The main manifestations are aversion to cold, cold extremities caused by yang deficiency.

5. Incidence Tendency   They are susceptible to phlegm, edema, swelling, diarrhea. It will change to cold type easily if the person catches a cold.

6. Ability to Adapt to External Environment   They can tolerant to summer but not winter and easily catch the pathogenic factors of wind, cold, and dampness.

iv. Constitution of Yin Deficiency

1. Characteristics of Body   The people with this constitution have slim body and dry skin.

2. Psychological Features   Their personalities are quick temper, outgoing, active, and lively.

3. Signs and Symptoms   They present as feverish sensation in the soles and palms, dysphoria, dry mouth and throat with no drinking, or preference to cold drinks, slightly dry nose, and dry stool, red small body of the tongue, few coating and partial dry, thread and rapid pulse.

4. General Characteristics   The main manifestations are dry mouth, throat and feverish sensation in the soles and palms caused by yin deficiency.

5. Incidence Tendency   They are susceptible to fatigue, insomnia and consumption of essence. It will change to heat type easily if the person catches a cold.

6. Ability to Adapt to External Environment   They are more likely to tolerate to winter but not to summer. On the other hand, they cannot stand pathogenic

现为主要特征。

5. **发病倾向**　易患感冒、胃下垂、肾下垂、脱肛等内脏下垂病，女性则易患子宫脱垂；自愈能力差，病后康复缓慢。

6. **对外界环境适应能力**　不耐受风、寒、暑、湿之邪。

（三）阳虚质

1. **形体特征**　肌肉松软不实。

2. **心理特征**　性格多沉静、内向。

3. **常见表现**　平素畏寒恶风，手足不温，冬天四肢冰冷，喜热饮食，精神萎靡，舌质淡胖嫩，脉沉迟弱。

4. **总体特征**　该类人群阳气不足，以畏寒怕冷、手足不温等虚寒表现为主要特征。

5. **发病倾向**　易患痰饮、肿胀、泄泻等病；感邪易从寒化。

6. **对外界环境适应能力**　耐夏不耐冬；易感风、寒、湿邪。

（四）阴虚质

1. **形体特征**　体形偏瘦、肌肤偏干。

2. **心理特征**　性情急躁，外向好动，活泼。

3. **常见表现**　胸前区、手足心热，心烦，口燥咽干、但不欲饮，或喜冷饮，鼻微干，大便干燥，舌体瘦小，舌红少苔，舌面偏干，脉细数。

4. **总体特征**　该类人群阴津不足，以咽干口燥、胸前区、手足心热等虚热表现为主要特征。

5. **发病倾向**　易患虚劳、失精、不寐等病；感邪易从热化。

6. **对外界环境适应能力**　耐冬不耐夏；不耐受暑、热、燥邪。

factors of heat, summer heat and dryness.

v. The Constitution of Phlegm-damp

1. Characteristics of Body   The people with the constitution of phlegm-damp usually have fat and potbellied body.

2. Psychological Features   The personalities of this kind of people are gentle, steady, and patient.

3. Signs and Symptoms   This kind of people present as oily facial skin, sweating and sticky body, chest tightness, excessive phlegm, sticky greasy or sweet taste in the mouth, thick-greasy tongue coating and taut-slippery pulse. What's more, they prefer greasy and sweet food.

4. General Characteristics   The main manifestations of phlegm-damp are potbellied, over weight, greasy coating of the tongue.

5. Incidence Tendency   They are susceptible to stroke, heart diseases, and diabetes.

6. Ability to Adapt to External Environment   They have difficulties to adapt to humid environment and the rainy season.

vi. Constitution of Damp-Heat

1. Characteristics of Body   The bodies of people with the constitution of damp heat are often moderate or thin.

2. Psychological Features   This kind of people tends to feel upset and irritable easily.

3. Signs and Symptoms   They present as dirty and oily complexion, prone to acne, dry bitter taste in the mouth, heavy breath, tired body, poor bowel movement, loose stools or constipated, short dark urine, or have peculiar smell, scrotum wet for male, leucorrhea for female, red body of the tongue, yellow greasy coating, slippery and rapid pulse.

4. General Characteristics   The main manifestations are oily complexion, bitter taste in the mouth, and yellow greasy coating caused by accumulation of damp heat.

5. Incidence Tendency   They are susceptible to epigastric pain, jaundice, urinary tract infection, sores and beriberi.

6. Ability to Adapt to External Environment   They have difficulties to adapt to the hot and humid climate in the late summer and early autumn as well as high temperature environment.

vii. Constitution of Blood Stasis

1. Characteristics of Body   This kind of people could have thin or fat body.

2. Psychological Features   They are easily

（五）痰湿质

1. **形体特征**　体形肥胖，腹部肥满松软。

2. **心理特征**　性格偏温和、稳重，多善于忍耐。

3. **常见表现**　面部皮肤油脂较多，多汗且黏，胸闷，痰多，口黏腻或甜，喜食肥甘厚味、甜食，苔腻，脉滑。

4. **总体特征**　该类人群痰湿凝聚，以形体肥胖、腹部肥满、口黏苔腻等痰湿表现为主要特征。

5. **发病倾向**　易患中风、胸痹、消渴等病。

6. **对外界环境适应能力**　对梅雨季节及潮湿环境适应能力差。

（六）湿热质

1. **形体特征**　形体中等或偏瘦。

2. **心理特征**　容易心烦急躁。

3. **常见表现**　面垢油光，易生痤疮，口苦、口干或口气重，肢体困重倦力，排便欠畅，大便黏滞不爽或燥结，小便短、黄或有异味，男性易阴囊潮湿，女性易带下黄浊、有异味，舌质偏红，苔黄腻，脉滑或偏数。

4. **总体特征**　该类人群湿热内蕴，以面垢油光、口苦、苔黄腻等湿热表现为主要特征。

5. **发病倾向**　易患胃脘痛、黄疸、热淋、带下、疮疡、脚气等病。

6. **对外界环境适应能力**　对夏末秋初湿热气候，湿重或气温偏高环境较难适应。

（七）血瘀质

1. **形体特征**　胖瘦均可见。

2. **心理特征**　易心烦，健忘。

irritable and forgetful.

3. Signs and Symptoms This people present as dark complexion, serious scaly and dry skin, pigmentation, easy bruising, dark lips, dark or petechiae tongue, enlarged and dark sublingual vein, as well as unsmooth pulse.

4. General Characteristics Due to the poor blood circulation, the main features of this kind of people are dark complexion, dry skin, and dark purple body of the tongue.

5. Incidence Tendency They are susceptible to abdominal masses, irregular menstruation, headache, dysmenorrhea, and other pain syndrome and blood syndrome.

6. Ability to Adapt to External Environment This people cannot tolerate to cold.

viii. Constitution of Qi Stagnation

1. Characteristics of Body This kind of people often has thin and slim body.

2. Psychological Features Their personalities are introverted instability, sensitive and full of anxiety.

3. Signs and Symptoms The expression of this people are depression, emotional vulnerability, suspicious, always melancholy and moody, unhappy, pale tongue, thin white fur, and string pulse.

4. General Characteristics The main manifestations are depression and anxiety caused by qi stagnation.

5. Incidence Tendency This kind of people are susceptible to hysteria, insomnia, the plum unclear syndrome, bulbous Lili syndrome (a kind of emotional disease), and depression syndrome.

6. Ability to Adapt to External Environment The ability to adapt to mental stimulation is poor, especially in the rainy weather.

ix. Constitution of Special Intrinsic Quality

1. Characteristics of Body There is no special feature for an allergic constitution person, but a person with congenital anomalies could present as abnormal or physiological defects.

2. Psychological Features There are various conditions with different intrinsic quality.

3. Signs and Symptoms There are vertical genetic, congenital and familial characteristics for people with hereditary diseases. The development of the fetus and the characteristics of the related diseases are affected by the maternal fetal transmission. People with allergic constitution are susceptible to allergic asthma, urticarial, itching throat, nasal congestion, and sneezing.

4. General Characteristics This kind of people presents as congenital disorders, with the main features of

3. 常见表现 面色晦黯，严重者肌肤甲错，色素沉着，容易出现瘀斑，口唇黯淡，舌黯或有瘀点，舌下络脉紫黯或增粗，脉涩。

4. 总体特征 该类人群血行不畅，以面色或肌肤晦黯、舌质紫黯等血瘀表现为主要特征。

5. 发病倾向 易患症瘕、月经不调、头痛、痛经以及其他痛证、血证等。

6. 对外界环境适应能力 不耐受寒邪。

（八）气郁质

1. 形体特征 形体瘦弱者为多。

2. 心理特征 性格内向不稳定、敏感多虑。

3. 常见表现 神情抑郁，情感脆弱，多愁善感，疑心重，烦闷不乐，舌淡红，苔薄白，脉弦。

4. 总体特征 该类人群气机郁滞，以神情抑郁、忧虑脆弱等气郁表现为主要特征。

5. 发病倾向 易患脏躁、不寐、梅核气、百合病及郁证等。

6. 对外界环境适应能力 对精神刺激适应能力较差；不适应阴雨天气。

（九）特禀质

1. 形体特征 过敏体质者一般无特殊；先天禀赋异常者或有畸形，或有生理缺陷。

2. 心理特征 随禀质不同情况各异。

3. 常见表现 过敏体质者常见哮喘、风团、咽痒、鼻塞、喷嚏等；患遗传性疾病者有垂直遗传、先天性、家族性特征；患胎传性疾病者具有母体影响胎儿个体生长发育及相关疾病特征。

4. 总体特征 该类人群先天失常，以生

physiological defects, allergic reactions and so on.

5. Incidence Tendency They are susceptible to asthma, urticarial, hay fever and drug allergy. Genetic disorders such as hemophilia and mongolism is popular. Fetal transmission of disease presents as five kinds of tardy growth (late standing, late walking, slow hair-growing, late teeth and late language), five flaccid syndromes (soft head, soft neck, soft limbs, soft muscle, soft mouth), fetal convulsion, and hydrocephalus due to non-closure of fontanel, *etc.*.

6. Ability to Adapt to External Environment The ability of adapting to external environment is poor. For example, people with this constitution are allergic to seasonal alternating periods and getting illness easily.

III. Regulation and Nursing of TCM Constitution

i. Constitution of Gentle Quality

1. Collocation the food of cold, hot, warm and cool, as well as whole grains and refined grains. Have the moderation diet. Do not often have too cold or too hot food and unsanitary food.

2. Adapt to climate change.

3. Do exercise properly and not to be excessive.

ii. Constitution of Qi Deficiency

1. Intake more food with the function of strengthening qi and spleen, such as chicken, pork , soybeans, white beans, *etc.*. Spinach and radish will be limited.

2. Pay attention to season alternates and try to go out as less as possible to avoid catching a cold.

3. Appropriate or gentle exercise is good for health, such as *tai chi*, *qigong*, slow walk *etc.*.

iii. Constitution of Yang Deficiency

1. More intake of food with the function of warming yang and warm property will be recommended such as lamb, quail, beef, chicken, ginger, onions, green onions, pepper, durian, litchi, and longan. The intake of food with cold property is limited, such as watermelon, pears, water chestnuts and green tea.

2. Keep warm in winter; go out as less as possible to avoid catching a cold.

3. Strengthen the body properly, and do exercise in the winter when there is plenty of sunshine.

iv. Constitution of Yin Deficiency

1. Intake more food with the function of nourishment

理缺陷、过敏反应等为主要特征。

5. 发病倾向 过敏体质者易患哮喘、荨麻疹、花粉症及药物过敏等；遗传性疾病如血友病、先天愚型等；胎传性疾病如五迟（立迟、行迟、发迟、齿迟和语迟），五软（头软、项软、手足软、肌肉软、口软），解颅，胎惊等。

6. 对外界环境适应能力 适应能力差，如过敏体质者对季节交替期间适应能力差，易引发宿疾。

三、体质调护

（一）平和质

1. 饮食方面，寒热温凉的食物要搭配食用，合理搭配粗细粮食，饮食要有节制，不宜经常食用吃过冷、过热或不干净的食物。

2. 适寒暑。

3. 适当锻炼身体，不宜过劳。

（二）气虚质

1. 饮食方面，多食用具有益气健脾作用的食物，如鸡肉、猪肉、山药、黄豆、白扁豆等。少食空心菜、生萝卜等。

2. 季节交替时节注意尽量少外出，避免感冒。

3. 适当锻炼身体，适宜做轻缓的运动，如打太极拳、练气功、慢步走等。

（三）阳虚质

1. 饮食方面，多食用温补阳气的食物，如羊肉、鹌鹑、牛肉、鸡肉，以及生姜、洋葱、大葱、花椒、榴莲、龙眼、荔枝等温性瓜果蔬菜。少食西瓜、梨、荸荠等生冷寒凉食物，少饮绿茶。

2. 冬天注意保暖，尽量少外出，避免感冒。

3. 适当锻炼身体，冬天选择阳光充裕的时候做运动。

（四）阴虚质

1. 饮食方面，多食鸭肉、瘦猪肉、绿豆、

and cool property, such as duck, lean pork, mung bean and wax gourd. The food with warm property is limited, such as lamb, leeks, garlic, pepper, and amomum tsao-ko.

2. Avoid outdoor activities and summer heat in summer and prevent to catch a cold.

3. Do exercise properly, such as *tai chi*, *tai chi sword*, *qigong* and other sports.

v. Constitution of Damp-Phlegm

1. Bland diet is good for this kind of people, such as yam, gourd melon, lotus seed, *qiàn shí etc.*. It is recommended to eat more food with warm property and function of warming yang, such as lamb, quail, beef, chicken, ginger, onions, green onions, pepper, durian, longan, as well as litchi. Avoid watermelon, pears, water chestnuts and other food with cold property. Drink less green tea.

2. This people should adapt to climate change and avoid living in damp places.

3. Most of people with constitution of damp phlegm are more likely over weight, and get sleepy easily. They should make exercise plan according to their own specific circumstances, step by step, and insist on doing exercise for a long time.

vi. Constitution of Damp-Heat

1. Bland diet is good for this kind of people. The food with sweet and cold properties will be recommended, such as mung beans, rice bean, mustard, watercress, white flowers, celery, cucumber, lotus root, pear, muskmelon, water chestnut and watermelon.

2. In summer, this people should have outdoor activities as less as possible in order to prevent summer heat stroke.

3. Some sports are recommended such as swimming, middle-distance race, mountain climbing, all kinds of ball games, martial arts, *etc.*.

vii. Constitution of Blood Stasis

1. Intake more of vinegar, hawthorn, roses, but the intake of greasy food should be limited.

2. This people should adapt to climate change.

3. For this people, dancing, walking and aerobics are recommended.

viii. Constitution of Qi Stagnation

1. Intake more food with the function of moving qi, alleviating qi stagnation, promoting digestion and inducing resuscitation, including hawthorn, roses, day lily, kelp, radish, and citrus. The intake of sweet food is limited.

2. This people should adapt to climate change,

冬瓜等甘凉滋润之品，少食羊肉、韭菜、辣椒、草果、大蒜等性温燥烈之品。

2. 夏天注意防暑，尽量少外出，避免感冒。

3. 适当锻炼身体，适合太极拳、太极剑、气功等项目。

（五）痰湿质

1. 饮食方面，以清淡为主，可多食山药、冬瓜、莲子、芡实等。不宜食用甜品、糕点。用温补阳气的食物，如羊肉、鹌鹑、牛肉、鸡肉，以及生姜、洋葱、大葱、花椒、榴莲、龙眼、荔枝等温性瓜果蔬菜。少食西瓜、梨、荸荠等生冷寒凉食物，少饮绿茶。

2. 适寒暑，避免居住在潮湿地方。

3. 此类人群体形多肥胖，容易困倦，故应根据自己的具体情况制订运动计划，循序渐进，长期坚持锻炼。

（六）湿热质

1. 饮食方面，以清淡为主，可多食绿豆、赤小豆、芥菜、西洋菜、白花菜、芹菜、黄瓜、藕等甘寒的食物，以及梨、香瓜、荸荠、西瓜等水果。

2. 夏天注意避暑，尽量少外出，避免高温中暑。

3. 锻炼身体，适合游泳、中长跑、爬山、各种球类运动、武术等。

（七）血瘀质

1. 饮食方面，多食醋、山楂、玫瑰花等，少食肥肉等滋腻之品。

2. 适寒暑。

3. 锻炼身体，可参加各种舞蹈、步行健身、徒手健身操等。

（八）气郁质

1. 饮食方面，多食山楂、玫瑰花、黄花菜、海带、萝卜、柑橘等具有行气、解郁、消食、醒神作用的食物。少食甜食。

2. 适寒暑，多与人沟通交流，避免独处。

communicate more with others, and avoid being alone.

3. Outdoor exercises are recommended, such as walking, swimming, as well as mountain climbing.

ix. Constitution of Special Intrinsic Quality

1. This people is requested to eat more food with the function of cultivating qi and strengthening exterior, and avoid to intake of buckwheat (containing sensitization material of buckwheat fluorescein), broad bean, *etc.*.

2. This kind of people has special constitutions and is allergic to medicine, food, gas, pollen and seasons. They should go out as less as possible during the time when season alternates. The bedroom should be well ventilated and provided with clean the sheet, bedding and mattress in order to prevent dust mite allergy.

3. Gentle exercise program are recommended including walking, shadow boxing, *etc.*.

(Xu-Dong-ying)

Section 6　Physical Exercise Care

Sports exercise can promote blood circulation and metabolism for the whole body. Regular physical exercise can help maintain health, enhance physique and delay aging. China is the first country to apply exercise to diseases prevention and treatment. *The Yellow Emperor's Inner Classic* states that people susceptible to flaccidity, atrophy, coldness of limbs and cold or heat syndrome can mostly be treated with *dǎo yǐn* (导引, exercises of breathing, hands and feet). Based on the ancient knowledge of physiology, traditional Chinese exercise emphasizes the development of physiological functions of the body organs so as to keep the well-being of both mind and body, and increase vigor and vitality. Traditional Chinese exercises include a variety of types, such as Tai ji quan, Tai ji sword, Ba Duan Jin (Eight-section exercise), Wu Qin Xi (Five-animal exercise), Yi Jin Jing (Channel-changing Scriptures), *etc.*. Each of these has its own characteristics with different styles and requirements. This section focuses on the basic principles of physical exercise care and the effects and essentials of Tai ji quan, Ba Duan Jin (Eight-section exercise), and Wu Qin Xi (Five-animal exercise).

3. 锻炼身体，适合慢步走、游泳、爬山等户外运动。

（九）特禀质

1. 饮食方面，多食益气固表的食物，少食荞麦（含致敏物质荞麦荧光素）、蚕豆等。

2. 适寒暑。此类人群体质特殊。过敏体质的人易对药物、食物、气味、花粉、季节过敏。季节交替时节尽量少外出。居室宜通风良好。保持室内清洁，被褥、床单要经常洗晒，可防止对尘螨过敏。

3. 锻炼身体，适合散步、太极拳等轻缓运动项目。

（徐冬英）

第六节　运动调护

运动可以促进人体气血流通，促进机体的新陈代谢。运动调护是指通过运动的方式达到维护健康、增强体质、延缓衰老的目的。中国是最早应用运动、锻炼防治疾病之一，《黄帝内经》记载："故其病多痿厥热寒，其治宜导引按跷"。运动调护方式众多，中国传统健身术为其中之一。中国传统健身术在中国古代生理知识的基础上，强调发展机体脏腑的生理功能，以精神旺健，神气充足，身心康乐为目标，增加人体内在的生命力。中国传统健身术的内容十分丰富，比较有代表性的有太极拳、太极剑、八段锦、五禽戏、易筋经等。因其种类不同，锻炼方式及要求也各有特色。本节重点介绍运动调护的原则以及太极拳、八段锦、五禽戏的作用和动作要领。

I. Basic Principle of Physical Exercise Care

i. Combination of Static and Dynamic, Stressing Moderate Exercise

It is imperative to properly combine static and dynamic when performing sports exercise. It should regulate respiration and balance mentality with the course of nature. Both the external physique and internal spirit should be involved in the whole process. It should move the body with a state of inner peace. Body exercise is for the physical health, and inner peace is for the mental health. Therefore, exercise can get both physique and spirit trained so as to ultimately benefit internal and external harmony. It reflects the ideas of "moving from dynamic to static" "integrating dynamic into static" "restricting dynamic with static" and "combining dynamic with static".

Physical exercise should be moderate, which is an important factor in maintaining health and prolonging life. Hua Tuo once pointed out that "human should exercise, but not excessively." In the reference from *Essential Recipes for Emergent Use Worth A Thousand Gold*, Sun Si-miao warned that "health maintenance should rely on regular and moderate exercise, and fatigue should be avoided in case of body damage." So what is the proper amount of exercise? Generally speaking, if one does not feel overtired after exercise, it indicates that the intensity is appropriate. It is also advised that if one feels a sense of soreness in muscles or has slightly bulging or heavy feeling, he/she should keep or increase the amount of exercise. If there is slight pain after exercise, the amount of exercise should be reduced. If there is a local numbness after exercise, one should stop the exercise immediately and identify the cause. Pulse rate and heart rate can also be used as indicators of exercise. One should monitor the heart rate during exercise. Subtract the age from 220, and the result is the maximum heart rate (beats/min). One should not go beyond his/her maximum heart rate while exercising. If one loses appetite, gets headache, feels exhausted and sweats excessively after doing exercise, it probably means that he/she takes too much exercise, exceeding the tolerance limit of body and will cause damage.

In short, it's better for the body to be dynamic and the mind to be static. Being dynamic does not mean fatigue and being static does not mean too ease. Keep the coordination and balance between dynamic and static so that the purpose of health maintenance can be achieved.

ii. Exercise Step by Step and in a Persistent Way

It's good for one to exercise step by step and increase

一、运动调护的原则

（一）动静结合，强调适度

运动调护时，要动静兼修，动静适宜。运动时，一切顺乎自然，进行自然调息、调心，神形兼顾，内外俱练，动于外而静于内，动主练而静主养神。这样，在锻炼过程中内练精神、外练形体，使内外和谐，体现由动入静、静中有动、以静制动、动静结合的整体思想。

身体的运动须适度，这是保持健康长寿的重要因素。华佗指出："人体欲得劳动，但不当极耳"；孙思邈在《备急千金要方》中告诫人们："养性之道，常欲小劳，但莫大疲及强所不能堪耳。"那么，如何掌握运动的量与度呢？一般情况下，以每次锻炼后不感觉到过度疲劳为宜；或参照"酸加、痛减、麻停"的原则予以调节，例如，如在运动后感觉肌肉酸楚，做抬举活动时稍有胀重感，可继续维持原来的运动量或者按原计划稍加大运动量；如运动后局部稍有疼痛，应减少运动量或更换为稍小的运动项目；如在运动后出现局部的麻木感，须立即停止运动，查明原因。也有人以脉搏及心跳频率作为运动量的指标，即运动时最高心率控制在：220- 自己的年龄 = 自己应控制的最高心率（次 /min）。若运动后食欲减退、头昏头痛、自觉劳累汗多、精神倦怠，说明运动量过大，超过了机体的耐受限度，会使身体因过劳而受损。

总之，在形体与心神的动静中，形体宜动，心神宜静，动静要适度。动不致大疲，静不致过逸，保持协调平衡，才能达到养生的目的。

（二）循序渐进，持之以恒

运动调护，应循序渐进，逐渐增加运动

the amount and degree of complexity gradually. For example, man shall run slowly and in a short distance at the beginning of exercise. After a period of time, the running speed and distance can be increased gradually.

There is an old saying in China "Running water would never stale, a door-hinge would never worm-eaten." It reveals a truth that moving things are unlikely to decline and also highlights the significance of regular exercise. If one exercises in a persistent way, it can help to keep healthy. Exercise regimen has a positive role on physical fitness, but no immediate effects. Rehabilitation and improvement of the physique is a slow process, so is the effects of exercise. Exercise regimen is not only a physical exercise but also exercise on one's will and perseverance. It is a process of self-defeat.

iii. Exercise at Right Time and by Right Person

1. Excercise at Right Time Generally, it is better to do exercise in the morning because of the fresh air. Doing exercise outsides helps us to exhale more carbon dioxide and inhale more oxygen to promote metabolism, enhance muscle strength, and increase lung capacity. However, strenuous exercise is not allowed before/after naps or before sleep at night in case of irritating the nervous system and affecting sleep quality. Furthermore, one should not take strenuous exercise before/after meals. Taking exercise before meals can lead to hypoglycemia, and exercise after meals may not only influence digestion, but also result in gastroptosis, chronic gastroenteritis, even hypotension.

2. Selection of Sports' Type by Right Person The selection of sports' type should also vary according to age, energy and stamina of different people. For the elderly, due to their declined muscle strength, slow response of nervous system and poor coordination ability, the best choice for them is slow and gentle exercise, such as walking, jogging, Tai ji quan, which can relax muscles and enable all parts of the body to participate. But young and strong people may choose vigorous and intensive activities such as long-distance running and football. Besides, exercises should also be chosen according to various occupations. For example, nurses, shop assistants, cook *et al.* may easily develop varicose veins of lower limbs due to longtime standing. Thus, they can choose leg lifting for exercise. Sedentary office staff can choose such excises as chest expanding, straightening up, heading up *etc.*. In a word, physical exercise should be selected according

量和动作的复杂程度。正确的锻炼方法是运动量由小到大，动作由简单到复杂。例如跑步，刚开始练跑时要跑得慢些、距离短些，经过一段时间锻炼，再逐渐增加跑步的速度和距离。

"流水不腐，户枢不蠹"，这句话一方面说明了动则不衰的道理，另一方面，也强调了不间断活动的重要性，只有持之以恒，才能达到健身效果。运动养生具有强身健体的作用，但不具有立竿见影之效。身体的康复和体质的改善是一个缓慢的过程，锻炼效果的出现需要日积月累。运动养生不仅是身体的锻炼，也是意志和毅力的锻炼，是一个战胜自我的过程。

（三）因时制宜，因人制宜

1. 运动锻炼因时制宜 一般而言，早晨运动较好，因为早晨阳光初照的时候，空气较新鲜，到室外进行运动锻炼，有助于将体内积聚的二氧化碳排出，吸入更多的氧气，增加机体的新陈代谢，增强肌肉，提高肺活量。午睡前后或夜晚临睡前不可做剧烈运动，以免引起神经系统的兴奋，影响睡眠。此外，进食前后也不宜剧烈运动，因进食前机体处于饥饿状态，易发生低血糖症；而饭后剧烈运动，不仅影响消化，还可引起胃下垂、慢性胃肠炎，甚至出现低血压等情况。

2. 运动项目因人制宜 根据年龄、精力和体力的不同，选择的运动项目也应该有所区别。老年人由于肌肉力量减退、神经系统反应较慢、协调能力差，宜选择动作缓慢柔和、肌肉协调放松、全身能得到锻炼的运动，如步行、慢跑、打太极拳等。年轻力壮、身体素质较好的人，可选择运动量较大的有氧运动，如长跑、踢足球等。此外，每个人工作性质不同，所选择的运动项目亦应有差别，如护士、营业员、厨师等行业，工作需要长时间站立，易发生下肢静脉曲张，可选择仰卧抬腿类运动；经常伏案工作者，可选择一些扩胸、伸腰、仰头的运动项目。总之，体

to one's interest as well as one's own physical condition. Suitable exercise may enhance the body immunity and contribute to health preservation.

育项目的选择，既要符合自己的兴趣爱好，又要结合自身特点，选择适合自己的运动，才能锻炼身体，达到增强身体免疫力和养生保健的效果。

II. Traditional Chinese Exercises

二、运动调护的方法

i. Tai Ji Quan

Tai ji quan is a treasured cultural legacy of China and it has gained an enthusiastic reception among people. It is characterized by graceful gestures, soft actions, and is suitable both for men and women, the old and the young. It is not restricted by season or time. Tai ji quan has been widely practiced in China for its benefits on improving physical fitness, preventing and treating diseases.

1. Function

(1) Improving respiratory function:When practicing Tai ji quan, one should breathe deeply down to the pubic region (dān tián, 丹田) with even, deep, long, slow breathing and enlarge chest and abdomen, which is conducive for maintaining flexibility of the lung tissues, increasing chest movement and vital capacity, and improving respiratory ventilation and air exchange function.

(2) Improving cardiovascular function:Tai ji quan involves movement of many muscles and joints in the body, which can relax the muscles and diastolize blood vessels simultaneously, thus improving blood and lymph circulation, and enhancing vessel flexibility. Regular practice of Tai ji quan can strengthen myocardial function, reduce vascular resistance, and play a positive role in cardiovascular disease prevention.

(3) Improving the function of nervous system: People are required to focus on the movement completely while practicing Tai ji quan. In this way, the brain concentrates on directing organs to coordinate the body actions. The self-control ability of the nervous system consequently is increased, so the nervous system functions are improved. Besides, it is favorable for resting the brain and eliminating fatigue.

(4) Dredging the meridians and nourish qi:As long as one keeps practicing Tai ji quan, it can help to dredge the ren mai, du mai, GB 26 (dài mài,) and chong mai. Subsequently, it will increase the qi in pubic region (dān tián), which keeps people energetic, vigorous and healthy.

（一）太极拳

太极拳是中华民族宝贵的民族遗产，深受人民大众的喜爱。它姿势优美，动作柔和，男女老幼皆宜，不受时间和季节限制，既能锻炼身体，又能防治疾病。

1. 作用

（1）调节呼吸系统功能：太极拳采用腹式呼吸方法，要求气沉丹田，呼吸匀、细、深、长、缓，保持腹实、胸宽的状态，可起到保持肺组织的弹性、改进胸廓活的动度、增加肺活量、提高肺的通气和换气功能的作用。

（2）调节心血管系统功能：太极拳动作包括各肌肉、关节的活动，其动作舒展，在放松肌肉的同时舒张了血管，有效地促进了人体血液及淋巴的循环，增强了血管的弹性。经常练习太极拳，可以提高心肌的功能、降低血管的阻力，能对心脑血管疾病起到良好的防治作用。

（3）调节神经系统功能：由于练太极拳时，要求精神贯注，意守丹田，不存杂念，即要心静用意。这样人的意念始终集中在动作上，故使大脑专注于指挥全身各器官、系统功能的变化和协调动作，提高了神经系统的自我意念控制能力，从而达到改善神经系统功能的作用，有利于大脑充分休息，消除机体疲劳。

（4）疏通经络，培补正气：坚持练习太极拳，达到一定程度便可通任、督、冲、带诸脉，增加丹田之气，使人精气充足、神旺体健。还可补益肾精、强壮筋骨、抵御疾病，

It also assists to nourish kidney essence, strengthen bones and muscles, and prevent diseases. In addition, it's beneficial for delaying aging and preventing spinal degenerative change in old people so as to prolong life ultimately.

2. Key Point

(1) Keep head up with neck straight: The head and neck should be lifted up, kept straight, and relaxed. This will help maintain the stability of the body's center of gravity.

(2) Keep chest held in with back straight, shoulder and elbow relaxed: All these refer to the gestures of the chest, back, shoulder and elbow. The chest should be held inward instead of being erect. The back should be straight. The shoulder and elbow should be relaxed in a natural way. Keep two sides of the shoulder on the same low level, and keep the elbow little curved and flexible, and be held when the arm stretches or shrinks.

(3) Keep eyes and hands coordinated with the waist as pivot, move feet quietly like a cat, differentiate empty steps and full ones: When practicing Tai ji quan, one must make upper and lower part coordinated with each other as a whole, which requires that the movements are initiated from the waist, the eyes move with hands, and that bow steps alternate with empty steps until the legs have force and can move steps slowly and softly.

(4) Guide movement with mind rather than strengthen: Induce the movements with mind first, then put forth one's strength to the extent that the strength is not shown externally, whereas, there is intense force internally.

(5) Correspond the mind with qi and make qi descend to pubic region (*dān tián*): It refers to coordinate breathing with mind. Abdominal respiration should be adopted. The inspiration and expiration should match with the opening and closing of the action.

(6) Seek static from dynamic, and combine dynamic and peace together: It means to move the body with a peaceful mind and concentrate.

(7) Keep every movement even and continuous: It means that the speed of each action should be even without interruption.

ii. Ba Duan Jin (Eight-Section Exercise)

Ba Duan Jin (eight-section exercise) consists of eight sections of movements, and that's why it is named "Eight-Section" exercise. It is also named as "Brocade", because the eight forms of movements are so smooth, soft and tender, just like a piece of brocade. It's a kind of aerobics

能防止早衰、延缓衰老，并可预防腰椎的退行性病变。

2. 动作要领

（1）虚领顶劲：头颈有上悬意念，并保持正直，松而不僵可转动，这样利于保持身体重心的稳定。

（2）含胸拔背、沉肩垂肘：是指胸、背、肩、肘的姿势。胸要舒松微含，不可外挺或故意内缩；背要松沉直竖，躯干正直，前后均要平正，不凹不凸；两肩平正松沉，不可上耸、前扣或后张；肘要松垂，肘关节微屈，手臂伸缩运转时，轻灵沉着而不飘浮。

（3）手眼相应，以腰为轴，移步似猫行，虚实分清：指打拳时必须上下呼应，融为一体，要求动作出于意，发于腰，动于手，眼随手转，两下肢弓步和虚步分清而交替，练到腿上有劲，轻移慢放没有声音。

（4）用意识导引动作，用意不用力：用意念引出肢体的动作来，随意用力，劲虽使得很大，外表却看不出来。

（5）意气相合，气沉丹田：就是用意与呼吸相配合，呼吸要用腹式呼吸，一吸一呼正好与动作一开一合相配。

（6）动中求静，动静结合：即肢体动而脑子静，思想要集中于打拳，所谓形动于外，心静于内。

（7）动作连贯均匀，连绵不断：指每一招一式的动作要快慢均匀，而各式之间又是连绵不断。

（二）八段锦

八段锦是由八段动作组成的健身术，故名"八段"，又因其动作舒展，如锦缎般柔和优美，故称为"锦"。它起源于北宋，是作用较好的一套健身操。八段锦有坐式和立式两

originating from the Song Dynasty. Traditionally, Ba Duan Jin (eight-section exercise) contains two forms of sets with eight postures: a standing set and a seated set. Generally speaking, there are two major schools of standing set: the Southern and Northern Schools. The former one prefers gentle actions, and the latter one prefers actions with strength. In the modern era, the standing set from Southern School is more widely practiced. Due to the simple actions and moderate motions, Ba Duan Jin (eight-section exercise) is suitable for all people, especially for the elderly and people with chronic diseases.

1. Function　Ba Duan Jin (eight-section exercise) is often viewed as a healthy exercise. It has been proved beneficial in many aspects. It can help to improve the function of neurohumoral regulation, strengthen blood circulation, and massage abdominal organs. It is also conducive to regulate the functions of nervous system, cardiovascular system, digestive system, respiratory system, immune system and motor organs, to strengthen tendon and bones, to activate muscles and meridians, to delay the aging and increasing longevity. Besides, Ba Duan Jin (eight-section exercise) also has preventive and curative effects on headache, dizziness, scapulohumeral periarthritis, lumbocrural pain, indigestion, neurasthenia, *etc.*.

2. Key Point　Ba Duan Jin (eight-section exercise) includes eight consecutive sections. Specific procedures are listed as follows: pressing up to the heavens with two hands to stimulate the "Triple Warmer" meridian (*sān jiāo*); drawing the bow to either side and letting the arrow fly when squatting in a lower horse stance; separating heaven and earth to especially stimulate the spleen and stomach; looking backwards to prevent sickness and strain; sway the head and shake the tail to remove excess heat (or fire) from the heart; two hands holding the feet to strengthen the kidneys and waist; clenching the fists and glare fiercely (or angrily) to increase general vitality and muscular strength; bouncing on the toes seven pieces to cure diseases. When practicing Ba Duan Ji (eight-section exercise), one should calm down and concentrate on the pubic region (*dān tián*) point, with the head up, mouth closed, tongue tip touching upper palate, eyes looking at the front horizontally, body relaxed and breathing naturally.

(1) Breathe evenly: The movement should be coordinated with breath and mind. The breathing should be natural, smooth, deep, long and calm with the use of mind to induce movement.

(2) Concentrate on pubic region (*dān tián*): The exercise requires to "induce actions with mind". The

种形式。立式八段锦在风格上一般分为南派和北派，南派以柔为主，北派以刚为主。现在比较流行的是南派站式八段锦。八段锦术式简单，易学易练，运动量适中，适合各类人群，尤其是老年人和慢性病患者。

1. 作用　八段锦能改善神经体液调节功能和加强血液循环，对腹腔脏器有柔和的按摩作用，对神经系统、心血管系统、消化系统、呼吸系统、免疫系统及运动器官都有良好的调节作用，可以柔筋健骨，通筋活络。八段锦除了具有强身健体的作用外，对于头痛、眩晕、肩周炎、腰腿痛、消化不良、神经衰弱诸症也有防治的功效。

2. 动作要领　八段锦包括八节连贯的动作，具体内容如下：双手托天理三焦；左右开弓似射雕；调理脾胃需单举；五劳七伤往后瞧；摇头摆尾去心火；两手攀足固肾腰；攒拳怒目增气力；背后七颠百病消。练习八段锦应精神安定，意守丹田，头似顶悬，闭口，舌抵上腭，双目平视，全身放松，呼吸自然。

（1）呼吸均匀：八段锦同样要配合呼吸，呼吸自然、平稳，做到呼吸深、长、匀、静。同时呼吸、意念与每个动作的要领相配合，利用意识引导练功。

（2）意守丹田：八段锦的运动要求用意引导动作。意到身随，动作不僵不拘。要心情

actions should be smooth and natural with a good mood and peaceful mind. It lays stress on "omphaloskepsis", so the mind training is more important than the body training.

(3) Combine relaxing and contracting: When one practices this exercise, he should fully relax muscles and nerves, stabilize the body gravity first and then move slowly and forcibly according to the movement essentials. One should pay attention to releasing and holding of force. When releasing the force, it should be natural. When exerting force, it should be well distributed and stable.

iii. Wu Qin Xi (Five-Animal exercise)

Wu Qin refers to tiger, deer, bear, ape and bird (crane). Xi means to play games or to juggle. Hence Wu Qin Xi (five-animal exercise) is a set of exercise forms by imitating the movements of the five animals. Each Xi contains two actions: raising the tiger's paws, tiger spring; bumping with antlers, running like a deer; bear massaging, bear wobbling; wrist curling and elbow el elvating like a ape, ape picking; bird stretching, bird flying. Each action should be done symmetrically in both left and right side with conscious breathing. It was created by Hua Tuo, a famous physician in the later Han Dynasty by summing up the experience of the predecessors. Keep practicing Wu Qin Xi can not only strengthen joints and bones, but also cure diseases.

1. Function

(1) For mental health: When doing five-animal exercise, exercisers should keep peace of mind before and within every session. Therefore, it can relieve mental nervousness and enhance mood stability so as to keep mental health.

(2) For physical health: Each of the five-animal exercise has its own advantage. The combination of those exercises forms a systematic whole. Regular practice of Wu Qin Xi can play a role in regulating qi and blood, reinforcing *zang-fu* organs, inducing meridians, stretching muscles, and lubricating joint.

(3) For respiration adjustment: Practicing five-animal exercise can dredge channels and meridians and promote the circulation of qi and blood, strengthen the lung function in controlling respiration and the function of kidney in governing qi reception. Only when qi can flow smoothly, blood can flow smoothly. Sufficient qi will make people energetic, and improve the health status.

2. Key Point

(1) Relax the whole body: completely relax, and keep in a good mood and a high spirit so as to make blood and qi flow freely. Be loose combined with tight, and soft

舒坦，精神安定，意识与动作配合融汇一体。姿势自如，强调意守丹田，意练重于体练。

（3）刚柔相济：在练习八段锦时要求全身肌肉、神经均放松，身体重心放稳，根据动作要领，轻缓、用力地进行。练功时始终注意松中有紧，松力时要轻松自然，用力时要均匀，稳定而且含蓄在内。

（三）五禽戏

五禽是指虎、鹿、熊、猿、鸟（鹤）五种动物。戏，即游戏、戏耍之意。所谓五禽戏，是指模仿虎、鹿、熊、猿、鸟五种动物的动作和神态，组编而成的一套保健强身的方法。每戏包含两个动作，即虎举、虎扑；鹿抵、鹿奔；熊运、熊晃；猿提、猿摘；鸟伸、鸟飞。每种动作左势、右势对称各做一次，并配以气息的调理。五禽戏是我国后汉著名医家华佗整理总结而成的："体有不快，起作禽之戏，怡而汗出"。坚持练习五禽戏，不但能强壮筋骨，还有祛疾除病之效。

1. 作用

（1）调心作用：五禽戏要求练功者在练功前和习练每一戏时都要进行心理调节，以缓解精神紧张的状况，提高情绪的稳定性，保持心理健康。

（2）调身作用：五禽戏每一戏都各具特色，连起来又浑然一体。经常练习可起到调气血、益脏腑、通经络、活筋骨、利关节的作用。

（3）调息作用：五禽戏可以疏通经络，调畅气血，使肺主呼吸，肾主纳气的功能得到加强，气通则血通，气足则神旺，气的功能改善，则整个人体的经络血脉畅通，从而促进身体健康。

2. 动作要领

（1）全身放松：练功时，首先要全身放松，情绪要轻松乐观。乐观轻松的情绪可使气

coupled with hard. Relax the whole body in case that it is over stiff or tense.

(2) Breathe evenly: breathe slowly, quietly and naturally with abdominal respiration. When breathing, the mouth should be closed with the tongue tip touching the upper palate. "Breathing in with the nose and out with the mouth."

(3) Be focused: concentrate on the movements without being distracted or interrupted and make sure to coordinate mind with qi.

(4) Act naturally: The five-animal exercise has their distinct characteristics in actions, such as slowness of a bear, lightness of a monkey, robustness of a tiger, softness of a deer, and activeness of a crane. People should stretch their body naturally and smoothly based on the characteristics of these five animals.

(Yang Jin-hua)

Section 7　Nursing during the Convalescent Phase

During the convalescent phase, healthy qi is gradually restored, pathogenic qi is weakened, function of the viscera is gradually improved and the disease is going to be cured. At this stage, the functions of the viscera are not yet fully restored and the circulation of qi and blood is not smooth yet. Thus proper treatment and nursing should be applied so that the pathogenic factors can be eliminated completely and the functions of the viscera can be fully restored. Contrarily, improper treatment and nursing will lead to renascence of pathogenic factors, dysfunction of qi and blood of the viscera, maladjustment of yin and yang and the relapse of disease. Therefore, during the convalescent phase of diseases, emphasis should be placed on the following aspects: moderate physical exercise, proper balance between work and rest, nursing according to the variations of the season and climate, reasonable diet, regulating emotions and avoiding excess of the five emotions, as well as preventing relapse due to improper drug application.

I. Preventing Relapse Due to External Pathogenic Factor

External pathogenic factors here generally refer to

血通畅，精神振奋；要求松中有紧，柔中有刚，全身放松可使动作不至过分僵硬、紧张。

（2）呼吸均匀：呼吸要平静自然，使用腹式呼吸，均匀和缓。吸气时，口要合闭，舌尖轻抵上腭，做到吸气用鼻，呼气用嘴。

（3）专注意守：要排除杂念，精神专注，根据各戏意守要求，将意志集中于意守部位，以保证意、气相随。

（4）动作自然：五禽戏动作各有不同，如虎之刚健、鹿之温驯、猿之轻灵、熊之沉缓、鹤之活泼等。练功时应根据动作特点，自然舒展，不宜拘紧。

（杨金花）

第七节　病证后期调护

病证后期调护是指对处于正气渐复，邪气已衰，脏腑功能逐渐恢复，病情好转，已趋于痊愈时期患者的调护。在这个时期，由于脏腑功能尚未完全恢复，气血尚未平复，应该注意合理的调养和护理，以使病邪彻底清除，脏腑功能完全恢复。若调护不当，可使病邪在体内复燃，导致脏腑气血紊乱，阴阳失调，而使疾病复发。因此，做好病证后期的调护十分重要，患者应适当锻炼以增强体质，劳逸适度；顺应四时气候变化，做好护理；合理调配饮食；调畅情志，防止五志过极。

一、防止因外邪复病

外邪，指六淫之邪。大病初愈之人，气

the six climatic factors. For the people who have newly recovered from the serious disease, the circulation of qi and blood is not smooth yet, the healthy qi is still insufficient and the defensive function of the body is weak. So they are prone to be attacked by the six climatic factors leading to the relapse of disease.

i. Cultivating Healthy Qi and Reinforcing Body Resistance

Defensive qi of the body distributes over the surface, circulates outside the vessels and has protective function for the body. It is the main safeguard of the body resistance against the invasion of the six climatic factors. So the exogenous factors are difficult to invade the body if the defensive qi is abundant. The defensive qi comes from the food essence transported and transformed by the spleen and stomach. It originates from the lower *jiao* and is dispersed by the *lung-qi*. Its main function is resisting the invasion of the exogenous pathogens. At the beginning of recovery, it is necessary to cultivate healthy qi, reinforce body constitution and strengthen body resistance. The methods are listed as follows:

1. The basic measure includes reasonable diet, sufficient nutrients and cultivating the kidney and spleen.

2. Have a sunbath for the back or the whole body to reinforce yang qi. The sunbath usually is carried out in the early morning when the sunlight is warm except in winter. This can make the body contact with air frequently so that the defensive qi is trained and has a smarter defensive function.

3. Take moderate physical exercises, such as taking a walk, jogging, doing *qigong* and Tai ji quan to strengthen body constitution.

4. Regulate daily life according to the climate. In spring and summer when it is gradually getting warmer and hotter, people should rise early in the morning and take a hike in the courtyard to make yang qi more abundant. In autumn and winter when it turns from hot to cool, then cold, people should rest early and rise late to make yang qi be stored inside and not escape.

ii. Avoiding Invasion of Pathogenic Factor

At the beginning of recovery, healthy qi is not yet fully restored, as well as qi and blood are not yet abundant and their defensive function and adapting ability are weak. So it is important to strictly prevent the invasion of the six climatic factors. The daily life should adapt to the climatic variations. The concrete measures are listed as follows.

1. Modifying the nursing methods according to seasonal climatic variations. One should not reduce clothes and quilts abruptly when it turns warm, and

血未复，正气尚虚，机体的卫外防御功能低下，常易感受六淫之邪而引起疾病的复发。

（一）扶正固卫

人体卫气分布于体表，运行于脉外，具有护卫机体作用，是抵御六淫之邪入侵的主要力量。卫气来源于脾胃运化的水谷精微，根于下焦，又依赖于肺气的宣发。病后初愈时要扶助正气，增强体质，提高机体卫外抗病的能力，具体措施如下：

1. 合理饮食，加强营养，补益脾肾是扶正固卫的根本措施。

2. 利用日光，晒浴背部或全身，以补养人体的阳气。一般除冬季外，以晨起阳光温煦不烈为日光浴的最佳时间，机体通过与外界空气经常接触，使卫气得到锻炼，卫外开合功能更为灵敏。

3. 适当的锻炼，如散步、慢跑、气功、太极拳等，以增强体质。

4. 制订合理的作息时间，春夏之季，天气由寒转暖、由暖转热，应早起床，广步于庭，使阳气更加充沛；秋冬之季，气候由热转凉而寒，应早卧晚起，使阳气内藏不致外泄。

（二）谨避风邪

患者在病后恢复阶段，正气尚虚，气血未充，卫外功能低下，适应能力较弱，应注意防止虚邪贼风的侵袭。生活起居应做到顺应四时，具体措施如下：

1. 根据四时寒热温凉气候变化而随时调护。如春季不可遇天气转暖而骤减衣被，春、

prevent contagions in spring and autumn. It is so hot in summer that people should pay attention to prevent sunstroke by lowering moderately indoor temperature and take medicine with effect of preventing sunstroke. One shouldn't be undressed in the wind when there is sweat, or take too much cold or iced drink and food, or enter into a cold room abruptly. One should keep warm in case of catching a cold when staying outdoors in cold winter, ventilate room timely to keep air fresh, and take medicine to avoid flu.

2. Keeping moderate indoor temperature and humidity in case pathogenic factors attaching other climatic factors to invade into the body.

3. Keeping environmental and personal sanitation. One should change clothes when it is wetted by sweat in case of incurring exogenous factors.

II. Preventing Relapse Due to Improper Diet

The spleen and stomach of the people who have just recovered from serious diseases are still weak. Improper diet is easy to incur relapse of the disease. The spleen and stomach are regarded as the root of life acquirement and the origin for qi and blood production. At the beginning of recovery, the residual pathogen is still not removed totally and the spleen and stomach are still weak. Improper diet is easy to incur the relapse of disease. The *Yellow Emperor's Inner Classic* says that "the intake of meat will lead to the relapse when the febrile disease is just cured. Eating too much will lead to the remaining of the febrile pathogen. This should be prohibited." So reasonable diet regulating is very important at this stage.

i. Reasonable Diet

For the patients at the beginning of recovery, the balance between yin and yang is unstable, healthy qi is insufficient and pathogenic factors still remains. One should prevent over-nutrition and retaining of pathogenic factors due to indulging in tonic food. So what one needs to do is as follows:

1. The diet should be reasonable, having a scientific proportion and be nutritious and various.

2. The diet should be bland and easy to be digested and absorbed. One should eat for more times with a small amount each time. One shouldn't eat too rapidly. Careful mastication and slow swallowing are advisable.

3. The diet should be healthy. One should avoid uncooked, cold food, hot food and unhygienic food, as well as prevent partiality to tonic.

秋季注意预防传染病；夏天炎热，注意防暑降温，适当降低室温，服用避暑药预防中暑，但不可袒胸露腹、贪凉饮冷或骤入凉室，汗出当风；冬季严寒外出应注意保暖，以免外感风寒，居室要定时开窗通气，保持空气新鲜，在感冒流行时可服药预防。

2. 保持居室内适宜的温、湿度，以防风邪相兼他邪而复感。

3. 注意环境以及个人清洁卫生，汗出后及时更衣，防止复感外邪。

二、防止因食复病

因食复病是指大病初愈，脾胃尚虚，因饮食不当，而导致疾病复发。脾胃为后天之本、气血生化之源。病后初愈，余邪未尽，脾胃虚弱，饮食不节极易导致疾病的复发，即所谓食复。《素问·热论》说："病热少愈，食肉则复，多食则遗，此其禁也。"可见合理的饮食调护在病证后期的重要性。

（一）合理膳食

由于病后初愈者具有阴阳平衡不稳及正虚邪恋的特点，应防止偏补太过与因补滞邪，因此，要求做到如下几个方面：

1. 饮食结构合理，科学搭配，营养丰富。

2. 饮食宜清淡、易消化，少食多餐，进食不可过急过快，宜细嚼慢咽。

3. 饮食应卫生，避免生冷、炙热、不洁饮食。

4. Differentiating syndromes to decide the food and tonic. The patients with cold syndrome should select warm-natured but not too hot food and tonic. The patients with heat syndrome should select cool-natured but not too cold food and tonic. The patients with deficiency syndrome should not take too much tonic.

ii. Abstinence from Special Food

For the patients whose diseases are newly cured, their pathogenic factor is still retained inside. It is advisable to keep away from the food that can strengthen the pathogenic factor and consume the healthy qi in case of relapse of disease. For example, the patients recovering from febrile illness should not take warm, hot or spicy food. The patients recovering from edema should abstain from salt. The patients recovering from diarrhea should abstain from fat and sweet food which all increases dampness. The patients recovering from skin rash should abstain from seafood. Besides, alcohol can increase heat and dampness so it is not fit for any disease.

III. Preventing Relapse Due to Overstrain

Relapse due to overstrain usually occurs in three aspects, which are physical overstrain, mental overstrain and sexual overstrain.

i. Abstinence from Physical Overstrain

During the rehabilitation, it is necessary to take moderate physical training such as taking a walk or doing Tai ji quan to promote the circulation of qi and blood, improve appetite and enhance constitution. It is helpful for the thorough recovery. The patients should not only persevere in physical labor or training but also avoid physical overstrain according to the principle of "a light labor without fatigue".

ii. Abstinence from Mental Overstrain

Mental overstrain may impair the heart and spleen and consume qi and blood. It is advisable to abstain from excess mental labor. The patients should regulate their style of life, combine moderate physical labor and mental labor, as well as keep in a pleasant mood.

iii. Abstinence from Sexual Overstrain

Sexual overstrain always impairs the kidney and leads to the consumption of kidney essence. When one is recovering from serious disease, one's kidney essence is quite deficient. Excessive sexual activity would make it more deficient. So during the stage of rehabilitation, the patients and spouses should be told to abstain from excessive sexual activity before thorough recovery so as to

4. 辨证施养，如寒病者，偏于温养，但不宜过燥；热病者，宜清养，但应防其过寒；虚证者不宜大补等，防止伤及脾胃。

（二）注意忌口

对于病后初愈之人，由于病邪余焰未熄，故凡能增邪伤正的饮食，皆应注意忌口，以免因食复病。如热病瘥后忌食温燥辛辣之品，水肿者忌盐，泻痢者忌滋腻增湿之物，瘾疹者忌食鱼虾海鲜等。又如醇酒助热增湿，诸病愈后，皆不相宜。

三、防止因劳复病

劳复是指病后初愈，因形体劳倦、劳神劳心及房劳过度等引起疾病的复发。

（一）防形体劳倦

病后初愈之时，应量力进行必要的形体活动，使气血流畅，增进食欲，增强体质，有助于彻底康复，如散步、打太极拳等。患者既要坚持劳动或运动锻炼，又要避免体劳过度，应以小劳不倦为原则。

（二）防劳神劳心

劳神劳心过度，会伤及心脾两脏，耗尽气血。应避免用脑过度。患者应调整生活方式，适度的体力劳动和脑力劳动相结合，保持心情舒畅。

（三）防房劳复病

房劳多累及肾，肾精耗损。大病之后，肾精本亏，再加房劳必令其更虚，故病后初愈，应分别对患者及配偶强调在身体完全康复之前宜静养，防止房劳耗伤肾精而致疾病复发。

prevent relapse due to consumption of kidney essence.

IV. Preventing Relapse Due to Extreme Emotion

Extreme emotions will cause disorder of qi activity and disharmony of visceral yin and yang, qi and blood or directly affect the viscera, and then lead to occurrence of diseases. At the late stage of disease, attention should be paid to regulate emotions in case of the relapse of disease.

i. Regulating Emotion

During the convalescent phase of diseases, it still needs a period of time to rehabilitate the visceral function. The patients are easy to be impatient. Improper emotional stimulations would affect the visceral function and lead to exacerbation or deterioration of diseases. Therefore, it is necessary to enlighten these patients actively and offer psychological nursing to them purposefully. The patients should build up optimism, remain a pleasant mood and avoid excessive emotional activities. It is beneficial for health to cultivate a pleasing temperament according to the personal character.

ii. Avoiding Extreme Emotion

When they impair the internal organs, the seven emotions mainly affect the activity of visceral qi and lead to disorder of the activity of qi. At the stage of rehabilitation, the extreme emotions of the patients would lead to exacerbation or deterioration of diseases. Therefore, at the late stage of diseases, the patients should avoid various unfavorable environmental and mental stimulations. The patients should remain optimistic, open-minded and self-confident, as well as be ready to adapt to the various discomfort conditions, so that the viscera would be sedate and the activity of qi would be in order. Then the disease would be cured thoroughly.

V. Preventing Relapse Due to Improper Drug Application

The spleen and stomach of the people who have just recovered from serious diseases are still weak. Improper drug application is easy to incur the relapse of disease. The spleen and stomach are regarded as the root of life acquirement and the origin for qi and blood production. At the beginning of recovery, the residual pathogen is still not removed totally and the spleen and stomach are still weak. Improper drug application is easy to incur the relapse of disease, especially for patients who suffer from peptic diseases. Therefore, rational intake of drug is very

四、防止因情复病

情志过极，可致气机紊乱，脏腑气血阴阳失调，也可直接影响脏腑发生疾病。在病证后期应注意调畅情志，防止五志过极，以免因情复病。

（一）调畅情志

病证后期，脏腑功能恢复需要一段时间，患者容易产生急躁等不良情志，这些不良刺激都可以影响脏腑功能，而使病情加重或恶化，因此，要给予积极的开导，有针对性地进行心理治疗，使患者树立乐观情绪，保持心情舒畅，避免七情过度。根据性格和情趣怡情悦志，以益于身体健康。

（二）避免情志过激

七情变动影响脏腑气机，导致气机紊乱，损伤五脏。患者在休养期间，如果出现情志变动和过激，可使病情加重，或迅速恶化。因此，在病证后期，应使患者避免各种不良环境、精神因素的刺激。应使患者保持乐观情绪，胸怀开阔，树立信心，主动适应各种不适情况，以使五脏安和，气机调畅，促进疾病痊愈。

五、防止因药复病

因药复病是指大病初愈，脾胃尚虚，因服药不当，而导致疾病复发。脾胃为后天之本、气血生化之源。病后初愈，余邪未尽，脾胃虚弱，服药不节极易导致疾病的复发，尤其是胃肠疾病的患者，因此病后合理服药很重要。

important for the people recovering from diseases.

i. Reasonable Drug Application

For the patients at the beginning of recovery, the balance between yin and yang, qi and blood is unstable. Over eating herbs with bitter-cold or bitter-dryness can result in the injury of patient's spleen and stomach with the manifestation of epigastric pain or diarrhea. So, the intake of the neutral herbs and herbs strengthening spleen and stomach are recommended for this kind of patients to keep healthy.

ii. Avoid over Intake of Tonic

For the patients whose diseases are newly cured, the intake of proper tonics is important. But improper intake of tonics can result in adverse reactions. For example, over intake of yang-tonifying herbs or qi-tonifying herbs can cause yin-fluid injury and heat accumulation. Over intake of blood-tonifying herbs or yin-nourishing herbs can result in poor digestion. So for this kind of patients, gentle neutral-tonifying herbs are recommended to avoid secondary diseases.

(Xu Dong-Ying)

（一）合理用药

由于病后初愈者身体出现气、血、阴、阳偏虚，服药时应避免苦寒、辛燥之品，因苦寒败胃、苦燥伤阴，易造成脾胃损伤，可出现胃脘痛、腹泻等病证。因此在此阶段，患者应根据身体情况，选择药性温和的药物和健脾胃的药物进行调理身体。

（二）避免过补

病后初愈之人，由于正气不足，应适当选用补益之品，补益药虽然能增强体质，但如果误投错用，危害亦大。补气、补阳药性多温燥，过用可伤阴助火，补血、补阴药，性多黏滞，过用妨碍消化功能。因此，对病后初愈，应选用清淡平补之品缓缓调理，以防过补滋生他病。

（徐冬英）

Key Points

1. People should follow the basic principle of "nourishing yang in spring and summer while nourishing yin in autumn and winter" in seasonal health preservation.

2. In spring and summer, people should go to bed later at night and get up earlier in the morning. In autumn, people should go to bed earlier at night and get up earlier in the morning. In winter, people should go to bed earlier at night and get up later in the morning.

3. Excessive joy damages the heart; excessive anger damages the liver; excessive thinking damages the spleen; excessive grief damages the lung; excessive fear damages the kidney.

4. Anger causes qi to rise; excessive joy causes qi to slacken; sorrow consumes qi; fear causes qi to sink; fright causes qi to be chaotic; excessive thinking causes qi to knot.

5. Principles of emotional nursing includes being sincere and considerate, nursing based on the people and avoiding stimuli.

6. The nursing of inter-restriction among emotions also known as mutual restriction between seven emotions, is to use one emotion to restrict another emotion in order to relieve or eliminate bad mood and to keep good mental state.

7. Empathic Therapy means a series of methods to transfer or change one's emotion and attention with certain measures to dispel bad emotion.

重点

1. 四时养生必须遵循"春夏养阳，秋冬养阴"的基本原则。

2. 春季和夏季应夜卧早起，秋季应早卧早起，冬季应早卧晚起。

3. 喜伤心，怒伤肝，思伤脾，悲、忧伤肺，恐伤肾。

4. 怒则气上，喜则气缓，悲（忧）则气消，恐则气下惊则气乱，思则气结。

5. 情志调护的原则包诚挚体贴、因人施护和避免刺激。

6. 以情胜情法又叫情志制约法，指以一种情志抑制另一种情志，以淡化或消除不良情绪，保持良好精神状态的一种方法。

7. 以情胜情法是通过一定的方法和措施转移或改变人的情绪和注意力，以解脱不良情绪

8. The method of persuasion means persuading patients by using correct and wise words to correct one's viewpoint, realize the harm brought by one's behavior, relieve one's unnecessary worry, boost one's confidence in fighting against the disease, follow doctors and nurses' advice to achieve early recovery.

9. Restraining is a method to prevent drastic emotions through regulating feelings and controlling sentiments to achieve psychological balance.

10. Dietary nursing is a vital part in health promotion and disease treatment, guided by the theory of pattern differentiation, the essence of which is to provide strategies for nursing care on nutrition and dietary, thus to supplement the *zang-fu* organs, dispel pathogen and balance yin and yang.

11. The performance of foods includes property, flavor and channel entry are the key to the specific performance. The properties of foods include coldness, hotness, warmness, and coolness, generally called four properties. The flavors of foods include acrid, sweet, sour, bitter and salty flavor. And the channel entry of foods is defined as the obvious function on the *zang-fu*, channels and collaterals.

12. Function of dietary nursing includes reinforcing healthy qi and supplementing deficiency, expelling excess to dispel pathogen, preventing disease and prolonging life.

13. The basic principle of dietary nursing includes adhering to an abstemious and regular diet, balancing the performance of foods, guaranteeing the dietary sanity, keeping delicate diet and reasonable processing, adhering to pattern differentiation and keeping good eating habits.

14. Food selection should take individual health condition, the specific function of foods and their combination into account.

的方法。

8. 说理开导法是指通过运用正确、巧妙的语言，对人进行劝说开导，端正人对事物的看法，认识自己的行为所造成的危害，解除不必要的忧愁顾虑，提高战胜疾病的信心，积极配合治疗，使机体早日康复。

9. 节制法指调节情绪，节制感情，防止七情过激，从而达到心理平衡的方法。

10. 饮食调护是指在治疗疾病的过程中，根据辨证施护的原则，利用食物自身的特性，对患者进行营养和膳食方面的指导和护理，以补益脏腑，祛邪扶正，调整阴阳，从而防病治病，促进健康。

11. 食物的性味归经决定着食物的功能效应。食物按其"性"可分为寒、热、温、凉，即"四性"；按其"味"可分为辛、甘、酸、苦、咸，即"五味"。食物的归经，为食物对人体脏腑及经络产生的明显作用。

12. 饮食调护的作用包括扶正补虚、泻实祛邪、防病益寿。

13. 饮食调护的基本原则包括饮食有节、搭配相宜、洁净卫生、饮食清淡、加工合理、辨证施食、习惯良好。

14. 食物的选择应权衡患者的体质及食物的性能与调和。

Chapter 5　Medication and Nursing of TCM

第五章　中医用药及护理

Learning Objectives

Mastery

1. To repeat the contraindications and indications of Chinese herbs.

2. To repeat the basic requirements of decocting methods of Chinese herbs.

3. To repeat all special decocting methods and its corresponding types of Chinese herbs.

4. To repeat the eight therapeutic methods of TCM and its corresponding nursing requirements.

Comprehension

1. To explain the common dosage forms of Chinese herbs.

2. To explain the principles of Chinese herbs medication.

Application

To apply resue and nursing methals of common Chinese herbal medicine poisoning.

学习目标

识记

1. 能复述中药用药禁忌。

2. 能复述中药煎煮法的基本要求。

3. 能复述特殊煎药法的种类及适用的药物。

4. 能复述中医用药八法及其护理要求。

理解

1. 理解中药常用剂型。

2. 理解中药给药规则。

应用

常用中草药进行中毒解救及护理方法。

Chapter 5

Case Study

Guì Zhī Tāng is the most primary prescription of *Treatise on Cold Damage and Miscellaneous Diseases*. It's called the Crown of Zhong Jing's all Prescriptions. In the annotation of *Guì Zhī Tāng*, it expatiates the herbal decocting methods and medication nursing. For example, it requires that the herbs should be chopped into small pieces with teeth. It also notes that "one may use seven liters (1 ancient liter is equal to 1.5kg) of water to decoct the herbs with weak fire and stop decocting when the decoction becomes three liters, then get rid of the dreg and drink one liter." It requires that after taking the decoction one may "eat one liter hot gruel to help exert the power of the decoction" and "keep warm with quilt for about two hours and mildly sweat all over to get better effect," but the diaphoresis "should not be too heavy, or the illness wouldn't be cured." For those seriously-ill patients, it needs 24 hours monitoring. Besides, it advises that one should "keep away from the food that is raw or cold, sticky or slippery, meaty or starchy, pungent or spicy, alcoholic, milky or effluvial after taking *Guì Zhī Tāng*".

Question: How many kinds of medication and nursing of TCM are involved in the case?

导入案例与思考

桂枝汤为《伤寒论》第一方，乃"仲景群方之冠"，其方中药物的用法及服药后护理方面的内容相当丰富。例如要求将药物"㕮咀（是指将药用口咬碎成小块）""以水七升，煮取三升""微火煮取"，其次，对于汗出的效果描述是"遍身絷絷微似有汗者益佳，不可令如水流漓，病必不除。"简言之，即周身连续微汗，而非大汗淋漓。此外，还要"啜粥"或"温覆"，对于病重者还需要"周时观之"。并主张服桂枝汤后要"禁生冷、黏滑、肉面、五辛、酒酪、臭恶等物"。

问题：分析本案例所涉及的中医用药护理有哪些？

Section 1   Dosage Form and Usage of Chinese Herb

第一节　中药剂型与用法

The forms of TCM preparations refer to the definite forms of drugs processed according to their properties and the purpose of medication. Different forms of preparations have their own characteristics and indications. There are more and more new forms invented with the development of TCM. The following are several widely used forms.

方剂在使用前，根据药性特点和治疗需要加工成一定的制剂形式，称为剂型。不同的剂型有其特点和适用范围。随着祖国医学的发展，新的剂型不断出现。现将常用的中药剂型介绍如下。

I. Decoction

一、汤剂

Decoctions are obtained by boiling the selected drugs which have been soaked in an appropriate amount of water or yellow rice wine for some time and then removing the residual masses. It is the most commonly used form of prepared drugs with the characteristics of quick absorption and action. The recipe can be modified to meet the needs of therapeutic purpose and is applicable to both acute and chronic illness. The decoction can be used internally or

汤剂系指将药物配成方剂后，加水或黄酒浸泡后，煎煮一定时间，去渣取汁，成为汤剂。其特点是吸收快，作用迅速，加减灵活，适用于慢性和急性病证。内服、灌肠、熏洗均可。

externally or for the purpose of fumigant and lotion.

II. Pill and Bolus

Pills and boluses are round solid form of preparations obtained by grinding drugs into powder, and mixing them with excipients such as water, honey, rice paste, flour paste, wine, vinegar and drug juices. Characterized by slow absorption, long efficacy, convenient taking, carrying and storage, they are the ideal forms for chronic diseases. The commonly used forms are described as follows:

i. Honeyed Bolus or Pill

Honeyed boluses or pills are made by grinding medicinal materials into fine powder, and mixing it with refined honey. Because honey is used as excipient, honeyed boluses or pills share the same functions as honey. They have the functions of benefiting vital energy, strengthening the middle warmer, reliving spasm, alleviating pain, relieving a cough, lubricating large intestine, detoxicating, harmonizing properties of herbs, modifying the taste and smell of herbs. They are applicable to various acute and chronic diseases, such as *Shèn Qì Wán* and *Ān Gōng Niú Huáng Wán*.

ii. Water-Paste Pill

Water-paste pills are made by fine powder of medicinal materials mixed with soluble liquid as excipients including water, wine, vinegar, some drug extracts and sugar liquid, characterized by easy absorption and quick effects, such as *Bǎo Hé Wán* and *Liù Shén Wán*.

iii. Paste-Pill

Paste-pills are medicinal mass made by grinding medicinal materials into fine powder mixed with paste of rice or flour as excipients. Paste-pills are hard in quality when they are dry, so the pills are decomposed and absorbed more slowly than honeyed boluses or pills and water-paste pills. These are very potential dosage form for strong irritants or poisonous medicinal materials which require being absorbed slowly, thus prolonging the therapeutic effect and reducing the gastro-intestinal irritation, such as *Xī Huáng Wán*.

iv. Concentrated Pill

Concentrated pills are made by decocting certain medicinal materials in a recipe and concentrating them into paste, mixing the extract with the powder of rest ingredients, drying and grinding the mixed materials into powder, mixing the powder with water, wine, or decoction of specific ingredients in the recipe as excipients. The concentrated pills are small in size, easy to take and store,

二、丸剂

丸剂系指根据配方要求，将药物研细，用水或蜂蜜、米糊、面糊、酒、醋、药汁等作为赋形剂制成圆形固体制剂。具有吸收慢，药力持久，服用、携带及贮存方便等特点，多用于慢性疾病的治疗。临床上常用的有以下几种：

（一）蜜丸

蜜丸系指以炼制过的蜂蜜为黏合剂将药材细粉制成的丸剂。因蜜丸中含有蜂蜜，故能益气补中，缓急止痛；滋润补虚，止咳润肠；还能起解毒、缓和药性、矫味矫臭等作用，适用于多种急慢性疾病，如肾气丸，安宫牛黄丸。

（二）水丸

水丸系指以水或水性液体（黄酒、醋、稀药汁、糖液等）为黏合剂将药材细粉制成的丸剂。水丸的特点是服用后在体内易于吸收，显效较快，如保和丸和六神丸。

（三）糊丸

糊丸系指以米糊或面糊等为黏合剂将药材细粉制成的丸剂。糊丸黏性大，干燥后较坚硬，服用后崩解和吸收较蜜丸、水丸缓慢。某些毒性药物或刺激性强的药物宜制成糊丸使用，使其服用后在体内徐徐吸收，既可延长药效，又减少药物对胃肠道的刺激，如犀黄丸。

（四）浓缩丸

浓缩丸系指将方中某些药物煎汁浓缩成膏，再与方中其他药物的细粉混合，经干燥、粉碎，以水或酒或方中部分药物的煎出液为赋形剂制成的丸剂。其特点是体积小，易于服用和吸收，发挥药效好，同时利于保存，

quickly digestive, effective and away from mildew and rot. But they have the risk of losing the active chemicals due to process in high temperature for long time.

v. Minute Pellet

Minute pellets are medicinal pills that are less than 2.5mm in diameter, with spherical or ellipsoidal shape, characterized by good appearance and fluidity, high content, low dose, stable and reliable release, well-distributed, large specific surface area, rapid dissolution and high bioavailability. Some of the TCM preparations had characteristics of minute pellet as early as in ancient times, such as *Liù Shén Wán* and *Hóu zhèng Wán*.

vi. Wax Pill

Wax pills are medicinal pills made by fine powder of medicinal materials mixed with beeswax as adhesive. The main components normally have low polarity and water undissolved properties. The pills can extend activity, release drugs slowly and prevent poisoning and harmonizing strong gastrointestinal irritation. But the variety is insufficient due to the difficultly in controlling release rate.

vii. Drop Pill

Drop pills refer to medicinal pills made by extracts mixed with medium, then dripped into undissolved condensate. These pills have quick action, and high bioavailability. They can be both applied internally, externally or in body cavities with large dose for low drug loading dosage.

III. Powder

Powders are dry intimate mixtures, which are further divided into internal (oral powders) or external (topical powders) use. They are quick in effect, simple in manufacture, easy in administration and convenient in storage. Therefore, powder is one of the commonly used dosage forms in clinic.

IV. Paste

They are medicinal preparations made by concentrating after decocting drugs in water or vegetable oil. These preparations are divided into two kinds, extract for oral administration and ointment and adhesive plaster for external application. Extract for oral administration is subdivided into semisolid or dry extracts, fluidextract and soft extracts while those for external application are

不易霉变，但是由于制作过程中受热时间较长，有些成分可能会受到影响，使药效降低。

（五）微丸

微丸系指直径小于 2.5mm 的各类球形或类球形的药剂。微丸具有外形美观，流动性好；含药量大，服用剂量小；释药稳定、可靠、均匀；表面积大，溶出快，生物利用度高等特点。中药制剂中很早就有微丸的特征，如六神丸，喉症丸等制剂均有微丸的特征。

（六）蜡丸

蜡丸系指以蜂蜡为黏合剂将药材细粉制成的丸剂。蜡丸的主要成分极性小，不溶于水，制成丸剂后在体内释放药物极慢，可延长药效，并能防止药物中毒或防止对胃肠道的强烈刺激，由于无法控制蜡丸释放药物的速率，目前其品种不多。

（七）滴丸

滴丸系指药材提取物与基质用适宜方法混匀后，滴入不相混溶的冷凝液中，收缩冷凝制成的丸剂。中药滴丸剂的主要特点是起效迅速，生物利用度高；滴丸用药部位多，可口服，腔道用和外用；滴丸载药量小，含药量低，服药剂量大。

三、散剂

散剂系指将一种或多种药材混合而成的干燥粉末状制剂。按医疗用途可将其分为内服散剂与外用散剂。散剂因奏效快，制法简便，剂量可随意增减，运输携带方便，亦是临床常用剂型之一。

四、膏剂

膏剂系指将药物用水或植物油煎熬浓缩而成的剂型，分内服和外用两种。内服膏剂有浸膏、流浸膏、煎膏三种；外用膏剂有软膏剂、硬膏剂两种。

subdivided into two kinds, ointments and plasters.

i. Semisolid or Dry Extract

They are semisolid or solid forms of preparation made by extraction of the effective components from drugs with solvents and by distillation of the solvents at low temperature. In accordance with the formulated standard, 1g extract is as effective as 2g to 5g drugs and the water content of semisolid or dry extracts is 15%-20% and 5% respectively. They tend to be served to make tablets, powders, capsules, granules, and pills.

ii. Fluidextract

Fluidextract is liquid preparations made by extraction of the effective components from drugs with solvents and by distillation of the solvents at low temperature, and by adjusting the concentration of extraction and alcohol to certain standard. Unless otherwise specified, 1ml fluidextract contains the therapeutic constituents of 1g of the standard drug that it represents. Fluidextract may be served as ingredients for other preparations such as tincture, syrup and mixture. The commonly used are *Gān Cǎo Liú Jìn Gāo* and *Yì Mǔ Cǎo Liú Jìn Gāo*.

iii. Soft Extract

Soft extract, also known as Caozi, refers to the thick semi-solid extraction dosage form (such as loquat paste) made by repeatedly decocting medicinal materials to a certain degree, removing dregs, extracting juice, and then concentrating, adding appropriate amount of honey or sugar. The decoction has the advantages of high concentration, small volume, good stability and easy to take. The effect of soft extract is mainly aimed to strengthen the weak body with calm therapeutic effects, so it is suitable for many kinds of chronic diseases.

iv. Ointment

Ointments are semisolid preparations intended for external application to the skin or mucous membranes. They are made by mixing drug powder and extract with suitable bases. Ointments act to protect and lubricate the skin for local treatment. They are applicable to chronic skin diseases but prohibited in acute skin diseases, such as *Sān Huáng Ruǎn Gāo*.

v. Plaster

Plasters refer to a form of preparations made by mixing drugs with stick bases or dissolving drugs in bases. They remain in a solid state at normal temperature, while at 36℃ or 37℃, they change to be softer and act on the affected local region or on the whole body, such as *Gǒu Pí Gāo* and *Shāng Shī Zhǐ Tòng Gāo*.

（一）浸膏

浸膏系指用溶媒将药物中的有效成分浸出后，低温将溶媒全部蒸发除去而成的半固体或固体浸出剂型。按规定标准，每1g浸膏相当于2~5g药物。浸膏又分为干浸膏和稠浸膏两种，其中干浸膏含水量为5%，稠浸膏一般的含水量为15%~20%。浸膏剂一般多用于配制片剂、散剂、胶囊剂、颗粒剂、丸剂等。

（二）流浸膏

流浸膏系指用适当溶媒浸出药物中的有效成分后，将浸出液中部分溶媒用低温蒸发除去，并调整浓度及含醇量至规定的标准而成的液体浸出剂型。除特殊规定外，流浸膏剂每1ml相当于原药材1g。流浸膏除少数品种可直接供临床使用外，大多作为配制其他制剂的原料。流浸膏剂一般多用于配制酊剂、合剂、糖浆剂等。常用的有甘草流浸膏、益母草流浸膏等。

（三）煎膏

煎膏又称膏滋，系指药材反复煎煮至一定程度，去滓取汁，再浓缩，加入适量蜂蜜或糖熬制而成的稠厚半固体浸出剂型（如枇杷膏）。煎膏剂具有药物浓度高，体积小，稳定性好，便于服用等优点。煎膏剂的效用以滋补为主，兼有缓和的治疗作用，多用于慢性疾病。

（四）软膏剂

软膏剂又称为药膏，系指药物、药材细粉、药材提取物与适宜基质混合制成的半固体外用剂型（如三黄软膏）。软膏剂主要用于保护皮肤、润滑皮肤和局部治疗，多用于慢性皮肤病，禁用于急性皮肤疾患。

（五）硬膏剂

硬膏剂系指将药物溶解或混合于黏性基质中制成的一类近似固体的外用剂型（如狗皮膏、伤湿止痛膏）。常温时呈固体状态，36~37℃时则软化释放药力，起到局部或全身治疗作用。

V. Pellet

Pellets refer to a form of preparations made by heating the medicinal minerals containing mercury and sulphur to sublimation. The advantages are that they are small in dosage but very effective and economic as a preparation for external application for chronic infective diseases, psoriasis, and chronic nasal sinusitis. Internal application should be prohibited because of the heavy metal toxicity.

VI. Gelatin

Gelatin or glue refers to a form of preparations made by decocting animal skin, bone, shell and horn in water until the material is condensed to a dry mass. With the functions of nourishing blood, stopping bleeding, dispelling wind evil and regulating menstruation, it is often indicated for fatigue, debility, consumptive diseases, haematemesis hemorrhage, uterine bleeding, soreness of lower back and knees, such as *ē jiāo* and *lù jiǎo jiāo*.

VII. Medicinal Wine

Wine preparation refers to transparent medicated liquid obtained by removal of the effective components from drugs in wine as a solvent. With the function of expelling wind, activating blood flow, dispelling stasis and alleviating pain, the wine preparation is served for the treatment of rheumatic pain and traumatic injury. But it may not be suitable for patients with hypertension and coronary heart disease, children and pregnant women. The commonly used are *Shí Quán Dà Bǔ Jiǔ* and *Fēng Shī Yào Jiǔ*.

VIII. Distilled Medicinal Liquid

Distilled medicinal liquid is obtained by distilling fresh drugs containing volatile oil in water by heating. It is bland in flavor, delicately aromatic and colorless and convenient to take orally. Usually it is served as beverage, especially in summer, such as *Jīn Yín Huā Lù*.

IX. Medicated Tea

It is a solid preparation made by pulverization of

五、丹剂

丹剂系指用含有汞、硫磺等成分的矿物药进行加热升华所得到的化合制剂。其特点是用量少，廉价易得，药效确切，用法多样化。临床上常用于治疗体表及慢性化脓感染、慢性鼻窦炎、牛皮癣等外科疾病。但其毒性较大，一般不可内服，并在使用中要注意剂量和应用部位，以免引起重金属中毒。

六、胶剂

胶剂系指用动物皮、骨、甲、角等为原料，以水煎提取胶质，浓缩成稠胶状，干燥后制成的固体块状（如阿胶，鹿角胶）。胶剂多供内服，其功能为补血、止血、祛风以及妇科调经等，以治疗虚劳、羸瘦、吐血、衄血、崩漏、腰腿酸软等症。

七、酒剂

酒剂又称药酒，系指用蒸馏酒浸泡药材，去渣提取澄清液体而制得的剂型（如十全大补酒、风湿药酒）。药酒多供内服，并加糖或蜂蜜矫味和着色。酒剂有祛风活血、散瘀止痛的功效，适用于治疗风湿痹痛、跌打损伤，但儿童、孕妇、心脏病及高血压患者不宜使用。

八、药露

药露又称露剂，系指将新鲜的含挥发性成分的药材用蒸馏法制成的芳香水剂（如金银花露）。药露气味清淡，芳香无色，便于口服。一般用作饮料，夏季尤为常用。

九、茶剂

茶剂系指将药物粉碎、加工而制成的粗

vegetable drugs, or by compressing drugs into square mixed with excipients. It can be served as decoction or infusion. The medicated tea is often applicable to food accumulation and common cold with cough.

末制品或加入适宜的黏合剂制成的方块状制剂。在使用时用沸水泡服或煎服。传统记载茶剂多应用于治疗食积停滞、感冒咳嗽等症。

X. Purified Mixture

It is a liquid preparation made by extracting and concentrating the active ingredients from medicinal materials in water or suitable solvent. The unit dose package is known as oral solution. Mixture is characteristic of synthetic effects, quick absorption and rapid action with convenient use. Other advantages are that it is possible to extract active multi-ingredients and produce in a great quantity. The commonly used is *Xiǎo Qīng Lóng Hé Jì*.

十、合剂

合剂系指药材用水或其他溶剂，采用适宜方法提取，经浓缩制成的内服液体剂型（如小青龙合剂）。单剂量包装者称口服液，是在汤剂的基础上改进和发展起来的中药剂型。合剂能综合浸出药材中的多种有效成分，保证制剂的综合疗效，吸收快，奏效迅速，可大量生产，免去煎煮中药的麻烦。

XI. Tablet

Tablets are solid forms containing medicinal substances with or without suitable binders and fillers and usually prepared by compression. Tablets may be coated for a variety of reasons, including protection of the ingredients from moisture or light, masking of unpleasant tastes and odors, and control of the site of drug release in the gastrointestinal tract. They may have advantages of convenient administration, low cost, easy storage, and accurate content of drugs, such as *Sāng Jú Gǎn Mào Piàn* and *Yín Qiào Jiě Dú Pi àn*.

十一、片剂

片剂系指药材提取物或药材细粉与适宜的辅料混匀压制而成的大小形状各异的固体剂型（如桑菊感冒片、银翘解毒片）。片剂可根据需要外表加包衣，如防潮、避光，味苦或者气味不佳的药物，还可外加糖衣；如需要在肠道内起作用或遇胃酸有效成分易被破坏的药物，可外包肠溶衣，使之在肠道内溶解。片剂具有使用方便、含量准确、生产成本低、易于贮运等优点。

XII. Syrup

Syrup is a saturated solution of sugar with drugs, extraction or aromatic ingredients. The sugar or aromatic ingredients may mask unpleasant tastes and odors. So it is also a pleasant form for children.

十二、糖浆剂

糖浆剂系指含有药物、药材提取物或芳香物质的浓蔗糖水溶液。糖和芳香剂能够掩盖某些药物的苦、咸等不适气味，改善口感，故糖浆剂深受儿童欢迎。

XIII. Granule

Infusion granule is made by making an extract of the drugs into medicated granule and mixing the granule with an appropriate amount of excipients. It is a new form for oral administration developed from decoction and syrup. The advantages of infusion include quick action, convenient use, easy carrying and wide indications, such as

十三、冲剂

冲剂又称颗粒剂，系指药材的提取物与适宜的辅料或药材细粉制成的干燥颗粒状制剂（如板蓝根冲剂、感冒灵冲剂）。它是在汤剂和糖浆剂的基础上发展起来的一种新型内服剂型，具有作用迅速、服用方便、便于携

Bǎn Lán Gēn Chōng Jì and *Gǎn Mào Líng Chōng Jì*.

带等优点，适用于多种疾病。

XIV. Injection

十四、注射剂

Injection is a kind of sterile solution obtained by refining the drugs. It is used for subcutaneous, muscular or intravenous injection. It is accurate in dosage, quick in action, convenient to use. There is no risk of influence of food and peptic juice, such as *Fù Fāng Dān Shēn Zhù Shè Yè*.

注射剂系指药物制成的供注入体内的无菌溶液、乳浊液和混悬液，以及供临用前配成溶液或混悬液的无菌粉末或浓缩液（如复方丹参注射液）。可用于皮下、肌内、静脉注射。它具有剂量准确、作用迅速、给药方便、药物不受食物或消化液的影响等优点。

XV. Suppository

十五、栓剂

Suppository is a solid form with various weights and shapes, adopted for introduction into the rectal, vaginal, or urethral orifice of the human body. They usually melt, soften, or dissolve at body temperature to release medicinal ingredients for general or local action. One commonly used is *Sān Huáng Shuān*.

栓剂是一种供腔道给药的固体剂型（如三黄栓），重量和形状各异，在常温下为固体，纳入人体腔道后，在体温下能迅速软化熔融或溶解于分泌液，逐渐释放药物而产生局部或全身作用。

XVI. Capsule

十六、胶囊剂

Capsules are solid dosage forms in which the drug is enclosed within either a hard or soft soluble container or "shell". The unpleasant odor of contained medicament can be covered with the shells. Capsules have the possibility to make the contained medicament available over an extended period of time following ingestion, to delay the release of medicament until the capsule has passed through the stomach and to maximize the bioavailability, such as *Yún Nán Bái Yào Jiāo Náng* and *Huò Xiāng Zhèng Qì Ruǎn Jiāo Náng*.

胶囊剂系指将药物直接分装在硬质空胶囊或有弹性的软质胶囊中制成的固体制剂（如云南白药胶囊、藿香正气软胶囊）。这种制剂能够掩盖药物的不良气味，其生物利用度高，可提高药物的稳定性，定时、定位释放药物。

(Wang Shi-yuan)

（王诗源）

Section 2　Contraindication for Medication of TCM

第二节　中药用药禁忌

There are three main different kinds of contraindications for TCM medication, prohibited combination, contraindication during pregnancy and dietary incompatibility.

中药用药禁忌主要有配伍禁忌、妊娠用药禁忌和饮食禁忌。

I. Prohibited Combination

i. Compatibility

Compatibility of drugs is based on the specific needs of syndromes and diseases and guided by certain rules, in which two or more drugs are selectively combined together for the purpose of appropriate clinical application. The combinational relationships between drugs are categorized into seven groups. They are single application, mutual reinforcement, mutual assistance, mutual restraint, mutual suppression, mutual inhibition and mutual antagonism. Single application means to use one drug alone. The other six relationships can be explained as follows:

1. Compatibility Reinforcing Effect Drugs can cooperate to reinforce the overall medicinal effects. These include mutual reinforcement and mutual assistance. When drugs which are similar in certain properties and efficacies are combined together to reinforce specific effects, it is referred to as mutual reinforcement. When combining drugs with similar properties and efficacies, or combining drugs with different properties and efficacies which are able to treat the same syndrome or disease, it is referred to as mutual assistance. As a matter of fact, one drug takes on the major role, while the others as an assistant to the major drug. This increases the treatment effect of the main drug.

2. Compatibility Reducing Toxicity or Side-effect These include mutual restraint and mutual suppression, which are actually the same, but expressed in two different ways. Mutual restraint means to use two drugs, in which the toxicity or side-effect of one drug can be reduced or removed by the other drug. When one drug can reduce or remove toxicity as well as the side effect of the other drug, it is called mutual suppression.

3. Compatibility Conducting Toxicity or Side-effect These include mutual inhibition and mutual antagonism. When two drugs are combined together, one can restrict the other, and that is, one drug can reduce or even totally neutralize the other drug's efficacy, which is referred to as mutual inhibition. When two drugs used together result in or reinforce toxicity, or increase side effects, this is referred to as mutual antagonism.

ii. Prohibited Combination

Drugs in specific compatibility which should be avoided are known as prohibited combination. The prohibited combination mainly refer to drugs which are in mutual inhibition and mutual antagonism. Presently, the commonly acknowledged prohibited combinations in TCM are the

一、配伍禁忌

（一）配伍

配伍是指按照病情需要和药性特点，有选择地将两种或两种以上的药物配合同用。前人把单味药的应用和药与药之间的配伍关系称为药物的"七情"，包括单行、相须、相使、相畏、相杀、相恶、相反。除单行外，其他六种配伍关系可概括为三类：

1. 增强疗效的配伍 药物经过配伍后，疗效比原来增强，包括相须和相使。相须是指性能功效相类似的药物配合应用，可以增强原有的疗效。相使是指性能功效方面有某些共性，或性能功效虽不相同，但是治疗目的一致的药物配合应用，以一种药物为主，另一种药物为辅，能提高主药疗效。

2. 减轻毒副作用的配伍 包括相畏和相杀。这两种配伍关系实际上是同一种配伍关系的两种提法。相畏是指一种药物的毒性反应或副作用，能被另一种药物减轻或消除。相杀是指一种药物能减轻或消除另一种药物的毒性反应或副作用。

3. 产生或增强毒副作用的配伍 包括相恶和相反。相恶是指两种药物合用，一种药物能使另一种药物原有的功效减弱、甚至丧失。相反是指两种药物合用，能产生或增强毒性反应或副作用。

（二）配伍禁忌

在选药组方时，有些药物应避免合用，称为配伍禁忌。在以上六种配伍关系中，相恶和相反属于此范畴。目前医药界普遍认可的配伍禁忌有前人提出的"十八反"和

eighteen antagonisms and nineteen incompatibilities.

Eighteen antagonisms: *wū tóu* with *bàn xià*, *guā lóu*, *bèi mǔ*, *bái liǎn* and *bái jí*. *Gān cǎo* with *hǎi zǎo*, *dà jǐ*, *gān suì* and *yuán huā*. *Lí lú* with *rén shēn*, *xuán shēn*, *shā shēn*, *dān shēn*, *kǔ shēn*, *xì xīn* and *sháo yào*.

Nineteen incompatibilities: *liú huáng* with *pò xiāo*, *shuǐ yín* with *pī shuāng*, *láng dú* with *mì tuó sēng*, *bā dòu* with *qiān niú zǐ*, *dīng xiāng* with *yù jīn*, *yá xiāo* with *sān léng*, *chuān wū* and *cǎo wū* with *xī jiǎo*, *rén shēn* with *wǔ líng zhī*, *guān guì* with *chì shí zhī*.

II. Contraindication during Pregnancy

Some drugs that can cause miscarriage, or have a negative effect on the gravida, or the growth and development of the fetus, are forbidden. They can be classified into two types as follows: to be given cautiously or to be avoided completely. The drugs to be given cautiously usually refer to blood-activating and stasis-dispelling, qi-moving, drastic hydragogues, and interior warming drugs. The drugs to be avoided usually have severe toxicity and powerful efficacy or cause miscarriage.

i. Drugs Given Cautiously during Pregnancy

Niú xī, *chuān xiōng*, *hóng huā*, *táo rén*, *jiāng huáng*, *mǔ dān pí*, *zhǐ shí*, *zhǐ qiào*, *dà huáng*, *fān xiè yè*, *lú huì*, *máng xiāo* and *fù zǐ*.

ii. Drugs Avoided during Pregnancy

Pī shí, *shuǐ yín*, *mǎ qián zǐ*, *chuān wū*, *bān máo*, *qīng fěn*, *xióng huáng*, *bā dòu*, *gān suí*, *dà jǐ*, *yuán huā*, *qiān niú zǐ*, *guā dì*, *gān qī*, *shuǐ zhì*, *méng chóng*, *sān léng*, *é zhú* and *shè xiāng*.

III. Dietary Incompatibility

During the period of taking medicine, the taboo of special food is called the dietary incompatibility when taking medicine, which is called the taboo of taking medicine for short, commonly known as taboo. Firstly, it is to avoid food that may hinder the function of spleen and stomach and affect the absorption of drugs. Secondly, avoid food that is harmful to certain diseases. For example, raw and cold food is unfavorable to cold syndrome, especially spleen and stomach deficiency cold syndrome; spicy and hot food is unfavorable to heat syndrome; too much cooking oil will aggravate fever; too much salt will

"十九畏"。

"十八反"是指乌头反半夏、瓜蒌、贝母、白蔹、白芨；甘草反海藻、大戟、甘遂、芫花；藜芦反人参、玄参、沙参、丹参、苦参、细辛、芍药。

"十九畏"是指硫黄畏朴硝，水银畏砒霜，狼毒畏密陀僧，巴豆畏牵牛子，丁香畏郁金，牙硝畏三棱，川乌、草乌畏犀角，人参畏五灵脂，官桂畏赤石脂。

二、妊娠用药禁忌

某些药物能引起流产或影响胎儿和孕妇的安全，应慎用或禁用。慎用药主要是活血化瘀药、行气药、攻下导滞药及温里药等。禁用药包括剧毒药、堕胎作用较强的药及作用峻猛的药。

（一）慎用药

牛膝、川芎、红花、桃仁、姜黄、牡丹皮、枳实、枳壳、大黄、番泻叶、芦荟、芒硝、附子等。

（二）禁用药

砒石、水银、马钱子、川乌、斑蝥、轻粉、雄黄、巴豆、甘遂、大戟、芫花、牵牛子、商陆、藜芦、胆矾、瓜蒂、干漆、水蛭、虻虫、三棱、莪术、麝香等。

三、饮食禁忌

服药期间禁忌进食某些食物，称为服药时的饮食禁忌，简称服药食忌，俗称忌口。一是忌食可能妨碍脾胃功能、影响药物吸收的食物。二是忌食对某种病证不利的食物。如生冷食物对于寒证，特别是脾胃虚寒证不利；辛热食物对热证不利；食油过多，会加重发热；食盐过多，会加重水肿等。三是忌食与所服药物之间存在类似相恶或相反配伍关系的食物。主要是避免药物与食物之间相

aggravate edema, *etc.*. Thirdly, there is a similar or opposite compatibility between food and drugs. It is mainly to avoid the interaction between drugs and food to reduce the curative effect or affect the absorption of drugs. For example, patients with Qi deficiency should not eat radish when taking ginseng or ginseng preparations. Because radish can promote qi, ginseng can replenish qi, one tonifying and one releasing, which reduces the effect of ginseng on Qi replenishment, so it is not suitable to take it at the same time. Others are Polygonum multiflorum avoid onion, garlic, radish, mint avoid turtle meat, Poria avoid vinegar, and so on.

(Wang Shi-yuan)

互作用而降低疗效或影响药物的吸收。例如气虚患者服用人参或人参制剂应忌食萝卜，因为萝卜行气，人参补气，一补一泄，降低了人参补气的作用，故不宜同时服用。其他还有何首乌忌葱、蒜、萝卜，薄荷忌鳖肉，茯苓忌醋等。

（王诗源）

Section 3　Method of Decocting

Decoction is the most commonly used dosage form. The following points are important in the decocting process and they are described as follows.

I. Utensil

First, choose the ceramic utensils with covers as decocting utensils, such as earthenware pot and jar. They do not create chemical reactions with the medicinal ingredients for their stable chemical property. Also, they conduct heat evenly and they are of high thermal insulation property. Second, the utensils made from enamelware and stainless steel can be selected. The metal utensils made from iron, copper and aluminium should be avoided to decoct drugs, as metal tends to create chemical reactions with medicinal ingredients, which may reduce the therapeutic effects and even cause toxicity or side effects.

II. Water

The water for decoction should be clear, pure and contain less mineral. Except for special requirement in prescription, well water, tap water, distilled water or purified water are suitable for decocting. Cool water or cool boiled water is used for first decoction, and boiled water should be avoided.

The volume of water is decided by the character, quantity, drinking degree and time of decocting of the

第三节　汤药煎煮法

汤药是临床上最常用的剂型，为了保证预期的疗效，应了解煎药时的注意事项。

一、煎药器具

首选有盖的陶瓷器皿如砂锅、砂罐。因其化学性质比较稳定，能避免在煎煮过程中与药物发生化学反应，从而保证了药物功效，且导热均匀，保暖性能好。其次是白色的搪瓷罐或不锈钢锅。煎药忌用铁、铜、铝等金属器皿，以免金属元素与药液发生化学反应，从而降低疗效，甚至产生毒副作用。

二、煎药用水

煎药用水以水质纯净、矿物质少为原则，除处方有特殊规定用水外，一般用井水、自来水、蒸馏水或纯净水。另外第一煎须用凉水或凉开水，忌用开水。

加水量应根据药物的性质、药量、吸水程度、煎煮时间而定。一般汤剂经水煎两次，

herbs. 70%-80% active ingredients of the herbs have been abstracted after being decocted twice. Traditionally, the water should be 3-5cm, 2-3cm above the drugs which are pressed into the pot respectively for the first decoction and the second decoction. The other way is that the total volume of water figures out according to 10ml water for 1g herbs. 70% of total volume of water is for the first decoction, 30% else is for the second decoction. The volume of water should be properly increased for decocting flowers, leave and grass. The volume of water should be reduced a bit for decocting minerals and shells. Add enough water into the pot for decocting. Avoid adding water frequently in the process of decocting. If the herbs are decocted parchingly, the decoction should be thrown away.

III. Herb Marinating

Medicinal materials should be marinated into cold water before being decocted. It is helpful to make medicinal materials soft and dissolve the active ingredients. General compound decoction should be marinated for 30-60 minutes. Prescription composed of flowers, leaves or glass ought to be marinated for 20-30 minutes. Prescription composed of roots, stems, seeds or fructification is marinated for 60 minutes. Medicinal materials should not be washed by water. Active ingredients of some medicinal materials are easy to dissolve and lose if washed.

IV. Decocting Fire

General medicinal materials are first decocted with strong fire and then with slow fire after the water boils. Exterior-releasing drugs or other aromatic drugs are not suitable to decoct with strong fire in order to prevent active ingredients from volatilizing. Invigorants should be first decocted with strong fire and then decocted with slow fire to make active ingredients sufficiently extracted.

V. Decocting Time

Decocting time is decided by the character of drugs and diseases and it is recorded when water is boiling. As

其中 70%~80% 的有效成分已析出，因此临床采用两煎法。传统的加水方法是将药物均匀放入药锅内，看准药物表面的位置，第一煎（头煎）加水至高出药面 3~5cm 处，第二煎（返渣再煎）加水至高出药面 2~3cm 处为宜。另一种加水方法是按平均每 1g 药加水约 10ml，计算出该方总的需水量，一般将全部用水的 70% 加到第一煎中，余下的 30% 留待第二煎用。煎花、叶、全草类药物，加水量要适当增多些；煎煮矿物类、贝壳类药物，加水量稍减。煎药时应一次将水加足，煎药过程中不可频频加水，如不慎将药煎糊后，应弃去，不可加水再煎后服用。

三、煎前泡药

煎药前，宜先用冷水将药材泡透。因中药大多数是干品，且含有淀粉、蛋白质，通过加水浸泡可使药质变软，煎药时有效成分易于析出。一般复方汤剂加水搅拌后应浸泡 30~60min；以花、叶、草类为主的方剂，需浸泡 20~30min；以根、茎、种子、果实类等药材为主的方剂，需浸泡 60min。煎药前亦不可用水洗药，因为某些中药成分中含有糖等易溶于水的物质；还有些中药是经过炮制的，如添加蜜、醋和酒等，若用水洗，会丧失一部分有效成分，降低药效。

四、煎煮火候

一般药物煎煮时宜先武火后文火，即在煎药开始用武火，至水沸后再改用文火。解表药及其他芳香性药物不宜久煎，以防有效成分挥发；滋补药宜先用武火煮沸后，改用文火久煎，使有效成分充分煎出。

五、煎药时间

煎药时间主要根据药物和疾病的性质而定。煎药时间从水沸时开始计算。一般药物一

for general drugs, first decoction and second decoction need to be 20-30 minutes and 10-20 minutes respectively. As for exterior-releasing drugs and other aromatic drugs, first decoction and second decoction need to be 15-20 minutes and 10-15 minutes respectively. As for invigorators, first decoction and second decoction need to be 40-50 minutes and 30-40 minutes respectively. Poisonous drugs should be decocted for about 60-90 minutes. Decoction is filtrated with gauze.

VI. Special Method

i. Decocting First

Shells such as *mǔ lì*, and minerals such as *shēng shí gāo*, *cí shí* are difficult to dissolve, so they should be crushed into pieces and decocted for 30 minutes before being mixed with other drugs in the decoction. Poisonous herbs, such as *fù zǐ*, *chuān wū*, ought to be first decocted for 1-3 hours in order to reduce or eliminate toxicity. Muddy or sandy herbs such as *zào xīn tǔ*, and herbs with light character and large quantity such as *lú gēn*, *máo gēn* should be decocted first, then its clear liquid should be utilized to decoct other herbs.

ii. Decocting Later

All the drugs with aromatic smell and volatile active ingredients, such as mint, Huoxiang, Amomum villosum, etc., should be added into pot 5-10 minutes before other drugs are finished decocting and decocted together with other drugs to prevent the effective components from volatilizing. The drugs that are easy to be damaged by long-term decocting, such as *rhubarb and Uncaria*, should be added in pot 10-15 minutes before other drugs are finished decocting.

iii. Wrap-Decocting

Some farinose herbs or herbs with floss, such as *huá shí*, *qīng dài*, *chē qián zǐ*, *xuán fù huā* should be wrapped with gauze for decoction to prevent turbidity and reduce irritation to the throat and digestive tract.

iv. Decocting Separately

Expensive drugs, such as *rén shēn*, *xī yáng shēn* should be decocted alone for 2-3 hours and be taken alone or with other decoction. Otherwise, the active ingredients tend to be absorbed into dregs of the other drugs, which is wasteful.

v. Melting

Some glial or viscous and soluble medicaments are easy to stick cooking pot or stick to other drugs when decocted with other drugs and lead to dissolution of the

煎需 20~30min，二煎需 10~20min；解表、芳香类药物，一煎需 15~20min，二煎需 10~15min；滋补类药物，一煎需 40~50min，二煎需 30~40min；有毒药物需久煎，约 60~90min。药煎好后，用纱布将药液过滤取汁。

六、特殊煎药法

（一）先煎

难溶于水的药物，如贝壳类（珍珠、牡蛎等）、矿石类（生石膏、磁石等）等，因其有效成分难以煎出，故应打碎先煎煮 30min，再下其他药物。有毒药物，如附子、川乌等，为降低或消除毒性，应先煎 1~3h。泥沙多的药物（如灶心土等）和质轻量大的药物（如芦根、茅根等）应先煎，澄清后取汁，以其药汁代水再煎其他药物。

（二）后下

凡气味芳香、有效成分易挥发的药物，如薄荷、藿香、砂仁等，宜在其他药物即将煎好前 5~10min 放入，再与其他药物同煎，防止有效成分挥发；其他久煎有效成分易被破坏的药物，如大黄、钩藤等，宜在煎好前 10~15min 放入。

（三）包煎

某些粉末状、有绒毛的药物，如滑石、青黛、车前子，旋复花等。宜用纱布包好入煎，以防止药液混浊及减少对喉咙、消化道的不良刺激。

（四）另煎

某些贵重的药材，为避免其有效成分在同煎时被其他药物吸附，可另煎 2~3h，煎好后，单独服用或兑入汤药中同服，如人参、西洋参等。

（五）烊化

胶质类或黏性大且易溶的药物，与其他药物同煎时易粘锅煮糊，或易黏附他药，以

active ingredient. So they should be separately heated and dissolved or placed in the liquid just filtered out, and cooked slightly or stirred while being still hot and drunk after dissolving, such as donkey-hide Gelatin, Caramel, and so on.

vi. Taking Infused

Some drugs which are not resistant to high temperature or tend to dissolve in water, such as *sān qī fěn, zhēn zhū fěn* should be infused with decoction or with boiled water for oral administration.

(Wang Shi-yuan)

Section 4　Principle of TCM Administration

The time and method of TCM administration have great effect on the therapeutic effects.

I. Time

i. Medication before Meal

The stomach is empty before meal. Taking drugs before meal can avoid drugs being mixed with food and promote drugs to move into the intestines for increasing therapeutic effect, so tonics, anti-acid drugs, drastic hydragogue and insect repellents should be taken before meal.

ii. Medication after Meal

After meal, the stomach is full of food, which can reduce irritative effect of the drugs on the stomach and intestines. Therefore, the stomachic drugs and stimulant drugs should be taken after meal.

iii. Medication before Sleep

Tranquilizers should be taken 30-60 minutes before sleep in order to treat insomnia. Drugs for seminal emission should be taken before sleep. Taking a laxative before sleep can promote defecation in the next morning.

iv. Others

Some drugs for certain diseases should be taken at a particular time. For example, anti-malaria drugs should be taken two hours before onset. But for acute diseases, the drugs should be taken immediately and many times a day.

致影响有效成分的溶解或药汁的滤出。故应单独加温溶化或将其置于刚煎好的去渣的药汁中，微煮或趁热搅拌，待溶解后服用，如阿胶、饴糖等。

（六）冲服

某些不耐高温且易溶于水的贵重药物，宜用开水或煎好的药液冲服。如：三七粉、珍珠粉等。

（王诗源）

第四节　中药给药原则

中药的服用时间和服用方法，对中药的疗效有很重要的影响。

一、服药时间

（一）饭前服用

饭前胃腑空虚，可避免药物与食物混合，有利于药物迅速进入肠道，充分发挥药效，故补益药、制酸药、峻下逐水药、攻积导滞药宜在饭前服用。

（二）饭后服用

饭后胃中存有较多食物，可减少药物对胃的刺激，故消食健胃药及对胃肠有刺激的药物宜在饭后服用。

（三）睡前服用

安神药宜在睡前 30min~1h 服用，助安眠；涩精止遗药宜在临睡前服，以便治疗梦遗滑精；缓下剂宜在睡前服，利于翌日清晨排便。

（四）其他

有些病定时发作，只有发病前某时服用才能见效，如截疟药应在疟疾发作前 2h 服用；当病情急险时，则当不拘时服，根据病情，可一天数服，也可煎汤代茶频饮。

II. Method

Usually, one dose can be taken two or three times per day. For the severe or acute disease, it can be taken once every four hours. When applying sweat-inducing drugs or purgatives, they should be stopped after accomplishing sweating and defecation. Patients with vomiting should take drugs in small dosage, but several times a day.

(Wang Shi-yuan)

二、服药方法

中药汤剂一般每日 1 剂，分 2~3 次温服，病重病急者可以每隔 4h 服药 1 次。应用发汗或泻药时，如药力较强，一般以得汗得下为度。呕吐患者宜小量频服，以免因量大再致吐，可浓煎药汁少量多次服用。

（王诗源）

Section 5　Eight Therapeutic Methods with Nursing Care

The eight therapeutic methods of TCM is summarized by Cheng Zhong-ling of the Qing Dynasty on the basis of the therapeutic principles of practitioners and specialists in the past dynasties, including sweat promotion, emetic therapy, purgative therapy, harmonizing therapy, warming therapy, heat-clearing therapy, dispelling therapy, and tonifying therapy.

I. Sweat Promotion and Nursing Care

i. Sweat Promotion

Sweating promotion therapy, also known as jiebiao method, is a kind of therapy that can help perspire through the functions of publicizing lung qi, regulating Ying and Wei, and opening and discharging the pathogenic factors of six evils on the muscle surface. It is recorded in *The Yellow Emperor's Canon of Internal Medicine* that if the body is hot like burnt charcoal, make it sweat and scatter the pathogenic factors. The purpose of sweating method is not to make people sweat. The main purpose of sweating method is to make the body surface open, and let ying and wei be harmonious again, let Lung Qi unobstructed and blood vessels unblocked, so as to dispel pathogenic factors. Therefore, in addition to treating the exterior syndrome of exogenous pathogenic factors of six evils, sweating method can be used to treat the patients with obstruction of the body's principle, barrier of Ying and Wei, and no sweating due to cold and heat. Such as exogenous wind cold, wind heat; measles at the beginning, the rash is not in full

第五节　中医用药"八法"及护理

中医用药"八法"是清代程钟龄根据历代医学家对治法归类总结而得来，"八法"通常是指汗法、吐法、下法、和法、温法、清法、消法、补法。

一、汗法及护理

（一）汗法

汗法又称解表法，是通过宣发肺气，调畅营卫，开泄腠理等作用，促使人体微微出汗，使肌表的外感六淫之邪随汗而解的一种治法。早在《黄帝内经》中已有记载，如《素问·生气通天论》："……体若燔炭，汗出而散"。汗法不是以使人出汗为目的，主要目的是使腠理开，营卫和，肺气畅，血脉通，从而能祛邪外出。故汗法除了主要治疗外感六淫之邪的表证外，凡腠理闭塞、营卫不通而寒热无汗者皆可以用汗法治疗。如外感风寒、风热；麻疹初起，疹未透发或透发不畅者；水肿实证兼有表证者；外感风寒兼有湿邪者；疮疡初起兼有恶寒发热等证。

bloom; edema syndrome with both exterior syndrome; exogenous wind cold with dampness evil; sores at the beginning of both cold and fever.

ii. Nursing Care

1. Dietary nursing   Light diet is recommended. Glutinous, greasy, acid and clod food should not be served for the patient. Because the acid food can restrain sweating and the cold food doesn't benefit to dispel cold.

2. Decocting method and administration   Diaphoretics should be decocted for a short time with strong fire and be taken hot. The patients should take hot congee, water or beverage to reinforce the effect of the decoction. They should lie on the bed covered with quilts to keep warm so as to assist perspiration.

3. Observation of sweating condition   Generally, stop taking the decoction when the patient perspires and defervesces. Light sweating is good for patients. The treatment should not be stopped until the patient is cured. The patient should be given with heavier sweating glucose and saline fluid or transfusion to avoid damaging healthy qi. If the patient sweats ceaselessly, the doctor should be informed immediately to take action to prevent damage of yin and loss of yang.

4. When the patient perspires and defervesces, the patient should be toweled off with dry or warm towels. The clothing for the patient who sweats ceaselessly shouldn't be changed. Towel should be put on the patient's chest and back to keep body dry and the clothing should be changed when he stops sweating. Attention should be paid to keep away from wind-cold pathogen.

5. Even the patient is still not sweating after taking medicine and the fever insists still, cold drinks and cold compress should not be given to avoid "door closed and thieves left inside", which means that the evil has no way out, and the heat is even worse when entering interior. We can acupuncture the points of Dazhui and Quchi to help sweat out the pathogenic factors.

6. The patients with exterior syndrome and wind-dampness syndrome should have several times of sweat promotion in order to dispel wind and eliminate dampness which is heavy and turbid in nature, and difficult to be eliminated.

7. Sweat promotion should be adapted according to different seasons and different health conditions of patients. For example, sweating in summer and for deficiency patients should be light, while sweating in winter and for strong patients should be heavy.

8. For prevention of heavy sweating, the diaphoretic herbs should not be used in combination with heat-relieving and pain-easing drugs such as Aspirin.

（二）护理方法

1. 饮食宜清淡，忌黏滑、油腻、辛辣、酸性和生冷食物。因酸性食物有敛汗作用，而生冷食物不易散寒。

2. 药宜武火快煎热服，饮热稀粥或热水、热饮料等，以助药力。服药后卧床加盖衣被，保暖以助发汗。

3. 观察出汗情况 一般是汗出热退即停药，以遍身微微汗出为宜、忌大汗。若汗出不彻，则病邪不解，需继续用药；而汗出过多，会伤津耗液、损伤正气，可给予患者口服糖盐水或输液；若大汗不止，易导致伤阴亡阳，应立即通知医师，及时采取措施。

4. 汗出热退后，应及时用干毛巾或热毛巾擦干，忌用冷毛巾擦拭，以防毛孔郁闭，不利病邪外达；大汗淋漓者，暂时不要给予更衣，可在胸前、背后铺上干毛巾，汗止时再更换衣被，注意避风寒，防止复感。

5. 病位在表者服药后仍无出汗，纵然热不退，也不可给予冷饮和冷敷，避免"闭门留寇"，使邪无出路，而入里化热，热反更甚；可针刺大椎、曲池穴位达到透邪发汗目的。

6. 对表证兼有风湿者，须多次微微发汗，以祛风除湿。因湿邪性质重浊，黏滞不爽，难以祛除。

7. 发汗要因人、因时而宜，如暑天炎热，汗之宜轻；冬天寒冷，汗之宜重；体虚者，汗之宜缓；体实者，汗之宜峻等。

8. 服发汗解表药时，禁用或慎用解热镇痛类西药，如阿司匹林等，防止汗出太过。

9. Blood pressure and heart rate should be observed for the patients treated with *má huáng* as remedy.

10. Sweat promotion is not applicable to the patients with such specific signs and symptoms as chronic stranguria, frequent ulcer, frequent bleeding, severe vomiting, diarrhea, edema, spontaneous perspiration, night sweat as well as low fever in later period.

II. Emetic Therapy and Nursing Care

i. Emetic Therapy

Emetic therapy is a treatment that phlegm, harmful substances remaining in the throat, esophagus and stomach are spit out with drugs. It is indicated for the patients with stroke, profuse sputum, mania, epilepsy, crapulent syncope, and disorder of qi activities, indigestive food or poisoning in the stomach. However, it should be used carefully for pregnant women, the aged and the infant.

ii. Nursing Care

1. Attention should be paid to the dose, application as well as rescue method. It is recommended that drugs should be taken in small dose increased gradually in order to prevent poisoning or severe vomiting. Further consultation from the doctor is necessary once the patients vomit after taking the remedy for the first time.

2. Stimulating the patient's palate and throat with spatula could help to induce vomiting. Sitting the patient and tapping the patient's upper back could be helpful when the patient is vomiting. The vomitus can be prevented inhaling into the respiratory tract by helping the patient to turn his head to one side for those lying in bed.

3. Patients should be given warm water for rinsing the mouth and clean vomitus, and the dirty clothes should be changed and bed should be made immediately.

4. Nurses should tell patient to keep away from wind blowing and prevent attack of common cold after vomiting.

5. Those patients vomiting repeatedly generally should take a little ginger juice or cold porridge or cold boiled water to detoxify the poison. If the vomiting couldn't still be relieved it can be treated according to the type of drug administration. For those who take bā dòu, they can be treated with cold porridge; if they ingest other poisons, they can be treated with mung bean soup; if the Qi is still in upward retrograde motion after vomiting, the medicaments with the effects of lending down abnormally ascending qi and harmonizing stomach should be recommended.

9. 服用含有麻黄的药物后，要注意患者血压及心率的变化。

10. 慎用汗法　凡淋家、疮家、亡血家和剧烈吐下之后均禁用汗法。对于表邪已尽或麻疹已透、疮疡已溃、虚证水肿、自汗、盗汗、热病后期津亏者均不宜用汗法。

二、吐法及护理

（一）吐法

吐法是通过药物，使停留在咽喉、胸膈、胃脘等部位的痰涎、宿食或毒物从口中吐出的一种治法。该法常用于中风、痰涎壅盛、癫狂、宿食、食厥、气厥、胃中残留毒物等。体虚气弱者，尤其是孕妇、老人、小儿均须慎用。

（二）护理方法

1. 使用涌吐药应注意用量、用法和解救方法。服药应小量渐增，以防中毒或涌吐太过。药物采取二次分服，服一次即吐者，需通知医生，决定是否继续服用。

2. 服药后可用压舌板刺激上腭、咽喉部，助其呕吐。呕吐时协助患者坐起，并轻拍患者背部促使胃内容物吐出。不能坐起者，协助患者头偏向一侧，避免呕吐物吸入呼吸道。

3. 吐后用温开水漱口，及时清除呕吐物、更换被污染的衣物，整理好床单位。

4. 服药得吐者，嘱患者坐卧避免风吹，以防吐后体虚，复感外邪。

5. 吐而不止者，一般可以服用少许姜汁或服用冷粥、冷开水解之。若吐仍不止者，可根据给药的种类分别处理；因服巴豆吐泻不止者，可用冷粥解之；误食其他毒物，可用绿豆汤解之；若吐后气逆不止，宜给予和胃降逆剂止之。

6. Nurses should observe and record the patient's body temperature, pulse, respiration, blood pressure, quantity, flavor and property of the vomitus. Fluid infusion is necessary for the patient with electrolyte disturbances.

7. After vomiting, the patients should not eat food until their digestive function gets recovered. Patients could take a few liquid diet or digestive food, but cold and greasy food is prohibited.

8. The vomitus should be reserved to do chemical examination in case of food poisoning.

III. Purgative Therapy and Nursing Care

i. Purgative Therapy

It is a treatment for eliminating the indigested food, excess heat-evil and fluid by the application of potent or mild purgatives. It is generally classified into purgation with drugs cold in nature, with drugs warm in nature, with drugs causing laxation, with drugs eliminating excess fluid and with drugs simultaneously purging and tonifying. However, it is contraindicated for weak patients and pregnant women.

ii. Nursing Care

1. Purgation by Drug Cold in Nature

It is indicated for excess syndrome with interior heat. The representative recipes are *Dà Chéng Qì Tāng* and *Zēng Yè Chéng Qì Tāng*.

(1) The patient with hyperpyrexia, dysphoria, thirsty and dry mouth should stay in a ward with good adjustment of temperature and humidity.

(2) Decocting *Dà Chéng Qì Tāng* correctly could benefit the purgative effect. The correct way is to decoct *zhǐ shí* and *hòu pǔ* first, then decoct *dà huáng* later, and then infuse *máng xiāo* in the decoction.

(3) Nurses should observe the patient's condition including vital signs, times of defecation, color, quantity and quality of bowels, as well as abdominal pain. Remedies should be available for the case with collapse.

(4) Patients should not eat food for 3-5 days during treatment. Congee and noodles are good for the case after defecating dry stools. Greasy, spicy food and wine should be avoided.

2. Purgation by Drug Warm in Nature

It is indicated for interior excess syndrome due to retention of cold evil. The representative recipes are *Dà Huáng Fù Zǐ Tāng* and *Wēn Pí Tāng*.

6. 严重呕吐者应注意体温、脉搏、呼吸、血压及呕吐物的量、气味、性质、性状并记录。必要时给予补液、纠正电解质紊乱等对症处理。

7. 患者吐后暂给予禁食，待胃肠功能恢复后再给予少量流质饮食或易消化食物以养胃气。忌食生冷、肥甘油腻之品。

8. 食物中毒或服毒患者，可根据需要保留呕吐物，以便化验。

三、下法及护理

（一）下法

下法是使用泻下药促进排便，以清除肠胃中饮食积滞、热结、水邪等的一种治疗方法。可分为寒下、温下、润下、逐下、攻补兼施。本法禁用于身体虚弱者和孕妇。

（二）护理方法

1. **寒下**　适用于里实热证。代表方有大承气汤、增液承气汤等。

（1）患者有高热、烦躁不安、口渴舌燥等表现，应安排在调节温湿度方面良好的病室，使患者感到凉爽、舒适，有利于静心养病。

（2）大承气汤正确煎煮方法是：先煎方中的枳实和厚朴，大黄后下，芒硝冲服，以发挥泻下作用。

（3）服药期间应密切观察病情变化及生命体征，观察排泄物的性质、量、次数、颜色、腹痛减轻的情况，若出现虚脱，应及时救治。

（4）在服药期间必要时应暂禁食3~5d。待燥屎泻下后再给患者服米汤、面条等易消化、养胃气的饮食，忌食油腻、辛辣食物及饮酒。

2. **温下**　适用于因寒成结之里实证。代表方有大黄附子汤、温脾汤等。

(1) The patient of excess syndrome with interior cold should stay in the ward located in sunny side and keep the body warm.

(2) The patient should take food of warm or hot in nature.

(3) The correct way to decoct *Wēn Pí Tāng* is that *dà huáng* is marinated in wine and then decocted with other drugs. The warm decoction should be administered before meals.

(4) Observation of patient's pain and masses in the abdomen is necessary in the period of treatment after the patient has taken the laxation. The condition should turn better if pain relieves and extremities become warm.

3. Purgation by Drugs Causing Laxation

It is indicated for dryness of the intestine, lack of body fluid, constipation in the aged, habitual constipation and constipation during pregnancy or after delivery. The representative recipes are *Wǔ Rén Tāng* and *Má Zǐ Rén Wán*.

(1) The drugs should be taken in the morning and evening with empty stomach. Dietary therapies, such as eating banana, honey and nutlet may benefit the defecation.

(2) The habit of bowel movement is very important for patients with habitual constipation while abdominal massage is also helpful.

4. Expelling Excessive Fluid with Potent Purgative

It is applicable to the excess type of fluid-retention disease including ascites and pleural effusion. It is contraindicated for the weak, pregnant women as well as patients with exterior cold syndrome. Attention should be paid to observe chest fullness and abdominal distention and pain after taking medicine.

5. Simultaneous Application of Purging and Tonifying

It is indicated for the patient with interior excess syndrome and constipation as well. Patients should stop taking the medication when the condition has been relieved.

IV. Harmonizing Therapy and Nursing Care

i. Harmonizing Therapy

Harmonizing therapy is a treatment for the elimination of evils in *shaoyang* meridian or the coordination of functions of viscera, vital energy and blood by the application of drugs with actions of dispersion and regulation. It is recorded in *Concise Supplementary Exposition on Cold Damage* (*Shāng Hán Míng Lǐ Lùn*, 伤寒

（1）里寒证患者宜住向阳病室，注意保暖。

（2）饮食上应给予温性或热性食品。

（3）温脾汤方中的大黄应先用酒浸泡后再与其他药同煎，药宜饭前温服。

（4）服药后应观察腹部疼痛减轻情况，宜连续轻泻。服药后，如腹痛渐减，肢温回缓，则病势好转。

3. **润下**　适用于热盛伤津，或病后津亏未复，或年老津涸，或产后血枯便秘，或习惯性便秘等。代表方有五仁汤、麻子仁丸等。

(1) 润下药一般宜早、晚空腹服用。在服药期间应配合食疗以润肠通便，如香蕉、蜂蜜、果仁等有助于通便。

(2) 对习惯性便秘患者应养成定时排便习惯，也可在腹部进行按摩疗法。

4. **逐水**　适用于水饮停聚体内，或胸胁有水气，或腹肿胀满，凡脉证俱实者，皆可逐水。由于此药有毒而力峻，易伤正气，所以体虚、孕妇忌用，有恶寒表证者不可服用。服药后要注意观察心下痞满和腹部胀痛情况。

5. **攻补兼施**　适用于里实证虚而大便秘结者。用药应中病即止，不可久服。

四、和法及护理

（一）和法

和法又称和解法，是通过和解疏泄作用的方药，祛除少阳病邪，调理脏腑气血，使表里、上下、脏腑、气血和调的一种治法。主要适用于邪犯少阳，肝脾不和，寒热错杂等病邪在半表半里之证。《伤寒明理论》说：

明理论) that "sweat promotion is used for treatment of pathogenic evil invading the exterior, purgative therapy for pathogenic evil in the interior and harmonizing therapy for pathogenic evil in the semi-superficial-interior". This therapy is not applicable to the case with interior excess or deficiency-cold syndrome.

ii. Nursing Care

1. *Xiăo Chái Hú Tāng* is a representative recipe for *shaoyang* syndrome which contains ginseng as major constituent. Thus radish should be excluded in the diet therapy because it can diminish *rén shēn*'s tonifying effect. Some medicines like calcium carbonate, magnesium sulfate and ferrisulphas should not be allowed to take with *Xiăo Chái Hú Tāng*, because the chemical interaction should result in toxic and adverse effects. The patient's body temperature, pulse and sweating should be observed and recorded during the treatment.

2. Medicine for regulating function of the liver and spleen is applied for the case manifested as distension and pain over the hypochondria, poor appetite, thin and whitish coating on the tongue, wiry and small pulse. Emotional nursing should benefit the treatment.

3. Medicine for regulating function of the stomach and intestine is applicable to the case manifested as epigastric lumpy stiffness, nausea, vomiting, abdominal distension, borborygmus and discharge of stools. The signs and symptoms mentioned above should be observed and recorded.

4. Light and digestive foods are good for strengthening the spleen, activating qi movement and promoting digestion, but foods with cold in nature as well as greasy or pungent foods are prohibited, such as melons and fruits.

V. Warming Therapy and Nursing Care

i. Warming Therapy

Warming therapy is a treatment for dispelling cold, resuming yang qi, smoothing channels and collaterals, and regulating blood as well. It is indicated for cold pathogen invading *zang-fu* organs, water-fluid retention, and yang qi declination. It is prohibited for patients with true heat and false cold syndrome or yin deficiency constitution.

ii. Nursing Care

1. It is very important to distinguish cold and heat syndromes. Misuse of the warming therapy for heat syndrome could result in worsened condition.

2. Daily life, diet, medication and other nursing therapies should all help the body to be warm, like keeping

"伤寒邪在表者，必渍形以为汗；邪气在里者，必荡涤以为利。其于不内不外，半表半里，既非发汗之所宜，又非吐下之所对，是当和解则可以矣。"禁用于病在表未入少阳或邪已入里之实证以及虚寒证。

（二）护理方法

1. 服和解少阳药（如小柴胡汤）期间，应忌食萝卜。因方中有人参，而萝卜可破坏人参的药效。亦忌同时服用碳酸钙、硫酸镁、硫酸亚铁等西药，以免相互作用产生毒副作用。服和解少阳药后，要仔细观察患者的体温、脉象以及出汗情况。

2. 调和肝脾药适用于肝气郁滞而导致胁肋胀痛，食欲缺乏，苔薄白，脉弦细等症。服药期间应配合情志护理，使患者心情舒畅，有利于提高治疗效果。

3. 调和肠胃药适用于邪犯肠胃，寒热夹杂，升降失常，致心下痞满，恶心呕吐，脘腹胀痛，肠鸣下利等证。服后应注意腹胀及呕吐情况，并注意排便的性质和量。

4. 服药期间宜给予清淡易消化的饮食，以健脾行气消食，忌食生冷瓜果、肥腻厚味及辛辣之品。

五、温法与护理

（一）温法

温法是通过温中、祛寒、回阳、通络等作用，使寒气去，阳气复，经络通，血脉和的一种治疗方法。适用于寒邪直中脏腑、寒饮内停、阳气衰微等证。真热假寒者、素体阴虚者忌用。

（二）护理方法

1. 辨别寒热真假，温法必须针对寒证，热证误用温热护法，可加重病情。

2. 生活起居、饮食、服药等护理均以

warm, drinking hot liquor, avoiding raw and cold food. It is suitable to eat warm food, such as mutton, longan, *etc.,* to promote the effect of medicine in dispersing cold and invigorating yang qi.

3. Drugs warming middle-jiao to dispel cold are indicated for deficiency syndrome due to protracted diseases. Nurses should ask the patient to persist in taking the medicine because the effects are relaxative and it takes effect for long time.

4. Drugs expelling cold by warming the meridians are applied for the case with cold pathogen attacking meridians. They should be used in combination with the herbs nourishing blood and activating meridians. *Dāng Guī Sì Nì Tāng* is the representative recipe. Attention should be paid to keep the extremities and abdominal region warm.

5. The patient with yang qi declination should be treated with herbs recuperating the depleted yang and rescuing the patient from danger. Nasal feeding is used for coma patients and the vital signs should be observed including consciousness, complexion, body temperature, blood pressure, pulse and blood circulation of extremities. The cases with ceaseless sweating, extreme cold limbs, dysphoria, and faint pulse should be rescued immediately.

6. The warming therapy involves drugs with dryness-heat in nature can result in consumption of yin and blood. So it is not suitable for pregnant women and the patients with yin deficiency or blood heat.

VI. Heat Clearing Therapy and Nursing Care

i. Heat Clearing Therapy

Heat clearing therapy is a treatment for clearing away the heat-evil with cold-natured drugs, and applicable to interior heat syndrome. The drugs promoting production of body fluid and benefiting vital energy are often used in combination with the drugs clearing interior heat. In later stage of febrile disease, both nourishing yin and clearing heat therapies are often used in cooperation.

ii. Nursing Care

1. Heat clearing therapy is applicable to interior heat syndrome. Comfortable clothing, fresh air, quite condition and soft light in ward can benefit the treatment.

2. Some drugs require special decocting. For example, gypsum prescribed in *Bái Hǔ Tāng* is decocted prior to other herbs for 15 minutes with strong fire and mint

"温"法护之，宜保暖，进热饮，忌生冷寒凉食物。宜食温性食物，如羊肉、桂圆等，以助药物的温中散寒、振奋阳气之功效。

3. 温中祛寒药适用于久病虚证，由于药力缓，见效时间长，嘱患者要坚持服药。

4. 温经散寒药适用于寒邪凝滞经脉之证。不宜单纯用辛热之品，应配伍养血通脉药同用。代表方有当归四逆汤。服药后，应注意保暖，尤以四肢及腹部切忌受凉。

5. 回阳救逆药主治阳气衰微、将亡之危证。昏迷患者可通过鼻饲法给药，服药期间应严密观察患者神志、面色、体温、血压、脉象及四肢回温的变化情况。如服药后，患者汗出不止、厥冷加重、烦躁不安、脉微欲绝等，为病情恶化，应及时通知医生，并积极配合医生抢救。

6. 温法所用药物，性多燥热，易耗阴血。凡阴亏、血热等证及孕妇不宜用温法。

六、清法与护理

（一）清法

清法又称清热法，是通过清热泻火，凉血解毒等作用，使邪热外泄，以清除里热证的一种治疗方法。适用于里热证。火热最易伤津耗液，大热又能伤气，所以清法中常配伍生津益气之品。若温病后期，热灼阴伤，或久病阴虚而热伏于里的，又当清法与滋阴并用，热并必除。

（二）护理方法

1. 清法适用于里热证，室温、衣被均宜偏凉，病房空气新鲜，光线柔和，环境安静，可根据病情调节室温。

2. 清热之剂，因药物不同，煎药方法亦应有区别，如白虎汤中的生石膏应打碎，用

prescribed in *Pǔ Jì Xiāo Dú Yǐn* should be decocted posterior to other herbs, for its active ingredients tend to volatilize or be destroyed during the process of decocting. All the decoctions for interior heat should be taken when it becomes cool or warm.

3. It is necessary to observe the patient's condition. The signs and symptoms of fever, thirst, consciousness and pulse should be observed. The alleviation of the above symptoms indicates relief of the condition. High fever and excessive thirst exist with coma, delirium, purple-red body of the tongue, this means heat blazing of both qi and nutrient systems. It is necessary to report to physicians and take special interventions in the case of convulsion. For ulcers and carbuncles, reduced swelling and decreased body temperature indicate relief of the disease. The operation is adapted for the case of pus. For those who suffer from heat blazing of both blood and nutrient systems, observation of consciousness becomes very important. Once convulsion occurs, the rescue should be given immediately.

4. Food with cold nature benefits the treatment for clearing interior heat. Vegetables and fruits are recommended, such as balsam pear, cucumber, mung bean, lotus root, pear and lettuce. The patients should be encouraged to drink water and juice of watermelon, pear and orange in order to promote fluid production to quench thirst.

5. Overdose and long term use of drugs with bitter and cold properties or drugs nourishing yin could result in injury of the stomach or deficiency of spleen and stomach yang. Therefore, this kind of drug should be stopped as soon as heat is cleared away. Sometimes it is necessary to prescribe drugs which can promote digestion during the treatment. Thus drugs with bitter and cold properties should be carefully used or the dose should be reduced for the old, weak, and the patients with spleen cold syndrome.

VII. Dispelling Therapy and Nursing Care

i. Dispelling Therapy

It is a treatment for dispelling tangible excess pathogens due to stagnated qi or blood, phlegm-dampness, indigested foods and parasites. It is mainly indicated for retention of food, fluid, phlegm, qi obstruction and blood stasis.

ii. Nursing Care

1. Drugs with different properties require different

武火先煎 15min，后入其他诸药，改用文火，煎至粳米熟；普济消毒饮中的薄荷气味芳香、含挥发油，应后下以减少有效成分挥发或分解破坏而损失。凡清热解毒之剂，均以取汁凉服或微温服。

3. 服药后需观察病情变化。如服白虎汤后，患者体温渐降，汗止渴减，神清脉静，为病情好转。若患者服药后高热烦渴不减，并出现神昏谵语，舌质红绛，提示病由气分转为气营两燔。若药后高热不退而出现四肢抽搐或惊厥者，提示热盛动风，应立即报告医师采取救治措施。对疮疡肿毒之证，在服药过程中若肿消热退，为病退之象。若疮疡已成脓，则应切开排脓；对热入营血者，要观察神志，出血及热极动风之兆，一旦发现，立即处理。

4. 饮食上应给予寒凉性食品以清除内热，多食蔬菜、水果，如苦瓜、黄瓜、绿豆、藕、梨、莴苣等。鼓励患者多饮水、西瓜汁、梨汁、柑橘汁等生津止渴之品。

5. 苦寒滋阴药久服伤胃或内伤中阳，热清邪除后宜停药，必要时添加和胃药。年老体弱、脾胃虚寒者慎用，或减量服用。

七、消法与护理

（一）消法
消法是指通过消食导滞和消坚散结作用，对气、血、痰、食、水、虫等积聚而成的有形之邪逐渐消散的一种治法。适用于饮食停滞，气滞血瘀，水湿内停，痰饮不化等证。

（二）护理方法
1. 消导之剂，要根据其方药的气味清淡、

decocting methods. Light flavor drugs should be decocted for a short time but those with heavy property require longer time.

2. Drugs of relieving dyspepsia are applicable to indigestion. Light and digestive foods, such as, *shān zhā* radish and vinegar are recommended during the course of treatment. For infants, it is very important to reduce dose of milk and milk feeding should be stopped if necessary.

3. During the treatment, the patient's signs and symptoms including quantity and quality of stools, abdominal pain and distention, and vomiting should be observed, especially for patients with diarrhea caused by dampness and heat pathogen and be prescribed with *Zhǐ Shí Dǎo Zhì Wán* in accordance with the principle of "treating diarrhea with purgatives". The case with dehydration originated from serious diarrhea should be reported to the doctor. If the patient is treated with drugs relieving and eliminating mass, it should be observed and recorded that the local symptoms such as pain, swelling and mass in size, shape, location, activity, tenderness, and whether the borderline of the mass is smooth or not for the case. If the patient manifests abruptly abdominal pain, nausea, hematemesis, pale complexion, sweating, cold extremities and minute pulse, it need to inform the doctor immediately and assist the doctor to save the patient.

4. The drugs with purgative or dispelling effect should be used temporarily and the medication should be stopped when the patients' condition have been relieved.

5. The drugs with dispelling effect should be taken after meals. Acid drugs such as hawthorn are forbidden to take with alkaline drugs such as compound aluminium and sodium bicarbonate to avoid neutralization reaction that decreases the therapeutic effect.

6. The drugs with dispelling effect should not be used in compatibility with tonics and astringents which can decrease the therapeutic effect.

7. The drugs with dispelling effect should be used cautiously for the old and the weak, while they are contraindicated for pregnant women and patients with deficiency of the spleen and stomach.

VIII. Supplementing Method and Nursing Care

i. Supplementing Method

Supplementing method is a therapeutic method for keeping the balance between *zang-fu* organs, qi and blood

厚重之别，采用不同的煎药法。如药味清淡，临床取其气者，煎药时间宜短；如药味厚重，取其质者，煎药时间宜延长。

2. 消食导滞剂常用于食积为病，服药时饮食宜清淡易消化，勿过饱，常用食物如山楂、萝卜、醋等；婴幼儿应注意减少乳食量，必要时可暂时停止喂乳。

3. 服用消食导滞剂时，应注意观察患者大便的性状、次数、质、量、气味、腹胀、腹痛及呕吐等情况。如果治疗因湿热滞食，内阻肠胃的患者，在选用枳实导滞丸治疗泻泄、下利时，属"通因通用"之法，须特别注意排便及腹痛情况，若泻下如注，次数频繁或出现眼窝凹陷等伤津脱液表现时，应立即报告医生。应用消痞化积药，注意患者的局部症状，如疼痛、肿胀、包块等，详细记录癥块大小、部位、性质、活动度、有无压痛、边缘是否光滑。此类药常以行气活血、软坚散结等药组方，如果患者突然腹部疼痛、恶心、吐血、便血、面色苍白、汗出厥冷、脉微而细，则病情加重，已变生他证，立即报告医生，并配合医生采取抢救措施。

4. 消导类药物有泻下或导滞之功效，不可久服，中病即止。

5. 凡消导类药物，均宜在饭后服用。与西药同服时，应注意配伍禁忌，如山楂含有机酸，忌与复方氢氧化铝、碳酸氢钠等碱性药物同服，以免酸碱中和反应，降低药效。

6. 该类药一般不与补益药和收敛药同用，以免降低药效。

7. 本类药对于年老、体弱者慎用；脾胃虚弱或无食积者及孕妇禁用。

八、补法与护理

（一）补法

补法又称补益法，是通过药物的补益作用，恢复人体脏腑或气血阴阳之间平衡的一

as well as yin and yang of the body with medicines of restorative effect. It is indicated for all kinds of deficiency syndrome. It is avoided for all kinds of excess syndrome.

ii. Nursing Care

1. Both the room temperature and humidity should be adjusted with the patient's condition as most of the patients with yang deficiency manifest cold symptoms, and most of the patients with yin deficiency manifest hot symptoms.

2. It should advise the patient to keep regular daily life, have sufficient sleep, do proper body exercises, and avoid fatigue, which can increase body's immunity.

3. Most of tonics with the properties of greasy taste or heavy quality should be decocted with small fire for long time to dissolve the ingredients thoroughly. *Ē jiāo* should be first melted and later mixed with the decoction for oral administration. Expensive tonics should be decocted alone or infused with a decoction or with boiled water for oral administration. The tonics are often taken before meal or on empty stomach.

4. Different kinds of foods are applicable to different conditions. Foods with warm nature are the good choice for patients with yang deficiency, such as beef, mutton, longan, but vegetables and fruits with cold nature should not be allowed. White tremella, agaric and soft-shelled turtle are applicable to patients with yin deficiency but foods which have pungent and warm nature such as cigarette, alcohol and pepper should not be allowed because they may damage yin. Chinese yam, chicken soup and *huáng qí* congee is applicable to patients with qi deficiency but cold nature foods should not be allowed. Foods nourishing blood and the heart such as animal blood and livers, Chinese dates, and spinach are applicable to patients with blood deficiency. Warming and tonifying therapies are applicable to people in winter while clearing and tonifying therapies are applicable to people in summer.

5. Emotional nursing can be very helpful for patients who suffer from chronic or severe diseases in the early recovery phase with symptoms of stress, pessimism, anxiety and sadness. Nursing staffs should encourage and soothe them to correctly deal with the diseases and build up their confidence and optimism in conquering the diseases.

6. Drugs with warm nature to tonify qi and assist yang should not be used for patients with yin deficiency and interior heat or hyperactivity of liver-yang. The drugs which have greasy nature and the function of nourishing yin and blood should be prescribed with those that can strengthen the spleen and stomach.

种治法。适用于各种虚证。凡实证及实证而表现虚证假象者禁用。

（二）护理方法

1. 由于阳虚多寒，阴虚多热，因此病室的温、湿度应根据患者的临床症状进行调节。

2. 嘱患者注意生活要有规律，做到起居有常，保持充足睡眠，适当锻炼身体，提高抗病能力，避免劳累。

3. 补益药大多质重味厚，煎药时宜文火久煎，阿胶需烊化，贵重药品应另煎或冲服。补益药宜空腹或饭前服下。

4. 由于虚证有阴、阳、气、血之别，饮食上应辨证进补。阳虚者，可选用牛、羊肉和桂圆等温补之品，忌生冷瓜果和凉性食品；阴虚者，应选用银耳、木耳、甲鱼等清补之品，忌烟、酒，辣椒等辛温香燥、耗津伤液之品；气虚者，可选用山药、母鸡人参汤、黄芪粥等健脾、补肺、益气之品，忌生冷饮食；血虚者可选用动物血、猪肝、大枣、菠菜等补血养心之品；冬季宜温补，夏季宜清补。

5. 虚证患者大多处在大病初愈或久病不愈等情况，易产生紧张、悲观、焦虑等不安情绪，护理人员应做好患者的心理疏导工作，给予精神上的安慰和鼓励，引导患者正确对待疾病，保持乐观情绪树立战胜疾病的信心。

6. 补气助阳药品，性多温燥，肝阳上亢、阴虚内热患者应慎用；滋阴养血药品性多滋腻，脾胃虚弱者应配合健脾益胃药。

7. The patients with deficiency syndrome which is difficult to cure should be instructed to persist in taking medicine accurately.

(Wang Shi-yuan)

Section 6　Rescue and Nursing Care for Chinese Medicinal Herb Poisoning

TCM has rich knowledge and cognition about the toxicity of Chinese medical herb. In ancient times, people frequently got poisoned in the process of looking for food and herbs. With the accumulation of experience, people gradually began to recognize the toxicity of Chinese medical herb. *Shennong's Classic of Materia Medica,* which divided herbs into three categories: superior, middle and inferior. It pointed out that the inferior grade herbs were deleterious and weren't appropriate for a long term usage. It also emphasized the necessity to eliminate or reduce the toxicity of toxic Chinese medical herb by a variety of processing methods. Some remedies for traditional Chinese material medica poisoning were recorded in *Treatise on Cold Febrile and Miscellaneous Diseases*（at the end of the Eastern Han Dynasty）. Many remedies for Chinese medical herb poisoning were specifically introduced in the *Handbook of Prescriptions for Emergency* which was written in the Jin Dynasty. Some diagnostic methods of Chinese medical herb poisoning, for instance, using a silver fork to test whether the arsenic was taken in or not, were firstly narrated in the *Record of Redressing Mishandled Cases* (*Xǐ Yuān Jí Lù,* 洗冤集录) written by a medicolegist called Song Ci (AD 1186—1249) in the Nan song Dynasty, which greatly enriched the toxicology of Chinese medical herb. Up to the modern times, the further research of the toxicity of Chinese medical herb has aroused people's concern and attention.

I. Concept of the Toxicity of Chinese Medical Herb

TCM has a variety of different cognition about the concept of the toxicity of Chinese medical herb in the history. In general, it has the following three aspects:

1. Generic Term Revering to the Entire Chinese

第六节　常用中草药中毒解救及护理

中医学对中药毒性的认识已有悠久的历史。上古时代，人们在寻觅食物及草药的过程中常发生中毒现象，随着经验的积累，人们渐渐开始对中药的毒性有所了解。《神农本草经》把中药分为上品、中品、下品三类，并指出下品"多毒，不可久服"，且指出需用各种炮制方法来消除或减弱有毒中药的毒性。东汉末年的《伤寒杂病论》记载了一些中药中毒的解救方法。晋代的《肘后备急方》具体介绍了不少中药中毒的解救方法。南宋法医学家宋慈撰写的《洗冤集录》中首次叙述了中药中毒的一些诊断方法，如"用银叉验服毒（砒霜）"等，大大地充实了中药毒理学的内容。至近代，中药的毒性得到更进一步的研究，并引起了人们的关注与重视。

一、中药的毒性概念

中医药对中药的毒性概念的认识，古今有很大的差异，归纳起来大致有以下三个方面：

1. **泛指一切中药的总称**　在古代医药文献

Medical Herb in General   In the ancient medical literatures, toxicity means the generic term of all the drugs. For example, "putting the poisons together to achieve the purpose of treating and curing patients", quoted from *Zhou Li Tian Guan* (*Zhōu Lǐ Tiān Guān,* 周礼·天官) which indicated that the poison means all the drugs.

　　2. Preference of Drug's Nature   Zhang Jing-yue (AD 1563-1640) once said that, "The drug's function relies on its toxicity. Anything that posses the effect to strengthen healthy qi and eliminate pathogenic factor can be entitled as toxicity. So it is acknowledged that poisonous drugs can eliminate pathogenic factors." He demonstrated the broad sense of the toxicity, and indicated that the toxicity of Chinese medical herb which is one of the drug's natures is a preference, and the basic principle of drug's treatment is to use the preference of drugs to regulate the imbalance of the body condition.

　　3. Toxic and Side effect   Chao Yuan-fang in the Sui Dynasty who said that all the toxic and hypertonic drugs could produce disorder and might kill people in the *General Treatise on Causes and Manifestations of All Diseases*. Many materia medica literatures of later ages had toxic or nontoxic recordation following the specific drugs. They also summarized some considerations about medicine compatibility, such as "eighteen clashes" "nineteen incompatibilities" "contraindications during pregnancy" "contraindications during medication" and so on.

　　The modern concept of toxic Chinese medical herb is always in a narrow sense, mainly referring to drugs which contain fiercely toxic components and have toxic and side effects, even cause the patient to death. Chinese medical herb with toxic and side effects is the focus of this section.

II. Route of Chinese Medical Herb Poisoning

i. Poisoning by Digestive Tract

　　It's major way of poisoning that the highly poisonous drugs are taken by oral and assimilated by gastrointestinal tract.

ii. Poisoning by Skin

　　Many medicines contain toxic components which have a characteristic of fat-solubility and water-solubility. These components can permeate skin and cause local inflammation, or even lead to systemic poisoning if they enter internal organs.

iii. Poisoning by Respiratory Tract

　　Vapour or powder which are produced in the process

中，毒药常是药物的总称。如《周礼·天官》所述"聚毒药以共医事"，就是指一切药物。

　　2. 指药物的性能偏胜   张景岳谓："药能治病，因毒为能……是凡可辟邪安正者，均可称为毒药，故曰毒药攻邪也。"论述毒药的广义含意，并阐明了毒性作为药物性能之一，是一种偏性，以偏治偏也就是药物治病的基本原理。

　　3. 指具有毒副作用的中药   隋代巢元方在《诸病源候论》中称："凡药物云有毒及有大毒者，皆能变乱，于人为害者，亦能杀人。"后世许多本草书籍在具体的药物项下，均有有毒无毒的记载，并总结了配伍用药的"十八反""十九畏""妊娠禁忌""服药禁忌"等注意事项。

　　近代概念之毒性中药，多为狭义，专指那些含有有毒成分，药性峻猛，进入机体易致毒副作用甚至使人致死者。本节所述侧重具有毒副作用的中药。

二、中草药中毒的途径

（一）经消化道中毒

　　口服剧毒中药，经胃肠道吸收后而致中毒，这是中草药中毒的主要途径。

（二）经皮肤中毒

　　许多药物所含的有毒成分具有脂溶性兼有适当的水溶性的特性，故能透入皮肤，轻则引起局部炎症，重则进入体内而引起和口服类似的全身性中毒。

（三）经呼吸道中毒

　　某些中草药在煎煮、加工炮制或制剂时，

of decoction. processing and preparing can enter the lung through mouth and nose, and quickly enter the blood circulation to cause poisoning.

iv. Poisoning by Mucous Membrane

Some poisonous Chinese medical herb solution can enter the internal of the body through eyes, mouth, anus and vaginal mucosa. Because the toxic components are absorbed quickly, the poisoning symptoms occur more early.

III. Common Causes of Chinese Medical Herb Poisoning

The causes are generally includes two categories.

i. Conscious Poisoning

It means intentional overdose of toxic drugs which could cause death, such as suicide or murder. Highly poisonous drugs, such as *pī shuāng, xióng huáng, mǎ qián zǐ, bā dòu, chán chú, bān máo*, and *shēng cǎo wū* are used commonly.

ii. Unconscious Poisoning

1. Inappropriate Processing and Dosage Toxic drugs especially highly poisonous drugs can be used after processing, such as *tiān nán xīng, fù zǐ, mǎ qián zǐ* and aconitum drugs. Otherwise, they tend to cause poisoning.

2. Overdose People should abide by strict dose to prevent the negative effects which are caused by overdose. For example, the overdose of herbs like *guā dì, cháng shān* and others can lead to death, and the overdose of *huáng qí* can cause fierce limb-pain.

3. Inappropriate Compatibility Some drugs with light toxicity may generate restrictive or adverse effects and even further aggravate their original toxicity, while some drugs without toxicity may become toxic because of inappropriate compatibility. For example, *gān cǎo* can aggravate the toxicity of adrenal and ephedrine, while *gān cǎo* can reduce the toxicity of *gān suí* in a small dose, but it can increase the toxicity in a large dose.

4. Constitution Factor Different individual always reacts differently to poisoning, especially the old and weak or susceptible patients.

5. Misuse of Drug Similar drug names, homonym, synonym, and similar drug appearances can lead to misusage and cause poisoning.

6. Long Term Use Long term use of *léi gōng téng*

其升腾的蒸汽或飞扬的粉末，经口鼻吸入肺部，并迅速进入血液循环，导致中毒。

（四）经黏膜中毒

有毒中草药溶液经眼、口腔、肛门、阴道黏膜等进入体内，可引起中毒，且毒物吸收较快，症状发生较早。

三、中草药中毒的常见原因

中药中毒的原因一般分两大类。

（一）有意识中毒

常见自杀和谋杀，即有意识过量服用有毒中药，引起中毒身亡。所用药物大多是砒霜、雄黄、马钱子、巴豆、蟾蜍、斑蝥、生草乌等毒剧中药。

（二）无意识中毒

1. **炮制与服法不当**　有毒中药尤其是毒性较强的中药，一般要经过炮制后才能使用。如天南星、附子、马钱子及乌头类药物，须加工炮制后使用，否则易引起中毒。

2. **剂量过大**　应掌握正确的用药剂量，防止超量而导致不良后果。如超剂量内服瓜蒂、常山等会致人中毒死亡，大剂量黄芪会引起剧烈肢痛等。

3. **配伍不当**　有些毒性不大的药物可因配伍不当产生制约或相反作用而加剧其原有毒性，甚至一些单用无害的药物可因配伍不当而产生毒性。如肾上腺毒及麻黄碱中毒时，使用甘草会加重毒性；甘草与甘遂配伍，小剂量能降低其毒性，大剂量会增强其毒性。

4. **体质因素**　人体对毒物的反应，往往因个体差异，年老体弱或过敏体质而有极大的不同。

5. **误用误食**　药名相似，异物同名，异名同物或物形相像，导致误用。

6. **长期服用**　如久服雷公藤可导致再生

can result in aplastic anemia. Long term use of *fān xiè yè can* lead to drug dependence.

7. Blind Medication　Some people who have incompliance and drug abuse think that Chinese herb is quite safe and can be applied to medical treatment and health care. They abuse folk recipes, simple recipes, and secret recipes and so on, which leads to poisoning too.

IV. Preventive Measure of Chinese Herb Poisoning

The fundamental preventive measure for Chinese herb poisoning is to eliminate the cause of the poisoning. Synthesizing the literature and reports, the following measures should be mainly adopted.

i. Appropriate Dosage

The main cause of poisoning is overdosed intake of drugs in a short time. A research reported that this reason accounted for about 89.68% of patients with renal damage caused by poisoning. So the dosage of Chinese herbs should strictly follow the recommendations in some authoritative reference books, such as *Chinese Pharmacopoeia (Zhōng Huá Rén Mín Gòng Hé Guó Yào Diǎn,* 中华人民共和国药典*).*

ii. Stop Medication as soon as Cured

Although some drug's single dose is normal or within the prescribed limit, it can cause cumulative intoxication due to the long-term use. Some data showed that the number of patients with renal damage caused by cumulative intoxication accounted for about 3.57%. Hence, TCM traditionally emphasizes the principle of stopping medication as soon as cured.

iii. Reducing Drug Toxicity and Side Effect by Rational Compatibility

The key to reducing and preventing drug poisoning is the proper compatibility between different Chinese herbs and Western medicine.

iv. Abide by Processing Technology and Prevent Misusage

An important measure to ensure safety and affectivity of clinical medication is the standard processing of Chinese herbs. Especially the drugs which contain certain toxicity, even in a correctly conventional dosage, can also cause severe poisoning without standard processing.

v. Pay Attention to the Individual Difference of Patient

Different individual always reacts differently to

障碍性贫血，长期服用番泻叶可导致药物依赖等。

7. 盲目用药　认为吃中药安全，有病治病，无病健身，不遵医嘱，滥用中药，迷信偏方、单方、秘方等，也可能会引起中毒。

四、中草药中毒的预防措施

预防中草药中毒的关键在于杜绝发生中草药中毒的原因，综合文献资料、报告，应主要采取以下措施。

（一）正确掌握药物用量

在短时间内大剂量或超大剂量用药是引起中毒的主要原因。有报告称由于该原因中毒造成肾损害者约占 89.68%。因此中药的用量一般应遵循《中华人民共和国药典》等权威性的参考书推荐的剂量。

（二）中病即止，防止长期用药

有些中草药单次应用剂量并不大（或在规定的剂量范围内），但如果长期服用，则可造成蓄积中毒。有资料显示：因药物蓄积中毒造成肾损害者约占 3.57%。因此中医历来强调"中病即止"的用药原则。

（三）合理配伍，降低药物毒性和不良反应

中药与中药、中药与西药之间，在临床应用时的合理配伍，是降低与防止药物中毒的关键。

（四）遵守炮制工艺，注意正确用法

中药材按标准炮制是临床用药安全有效的重要措施。特别对具有一定毒性的中草药，如未经炮制或炮制不当，即使服用常量，亦可出现严重中毒。

（五）重视患者的个体差异

人体对毒物的反应，常因个体差异而有

poison. As for drug use, TCM greatly emphasizes the principle of theory of *sān yīn zhì yí*, which means climate-concerned, environment-concerned and individuality-concerned idelogy. The young, the old, the maternal and the weak should cautiously use the toxic drugs.

vi. Strength the Health Publicity and Education to Prevent Blind Medication

To prevent poisoning which is caused by erroneous folk prescriptions, the intensified publicity is necessary.

vii. Improve Management Level and Establish Monitoring System of Adverse Drug Reaction

Establishing monitoring system of adverse drug reactions and conducting the modernized research of Chinese herb are the technical requirements of drugs' poisoning reduction. People should obey the *Measures for the Control of Poisonous Drugs for Medical Use* (*Yī Liáo Yòng Dú Xìng Yào Pǐn Guǎn Lǐ Bàn Fǎ*, 医疗用毒性药品管理办法), which establishes the supervisory system, analyzes the causes of poisoning to define the responsibility and takes preventative measures.

V. Clinical Manifestation of Chinese Herb Poisoning

i. Allergic Reaction

The clinical symptoms are mild in general, such as urticaria or herpes. Besides, patients can also have oppressed feeling in chest, shortness of breath, dyspnea or irritability. Some patients may have gastrointestinal symptoms like nausea, vomiting, abdominal pain and diarrhea. It can also cause allergic shock, which is mortiferous. The allergic reaction occurs shortly after medication. In general, the injection reaction is more severe than oral agents.

ii. Toxic Reaction

The severity of clinical symptoms varies with the dosage. Patients who are toxic due to a high dose often have an acute onset and urgent development. It may cause death if emergency treatment is not given timely. Different herbs can cause different clinical symptoms according to their different toxic action points.

1. Neurological Symptoms The toxic effects of herbs can affect the whole nervous system. Its toxic symptoms represent as disturbance and loss of sensory function, motor function and thinking function. Patients often die because of severe state of illness.

2. Gastrointestinal Symptoms It can cause different alimentary system reactions, like dry mouth,

很大不同。传统中医在药物应用上特别强调三因制宜，年幼、年老、孕产妇、重要脏器功能不佳者应慎用有毒中药。

（六）加强健康宣教，防止盲目用药

加强宣传教育，避免患者擅自或轻信游医偏方服用中药而致中毒。

（七）提高管理水平，建立药物不良反应监测制度

提高管理水平，建立药物不良反应监测制度及深入进行中药现代化研究，这是减少中草药中毒的组织措施与规范化的技术要求。对有毒中药要严格遵守国家关于《医疗用毒性药品管理办法》，建立监察制度，分析中毒的原因，明确责任，防患于未然。

五、中草药中毒的临床表现

（一）过敏反应

一般临床症状较轻，常见皮肤荨麻疹或疱疹，此外兼见胸闷气短、咳喘、烦躁不安，部分患者表现为恶心、呕吐、腹痛、腹泻等消化道症状，亦有因过敏性休克致死者。过敏反应多在用药后短期内出现，一般注射剂反应重于口服剂。

（二）中毒反应

根据剂量的不同临床症状亦有轻重之差异，一次大剂量应用而中毒者多起病急、发展迅速，若不及时抢救，常可导致死亡。根据药物的毒性作用部位不同，临床表现有以下几方面。

1. 神经系统症状 药物的毒性作用于整个神经系统，其中毒的症状包括感觉功能、运动功能和思维功能的障碍或丧失，患者常因病情严重而死亡。

2. 消化系统症状 可引起口干、流涎、恶心、呕吐、腹痛、腹泻、血便、烦躁乏力

salivation, nausea, vomiting, abdominal pain, diarrhea, bloody stool, restlessness and tiredness.

3. Respiratory Symptoms It can cause bronchospasm, asthma, dyspneic respiration, and so on. Severe cases can also have drop of blood pressure, which finally leads to the death of patiens.

4. Urinary Symptoms It can cause frequency of urinatior, urgent urination, urodynia, hematuria, oliguria or anuria and acute renal failure.

5. Circulatory System Symptoms It can cause chest oppression, dyspnea, fluster and arrhythmia.

6. Toxic Shock It can cause coma, drop of blood pressure, unconsciousness and weak pulse.

7. Others It can also cause pigmentation, hydroderma and hardening of the whole body skin, and drug-induced hepatitis.

VI. Rescue and Nursing Care for Chinese Herb Poisoning

i. Rescue for Chinese Herb Poisoning

Once the toxic reaction is diagnosed, rescue should be taken immediately by the intergration of Chinese and western medicine according to the following principles.

1. Stop Contacting the Toxicant Immediately

(1) Leave the poisoning scene: For aspirational poisoning, it needs to get the patients out of the poisoning scene immediately and remove their contaminated clothing.

(2) Flush the body surface: It should wash the contaminated parts, such as the surface of skin or mucosa thoroughly using clear water.

(3) Local treatment: If the toxic herbs directly contact with some local part of body in the process of their collection, production, medical processing, reserve, transportation or use, it should take the local treatments immediately, and expel the toxins as much as possible.

2. Rapid Elimination of Toxin that hasn't Been Absorbed yet

(1) Emetic therapy: Emetic therapy is the fastest effective way to resolve toxins, for those who have taken the toxins within 2 to 3 hours and gastrolavage isn't available or those whose condition are mild and could have active cooperation with the doctors consciously.

1) Simple emetic action: To use spatula, chopstick, finger or feather to stimulate the laryngeal part of pharynx to make them vomit.

2) Emetic action by using western medicine: To dissolve sodium sulfate or potassium antimony tartrate in

等不同消化系统反应。

3. 呼吸系统症状 可引起支气管痉挛、哮喘、呼吸困难等症状，严重者还可出现血压下降等，最后导致患者死亡。

4. 泌尿系统症状 可引起尿频、尿急、尿痛、血尿、少尿或无尿、急性肾功能不全。

5. 循环系统症状 可引起胸闷、气短、心慌、心律不齐等。

6. 中毒性休克 可引起昏迷、血压下降、不省人事，脉搏细弱。

7. 其他 可引起色素沉着、全身皮肤水肿、变硬，药物中毒性肝炎等。

六、中草药中毒的解救及护理

（一）中草药中毒的解救

中毒反应一旦确诊后，必须迅速根据以下原则采用中西医结合方法进行抢救。

1. 立即终止接触毒物

（1）脱离中毒现场：对吸入性中毒应及时脱离现场，去除污染衣物。

（2）体表的冲洗：清洗中毒部位如皮肤表面或黏膜，用清水充分洗涤。

（3）局部处理：中草药在其采集、生产、炮制、贮运和使用过程中，若是有毒物直接接触局部的应立即进行局部处理，以尽可能地排毒。

2. 快速排出尚未吸收的毒物

（1）催吐：催吐是即时最快而有效的解毒方法。对毒物入口在 2~3min 以内，无洗胃条件或病情轻而又合作的清醒患者，可采用催吐法：

1）简易催吐法，用压舌板、筷子、手指或羽毛等机械法刺激咽喉部，使之呕吐；

2）西药催吐法，可用硫酸钠或酒石酸锑钾等药，溶于水中，口服催吐；

water and take it orally to vomit.

3) Emetic action by using Chinese herbs: Oral administration of the herbs with the emetic effects can expel the toxin which is kept in the gastric cavity from mouth cavity following vomitus.

(2) Gastrolavage: Gastrolavage is the most effective way to resolve toxins. Generally speaking, within 4 to 6 hours after taking the highly poisonous herbs, there still left a large sum of toxins and is not totally absorbed by the organism. Gastrolavage is the most effective way to avoid the toxins being absorbed by the digestive canal. Whether the gastrolavage is thorough or timely is the key of the rescue.

(3) Purgation: In order to expel the toxins that already has entered or is still remained in the intestinal tract, people can adopt the method of relieving constipation by purgation.

1) Purgation of western medicine: Take 25%-50% sodium sulfate solution or magnesium sulfate solution orally or use normal saline or suds. Magnesium sulfate sometimes can be absorbed by the intestinal tract, so it's not suitable for the patients who are in a central inhibitory poisoning state.

2) Purgation of Chinese herbs: Chinese herbs can not only expel intracorporal toxins through stool, they can also induct the toxins to be expelled through urine.

3. Block the Adsorption of the Toxin After gastrolavage or emetic action, the patient should take medical charcoal, which can adsorb alkaloid, metal and other toxins. That can reduce the amounts of toxins absorbed by digestive canal. Some herbs can absorb toxins, or let some toxins have precipitation reaction, or become insoluble substance, which make the toxins being adsorbed easily and reduced its toxic effects.

4. Accelerate the Expelling of Absorbed Toxin and Resolving Toxin People can choose different kinds of methods and antidotes according to the quality, component and action area of the toxic herb, such as diuretic, antidotes, hemodialysis, peritoneal dialysis, antidotes of herbs and other ways. If people can confirm the toxic herbs definitely, they can use the prescription principles of herbs to resolve toxins, such as (mutual) suppression and mutual restraint between two drugs. People could use the opposite property of the two drugs to get rid of the toxicity and ill-effect.

5. Other Treatment Besides taking the measures of emetic action and gastrolavage, people can also take the auxiliary methods like needling treatment to cure

3）中药催吐法，通过内服催吐类中药而引发呕吐，使滞留于胃脘部的中毒中药随涌吐物一并从口腔中排出体外而达到解救目的的方法。

（2）洗胃：洗胃是即时最有效的解毒方法。一般在服下剧毒中药 4~6min 内，胃肠中尚有大部分未被吸收的毒物，洗胃是避免毒物从消化道吸收最有效的方法。洗胃是否彻底及时关系抢救的成败。

（3）导泻：为迅速排出已经进入肠道的毒素或残留于肠道的毒素，可采用泻下的方法：

1）西药导泻法，25%~50% 的硫酸钠或硫酸镁溶液口服导泻，或用生理盐水、肥皂水灌肠，因硫酸镁有时也会被肠道吸收，故中枢抑制性中毒反应者不宜使用；

2）中药导泻法，在通过大便排出体内毒物的同时，也可诱导有毒物质从小便排出体外。

3. 阻滞毒物的吸收 洗胃或催吐后给患者服用药用炭，可吸附生物碱及金属等毒物，减少毒物经消化道吸收。有些中药能够吸附毒物或使某些毒物产生沉淀反应或形成不溶性物质，使之不易吸收从而减轻其毒性反应。

4. 加速已吸收毒物的排出和解毒 可根据中毒药物的性质、成分、作用部位而选择不同的方法和解毒剂，如应用利尿剂、解毒剂、血液透析、腹膜透析、中药解毒剂等。如果明确知道中毒药物名称时，可根据中药的相杀、相畏配伍原则，使用中药解毒。利用药物药性的相互对峙解除其中一种药物的毒性和不良反应。

5. 其他疗法 中药中毒之解救，除了采取催吐、洗胃等措施外，亦可辅以针刺对症

the illness. Needling treatments can alleviate the toxic symptoms and help the organism to recover.

ii. Nursing Care for Chinese Herb Poisoning

1. Clinical Observation

(1) Nurses should observe the patients' variations of mentality, pupil and vital signs strictly, while take records in time, such as time of poisoning, symptoms and treatment process.

(2) If the toxic herb is uncertain, nurses should assist doctors to ask about the medical history carefully, take the specimen correctly and make qualitative and quantitative analyses of the toxicant aimed at the specimen.

(3) Nurses should observe patient's other accompanied symptoms carefully and assist the doctors to give expectant treatments and nursing care.

2. Dietary Nursing Care　Patients of food poisoning have a bad appetite at the early stage. Liquid diets are suitable for them at this time. Patients of oral poisoning often suffer from digestive canal damage, so it's suitable for them to eat food which has nutritional value, and easy to digest. Nurses should encourage them to have more meals a day but less food at each and avoid overeating. People should obey the alimentary taboos of the different herb poisoning.

3. Living Nursing Care　Patients of acute poisoning should have a bed rest. The ward should maintain good ventilation, comfortable temperature and humidity. Eclamptic patients should be placed in a quiet single room and the lighting of the room should be dim. All needed examinations and treatments should be arranged at one time. Nurses should keep quiet to avoid pessimal stimulation on patients. Patients with vexation and agitation should be given sedative with short half-life period. Guard bar should be put to avoid them falling down from bed.

4. Emotional Nursing　Most people believe that herbs are free of toxin or side effects and are safer than western medicine. Once patients would have toxic symptoms, they'll have bad emotions, such as anxiety, doubt, irritability and agitation. In addition, since lacking of the knowledge of poisoning, patients and their family members are all restless. At this time, nurses should communicate with them timely and initiatively and let them give active cooperation to the treatments and nursing care of the medical personnel after they have understood the state of illness and the prognosis.

(Wang Shi-yuan)

治疗，可减轻中毒症状，促进机体恢复正常。

（二）中草药中毒的护理

1. 病情观察

（1）应严密观察患者神志、瞳孔、生命体征变化并及时记录。同时，应记录中毒时间、中毒后出现症状、处理过程等。

（2）不明药物中毒时，应配合医生仔细询问病史，正确留取标本，针对标本作毒物定性或定量分析、鉴定。

（3）仔细观察患者的其他伴随症状，协助医生对症处理和护理。

2. 饮食护理　饮食中毒患者早期食欲缺乏，宜进流食。口服中毒者常有消化道的损害，在恢复期宜进营养丰富、易于消化的食物，并少食多餐，不宜过饱。遵守不同药物中毒的饮食宜忌。

3. 生活起居护理　急性中毒患者应卧床休息，保持通风，病室温度及湿度应适宜。惊厥患者宜安置于安静的单人房间，光线宜暗。各项检查、治疗尽量集中处置，保持安静，避免声响，以减少对患者的各种不良刺激。烦躁不安者给予半衰期较短的镇静剂，必要时加床边护栏，防止坠床。

4. 情志护理　多数人认为中草药无毒副作用、较安全。但患者一旦出现中毒症状后，会表现焦急、疑虑、烦躁、激动等不良情绪。加之对中毒知识的缺乏，患者及家属的心里充满了不安。护士要及时主动与患者及家属沟通交谈，让其了解病情及预后情况，配合医护人员的救治和护理。

（王诗源）

key points

1. There are many new forms invented with the development of TCM. The widely used forms include decoctions, pill and bolus, powder, gelatin or glue, wine preparation, distilled medicinal liquid, medicated tea, mixture, tablet, syrup, infusion granule, injection, suppository and capsule, and so on.

2. There are three main different kinds of contraindications for medication of TCM, namely: prohibited combination, contraindication during pregnancy and dietary incompatibility.

3. The combination relationships between drugs are categorized into seven groups. They are acting singly, mutual reinforcement, mutual assistance, mutual restraint, mutual suppression, mutual inhibition and mutual antagonism.

4. How to rescue poisoning of traditional Chinese Medicine. We should stop contacting the toxicant immediately and expel the toxins that are still not absorbed immediately. Gastrolavage is the most effective prompt way to resolve toxins. In order to expel the toxins that already has entered or is still remained in the intestinal tract, people can adopt the method of relieving constipation by purgation. We should block the adsorption of the toxins. After gastrolavage or emetic action, nurses should let the patient take medical charcoal, which can absorb alkaloid, metal and other toxins, so that it can reduce the amounts of toxins absorbed by digestive canal.

5. People should choose the ceramic utensils with covers as decocting utensils, such as earthenware pot and jar. The metal utensils made from iron, copper and aluminium are forbidden to decoct drugs, as metal tends to create chemical reactions with medicinal ingredients, which may reduce the therapeutic effects and even cause toxicity or side effects.

6. The water for decoction should be clear, pure, and contain less mineral. Except for special requirement in prescription, well water, tap water, distilled water or purified water are suitable for decocting. Cool water or cool boiled water is used for first decoction, and boiled water should be avoided. The water should be 3-5cm, 2-3cm above the drugs which are pressed into the pot respectively for the first decoction and the second decoction.

7. Medicinal materials should be marinated into cold water before being decocted. It is helpful to make medicinal materials soft and dissolve the active ingredients.

8. General compound decoction should be marinated for 30-60 minutes. Prescription composed of flowers or leaves or glass ought to be marinated for 20-30

要点

1. 随着中医药的发展，中药新剂型被研发应用。广泛应用的剂型有汤剂、丸剂、散剂、膏剂、酒剂、蒸馏药液、药茶、丹剂、片剂、糖浆、冲剂、注射液、栓剂、胶囊剂等。

2. 中药的禁忌证主要有三种，即配伍禁忌、孕期禁忌和饮食禁忌。

3. 中药药物之间的关系可分为七类，单行、相须、相使、相畏、相杀、相恶、相反。

4. 中药中毒抢救。立即停止接触毒物并排出尚未被吸收的毒素，洗胃是排出毒素最有效的方法，为了排除已进入或仍留在肠道内的毒素，人们可以采用泻下通便的方法。阻断毒素的吸附，在洗胃或催吐后，护士应让病人服用能吸收生物碱、金属和其他毒素的医用木炭，从而减少消化道吸收的毒素量。

5. 人们应该选择有盖的陶瓷器皿作为煎煮用具，铁、铜和铝制成的金属器皿被禁止煎药，因为金属倾向于与药物成分产生化学反应，这可能会降低治疗效果，甚至引起毒性或副作用。

6. 煎药应当用清澈、纯净、矿物质含量少的水。除处方中有特殊要求外，井水、自来水、蒸馏水或纯净水均可煎煮，头煎采用凉水或凉开水，切忌用开水，两次加水量应分别在药物上方 3~5cm 和 2~3cm 处。

7. 药材煎前应先用冷水浸泡。有助于药材的软化和有效成分的溶解。

8. 一般复方汤剂应浸泡 30~60min。由花、叶或草类为主的处方应浸泡 20~30min。由根、

minutes. Prescription composed of roots or stems or seeds or fructification is marinated for 60 minutes. Medicinal materials should not be washed by water. Active ingredients of some medicinal materials are easy to dissolve and lose if washed.

9. General medicinal materials are first decocted with strong fire and then with slow fire after the water boils.

10. Exterior-releasing drugs or other aromatic drugs are not suitable to decoct with strong flame in order to prevent active ingredients from volatilizing. Invigorant should be first decocted with strong flame and then decocted with mild flame to make active ingredients sufficiently extracted.

11. The stomach is empty before meals. Taking drugs before meal can avoid drugs being mixed with food and promote drugs to move into the intestines immediately to bring effects. So tonics, anti-acid drugs, drastic hydragogue and insect repellents had better be taken in this way. After meals, the stomach is full of food, which can reduce irritative effect of the drugs on the stomach and intestines. Therefore, the stomachic drugs and stimulant drugs should be taken after meal.

12. Tranquilizers should be taken 30-60 minutes before sleep in order to treat insomnia. Drugs to stop seminal emission should be taken before sleep. Taking a laxative before sleep can promote defecation in the next morning.

13. It is important to master special nursing methods for sweat promotion therapy, emetic therapy, purgative therapy, harmonizing therapy warming therapy, heat clearing therapy, dispelling therapy and tonifying therapy.

14. Preventive measures of Chinese herbs poisoning include appropriate dosage, stopping medication as soon as cured, reducing drug toxicity and side effects by rational combination of medicinals, abiding by processing technology and preventing misuse, paying attention to the individual difference of patients, strengthing the health publicity and education to prevent blind medication, improving management level and establishing monitoring system of adverse drug reactions.

茎、种子或果实组成的处方浸泡 60min。药材不能用水冲洗。有些药材的活性成分冲洗后容易溶解流失。

9. 一般药材先用武火煎，待水煮沸后用文火煎。

10. 中药通常要先用强火煎，再用弱火煎，使活性成分充分提取。发散类中药或其他芳香类药物不宜用强火焰煎煮，以防止活性成分挥发。

11. 饭前胃中空虚，饭前服用药物可以避免药物与食物混合，促进药物迅速进入肠道发挥药效。因此，补药、制酸药、催眠药、驱虫药等最好采用这种方法。饭后胃中存有较多食物，可以减少药物对胃的刺激作用，应在饭后服用消导药和抗风湿药。

12. 安神药、涩精止遗药、缓下药应在睡前 30~60min 应服用。睡前服用缓下药可以促进第二天早晨的排便。

13. 汗吐下和温清消补八法的护理。

14. 中药中毒的预防措施包括合理用药、尽快停药、减少用药毒副作用、监督中药炮制技术、防止误用、注重患者个体差异、加强卫生宣传教育，预防盲目用药，提高管理水平，建立药品不良反应监测体系。

Chapter 6　Commonly Used TCM Technique

第六章　常用中医护理技术及操作

<hr />

Learning Objectives	学习目标

Mastery

1. To repeat the meanings and functions of each commonly used TCM techniques.
2. To summarize the operation procedures of each commonly used TCM techniques.
3. To repeat the assessment, preventions and treatment of the possibility of accidents in using TCM techniques.

Comprehension

1. To explain the indications and contraindications of each commonly used TCM technique.
2. To understand how to choose the operating location of all of the operations by examples.
3. To give examples to explain the basic requirements of manipulations of each commonly used TCM technique.
4. To correctly understand the essentials operations of manipulations of each commonly used TCM technique.

Application

1. To implement the operation procedures of each commonly used TCM technique

识记

1. 能复述常用中医护理操作技术的各项操作技术的内涵、作用。
2. 能概述出常用中医护理操作技术的各项操作的程序。
3. 能复述各项常用中医护理操作技术意外情况的评价、处理和预防措施。

理解

1. 能理解常用中医护理技术的适应范围与禁忌证。
2. 能理解各项操作施术部位的选取。
3. 能举例解释各项操作施术的基本要求。
4. 能正确理解各种常见各项操作技术的重要操作要领。

运用

1. 能根据患者的情况，应用标准的护理操作程序为患者实施中医护理技术。

with standardized operation procedures according to individual's condition.

2. To exactly implement healthcare education of the commonly used TCM techniques.

2. 能做好常用中医护理技术的健康教育。

Case Study

The patient, female, 52 years old, a series of symptoms of menstrual disorder, insomnia, dreaminess, emotional lability occurred and is easy to be agitated recently. She always felt hot in the afternoon. She has a red tongue through the tongue diagnosis and thin pulse through the pulse diagnosis. She is diagnosed as perimenopausal syndrome. Now, it will apply auricular seeds taping therapy to the patient.

Question 1: Please find out the relevant auricular points according to the both of the patient's condition and the principles of selecting auricular points.

Question 2: Please explain the reason why select the points according to the both of the patient's condition and the principles of selecting auricular points.

Question 3: How to conduct health education to the patient, when a nurse implements the auricular seeds taping therapy for the patient.

TCM has thousands of years of history and accumulates abundant empirical experiences on treating disease and caring for patients. Techniques of TCM are the important composition of TCM nursing and embody the practical application of the TCM treatment. The characteristics of techniques are simple operation, economy, safety, definite efficacy, wide applicability, easy popularization and so on. This chapter mainly introduces approximately 21 kinds of techniques such as acupuncture, tuina, moxibustion, cupping therapy, scraping therapy, auricular seed taping therapy, hot compress therapy and so on.

导入案例与思考

患者，女，52 岁，近期出现月经紊乱，失眠，多梦，性情善变，易烦躁，午后潮热，舌红脉细。经诊断为围绝经期综合征，现采取耳穴压豆法治疗。

问题 1：根据以上病情及取穴原则，请正确选择相应的耳穴，并说明依据。

问题 2：实施此项操作，应如何向患者做好健康宣教。

从古至今，历代医家在长期医疗活动过程中积累了丰富的治疗方法。中医护理技术是以中医基础理论为指导，将中医传统的治疗方法在护理工作中的具体应用，是中医护理学重要组成部分，具有操作简单、经济安全、疗效确切、适用范围广、易于普及等特点。本章主要介绍针刺法、推拿法、灸法、拔罐法、刮痧法、穴位按压法、耳穴埋豆法、热熨法等二十一项操作技术。

Section 1   Acupuncture

Acupuncture refers to a therapeutic method under the guidance of TCM meridian theory that stimulates certain locations of the body by manipulating different metal needles to inspire qi of the meridian and collaterals, as well as regulate yin and yang in order to balance the body. Acupuncture techniques include filiform needle therapy, dermal needling therapy, electro-acupuncture therapy, hydro-acupuncture therapy, and auricular acupuncture therapy.

第一节   针刺法

针刺法，是在中医经络学说理论指导下，采用不同金属制成不同型号的针具，施以不同的手法，刺激人体的腧穴，以激发经络之气，调整阴阳，从而使机体恢复平衡，达到治疗疾病目的的方法。它包括毫针刺法、皮肤针法、电针法、水针法、耳针法等。

I. Filiform Needle Therapy

i. Structure and Gauge of the Filiform Needle

1. Structure of the Filiform Needle A filiform needle popularly used today is made of stainless steel which is of high hardness and elasticity, and is noncorrosive and inexpensive. A needle made of gold, silver or mixed alloy is expensive and is of low hardness and elasticity. However, it has higher conduction of electricity and heat, therefore, it is proper for warm needling.

A filiform needle is divided into 5 parts including needle tip, needle body (needle shaft), needle root, needle handle and needle tail (Fig.6-1).

Needle tip is the sharp part in the front of needle body. Needle body is the main part between needle tip and handle. Needle root is the connecting part between needle body and needle handle. Holding needle part is called needle handle. The ending part of the shank is called needle tail. Needle handle and needle tails are formed to many varieties of shapes such as spiral or cylinder *etc.*.

2. Gauge of the Filiform Needle The gauge of a needle is determined by its length and diameter. The traditional gauge measured by millimeters "mm" is listed as below (Table 6-1 and Table 6-2). The needle's hardness is related to its length and diameter. So the selection of needles is according to the patient's constitution, conditions of the disease, locations of the points and so on, to be treated by dialectical view on clinic. Generally, the length of needle body that the most commonly used range is 0.32-0.38 cm and the diameter is 25-50mm.

ii. Practicing Needling Skill

It is important to practice needling skill and the

一、毫针刺法

（一）毫针的构造、规格

1. 毫针的构造 现代临床所用的毫针多由不锈钢制成。不锈钢毫针具有良好的弹性和强度，不易生锈，并且价格便宜，因此最为常用。用金、银或合金制成的毫针强度和韧性稍差，价格昂贵，但其导电性和热传导性能明显优于不锈钢毫针，适合于温针。

毫针的结构可分为五个部分，即针尖、针身、针根、针柄、针尾（图 6-1）。

针尖是针身的尖端锋锐部分，亦称针芒；针身是针尖与针柄之间的主体部分，亦称针体；针身与针柄连接的部分称为针根；针体与针根之后执（持）针着力的部分称为针柄；柄的末梢部分称为针尾。针柄与针尾多缠绕呈螺旋状或圆筒状等多种形状。

2. 毫针的规格 毫针的规格主要以针身的长短和粗细来区分，以"mm"为计量单位，目前所用毫针的长短、粗细规格分别见表 6-1 和表 6-2。毫针的粗细与针刺的强度有关，所以在临床应根据患者的体质、病情和腧穴部位等进行辨证选用。一般粗细 28~30 号（0.32~0.38mm）和长短为 1~2 寸（25~50mm）者最为常用。

（二）毫针刺法的练习

毫针刺法的练习，主要是对指力和手法

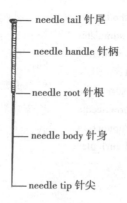

needle tail 针尾

needle handle 针柄

needle root 针根

needle body 针身

needle tip 针尖

Fig. 6-1　Structure of the Filiform Needle
图 6-1　毫针的构造

Table 6-1　Length of the Filiform Needle

Old gauge/cun	0.5	1	1.5	2	2.5	3	4	4.5	5	6
Length of needle body/mm	15	25	40	50	65	75	100	115	125	150

表 6-1　毫针长短的规格

规格 / 寸	0.5	1	1.5	2	2.5	3	4	4.5	5	6
长度 /mm	15	25	40	50	65	75	100	115	125	150

Table 6-2　Diameter of the Filiform Needle

Size	26	27	28	29	30	31	32	33	34	35
Diameter/mm	0.45	0.42	0.38	0.34	0.32	0.30	0.28	0.26	0.24	0.22

表 6-2　毫针粗细的规格

规格 / 号数	26	27	28	29	30	31	32	33	34	35
直径 /mm	0.45	0.42	0.38	0.34	0.32	0.30	0.28	0.26	0.24	0.22

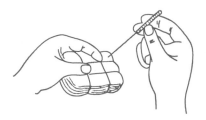

Fig. 6-2(a)　Practice Needling Skills
图 6-2(a)　指力练习

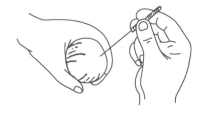

Fig. 6-2(b)　Practice Finger Force
图 6-2(b)　手法练习

Fig. 6-2　Practice
图 6-2　练习

finger force [Fig. 6-2(a), (b)]. Since its body is slender and flexible, the filiform needle will be difficult for an untrained clinician to insert without causing pain or to administer different manipulations skillfully. Therefore, adequate training of needling skill and finger force is essential for a beginner.

1. Practicing Finger Force　Finger force practice is to train the beginner to exert his or her fingers force on the needle tip so as to insert the needle into the human body smoothly. Finger force practice can be first conducted on a paper pad or cotton ball. It is suggested to hold a paper or cotton ball with the left hand and the needle with the thumb, index and middle fingers of the right hand. In doing so, the needle should be kept upright

的练习 [图 6-2（a）,（b）]。由于毫针针身细而软，如果没有一定的指力和熟练的手法，则很难顺利进针和进行各种手法的操作。这不仅会引起患者的疼痛，而且会影响治疗效果。因此，指力和手法的练习，是针刺初学者重要的基本技能训练。

1. 指力练习　指力，是指术者持针之手的力量和使力达针尖的技巧。指力的练习，可在纸垫或棉团上进行。练习时，一般左手持纸垫或棉团，右手持针，右手拇、示、中三指如持毛笔状挟持针柄，使针垂直于纸垫或棉团，当针尖抵达纸垫或棉团后，手指渐

as if holding a Chinese writing brush, and then hold the needle body vertically to the paper pad or cotton ball. Just after the needle tip touches the pad or the ball, finger force is gradually exerted to make the needle enter the pad or ball. Keep doing so until the needle can be inserted smoothly, dexterously and rapidly into the pad or ball.

2. Practicing Common Manipulation Practicing common manipulation is conducted based on practicing finger force. The commonly used practicing manipulation are as follows (Fig. 6-2).

(1) Practicing quick puncturing: To use the thumb, middle finger and index finger of the right hand to hold the needle, insert it quickly vertically into the appropriate point on the pad or ball for a depth of 2-3mm repeatedly. This is to train the beginner how to insert the needle quickly and without pain.

(2) Practicing lifting-thrusting manipulation: After the needle is inserted, lift and thrust the needle repeatedly and moderately at the insertion point. The needle should reach the desired and appropriate depth. Moreover, the needle body should always be kept vertical throughout the entire process.

(3) Practicing twirling-rotating manipulation: After the needle is inserted, use the thumb and index finger to hold the needle handle and twist it on the original spot clockwise with the thumb moving forward and the index finger moving backward, and then counter-clockwise with the thumb moving backward and the index finger moving forward. The twisting angle should be even and the manipulation should be dexterous and consistent in speed.

In the process of practice, lifting-thrusting and twirling-rotating manipulations can be done in a simultaneous operation untill it has been mastered finally. In order to improve the level of acupuncture technique and experiment with different feelings, it can be practiced on themselves or each other between classmates.

iii. Preparation Prior to Treatment

1. Assessment Prior to Treatment It needs to assess the patient's history, major symptoms, location of the disease, the points for treatment, skin condition of points and the patient's constitution, age, education background, psychological status, understanding of the disease, cognition degree of acupuncture, sensitivity degree of point and degree of cooperation with the doctor.

2. Selection of Needles Using appropriate needles is one of the most important components to

加压力，待针刺透纸垫或棉团后，再换一处如前法刺之，练习至针能灵活迅速刺入。

2. **手法练习** 针刺手法练习，是在指力练习的基础上进行的，主要有以下几种：

（1）速刺练习：术者以右手拇、示、中指持针，使针尖快速刺入 2~3mm，反复练习以提高进针速度，速刺可以减少疼痛。

（2）提插练习：术者以右手拇、示、中指持针，针刺入一定深度后做上提下插的动作。要求提插幅度适宜，针体垂直无偏斜。

（3）捻转练习：术者以右手拇、示、中指持针，针刺入后做来回捻转，针刺深度不变。要求捻转角度均匀，运用灵活，快慢自如。

在练习过程中，捻转与提插可以同时操作，最终达到捻转角度来去、提插幅度上下一致，快慢均匀。为了临床施术时做到心中有数，体验不同的针刺手法所产生的不同作用，可在自己身上进行练针，或与同学之间相互试针，以提高针刺手法的操作水平。

（三）针刺前的准备

1. **针刺前评估**

了解既往史、当前主要症状、发病部位及所刺腧穴皮肤情况；了解患者的体质、年龄、文化层次、精神状态、心理状态及对疾病的认识；了解患者对针刺法的认知程度、腧穴敏感程度和配合程度。

2. **针具选择** 正确选择使用不同规格的针具，是提高疗效和防止医疗事故的一个重

ensure good therapeutic effects and avoid possible medical accidents during acupuncture process. Needles are chosen based on patients gender, age, physique, somato types, the points and conditions of the treatment regions and different diseases. Generally speaking, thick and long needles are chosen for men, people with large body's structure, obese persons and people with a deep-seated disease. On the other hand, short and thin needles are selected for women, people with feeble body's structure, lean patients or people with a low-seated disease. As for the locations of the points, the areas with little muscles and points superficially inserted are treated with short and thin needles. Places with thick muscles and points deeply inserted are treated with long and relatively strong needles. It is strongly suggested that about 5 to10mm length of the needle body should be exposed over the skin after insertion of an appropriate depth in clinic.

3. Posture Selection of the Patient Proper posture selection of the patient takes a great effect on accurately locating points, manipulating the needle and treating results. Poor posture will cause difficulties in locating points, in manipulation and prolonged retention of the needle, and may cause tiredness or even fainting of the patient. The principle for selecting an appropriate posture is to conveniently locate the point, manipulate the needle and make the patient comfortable to endure the retained needle for a long time. In general, a lying down posture is recommended for the weak, nervous or first-time visitors and a change of position is not allowed during the operating.

There are lying posture and sitting posture. The lying down posture is further categorized into supine, lateral recumbent and prone positions, while the sitting posture is divided into supine sitting, sitting in flexion and lateral sitting. The postures and their indications are listed as follows (Fig. 6-3).

Supine posture: It is suitable for points on head, face, neck, chest, abdomen and limbs [Fig. 6-3(a)].

Lateral recumbent posture: It is suitable for points on the lateral side of head, chest and abdomen, arms and legs [Fig. 6-3(b)].

Prone posture: suitable for points on head, neck, shoulder, back, lumbar and sacrum and the posterior and lateral region of the lower limbs [Fig. 6-3(c)].

Sitting in supine posture: It is suitable for points on head, face, neck, upper chest and upper limbs [Fig. 6-3(d)].

Sitting in flexion: It is suitable for points on the top of head, back of head, neck, shoulder and back [Fig. 6-3(e)].

要因素。应根据患者的性别、年龄、体质、体型、针刺的部位和不同的疾病等因素，选择适宜的针具。一般来说，男性、体质强壮、体胖、病变部位较深者，可选用稍粗、较长的毫针；女性、体质较弱、体瘦、病变部位较浅者，可选用较短、较细的毫针。皮薄肉少之处和针刺较浅的腧穴，宜选细而短的毫针；皮厚肉丰之处和针刺较深的腧穴，应选稍长、稍粗的毫针。毫针长度的选择，临床上常以将针刺入应达深度后在皮肤外仍有5~10mm的针身外露为宜。

3. 体位选择 针刺时患者体位选择是否适当，对腧穴的正确定位、针刺的施术操作及治疗效果均有很大影响。如所选的体位不适当，可使术者取穴困难，不便于操作，也不宜留针，轻则引起患者疲劳，重则能使患者发生晕针。针刺时体位的选择，应以便于术者能正确取穴、进针，患者感到舒适自然，并能持久为原则。凡体质虚弱、年老、精神过度紧张和初诊患者，应首先考虑卧位，在针刺和留针的过程中应嘱患者切不可移动体位。

临床上常用的体位有两种，即卧位和坐位。卧位又分仰卧位、侧卧位、俯卧位；坐位又可分为仰靠坐位、俯伏坐位、侧伏坐位。

仰卧位：适用于取头、面、颈、胸、腹部和部分四肢部的腧穴 [图 6-3（a）]。

侧卧位：适用于取侧头、侧胸、侧腹、臂和下肢外侧等部位的腧穴 [图 6-3（b）]。

俯卧位：适用于取头、项、肩、背、腰、骶和下肢后面、外侧等部位的腧穴 [图 6-3（c）]。

仰靠坐位：适用于取前头、面、颈、胸上部和上肢的部分的腧穴 [图 6-3（d）]。

俯伏坐位：适用于取头顶、后头、项、肩、背等的腧穴 [图 6-3（e）]。

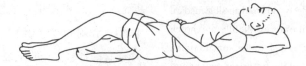

Fig. 6-3(a)　Supine Posture
图 6-3(a)　仰卧位

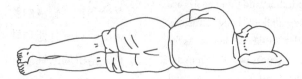

Fig. 6-3(b)　Lateral Recumbent Posture
图 6-3(b)　侧卧位

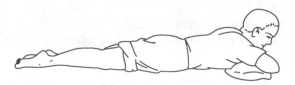

Fig. 6-3(c)　Prone Posture
图 6-3(c)　俯卧位

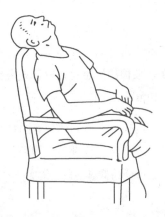

Fig. 6-3(d)　Sitting in Supine Posture
图 6-3(d)　仰靠坐位

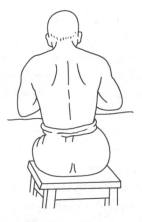

Fig. 6-3(e)　Sitting in Flexion
图 6-3(e)　俯伏坐位

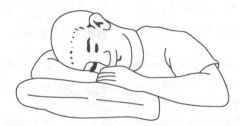

Fig. 6-3(f)　Sitting in Lateral Posture
图 6-3(f)　侧伏坐位

Fig. 6-3　Posture
图 6-3　体位

Sitting in lateral posture: suitable for points on the lateral sides of head and neck [Fig. 6-3(f)].

4. Sterilization Disinfection must be done before acupuncture. Sterilization in acupuncture includes sterilization of needles and instruments, disinfection of the hands of acupuncturist and disinfection of the area selected for needling.

(1) Sterilization of needles and instruments: The following methods of sterilization are indicated for non-disposable needles finished cleaning, in which the autoclave sterilization is the most effective one.

1) Autoclave sterilization: Needles wrapped up in gauze or stored in tubes or boxes are then put in an autoclave which with pressure at 98-147kPa and temperature in 115-123℃ for over 30 minutes.

2) Boiling sterilization: Put the needles and apparatus into the water and heat them until boiling for 10 to 15 minutes. This sterilization method is commonly applied since it is simple and easy. However, boiling water may cause corrosion to the metal apparatus and blunting of the blade and needle tip.

3) Medicinal sterilization: Soak the needles in 75% alcohol liquid for 30-60 minutes, then remove and wipe off the excess liquid from the needle with a piece of dry cloth. Other tools such as the tray and tweezers that contact with the needles directly should also be sterilized in the same way. Sterilized needles must be put in the sterilized trays.

Acupuncture needles can be reused after sterilization. Although it can save some costs, there still exists a risk of cross contamination. Sterilized reused needles have been gradually replaced by disposable needles in current clinical practice.

(2) Disinfection of the hands of the acupuncturist: Before acupuncture, the operator should wash his or her hands with soap, rinse with tap water, and then wipe with 75% alcohol-soaked cotton balls. The acupuncturist's fingers should try to avoid touching the needle body. If it can't avoid touching the needle body, the acupuncturist must use disinfection dry cotton ball as isolation to ensure that needle body is sterile.

(3) Disinfection of the area selected for needling: In general, it should wipe twice the area on the body surface selected for needling with a 75% alcohol-soaked cotton ball or 0.5% iodine-soaked cotton balls in a circular manner starting from the center and moving externally. In blood letting with three-edged needle, the local area should be first wiped with a 2% iodine-soaked cotton

侧伏坐位：适用于取侧头、侧颈部的腧穴 [图 6-3（f）]。

4. 消毒 针刺前必须做好消毒工作，其中包括针具消毒，术者手指的消毒和施术部位的消毒。

（1）针具消毒：如果使用非一次性针具，清洗后，可根据具体情况选择下列方法进行消毒，其中以高压蒸汽灭菌法为佳。

1）高压消毒：将毫针等器具用纱布包扎，或装在试管、针盒里，放在密闭的高压蒸汽消毒锅内，一般在 98~147kPa 的压力，115~123℃高温下保持 30min 以上，即可达到消毒的目的。

2）煮沸消毒：将毫针等应用器械放置清水中，加热沸腾后，再煮 10~15min。此法简便易行，无需特殊设备，故比较常用，但对锋利的金属器械，容易使锋刃变钝。

3）药物消毒：将针具放在 75% 乙醇内浸泡 30~60min，取出擦干使用。直接与毫针接触的针盘、镊子等也应进行消毒，已消毒的毫针必须放在消毒的针盘内。针具的重复使用，虽可节约部分费用，但存在交叉感染的可能性，目前临床多选用一次性针具取代针具消毒。

（2）术者手指的消毒：在针刺前，术者的手，需要用肥皂水洗刷干净，再用 75% 乙醇棉球涂擦后，才能实施针刺术。持针施术时操作者应尽量避免手指直接接触针身，如刺法需要触及针身时，必须用消毒干棉球作为隔物，以确保针身无菌。

（3）施术部位的消毒：在患者需要针刺的腧穴部位，用 75% 乙醇棉球，或用 0.5% 碘伏棉球擦拭即可。如使用三棱针放血时，应先用 2% 碘酒涂擦局部皮肤，待干后，再用 75% 乙醇脱碘。消毒之处皮肤应避免接触污染物，以防重新污染。

ball, followed by a 75% alcohol-soaked cotton ball to de-iodinate the area where is dried. Keep the disinfected area clean from dirt and contamination.

iv. Needling Method

1. Methods of Needle Insertion   It refers to the needles are inserted into the skin. In practice, the right hand is usually applied to hold the needle handle. The correct method is to hold the needle handle with the thumb, index and middle fingers as if holding a traditional Chinese writing brush (Fig. 6-4). Hence the right hand is named the "puncturing hand". The left hand is usually applied to press down the skin around the point or assisted in holding the needle handle to support the insertion of the needle. Hence it is named the "pressing hand".

The function of the puncturing hand is to hold the needle and administrate the needling manipulations. During the insertion of the needle, the finger force has to be gathered and passed down to the needle tip in order to puncture through the skin smoothly. During the manipulation of the needling, the fingers have to coordinate with each other to conduct various movements of the needle such as twirling and rotating, lifting and thrusting, vibrating, scraping, flicking, shaking, withdrawing the needle and so on.

The function of the pressing hand is to fix the location of the point and hold the needle handle to support the puncturing hand to insert the needle vertically and quickly in order to reduce pain caused by needling and regulate and control the needling sensation. The commonly used needle insertion methods are listed below (Fig.6-5).

(1) Inserting the needle with one hand: Usually the right hand (puncturing hand) is used. Hold the needle handle with the thumb and index finger. The tip of the middle finger gently touches the skin close to the point and the belly of the middle finger supports the lower part of the needle at the same time. The needle can be inserted

（四）针刺的方法

1. **进针法**   进针法是指将毫针刺入皮肤的操作方法。临床上一般多用右手持针，主要以拇、示、中三指挟持针柄，其状如持毛笔（图6-4）。故右手又称为"刺手"。左手爪甲按压所刺部位或辅助针身，故称左手为"押手"。

刺手的作用是掌持针具，施行手法操作，进针时运指力于针尖，使针刺入皮肤，行针时便于左右捻转、上下提插和弹刮搓震以及出针操作等。

押手的作用是固定腧穴位置，挟持针身协助刺手进针，使针身有所依附而保持针垂直，力达针尖，以利于进针，减少刺痛和协助调节、控制针感。具体的进针方法，临床常用的有以下几种。

（1）单手进针法：单手进针是指仅用单只手（刺手）将针刺入穴位的方法。通常是以右手拇指、示指挟持针柄，中指指端靠近穴位，指腹抵住针尖和针身下端，当拇、示指

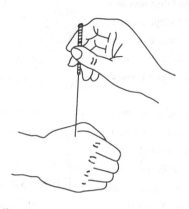

Fig. 6-4   Methods of Needle Insertion
图6-4   持针姿势

quickly by exerting finger force from the thumb and the index finger, meanwhile bending the middle finger [Fig. 6-5(a)].

(2) Inserting the needle with both hands: This means that the left and right hands (puncturing hand and pressing hand) work together to push the needle into the skin. There are four kinds of needle inserting methods for using both hands:

1) Inserting the needle with the aid of the finger of the pressing hand: Press on the point with the nail of the thumb or the index finger, or the middle finger of the pressing hand, then hold the needle with the right hand and insert it into the skin close to the edge of the nail of the finger of the left hand. This method is suitable for insertion of short needles [Fig. 6-5(b)].

2) Inserting the needle by gripping the needle: Grip the lower portion of the needle body with the thumb and index finger of the left hand with a dry sterilized cotton ball. Fix the needle tip on the skin where the point is located. Hold the needle handle with the right hand, and then quickly insert the needle into the skin with pressure exerted downward with the two hands simultaneously. This method is suitable for insertion of long needles [Fig. 6-5(c)].

3) Inserting the needle by stretching the skin: Put the thumb and index fingers or the index and middle fingers of pressing hand on the skin where the point is located. Separate the two fingers to stretch the skin tightly, then insert the needle with the right hand. This method is suitable for points where the skin is loose or has wrinkles [Fig. 6-5(d)].

4) Inserting the needle by pinching the skin: Pinch the skin upwards around the point with the thumb and index finger of the left hand. Hold the needle with the right hand and insert the needle into the pinched skin. This method is suitable for points where the skin and muscles are flabby and thin [Fig. 6-5(e)].

(3) Inserting the needle within the guide tube: Inserting the needle with a guide tube made of stainless steel or glass or plastic instead of inserting with the pressing hand. The length of the tube is usually 5 mm shorter than the selected needle, and the diameter is about 2 to 3 times that of the handle of the needle. Put the needle into the guide tube, put the tube with needle on the point, hold the tube with the pressing hand, and then quickly press the tip of the needle into the point with the index finger or middle finger of the right hand, while removing the tube to manipulate the needle [Fig. 6-5(f)].

2. Direction, Angle and Depth of Needle Insertion   In the process of acupuncture, correct direction, angle and depth of the needle are very important

向下用力时，中指随之屈曲，针尖迅速刺透皮肤［图6-5（a）］。

（2）双手进针法：即左右双手（刺手与押手）互相配合将针刺入皮肤，常用的方法有以下几种：

1）指切进针法：以左手拇指或示指或中指的爪甲切按在穴位上，右手持针，紧靠指甲将针刺入皮肤。适用于短针的进针［图6-5（b）］。

2）挟持进针法：以左手拇、示二指挟持消毒棉球，挟住针身下端，露出针尖，将针尖固定于针刺穴位的皮肤表面，右手持针柄，使针垂直，在右手指力下压时，左手拇、示指同时用力，两手协同将针刺入皮肤。适用于长针的进针［图6-5（c）］。

3）舒张进针法：用左手拇、示二指或示、中二指将所刺腧穴部位的皮肤向两侧撑开绷紧，使针从左手拇、示二指的中间刺入。适用于皮肤松弛部位腧穴的进针［图6-5（d）］。

4）提捏进针法：以左手拇指和示指将针刺部位的皮肤捏起，以右手持针从捏起部的上端刺入。适用于皮肉浅薄部位的进针［图6-5（e）］。

（3）针管进针法：针管进针法就是利用不锈钢、玻璃或塑料等材料制成的针管代替押手进针的方法。针管一般比针短5mm，针管直径约为针柄的2~3倍，选平柄毫针装入针管之中，将针尖所在的一端置于穴位之上，左手挟持针管，用右手示指或中指快速叩打针管上端露出的针尾端，使针尖刺入穴位，再提取针管，施行各种手法［图6-5（f）］。

2. 针刺的方向、角度、深度　针刺过程中，掌握正确的针刺方向、角度和深度，是

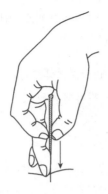

Fig. 6-5(a) Inserting the Needle with One Hand
图 6-5(a) 单手进针法

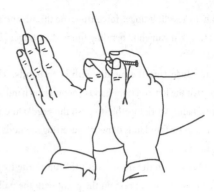

Fig. 6-5(b) Inserting the Needle with the Aid of the Finger of the Pressing Hand
图 6-5(b) 指切进针法

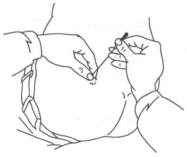

Fig. 6-5(c) Inserting the Needle by Gripping the Needle
图 6-5(c) 挟持进针法

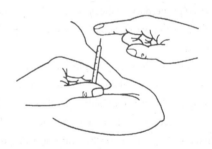

Fig. 6-5(d) Inserting the Needle by Stretching the Skin
图 6-5(d) 舒张进针法

Fig. 6-5(e) Inserting the Needle by Pinching the Skin
图 6-5(e) 提捏进针法

Fig. 6-5(f) Inserting the Needle within the Guide Tube
图 6-5(f) 针管进针法

Fig. 6-5 Methods of Needle Insertion
图 6-5 进针法

aspects for inducing the needling sensation, bringing about the desired therapeutic results and avoiding accidents. For the same point, different direction, angle or depth may cause different results. An appropriate direction, angle or depth is determined according to the location of the point, the specific disease condition, the patient's constitution, acupuncture, manipulation, and so on.

增强针感、提高疗效、防止意外事故发生的重要环节。临床上同一腧穴，由于针刺的角度、方向和深度不同，所产生针感的强弱、传感的方向和治疗效果常有明显的差异。针刺的角度、方向和深度根据施术腧穴所在的具体位置、患者体质、病情需要和针刺手法等具体情况而定。

(1) Direction of needle insertion: The direction of needle insertion depends upon the direction of the meridian, points and the therapeutic purpose.Generally speaking, for reinforcing purpose, the needle is inserted in the direction of the meridian, while for reducing purpose, the needle is inserted against it. To guarantee the safety, the needle has to be inserted in a specific direction for some points. For example, in inserting the RN 22 (*lián quán)*, the needle tip should face the root of the tongue and be inserted slowly. For points on the back, the needle tip should face the spine. In order to transmit the needling sensation to the diseased area, the needle tip usually faces the direction of the illness.

(2) Angle of needle insertion: The angle of needle insertion refers to the angle formed between the needle and the skin surface. It depends upon the anatomical location of the points and the therapeutic purpose. Generally speaking, there are three kinds of angles of needle insertion: perpendicular, oblique and horizontal insertion.

1) Perpendicular insertion: Keep the angle between the needle and the skin surface at 90° and insert the needle perpendicularly. It is used for most points especially where there are thick muscles such as on the limbs, abdomen and lower back.

2) Oblique insertion: Keep the angle between the needle and the skin surface at 45° and insert the needle obliquely. It is used for points located on the edge of bones, or where there are vital internal organs, or where the main arteries and scar should be avoided, such as points on the chest and upper back.

3) Horizontal insertion: It is also known as transverse insertion or insertion along the skin. Keep the angle between the needle and the skin surface at 15° and insert the needle transversely. It is applicable to areas where the muscles are very thin such as points on the head (Fig. 6-6).

（1）针刺的方向：针刺的方向一般应依经脉循行的方向、腧穴部位的特点和治疗的需要而定。一般而言，应用补法时，针尖朝向须与经脉循行的方向一致；应用泻法时，针尖朝向须与经脉循行的方向相反。根据针刺腧穴所在部位的特点，某些穴位必须朝向某一特定的方向或部位。如针刺廉泉穴时，针尖应朝向舌根方向缓慢刺入。针刺背部某些腧穴，针尖要朝向脊柱方向等。为使针刺的感应达到病变所在部位，针刺时针尖应朝向病所，以便达到"气至病所"的目的。

（2）针刺的角度：针刺的角度是指进针时针身与所刺部位皮肤表面形成的角度，主要依腧穴所在部位的解剖特点和治疗要求而定。一般分为直刺、斜刺和横刺三种。

1）直刺：针身与皮肤呈90°角，垂直刺入。适用于人体大部分腧穴，尤其是肌肉丰厚部位的腧穴，如四肢、腹部、腰部的穴位。

2）斜刺：针身与皮肤呈45°角，倾斜刺入。适用于骨骼边缘的腧穴，或内有重要脏器不宜深刺的部位，或为避开血管及瘢痕部位而采取此法，如胸、背部的穴位。

3）横刺：也称为平刺，或称沿皮刺，针身与皮肤呈15°角左右，横向刺入。适用于皮肤浅薄处腧穴，如头部的穴位（图6-6）。

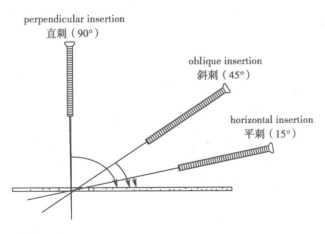

perpendicular insertion
直刺（90°）

oblique insertion
斜刺（45°）

horizontal insertion
平刺（15°）

Fig. 6-6　Angle of Needle Insertion

图6-6　针刺的角度

(3) Depth of needle insertion: Depth of needle insertion is chosen based on the specific condition, besides according to routine depth of needle insertion.

1) Constitution: For weak constitutions, insert the needle shallowly. For strong constitutions, insert the needle deeper.

2) Age: For elderly with a debilitating condition or for infants, shallow needle insertion is advisable, while for young or strong people, deep needle insertion is recommended.

3) Disease condition: For person with exterior syndrome, or yang syndrome, or deficiency syndrome, or new diseases, a shallow insertion is advisable. For person with interior syndrome, or yin syndrome, or excess syndrome, or protracted diseases, a deep insertion is suitable.

4) Location: For points on the face and head, chest and upper back where there are thin skin and muscles, shallow insertion is advisable. For points on the limbs, hip and abdomen where there are abundant muscles, deep insertion is suggested.

v. Needling Manipulation

Needling manipulations refer to kinds of operations conducted to promote arrival of qi, regulate the needling sensation, and promote the needling sensation diffuse or transmit after the needle is inserted into the point. They are divided into basic manipulations and assistant manipulations (Fig.6-7).

1. Basic Manipulations　Basic manipulations are the basic skills of acupuncture. Lifting and thrusting, twirling and rotating are commonly used.

(1) Lifting and thrusting: Lifting and thrusting refer to a basic manipulation that the needle is lifted from the point and thrust into the point after it is inserted into the body [Fig. 6-7(a)]. Lifting means the needle to move from the deep to the superficial. Thrusting means the needle to move from the superficial to the deep. The amplitude, frequency, and the duration of lifting and thrusting are decided by the constitution of the patient, condition of the disease, location of the point and the therapeutic purpose. When performing a lifting-thrusting manipulation, the finger force exerted onto the needle must be kept even and smooth in order to keep the amplitude of about 0.3-0.5 cun and a frequency of about 60 times *per* minute. Keep the needle vertical and maintain the original direction and angle of the needle.

(2) Twirling and rotating: Twirling and rotating refer to a basic manipulation to twist the needle handle

（3）针刺的深度：针刺的深度是指针身刺入腧穴部位的深浅而言。在临床上，针刺的深度除根据每个腧穴的常规刺入深度外，还应根据具体情况而定。

1）体质：身体瘦弱者，宜浅刺；身强体胖者，宜深刺。

2）年龄：年老体弱和小儿娇嫩之体，宜浅刺；中青年身强体壮者，宜深刺。

3）病情：表证、阳证、虚证、新病者宜浅刺；里证、阴证、实证、久病者宜深刺。

4）部位：头面和胸背及皮薄肉少处的腧穴，宜浅刺；四肢、臀、腹及肌肉丰满处的腧穴，宜深刺。

（五）行针手法

行针又名运针，是指将针刺入腧穴后，为得气、调节针感以及使针感向某一方向扩散、传导而施行的各种针刺操作方法，行针的手法可分为基本手法和辅助手法。

1. 基本手法　行针的基本手法，是针刺的基本动作，常用的有提插法和捻转法两种。

（1）提插法：是将针刺入腧穴的一定深度后，使针在穴位内进行上提、下插的操作方法。针由浅层向下刺入深层的操作谓之插，从深层向上退至浅层的操作谓之提[图6-7（a）]。

至于提插幅度的大小、层次的变化、频率的高低和操作时间的长短等，应根据患者的体质、病情和腧穴的部位以及术者所要达到的目的而灵活掌握。使用提插法时的指力一定要均匀一致，幅度不宜过大，一般以0.3~0.5寸为宜；频率不宜过高，每分钟60次左右；保持针身垂直，不改变针刺角度、方向。

（2）捻转法：将针刺入一定深度后，用拇指与示、中指挟持针柄作一前一后、左右

with the thumb, the index and middle fingers forward and backward alternately. The amplitude, frequency and the duration of the manipulation are decided by the constitution of the patient, location of the point, condition of the disease and the therapeutic purpose.

The two basic manipulations above listed can be used independently or jointly [Fig. 6-7(b)].

2. Assistant Manipulations

(1) Meridian pushing method: Massage and pat the skin and muscles with the fingers of the pressing hand gently along the course of the meridian of the point. This is applied to activate qi and blood, to excite the meridian-qi, to promote the needling sensation [Fig. 6-7(c)].

(2) Needle-scraping method: Hold the needle tail with the thumb or the middle finger and scrape the needle handle slightly with the nail of the thumb, or the index finger, or the middle finger starting from the lower to the upper portion. This may excite the meridian-qi and be used as a method to promote and move the needling sensation [Fig. 6-7(d)].

(3) Needle-flicking method: Flick the needle handle with the fingertips gently to make it vibrate. This may excite the meridian-qi, and promote the needling sensation [Fig. 6-7(e)].

(4) Needle-shaking method: Hold the needle handle with the hand and shake the needle left and right as if shaking a scull of boat. When the needle is inserted vertically, the shaking is often combined with lifting in order to expel evil qi. In an oblique or transverse insertion, the needle is shaken left and right as if a dragon is waving its tail, keeping the depth of the needle fixed. This can induce the one way spreading of the needling sensation [Fig. 6-7(f)].

(5) Wing-spreading method: Rotate the handle of the needle swiftly several times with the thumb and index finger in small amplitude, and then release the needle repeatedly. The twirling of the needle and finger releasing should be performed like the spreading of the wings of a flying bird. This may promote or strengthen the needling sensation [Fig. 6-7(g)].

(6) Needle-vibrating method: Hold the handle of the needle with the hand, then lift and thrust, twist and rotate the needle quickly in small amplitude in order to vibrate the needle. This method is used to promote the arrival of qi or reinforce the effect of eliminating the pathogen and supporting the vital [Fig. 6-7(h)].

vi. Arrival of Qi

The arrival of qi, which is also named the needle

交替旋转捻动的动作。捻转角度的大小、频率的高低和时间的长短,应根据患者的体质、病情、腧穴的特点及术者所要达到的目的而灵活运用[图6-7(b)]。

以上两种基本手法,既可单独应用,也可相互配合使用,在临床上必须根据患者的具体情况灵活掌握,才能发挥其应有的作用。

2. 辅助手法

(1)循法:是用手指顺着针刺穴位所属经脉循行路线上下轻轻地揉按抚摩或扣打的方法。此法可宣通气血、激发经气,促使针感传导或缓解滞针引发的疼痛[图6-7(c)]。

(2)刮法:也称刮柄法或划柄法。是将针刺入腧穴一定深度后,用拇指或示指的指腹抵住针尾,拇指、示指或中指爪甲,由下而上频频刮动针柄的一种方法。此法可激发经气,是一种催气、行气之法[图6-7(d)]。

(3)弹法:是将针刺入腧穴的一定深度后,以手指轻轻叩弹针柄,使针身产生轻微的震动,而使经气速行。此法亦有激发经气,催气速行的作用[图6-7(e)]。

(4)摇法:也称摇柄法,是将针刺入腧穴一定深度后,手持针柄进行摇动,如摇橹或摇辘轳之状。此法若直立针身而摇,多自深而浅的随摇随提,用以出针泻邪。若卧针斜刺或平刺而摇,一左一右,不进不退,如青龙摆尾,可使针感单向传导[图6-7(f)]。

(5)飞法:是用拇、示指持针柄,小幅度地捻搓针柄数次,然后放开两指,一搓一放,状如飞鸟展翅。此法用于气至之前,可促使得气;用于得气之后,则可增强得气感应[图6-7(g)]。

(6)震颤法:是将针刺入腧穴一定深度后,右手持针柄,用小幅度、快频率的提插捻转动作使针身产生轻微的震颤,以促使得气或增强祛邪、扶正的作用[图6-7(h)]。

(六)得气

得气,是指针刺入腧穴后,通过捻转提

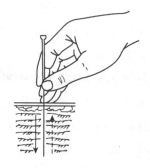

Fig. 6-7(a) Lifting and Thrusting
图 6-7(a) 提插法

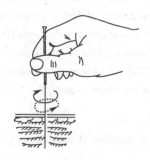

Fig. 6-7(b) Twirling and Rotating
图 6-7(b) 捻转法

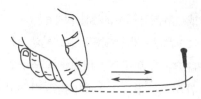

Fig. 6-7(c) Meridian Pushing Method
图 6-7(c) 循法

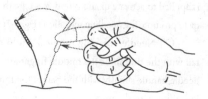

Fig. 6-7(d) Needle-Scraping Method
图 6-7(d) 弹法

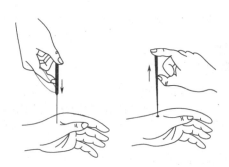

Fig. 6-7(e) Needle-Flicking Method
图 6-7(e) 刮法

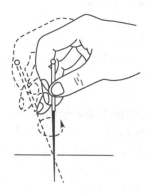

Fig. 6-7(f) Needle-Shaking Method
图 6-7(f) 摇法

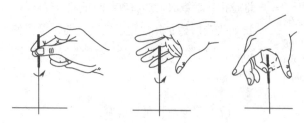

Fig. 6-7(g) Wing-Spreading Method
图 6-7(g) 飞法

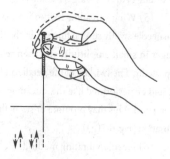

Fig. 6-7(h) Needle-Vibrating Method
图 6-7(h) 震颤法

Fig. 6-7 Needling Manipulation
图 6-7 行针法

sensation, refers to producing a special sensation in the area after acupuncture and certain manipulations. The needling sensation may be evaluated from two aspects. One aspect is the sensation of the point from the patient, and the other is the sensation of the needle from the operator. When qi appears, the operator may feel tightness around the needle, while at the same time, most the patients may feel soreness, numbness, distension, heaviness, and some appear hot, cold, itching, pain, line feeling and so on around the point, which may also transmit to other places along the distribution of the meridian. If qi doesn't appear, the operator will feel an empty sensation below the needle, and the patient will feel none of the sensations stated above.

There is a close relation between the arrival of qi and the therapeutic outcome. Just as *The Yellow Emperor's Inner Classic* states that "the rule of acupuncture is that when there is the arrival of qi, there is therapeutic efficacy". Generally speaking, if the needling sensation appears quickly, the therapeutic effect comes quickly too, and vice versa. There will be no effect if there is no needling sensation. In practice, failure of the arrival of qi may be caused by many factors such as inaccurate location of the point, inappropriate angle, depth of the needle and so on. Therefore, it needs to be managed with some other methods or to await or promote the arrival of qi.

Awaiting the needling sensation means retaining the needle peacefully in the point for a period of time. Promoting the needling sensation is to apply some manipulations such as lifting and thrusting, twisting and rotating, needle-flicking, meridian pushing, needle-scraping in order to induce the arrival of qi when the initial methods fail to produce it.

Box 6-1 Learning More

Reinforcing and Reducing Manipulations of the Filiform Needle

Reinforcing and reducing manipulations of the filiform needle is an important step of acupuncture treatment. It is also a core content of filiform needle. Reinforcing manipulation is a method which inspires healthy qi in human body and makes hypofunction recovery. Reducing manipulation refers to a method which expels pathogen to make abundantly pathogenic function return to normal. Reinforcing and reducing manipulations of the filiform needle is throughout the entire process of acupuncture, namely, from inserting the needle to withdrawing the needle. Factors related to the effect of reinforcing and reducing manipulation are the function conditions of the

插等手法，使针刺部位产生特殊的感觉，亦称为"针感"。针下是否得气，可以从两个方面分析判断，即患者对针刺的感觉和术者刺手下的感觉。当针刺腧穴得气时，术者会感到针下有徐和/或沉紧的感觉。同时，患者也会在针下出现相应的酸、麻、胀、重等感觉，也有的出现热、凉、痒、痛、抽搐、蚁行感等，或这种感觉可沿着一定部位、向一定方向扩散传导。若无经气感应而不得气时，术者则感到针下空虚无物，患者亦无酸、麻、胀、重等感觉。

得气与否与针刺疗效关系甚密，正如《灵枢·九针十二原》所说："刺之要，气至而有效。"一般而言，得气快，疗效出现也快；得气慢，疗效出现也慢；若不得气，就可能无治疗效果。在临床上若针刺不得气，多因取穴不准或针刺角度、深度不当所致。对此应根据不同原因作相应调整，或运用候气、催气等方法。

候气是将针留置于所刺腧穴之内，安静地、较长时间地留针，以候气至。针刺后若不得气，可进行提插、捻转及弹、循、刮等运针手法，以激发经气，促使气至，这种促使得气方法称为催气。

知识拓展 6-1

针刺补泻

针刺补泻是针刺治病的一个重要环节，也是毫针刺法的核心内容。补法是泛指能鼓舞人体正气，使低下的功能恢复旺盛的方法。泻法泛指能疏泄病邪使亢进的功能恢复正常的方法。补泻手法贯穿整个针刺过程，从进针至出针全过程。同时针刺补泻手法效应还受患者功能状态、体质和操作技巧影响，基础的手法有捻转补泻、提插补泻。

patient, characteristics of points, skill of the manipulation. Based methods of reinforcing and reducing are twirling and rotating the needle, lifting and thrusting the needle.

vii. Retaining and Withdrawing the Needle

1. Retaining the Needle　Retaining the needle means that the needle should be kept in the point after it is inserted up to a given depth in the point and manipulated. The aim of retaining the needle is to strengthen the needling effects or to do further manipulations. Retaining the needle for 10 to 20 minutes is recommended for most common diseases. The duration of the needle retention should be prolonged or be for a few hours in some special diseases, such as acute abdominal pain, tetanus, cold or intractable pain, spastic case, so as to do intermittent manipulations to strengthen and solidify the effect. If qi doesn't arrive, the needle can be retained to await the arrival of qi. Whether the needle is retained or not and the duration of the needle retention should be determined by certain conditions.

2. Withdrawing the Needle　Withdrawing the needle means that the needle is taken out when the manipulation is completed. Press the skin around the needle with the thumb and index finger or the index and middle fingers of the pressing hand, rotate the needle gently and lift it up slowly to skin level, then withdraw it quickly with the puncturing hand. The bleeding should be managed by applying pressure on the area with a dry sterilized cotton ball. Patients should take a rest after the needle is withdrawn. The number of needles should be counted after each acupuncture treatment.

viii. Management and Prevention of Possible Accident

Acupuncture is a relatively safe therapy. However, careless administration, inappropriate acupuncture manipulation, or insufficient understanding of human anatomy will sometimes lead to accidents during treatment. The following common accidents in acupuncture are listed.

1. Acupuncture Syncope　Acupuncture syncope refers to the patient fainting during the course of acupuncture treatment.

(1) Causes: The patient is weak and nervous, or tired and hungry with profuse sweating, diarrhea or hemorrhage. Improper posture during acupuncture or excessive or violent manipulation can also cause acupuncture syncope.

(2) Manifestations: The patient suddenly presents symptoms of fainting, mental fatigue, pale complexion, dizziness, vertigo, nausea, profuse sweating, palpitations,

（七）留针与出针

1. **留针**　将针刺入腧穴并行针施术后，使针留置于腧穴内称为留针。留针的目的是为了加强针刺的作用和便于继续行针施术。一般病证只要针下得气后施以适当的补泻手法即可出针或留针 10~20min；但对一些特殊病证，如急性腹痛，破伤风，寒性、顽固性疼痛或痉挛性病证，可适当延长留针时间，有时留针可达数小时，以便在留针过程中作间歇性行针，以增强、巩固疗效。若不得气时，也可静置久留，以待气至。在临床上留针与否或留针时间的长短，不可一概而论，应根据患者具体病情而定。

2. **出针**　在行针或留针完毕后，将针拔出的操作称为出针。出针时一般先以左手拇、示指按住针孔周围皮肤，右手持针作轻微捻转，慢慢将针提至皮下，然后迅速将针拔出，再用消毒干棉球按压针孔，以防出血。出针后患者应休息片刻方可活动，术者应核对针数，以防遗漏。

（八）异常情况的处理与预防

针刺治疗疾病，虽然比较安全，但如果操作不慎，或针刺手法不得当，或对人体解剖部位缺乏全面的了解等，有时也会出现一些异常情况，常见针刺异常情况如下。

1. **晕针**　晕针是针刺过程中，患者发生的晕厥现象。

（1）原因：患者体质虚弱，精神紧张，或疲劳、饥饿、大汗、大泻、大出血之后，或体位不当，或术者在针刺时手法过重而致。

（2）症状：患者突然出现精神疲倦、面色苍白、头晕目眩、恶心欲吐、多汗、心慌、

cold limbs, decreased blood pressure, thread or indistinct pulse, pale and purple lips and nails, and urinary and fecal incontinence.

(3) Administration: Stop the needling immediately, and withdraw all the needles out of the body. Help the patient lie on a supine posture and keep the patient's body warm. In minor cases, ask the patient to have a rest, and give him or her some warm water or sugar water to drink. The symptoms will be removed shortly. For severe cases, the patient can be treated by pinching or puncturing certain points such as DU 26 (*shuǐ gōu, also called rén zhōng*), PC 6 (*nèi guān*), and ST 36 (*zú sān lǐ*), or administering moxibustion on the DU 20 (*bǎi huì*), RN 6 (*qì hǎi*), and RN 4 (*guān yuán*). Other first-aid methods should be administered as deemed necessary.

(4) Prevention: Give a thorough explanation of the procedure to the patient in order to dispel his or her fear of acupuncture, especially to someone who is going to experience acupuncture for the first time or nervous or weak. Select a comfortable posture for needling. Supine posture is better. Select as fewer points as possible and use gentle manipulation. Advise the patients to eat, rest, or drink if they are hungry, fatigued, or thirsty before receiving acupuncture. Keep observing the patient carefully during acupuncture, especially his or her complexion. When there are some pre-symptoms of acupuncture syncope, appropriate treatment should be applied as early as possible.

2. Sticking of the Needle   During or after manipulation the needle is retained in the point, the operator finds that the inserted needle is stuck and difficult to rotate, lift, insert or withdraw, while the patient feels a severe pain or discomfort in the needling area.

(1) Causes: Muscles strongly contract around the needle induced by a very nervous patient, or the muscle tissues twist around the body of the needle caused by an excessive unidirectional rotation of the needle by the acupuncturist.

(2) Manifestations: The inserted needle is stuck and difficult to move and induces a severe pain or discomfort to the patient.

(3) Administration: As for excessive contraction of the local muscles, needle retention can be prolonged slightly. Gently massage or tap the muscles around the needled point, or scrape and flick the needle handle, or insert one or more additional needles close to the stuck needle so as to move the stagnated qi and blood as well as release the localized muscle tension. A backward rotation

四肢发冷、血压下降、脉象沉细或神志昏迷、唇甲青紫、二便失禁、脉微细欲绝等。

（3）处理：立即停止针刺，将针全部起出。使患者平卧，注意保暖，轻者仰卧片刻，给饮温开水或糖水后，即可恢复正常。重者在上述处理的基础上，可刺人中、内关、足三里，灸百会、气海、关元等穴，必要时，配合其他急救措施。

（4）预防：对于初次接受针刺治疗或精神过度紧张、身体虚弱者，应先做好解释工作，消除其对针刺的顾虑；同时选择舒适持久的体位，最好采取卧位；选穴宜少，手法要轻。若饥饿、疲劳、大渴时，应令其进食、休息、饮水后再予针刺。术者在针刺治疗过程中，要精神专一，随时注意观察患者的神色，询问患者的感觉，一旦有不适等晕针先兆，可及早采取处理措施。

2. 滞针   滞针是指在行针时或留针后术者感觉针下涩滞，捻转、提插、出针均感困难，而患者感觉疼痛的现象。

（1）原因：患者精神紧张，当针刺入腧穴后，患者局部肌肉强烈收缩，或行针手法不当，向单一方向捻针太过，以致肌肉组织缠绕针体而成滞针。若留针时间过长，有时也可出现滞针。

（2）症状：针在体内捻转不动，提插、出针均感困难，若勉强捻转、提插时，则患者痛不可忍。

（3）处理：若患者精神紧张，局部肌肉过度收缩时，可稍延长留针时间，或于滞针腧穴附近进行循按或叩弹针柄，或在附近再刺一针，以宣散气血，缓解肌肉紧张。若单向捻针而致者，可向相反方向将针捻回，并用

of the needle should be conducted if the adverse needle retention is caused by unidirectional rotation. In addition, flick and scrap the needle handle gently in order to loosen the twisted muscle fibers.

(4) Prevention: Give an abundant explanation to the nervous patient in order to improve apprehension to acupuncture and remain relaxed. Select the proper manipulation method and avoid one direction rotation in case the muscle fibers twist over the body of the needle.

3. Bending of the Needle　It refers to the bending of the needle which is in the human body during the insertion or retention of the needle.

(1) Causes: an unskilled or inaccurate insertion, or a tough insertion, or the needle hits some tissues or bones. The patient changes his or her body posture during the retention of the needle. An accidental movement of the needle by an exterior object is another common reason.

(2) Manifestations: The needle body is bent and the original direction and angle of the needle are changed when it is inserted or retained. As a result, it causes difficulties in lifting, thrusting, twirling, or withdrawing of the needle that lead to further pain.

(3) Administration: Stop the manipulation immediately. If the needle is bent at a smaller angle, withdraw the needle gently following the bend of the curve of the needle. If the needle is bent at a greater angle caused by a change in posture, restore it to the original position and withdraw the needle gently after the local muscles have relaxed. Avoid withdrawing the needle forcefully otherwise it may break.

(4) Prevention: The practitioner should manipulate skillfully, and use steady finger force to insert the needle instead of a sudden or tough insertion. Ask the patient to select comfortable posture and remain it during the needle retention. Keep the needle away from exterior objects that may compress them.

4. Breaking of the Needle　This refers to the situation when a needle is broken and a part of the needle is left in the body during needling.

(1) Causes: It can be caused by a poor quality needle, such as one that has corrosion on the root or the needle body. It can also be caused by incorrect needling manipulation such as tough lifting, thrusting, and twisting the needle with improper force which induces muscle spasms. A sudden change in body position by the patient, bending or sticking of the needle may induce needle breaking as well.

(2) Manifestations: The needle body is suddenly broken during needling. The inside part of the broken needle may have an exposed end externally or it may

刮柄、弹柄法，使缠绕的肌纤维松弛，即可消除滞针。

（4）预防：对精神紧张者，应先做好解释工作，消除患者不必要的顾虑。注意行针的操作手法要适当，避免单向捻转以避免肌纤维缠绕针身而防止滞针的发生。

3. 弯针　弯针是指进针时或将针刺入腧穴后，针身在体内形成弯曲的现象。

（1）原因：术者在进针时，手法不熟练，用力过猛、过速；针尖碰到坚硬组织；患者在针刺或留针时移动体位；因针柄受到某种外力压迫、碰击等。

（2）症状：针柄改变了进针或刺入留针时的方向和角度，提插、捻转及出针均感困难，而患者感到疼痛。

（3）处理：出现弯针后不得再行提插、捻转等手法。如针轻微弯曲，应慢慢将针起出。若弯曲角度过大时，应顺着弯曲的方向将针起出，切忌强行拔针，以免将针断入体内。

（4）预防：术者进针手法要熟练，指力要均匀，并要避免进针过速、过猛。选择适当体位，在留针过程中，嘱患者不要随意变换体位，注意保护针刺部位，针柄不得受外物碰撞和压迫。

4. 断针　断针又称折针，是指针体折断在人体内。若术前能做好针具的检修和施术时加以注意，是可以避免的。

（1）原因：针具质量欠佳，针身或针根有损伤剥蚀，进针时强力提插、捻转，肌肉强烈收缩，留针时患者随意变更体位，或弯针、滞针未能进行及时的正确处理等。

（2）症状：行针时或出针后发现针身折断，其断端部分针身尚露于皮肤外，或断端

completely merge into the body.

(3) Administration: The practitioner should keep calm and ask the patient not to shift his or her original position so as to prevent the needle fragment from sinking deeper into the tissues. Pull the broken fragment of the needle out with fingers or tweezers if the fragment exposes is exposed externally. If the broken end of the needle is at skin level, press the skin around the needle with the thumb and index finger of the left hand vertically in order to expose it, and then pull it out with tweezers using the right hand. In case the broken fragment is submerged under the skin surface or is seated deeply in the muscle, it needs to be located via radiographs or ultrasound and be removed surgically.

(4) Prevention: Check the needle carefully prior to manipulations and do not use poor quality needles. Operate the needle skillfully and properly to avoid forceful manipulations. Ask the patient for full cooperation during acupuncture and not to change body posture. In acupuncture, a certain part of the needle body should be exposed above the skin, which means avoiding inserting the needle shaft entirely into the body. If needle bends, don't insert and manipulate. If sticking of the needle occurs, it should be taken care of properly and immediately.

5. Hematoma This refers to the swelling and pain caused by subcutaneous bleeding after needling.

(1) Causes: A poor quality needle hurts the blood vessels.

(2) Manifestations: A localized, distended and painful bruise with a black purplish color usually appears after the needle is withdrawn.

(3) Administration: No management is necessary for a small hematoma which will disappear by itself within a few days. If the hematoma is moderately severe with obvious swelling and pain that inhibits normal activities, it needs to be managed by applying cold compresses early to stop bleeding, and applying hot compresses or mildly massaging the area to dissipate the stagnated blood.

(4) Prevention: Check or examine the needle carefully. Be familiar with the anatomy of the human body and avoid pricking the blood vessels. Press on the point with a dry sterilized cotton ball immediately after the needle is withdrawn.

6. Post-needling Sensation It means the patient feel sensation of soreness, numbness, distension, heaviness, and even pain in point parts for a while after needling.

(1) Causes: Most conditions are due to excessive

全部没入皮肤之下。

（3）处理：术者态度必须从容镇静，嘱患者切勿变动原有体位，以防断针向肌肉深部陷入。若残端部分针身显露于体外时，可用手指或镊子将针起出。若断端与皮肤相平或稍凹陷于体内者，可用左手拇、示二指垂直向下挤压针孔两旁，使断针暴露体外，右手持镊子将针取出。若断针完全深入皮下或肌肉深层时，应在X线下定位，手术取出。

（4）预防：为了防止断针，针刺前应认真仔细地检查针具，对不符合质量要求的针具，应剔除不用。避免过猛、过强的行针。在行针或留针时，应嘱患者不要随意更换体位。针刺时更不宜将针身全部刺入腧穴，应留部分针身在体外，以便于针根断折时取针。在进针行针过程中，如发现弯针，应立即出针，切不可强行刺入或行针。对于滞针等亦应及时正确地处理。

5. **血肿** 血肿是指针刺部位出现的皮下出血而引起肿痛的现象。

（1）原因：针尖弯曲带钩，使皮肉受损，或刺伤血管所致。

（2）症状：出针后，针刺部位肿胀疼痛，继则皮肤呈现青紫色。

（3）处理：若微量的皮下出血而局部小块青紫时，一般不必处理，可以自行消退。若局部肿胀疼痛较剧，青紫面积大而且影响到活动时，可先冷敷止血后，再热敷或在局部轻轻揉按，以促使局部瘀血消散吸收。

（4）预防：仔细检查针具，弯曲带钩的针应剔除；熟悉人体解剖部位，避开血管针刺，出针时立即用消毒干棉球按压针孔。

6. **后遗感** 针刺后持续一段时间出现酸、麻、重、涨，甚至疼痛感。

（1）原因：多数由于操作手法过重；亦可

needling manipulation or some may be caused by too longer needle retention time.

(2) Manifestations: The patient presents as soreness, numbness, distension, heaviness, and even pain in point parts after needling.

(3) Administration: If it is not serious, it will be improved by massaging the point or along the course of the meridian of the point gently. In addition to massage the local skin and muscles, also cooperate with moxibustion to remove and improve the bad feelings, if the post-needling sensation is strong.

(4) Prevention: Avoid the forceful excessive manipulations. Do not prolong the needle retention time. It will avoid the risk of post-needling sensation by massaging the local skin and muscles up and down with the fingers gently along the course of the meridian of the point after needling.

7. Peripheral Nerve Stabbed It refers to the patients with a feeling of numbness, sensory disability or obstacle even hypofunction on the area of acupuncture after needling.

(1) Causes: It is inappropriate to do needling manipulation, or prolong the stimulation time of needling in the points where there distributes nerve trunk or the main nerve branch.

(2) Manifestations: The patients have a feeling of electric shock or sensory disability including numbness, hot feeling, pain and even hypofunction of touch or warmth in the nerve distribution area after needling.

(3) Administrations: Take the massage treatment, and encourage patients to strengthen functional exercise within 24 hours after injury. In some severe cases, it should be treated by point injection with B vitamins drugs on the corresponding points.

(4) Preventions: The practitioner should manipulate skillfully, especially they should pay attention to the depth of needle insertion, the degree of needle manipulation, the time of needle retaining in the points where there distributes nerve trunk or the main nerve branch. It should stop and withdraw the needle at once when the patients have a feeling of electric shock as the needle is inserting.

ix. Precaution and Contraindication for Acupuncture

Since there are various physiological states present in different people due to living environments and conditions

留针时间过长所致。

（2）症状：在出针后，局部遗留酸痛、胀重、麻木等不适感。

（3）处理：轻者用手指在局部上下循经按揉，即可消失或改善；重者除在局部上下循经按揉外，并可用艾条施灸，也可很快消除。

（4）预防：针刺手法不宜过重；留针时间不宜过长。一般病证，出针后循经按揉，避免出现后遗感。

7. 刺伤周围神经 针刺后出现针刺部位麻木感，或感觉减退或障碍，甚至功能障碍。

（1）原因：在有神经干或主要分支分布穴位上，行针手法过重，刺激手法时间过长；或操作手法不熟练；或留针时间过长。

（2）症状：当即出现触电样针感，或向末端分散的麻木感，甚则神经分布区可出现感觉障碍，包括麻木、发热、痛觉、触觉及温觉减退等。同时，有程度不等的功能障碍、肌肉萎缩。

（3）处理：应用 B 族维生素类药物治疗，严重者可在相应经络腧穴上进行 B 族维生素类药物穴位注射，可应用激素冲击疗法。损伤后 24h 内即采取按摩治疗措施，并嘱患者加强功能锻炼。

（4）预防：在有神经干或主要分支分布的腧穴上，行针手法不宜过重，刺激手法时间不宜过长，操作手法要熟练，留针时间不宜过长。出现触电感时，不可再行操作。

（九）针刺注意事项

由于人的生理功能状态和生活环境条件等因素，在实施针刺术时，还应注意以下几

that do not match the general principles of acupuncture, it is advisable for the acupuncturist to pay attention to the following circumstances.

1. Do not do acupuncture immediately when a patient is famished, tired, or nervous. Do not apply a strong manipulation to a patient who is dually deficient of qi and blood. Supine posture is advisable to the person when acupuncture is conducted.

2. Do not choose points in the lower abdominal region for pregnant women in the first trimester. For pregnant women over 3 months, acupuncturing points of the abdominal and lumbosacral areas should be avoided. Certain points including SP 6 (*sān yīn jiāo*), LI 4 (*hé gǔ*), BL 60 (*kūn lūn*), and BL 67 (*zhì yīn*), which intensively promote blood circulation, are contraindicated during the entire pregnancy. Acupuncture should not be applied to women during their menstrual periods, unless they are treated for irregular menstrual periods.

3. Do not select points on the crown of the head of an infant since his or her fontanelle has not closed yet.

4. Do not provide acupuncture for patients who suffer from autogenous hemorrhage.

5. Do not apply acupuncture to the infected, ulcerated, or scarred skin or tumors.

6. Do not insert the needle vertically and deeply to points on the chest, hypochondriac and lumbar regions and back where *zang-fu* organs are located. Patients suffering from splenohepatomegaly, emphysema should be paid more attention to.

7. When performing acupuncture in the ocular region and neck, choosing points such as DU 16 (*fēng fǔ*) and DU 15 (*yǎ mén*), along with points on the spinal region, the angle and depth of needle insertion, amplitude of manipulation, duration of needle retention and so on need to be considered very carefully to avoid damage to vital organs.

8. For patients with urinary retention, the direction, angle and depth of needle insertion should be strictly monitored when one applies acupuncture in the lower abdomen so as not to damage the bladder.

x. Operating Procedure

1. Assessment　Check the doctor's prescription, the patient's name, bed number, patient's condition; skin condition of operation area; tolerance to acid bilges feeling; psychological status, environment and so on. Make a certain explanation to the patient in order to cooperate with.

2. Preparation　Prepare supplies which include

个方面：

1. 患者在过于饥饿、疲劳、精神过度紧张时，不宜立即进行针刺。对于气血虚弱者，进行针刺时，手法不宜过强，并应尽量选用卧位。

2. 妇女怀孕 3 个月以内者，小腹部的腧穴不宜针刺。若怀孕 3 个月以上者，其腹部、腰骶部腧穴也不宜针刺。至于三阴交、合谷、昆仑、至阴等一些通经活血的腧穴，在怀孕期禁刺。如妇女行经期，若非为了调经，亦不应针刺。

3. 小儿囟门未合时，头顶部的腧穴不宜针刺。

4. 常有自发性出血或损伤后出血不止的患者，不宜针刺。

5. 皮肤有感染、溃疡、瘢痕或肿瘤的部位，不宜针刺。

6. 对胸、胁、腰、背脏腑所居之处的腧穴，不宜直刺、深刺。肝、脾大，肺气肿患者更应注意。

7. 针刺眼区和项部的风府、哑门等穴和脊椎部的腧穴，要注意掌握一定的角度，更不宜大幅度地提插、捻转和长时间地留针，以免伤及重要组织器官。

8. 对于尿潴留的患者，在针刺小腹部腧穴时，也应掌握适当的针刺方向、角度、深度等，以免误伤膀胱等器官，出现意外的事故。

（十）操作程序

1. **评估**　核对医嘱，核对患者姓名、床号，评估患者病情、施术皮肤状况、对酸胀感的耐受度、心理状况、环境等。

2. **准备**　用物准备（治疗盘、一次性毫

disposable and sterile needles, skin disinfection solution, sterile swabs, bending plate, hand sanitizers. Necessary for sterile cotton ball, pad, folding screen, blankets. Bring all materials to the patient's bedside.Patient Preparation: Get and keep the position comfortable, which is easy to be acted by the operator. Expose the operation site and choose acupuncture point according to the need of treatment. Pay attention to keep warm.

3. Location of Acupoint　　Choose and find out acupoint according to acupoint positioning method, ask patients' feel, then determine acupoints at last. Disinfect operator's hands and local skin of patients.

4. Skin Degerming　　Disinfect operator's hands and local skin of patients.

5. Selection and Examination of Filiform Needle　　Select and examine filiform needle to ensure safety according to depth of acupoint, patients' condition and habitus.

6. Inserting Needle　　Select suitable inserting needle methods and apply correct direction, angle and depth of the needle to inserting needle on the basis of the acupuncture position, patients' condition and so on.

7. Manipulation of the Needles　　By Lifting and thrusting, twirling and rotating, or the others needle manipulations to promote or regulate the needling sensation which are the feeling of acid, hemp, bilge, heavy, distal to the diffusion, and it named after "de qi" too. Keep the needle in the place.

8. Observation　　Ask and observe the patient's reaction to know whether needling accidents happen to the patient which include bent needle, stuck needle, broken needle, fainting in the process of operation.

9. Withdrawing of Needle　　When the manipulation is completed, grab the skin around the needle with the thumb and index finger or the index and middle fingers of the pressing hand, rotate the needle gently and lift it up slowly to skin level, then withdraw it quickly with the puncturing hand. Press pinhole with swab lightly. The number of needles should be counted after the operation finished.

10. Tidy　　When the operation ends, assist patients to dress and get comfortable lying position, tidy bed unit and supplies, wash hands and perform health education.

11. Evaluation　　Evaluate whether the acupoint location is accurate, technique is skillful, patient's symptoms are being improved or there is any other discomfort. Evaluate whether communication and humanistic care are better, and whether there is any acupuncture accident.

针、2% 碘酊、75% 乙醇、无菌棉签、弯盘、治疗本、手消毒液，必要时备无菌棉球、垫枕、围屏、毛毯），备齐用物，携至床旁；患者准备，取舒适体位，暴露施术部位，注意保暖。

3. **定位**　　按取穴方法取穴，询问患者感觉，确定穴位。

4. **皮肤消毒**　　操作者手消毒，患者局部皮肤消毒。

5. **选检毫针**　　根据腧穴深浅、患者的病情、体质选择毫针，检查毫针。

6. **进针**　　根据针刺部位、患者病情等，选择正确的进针方向，角度、深度进针。

7. **行针**　　提插捻转，调节针感，产生酸、麻、胀、重感觉，并向远端扩散即得气，留针。

8. **观察**　　有无晕针、弯针、滞针、断针等不适感。

9. **起针**　　一手按住针孔周围皮肤，一手持针缓慢退出皮下后快速拔出，用棉签轻压针孔，防出血，核对针数。

10. **整理**　　协助患者穿好衣着，安排舒适体位，整理床单位，整理用物，做好健康教育。

11. **评价**　　选穴是否准确，操作方法是否正确、熟练，是否沟通到位、是否做到人文关怀。患者是否有得气感，症状是否缓解。是否发生针刺意外。

12. Record   Record the acupoints, method, retaining needle time, efficacy, signature and so on.

II. Auricular Acupuncture Therapy

Auricular acupuncture therapy is one of the acupuncture therapies used to prevent and treat diseases. It is done by needling or stimulating areas on the ear. It is simple and convenient for daily use and has a wide range of indications. It can also be used as a supplementary diagnostic approach with a considerable clinical significance.

i. Relationship between the Ear, Channel and *Zang-fu* Organs

There are intimate relationships between the ear and channels. The channels of hand *taiyang*, hand *shaoyang*, foot *shaoyang*, and hand *yangming* all enter the ear. The channels of foot *yangming* and foot *taiyang* travel to the front and the superior cornu of ear respectively. The branch of hand *jueyin* channel goes out of the post aurem. The *yinqiao* and *yangqiao* channels run into the post aurem. Though the six yin channels do not enter the ear directly, they connect with the ear by their divergent channels that separate, enter, resurface and finally join their interior-exterior related yang channels respectively. Therefore, it is said that all the twelve channels connect with the ear directly or indirectly.

The ear has close relations with *zang-fu* organs as well. *The Yellow Emperor's Inner Classic* records that the ear links to the five *zang* organs physiologically. *The Extensive Techniques of Massage* (*Lǐ Zhèng An Mó Yáo Shù*, 厘正按摩要术) says that the back of the ear is divided into five parts that correspond to the five *zang* organs respectively. This shows the close relationship between the ear and the *zang-fu* organs.

ii. Anatomical Nomenclature of the Surface of the Auricle

Auricle is the part of external ear. The anatomical nomenclature of the Auricle is as follows (Fig. 6-8):

1. The Auricle

(1) Helix: It is the curved free rim of the auricle.

(2) Helix tubercle: The tubercle is located on the posterior-superior portion of the helix.

(3) Helix cauda: The inferior part of the helix is at the junction of the helix and the lobe.

(4) Helix crus: It is the transverse ridge of the helix that continues backward into the concha of the ear.

(5) Antihelix: It refers to the "Y" shaped prominence

12. 记录   穴位、方法、留针时间、疗效并签名。

二、耳针法

耳针是用针刺刺激耳郭穴位以防治疾病的一种方法。其治疗范围较广，操作简便，并对疾病的诊断也有一定的参考意义。

（一）耳与经络脏腑的关系

耳与经络的联系是相当密切的，手太阳、手足少阳经脉及手阳明络脉均入耳中；足阳明、足太阳经脉分别上耳前、至耳上角；手厥阴经别出耳后；阴跷、阳跷脉入耳后。六阴经虽不入耳，但都通过经别离、入、出、合与阳经相合，而与耳相联系。因此，十二经脉都直接或间接上达于耳部。

耳与脏腑的关系亦相当密切，据《内经》《难经》等记载，耳与五脏均有生理功能上的联系。《厘正按摩要术》进一步将耳郭分为心肝脾肺肾五部，说明耳与脏腑在生理功能上是息息相关的。

（二）耳郭表面解剖

耳郭是外耳的部分，为了熟悉耳穴的分布情况，介绍耳郭的主要表面解剖结构（图6-8）。

1. 耳郭

（1）耳轮：耳郭卷曲的游离部分。

（2）耳轮结节：耳轮外上部的膨大部分。

（3）耳轮尾：耳轮向下移行于耳垂的部分。

（4）耳轮脚：耳轮深入耳甲的部分。

（5）对耳轮：与耳轮相对呈"Y"形的隆

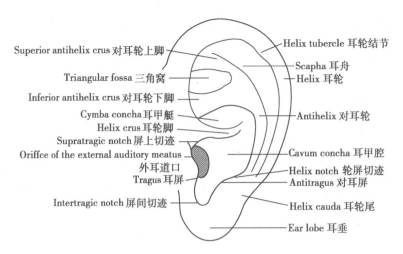

Fig. 6-8 Anatomical Nomenclature of the Surface of the Auricle

图 6-8 耳郭表面解剖图

that is roughly parallel to the helix, including the body of the antihelix, superior antihelix crus and inferior antihelix crus.

(6) Body of the antihelix: It refers to the main part of the antihelix that extends in a vertical direction.

(7) Superior antihelix crus: It is the superior branch of the bifurcation of the antihelix.

(8) Inferior antihelix crus: It is the inferior branch of the bifurcation of the antihelix.

(9) Triangular fossa: This refers to the triangular depression formed by superior and inferior antihelix crus and the corresponding helix.

(10) Scapha: This refers to the depression between the helix and the antihelix.

(11) Tragus: It is the flap-shaped tubercle in front of the auricle.

(12) Upper-tragic notch: This is the depression between the tragus and helix.

(13) Antitragus: This refers to the flap-shaped tubercle opposite of the tragus and superior to the ear lobe.

(14) Intertragic notch：This refers to the depression between the tragus and antitragus.

(15) Helix notch: This refers to the depression between the antihelix and antitragus.

(16) Ear lobe: This is the lowest part of the auricle devoid of cartilage.

(17) Concha: This is the hollow area formed by parts of the helix and antihelix, tragus, antitragus and the orifice of the external auditory meatus.

(18) Cavum concha: This is the concha inferior to the helix crus.

起部，由对耳轮体、对耳轮上脚和对耳轮下脚三部分组成。

（6）对耳轮体：对耳轮向下部呈上下走向的主体部分。

（7）对耳轮上脚：对耳轮向上分支的部分。

（8）对耳轮下脚：对耳轮向下分支的部分。

（9）三角窝：对耳轮上、下脚与相应耳轮之间的三角形凹窝。

（10）耳舟：耳轮与对耳轮之间的凹沟。

（11）耳屏：耳郭前方呈瓣状的隆起。

（12）屏上切迹：耳屏与耳轮之间的凹陷处。

（13）对耳屏：耳垂上方、与耳屏相对的瓣状隆起。

（14）屏间切迹：耳屏与对耳屏之间的凹陷处。

（15）轮屏切迹：对耳轮与对耳屏之间的凹陷处。

（16）耳垂：耳郭下部无软骨的部分。

（17）耳甲：部分耳轮和对耳轮、对耳屏及外耳门之间的凹窝。由耳甲艇、耳甲腔两部分组成。

（18）耳甲腔：耳轮脚以下的耳甲部。

(19) Cymba concha: This is the concha superior to the helix crus.

(20) Orifice of the external auditory Meatus: It is the opening in front of the cavum concha.

2. Reverse of Auricle

(1) Reverse of helix: It is the flat part of the reverse of helix.

(2) Reverse of helix cauda: It is the flat part of the reverse of helix cauda.

(3) Reverse of ear lobe: It is the flat part of the reverse of ear lobe.

(4) Apophysis of scapha: It is the apophysis part of the reverse of scapha.

(5) Apophysis of triangular fossa: It is the apophysis part of the reverse of triangular fossa.

(6) Apophysis of cymba concha: It is the apophysis part of the reverse of cymba concha.

(7) Apophysis of cavum concha: It is the apophysis part of the reverse of cavum concha.

(8) Groove of superior antihelix crus: It is the groove of the reverse of superior antihelix crus.

(9) Groove of inferior antihelix crus: It is the groove of the reverse of inferior antihelix crus.

(10) Groove of body of the antihelix: It is the groove of the reverse of body of the antihelix.

(11) Groove of helix crus: It is the groove of the reverse of helix crus.

(12) Groove of antitragus: It is the groove of the reverse of antitragus.

iii. Distribution of Auricular Point

Auricular points are the specific areas distributed over the ear. When there is an illness in the body, on the corresponding area of the ear occur obvious tenderness, disturbances in the skin electrical properties, and it may manifest positive changes of deformities or discoloration including pimples, desquamation, nodules, congestion, blisters and so on. All these changes and manifestations can be used for diagnosis as well as for treatment.

There exists some regularity in the distribution of auricular points. They are based on the upside down fetus distribution theory, which is explained below. Points related to the portions of the head are located on the ear lobe. Points related to the upper limbs are located on the scapha. Points related to the lower limbs are located on the superior and inferior antihelix crus. Points related to

（19）耳甲艇：耳轮脚以上的耳甲部。

（20）外耳门：耳甲腔前方的孔窍。

2. 耳郭背面

（1）耳轮：耳轮背部的平坦部分。

（2）耳轮尾背面：耳轮尾背部的平坦部分。

（3）耳垂背面：耳垂背部的平坦部分。

（4）耳舟隆起：耳舟在耳背呈现的隆起。

（5）三角窝隆起：三角窝在耳背呈现的隆起。

（6）耳甲艇隆起：耳甲艇在耳背呈现的隆起。

（7）耳甲腔隆起：耳甲腔在耳背呈现的隆起。

（8）对耳轮上脚沟：对耳轮上脚在耳背呈现的凹沟。

（9）对耳轮下脚沟：对耳轮下脚在耳背呈现的凹沟。

（10）对耳轮沟：对耳轮体在耳背呈现的凹沟。

（11）耳轮脚沟：耳轮脚在耳背呈现的凹沟。

（12）对耳屏沟：对耳屏在耳背呈现的凹沟。

（三）耳穴的分布

耳穴是指分布在耳郭上的一些特定穴位。人体的内脏或躯体发生病变时，往往在耳郭的相应部位出现压痛敏感、皮肤电特异性改变和脱屑、水疱、丘疹、充血、硬结、疣赘、色素沉着等变形、变色的阳性反应点。参考这些现象来诊断疾病，并通过刺激这些部位可防治疾病。

耳穴在耳郭的分布有一定的规律，根据形如胚胎的耳穴分布图看到：与头面相应的穴位在耳垂，与上肢相应的穴位居耳舟，与下肢相应的穴位在对耳轮上下脚，与胸腔内脏相应的穴位集中在耳甲腔，与腹腔内脏相

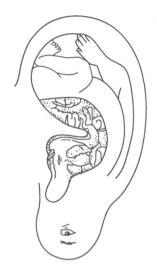

Fig.6-9　Distribution of Auricular Points
图 6-9　耳穴分布图

the organs in the chest are located on the cavum concha. Points related to the organs in the abdomen are located on the cymba concha. Points related to the spine and trunk are located on the antihelix. Points related to the pelvic cavity are located in the triangular fossa. Points related to the digestive tract are distributed around the helix crus. Points related to the urinary tract are located at the junction of the inferior antihelix crus and the cymba concha. Points related to the nasopharynx are distributed around the tragus (Fig. 6-9).

应的耳穴分布在耳甲艇，与脊柱和躯干相应的耳穴分布在对耳轮上，与盆腔相应的耳穴分布在三角窝，与消化道相应的耳穴分布在耳轮脚周围，与泌尿道相应的耳穴分布在耳轮下脚与耳甲艇交界处，与鼻咽部相应的穴位分布在耳屏四周（图 6-9）。

Box 6-2 Learning More

Knowledge of Distribution of Auricular Points

In the 1950s, auricular acupuncture therapy was sprung up in Europe. P. Nogier, who is a French Doctor of Medicine (M. D.), published an unabridged figure of auricular points which shows distribution of the auricular points that is like the upside down fetus, and introduced more than forty acupuncture therapies. Currently, some professors put forward to biological holographic theory to explain distribution of auricular points.

知识拓展 6-2
耳穴分布的认识

20 世纪 50 年代，耳针疗法在欧洲兴起。1957 年，法国医学博士诺吉尔（P. Nogier）发表了形如胚胎倒影较为完整的耳穴图，认为耳朵穴位分布恰像一个倒置的胎儿，并记载耳穴 40 多个。当前还提出生物全息理论来说明解释耳穴的分布。

iv. Location and Indication of Auricular Point

For the locations of auricular points, please Fig. 6-10.

1. Point on the Helix (12 Areas, HX1-HX12) The whole helix is divided into 12 regions. The helix crus are HX1. The part of the helix from the helix notch to the upper edge of the inferior antihelix crus is divided into 3 equal areas, which are HX2, HX3, and HX4 counting from below to above. The helix between the two crura of the

（四）耳穴的部位和主治

耳穴的部位见图 6-10。

1. **耳轮穴位部位及主治**　耳轮分为 12 个区。耳轮脚为耳轮 1 区。耳轮脚切迹到对耳轮下脚上缘之间的耳轮分为 3 等份，自下向上依次为耳轮 2 区、3 区、4 区；对耳轮下脚上缘到对耳轮上脚前缘之间的耳轮为耳轮 5 区；对

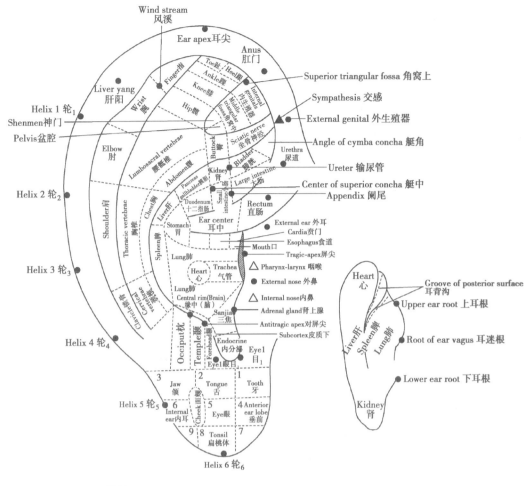

Note: 图例：
---- Points on the surface 示表面穴区
● Points on the surface 示表面穴区
△ Points on the inner aspect 示内侧面穴区

Fig. 6-10 Distribution of Auricular Points
图 6-10 耳穴分布图

antihelix is HX5. HX6 extends from the anterior edge of the superior crus of the antihelix to the apex of ear. HX7 extends from the apex of ear to the upper edge of the helix tubercle. The area from upper edge to the lower edge of the helix tubercle is HX8. The part from the lower edge of the helix tubercle to the notch of helix-lobe is equally divided into 4 areas, which from above to below are HX9, HX10, HX11, and HX12 respectively (Table 6-3).

2. Point on the Scapha (6 Areas, SF1-SF6) The scaphoid fossa is separated horizontally into 6 equal sections, which from upper to lower part of the scapha are SF1, SF2, SF3, SF4, SF5, and SF6 respectively (Table 6-4).

3. Point on the Antihelix (13 Areas, AH1-AH13) Both the superior and inferior crus of antihelix are separated into 3 equal sections. The lower 1/3 of the superior crus of the antihelix is AH5. The middle 1/3 is

耳轮上脚缘到耳尖之间的耳轮为耳轮 6 区；耳尖到耳轮结节上缘为耳轮 7 区；耳轮结节上缘到耳轮结节下缘为耳轮 8 区。耳轮结节下缘到轮垂切迹之间的耳轮分为 4 等份，自上而下依次为耳轮 9 区、10 区、11 区和 12 区（表 6-3）。

2. 耳舟穴位部位及主治 耳舟分为 6 等份，自上而下依次为耳舟 1 区、2 区、3 区、4区、5 区、6 区（表 6-4）。

3. 对耳轮穴位部位及主治 将对耳轮分为 13 区。对耳轮上脚分为上、中、下 3 等份；下 1/3 为对耳轮 5 区，中 1/3 为对耳轮 4 区；

Table 6-3　Locations and Indications of Points on the Helix

Name	Location	Indications
Ear Center (HX1)	on the helix crus, on HX1	hiccups, urticaria, pruritus, infantile enuresis, hemorrhagic diseases
Rectum (HX2)	on the helix close to the notch superior to the tragus, on HX2	constipation, diarrhea, prolapse of the anus, haemorrhoids
Urethra (HX3)	on the helix superior to Rectum, on HX3	frequent, painful, or dripping urination; retention of urine
External Genitals (HX4)	on the helix superior to Urethra, on HX4	testitis, epididymitis, vulvar or scrotal pruritus
Anus (HX5)	on the helix anterior to the triangular fossa, on HX5	hemorrhoids, anal fissure
Ear Apex (HX6,7 i)	on the apex where the ear is folded forward at the juncture of HX6 and HX7	fever, hypertension, acute conjunctivitis, stye toothache, insomnicl
Node (HX8)	on the tubercle of the helix, on HX8	dizziness, headache, hypertension
Helix1 (HX9)	inferior to the helix tubercle, on HX9	fever, tonsillitis, upper respiratory tract infection
Helix2 (HX10)	inferior to the helix1, on HX10	fever, tonsillitis, upper respiratory tract infection
Helix3 (HX11)	inferior to the helix2, on HX11	fever, tonsillitis, upper respiratory tract infection
Helix4 (HX12)	inferior to the helix3, on HX12	fever, tonsillitis, upper respiratory tract infection

表 6-3　耳轮穴位部位及主治

穴名	部位	主治
耳中	在耳轮脚处，即耳轮 1 区	呃逆、荨麻疹、皮肤瘙痒症、小儿遗尿、出血性疾病
直肠	在耳轮脚棘前上方的耳轮处，即耳轮 2 区	便秘、腹泻、脱肛、痔疮
尿道	在直肠上方的耳轮处，即耳轮 3 区	尿频、尿急、尿痛、尿潴留
外生殖器	在对耳轮下脚前方的耳轮处，即耳轮 4 区	睾丸炎、附睾炎、外阴瘙痒症
肛门	在三角窝前方的耳轮处，即耳轮 5 区	痔疮、肛裂
耳尖	在耳郭向前对折的上部尖端处，即耳轮 6、7 区交界处	发热、高血压、急性结膜炎、睑腺炎、牙痛、失眠
结节	在耳轮结节处，即耳轮 8 区	头晕、头痛、高血压
轮 1	在耳轮结节下方的耳轮处，即耳轮 9 区	发热、扁桃体炎、上呼吸道感染
轮 2	在耳轮 1 区下方的耳轮处，即耳轮 10 区	发热、扁桃体炎、上呼吸道感染
轮 3	在耳轮 2 区下方的耳轮处，即耳轮 11 区	发热、扁桃体炎、上呼吸道感染
轮 4	在耳轮 3 区下方的耳轮处，即耳轮 12 区	发热、扁桃体炎、上呼吸道感染

AH4. The upper 1/3 is divided horizontally into 2 equal subparts, of which the lower half is AH3. The upper half is once again divided perpendicularly into 2 subparts, the posterior half is AH2 and the anterior half of which is AH1. The front and middle 2/3 of the inferior crus are AH6, and back 1/3 of which is AH7. The body of the antihelix is separated horizontally into 5 equal sections.

再将上 1/3 分为上、下 2 等份，下 1/2 为对耳轮 3 区，再将上 1/2 分为前、后 2 等份，后 1/2 为对耳轮 2 区，前 1/2 为对耳轮 1 区。对耳轮下脚分为前、中、后 3 等份，中、前 2/3 为对耳轮 6 区，后 1/3 为对耳轮 7 区。对耳轮体从对耳轮上、下脚分叉处至轮屏切迹分

Table 6-4　Locations and Indications of Points on the Scapha

Name	Location	Indications
Finger (SF1)	on the uppermost section of the scaphoid fossa, on SF1	paronychia, pain and numbness of the fingers
Wrist (SF2)	n the section inferior to SF1, on SF2	pain in the wrist
Wind Stream (SF1, 2 i)	between the sections of Fingers and Wrist, midpoint between SF1 and SF2	urticaria, pruritus, allergic rhinitis
Elbow (SF3)	on the third section from the top of the scaphoid fossa, on SF3	external humeral epicondylitis, pain in elbows
Shoulder (SF4, 5i)	on the fourth and fifth sections from the top of the scaphoid fossa, on SF4 and SF5	periarthritis of the shoulder, pain of the shoulder
Clavicle (SF6)	on the lowermost section of the scaphoid fossa, on SF6	periarthritis of the shoulder

表 6-4　耳舟穴位部位及主治

穴名	部位	主治
指	在耳舟上方处，即耳舟 1 区	甲沟炎、手指麻木和疼痛
腕	在指区的下方处，即耳舟 2 区	腕部疼痛
风溪	在耳轮结节前方，指区与腕区之间，即耳舟 1、2 区交界处	荨麻疹、皮肤瘙痒症、过敏性鼻炎
肘	在腕区的下方处，即耳舟 3 区	肱骨外上髁炎、肘部疼痛
肩	在肘区的下方处，即耳舟 4、5 区	肩关节周围炎、肩部疼痛
锁骨	在肩区的下方处，即耳舟 6 区	肩关节周围炎

Then it is also divided vertically into 2 sections, the medial side taking 1/4, and the lateral side taking 3/4. Thus the body of antihelix is divided into 12 areas. The anterior superior 2/5 are AH8, while the posterior superior 2/5 are AH9. The front intermediate 2/5 are AH10 while the back intermediate 2/5 are AH11. The front inferior 1/5 is AH12 while the back inferior 1/5 is AH13 (Table 6-5).

4. Point on the Triangular Fossa (5 Areas, TF1-TF5） The triangular fossa is separated into 3 equal sections. The middle 1/3 is TF3. The uppermost 1/3 is separated into 3 equal sections again. The upper 1/3 is TF1 and the middle and lower 2/3 are TF2. The lowest 1/3 section is separated into 2 equal sections, the upper half of which is TF4 and lower half of which is TF5 (Table 6-6).

5. Point on the Tragus (4 Areas, TG1-TG4) The external surface of the tragus is divided into 2 equal parts from above to below, the upper 1/2 is TG1 and lower 1/2 is TG2. The internal surface of the tragus is separated

为 5 等份，再沿对耳轮耳甲缘将对耳轮体分为前 1/4 和后 3/4 两部分，前上 2/5 为对耳轮 8 区，后上 2/5 为对耳轮 9 区，前中 2/5 为对耳轮 10 区，后中 2/5 为对耳轮 11 区，前下 1/5 为对耳轮 12 区，后下 1/5 为对耳轮 13 区（表 6-5）。

4. 三角窝穴位部位及主治 将三角窝分为 5 区。三角窝由耳轮内缘至对耳轮上、下脚分叉处分为前、中、后 3 等份，中 1/3 为三角窝 3 区；再将前 1/3 分为上、中、下 3 等份，上 1/3 为三角窝 1 区，中、下 2/3 为三角窝 2 区；再将后 1/3 分为上、下 2 等份，上 1/2 为三角窝 4 区，下 1/2 为三角窝 5 区（表 6-6）。

5. 耳屏穴位部位及主治 将耳屏分成 4 区。耳屏外侧面分为上、下 2 等份，上部为耳屏 1 区，下部为耳屏 2 区。将耳屏内侧面分为

Table 6-5　Locations and Indications of Points on the Antihelix

Name	Location	Indications
Heel (AH1)	on the anterosuperior portion of the superior antihelix crus, on AH1	heel pain
Toe (AH2)	on the posterosuperior portion of the superior antihelix curs inferior to the apex, on AH2	paronychia, toe pain
Ankle (AH3)	at the part inferior to heel and toe, on AH3	sprained ankle
Knee (AH4)	at the middle 1/3 of the superior antihelix crus, on AH4	pain of the knee joint, sciatica
Hip (AH5)	at the lower 1/3 of the superior antihelix crus, on AH5	hip joint pain or sprain, pain in lumbosacral area, sciatica
Sciatic Nerve (AH6)	at the inferior 2/3 of the inferior antihelix crus, on AH6	sciatica, lower limb paralysis
Sympathesis (AH6a)	on the juncture between the terminus of the inferior antihelix crus and the helix	spasms of the stomach and intestines, angina, biliary colic, ureterolith, functional disorders of autonomic nerves
Buttock (AH7)	on the posterior 1/3 of the inferior antihelix crus, on AH7	sciatica, gluteal fascitis
Abdomen (AH8)	on the upper 2/5 of the front part of the body of the antihelix, on AH8	abdominal pain or distension, diarrhea, acute lumbar muscle sprain, dysmenorrhea, labor pain
Lumbosacral Vertebrae (AH9)	posterior to AH8, on AH9	pain in the lumbosacral region
Chest (AH10)	on the central 2/5 of the front part of the body of the antihelix, on AH10	pain and fullness in the chest or rib-sides, intercostal neuralgia, oppression of the chest, mastitis
Thoracic Vertebrae (AH11)	posterior to AH10, on AH11	chest pain, distending pain of the breasts before menstruation, mastitis, postpartum hypogalactia
Neck (AH12)	on the lower 1/5 of the front part of the body of the antihelix, on AH12	stiff neck, pain of the neck
Cervical Vertebrae (AH13)	posterior to AH12, on AH13	stiff neck, cervical spondylopathy

表 6-5　对耳轮穴位部位及主治

穴名	部位	主治
跟	在对耳轮上脚前上部，即对耳轮 1 区	足跟痛
趾	在耳尖下方的对耳轮上脚后上部，即对耳轮 2 区	甲沟炎、趾部疼痛
踝	在趾、跟区下方处，即对耳轮 3 区	踝关节扭伤
膝	在对耳轮上脚中 1/3 处，即对耳轮 4 区	膝关节疼痛、坐骨神经痛
髋	在对耳轮上脚的下 1/3 处，即对耳轮 5 区	髋关节疼痛、坐骨神经痛、腰骶部疼痛
坐骨神经	在对耳轮下脚的前 2/3 处，即对耳轮 6 区	坐骨神经痛、下肢瘫痪
交感	在对耳轮下脚末端与耳轮内缘相交处，即对耳轮 6 区前端	胃肠痉挛、心绞痛、胆绞痛、输尿管结石、自主神经功能紊乱
臀	在对耳轮下脚的后 1/3 处，即对耳轮 7 区	坐骨神经痛、臀筋膜炎

穴名	部位	主治
腹	在对耳轮体前部上 2/5 处，即对耳轮 8 区	腹痛、腹胀、腹泻、急性腰扭伤、痛经、产后宫缩痛
腰骶椎	在腹区后方，即对耳轮 9 区	腰骶部疼痛
胸	在对耳轮体前部中 2/5 处，即对耳轮 10 区	胸胁疼痛、肋间神经痛、胸闷、乳腺炎
胸椎	在胸区后方，即对耳轮 11 区	胸痛、经前乳房胀痛、乳腺炎、产后泌乳不足
颈	在对耳轮体前部下 1/5 处，即对耳轮 12 区	落枕、颈椎疼痛
颈椎	在颈区后方，即对耳轮 13 区	落枕、颈椎综合征

Table 6-6　Locations and Indications of Points on the Triangular Fossa

Name	Location	Indications
Superior Triangular Fossa (TF1)	on the upper part of the superior 1/3 of the triangular fossa, on TF1	hypertension
Internal Genitals (TF2)	at the lower 2/3 part of the superior 1/3 of the triangular fossa, on TF2	dysmenorrhea, irregular menstruation, leukorrhagia, dysfunctional uterine bleeding, impotence, seminal emission, premature ejaculation
Middle Triangular Fossa (TF3)	in the middle 1/3 of the triangular fossa, on TF3	asthma
Shenmen (TF4)	on the upper part of the posterior 1/3 of the triangular fossa, on TF4	insomnia, profuse dreaming, withdrawal syndrome, epilepsy, hypertension, neurasthenia, pain disorders
Pelvis (TF5)	on the lower part of the posterior 1/3 of the triangular fossa, on TF5	pelvic inflammation, adnexitis

表 6-6　三角窝穴位部位及主治

穴名	部位	主治
角窝上	在三角窝前 1/3 的上部，即三角窝 1 区	高血压
内生殖器	在三角窝前 1/3 的下部，即三角窝 2 区	痛经、月经不调、白带过多、功能性子宫出血、阳痿、遗精、早泄
角窝中	在三角窝中 1/3 处，即三角窝 3 区	哮喘
神门	在三角窝后 1/3 的上部，即三角窝 4 区	失眠、多梦、戒断综合征、癫痫、高血压、神经衰弱、痛证
盆腔	在三角窝后 1/3 的下部，即三角窝 5 区	盆腔炎、附件炎

into 2 equal sections too. The upper part of which is TG3 and the lower part of which is TG4 (Table 6-7).

6. Point on the Antitragus (4 Areas, AT1-AT4)　Draw a vertical line from the apex of antitragus down to upper line of ear lobe. Draw another line from the midpoint between the apex of antitragus and antihelix-antitragus notch down to upper line of ear lobe. Therefore,

上、下 2 等份，上部为耳屏 3 区，下部为耳屏 4 区（表 6-7）。

6. 对耳屏穴位部位及主治　将对耳屏分为 4 区。由对屏尖及对屏尖至轮屏切迹连线之中点，分别向耳垂上线作两条垂线，将对耳屏外侧面及其后部分成前、中、后 3 区，前为

Table 6-7　Locations and Indications of Points on the Tragus

Name	Location	Indications
Upper Tragus (TG1)	on the upper 1/2 of the external surface of the tragus, on TG1	laryngitis, rhinitis, simple obesity
Lower Tragus (TG2)	on the lower 1/2 of the external surface of the tragus, on TG2	rhinitis, nasal obstruction, simple obesity
External Ear (TG1u)	anterior to the superior tragic notch nearby the helix, on the upper edge of TG1	otitis externa,, otitis media, tinnitus
Apex of Tragus (TG1p)	on the center of the upper eminence of the tragus, posterior to the edge of TG1	fever, toothache, squint
External Nose (TG1, 2)	at the middle part of lateral side of the tragus, the junction of upper and lower tragus	nasal vestibulitis, rhinitis
Adrenal Gland (TG2p)	on the center of the lower eminence of the tragus, on the posterior edge of TG2	hypotension, rheumatic arthritis, mumps, dizziness, asthma, shock, allergic diseases
Pharynx and Larynx (TG3)	on the upper 1/2 of the internal side of the tragus, on the TG3	loss of voice, pharyngitis, tonsillitis
Internal Nose (TG4)	on the lower 1/2 of the internal side of the tragus, on the TG4	rhinitis, maxillary sinuitis , nose bleeding
Anterior Intertragic Notch (TG2b)	at the lowest part of the front of the intertragic notch, the lower edge of the area of lower tragus	pharyngitis, stomatitis, eye disorders,

表 6-7　耳屏穴位部位及主治

穴名	部位	主治
上屏	在耳屏外侧面上 1/2 处，即耳屏 1 区	咽炎、鼻炎、单纯性肥胖
下屏	在耳屏外侧面下 1/2 处，即耳屏 2 区	鼻炎、鼻塞、单纯性肥胖
外耳	在屏上切迹前方近耳轮部，即耳屏 1 区上缘处	外耳道炎、中耳炎、耳鸣
屏尖	在耳屏游离缘上部尖端，即耳屏 1 区后缘处	发热、牙痛、斜视
外鼻	在耳屏外侧面中部，即耳屏 1、2 区之间	鼻前庭炎、鼻炎
肾上腺	在耳屏游离缘下部尖端，即耳屏 2 区后缘处	低血压、风湿性关节炎、腮腺炎、眩晕、哮喘、休克、过敏性疾病
咽喉	在耳屏内侧面上 1/2 处，即耳屏 3 区	声音嘶哑、咽炎、扁桃体炎
内鼻	在耳屏内侧面下 1/2 处，即耳屏 4 区	鼻炎、上颌窦炎、鼻衄
屏间前	在屏间切迹前方耳屏最下部，即耳屏 2 区下缘处	咽炎、口腔炎、眼病

the antitragus is separated into 3 sections on its external surface. The anterior area is AT1, the intermediate area of which is AT2 and posterior area of which is AT3. The internal surface of the antitragus is AT4 (Table 6-8).

7. Point on the Concha (18 Areas, CO1-CO18)　It is necessary to know the marker points and lines on the auricle firstly. The concha is separated into 18 areas by those marker points and lines. Point A is located at the medial edge of the helix, at the junction between the

对耳屏 1 区、中为对耳屏 2 区、后为对耳屏 3 区。对耳屏内侧面为对耳屏 4 区（表 6-8）。

7. 耳甲穴位部位及主治　将耳甲用标志点、线分为 18 个区。在耳轮的内缘上，设耳轮脚切迹至对耳轮下脚间中、上 1/3 交界处为 A 点；在耳甲内，由耳轮脚消失处向后作一

Table 6-8 Locations and Indications of Points on the Antitragus

Name	Location	Indications
Forehead (AT1)	on the anterior part of the outer side of the antitragus, on the AT1	frontal headache, dizziness insomnia, profuse dreaming
Posterior Intertragic Notch (AT1b)	on the anteroinferior part of the antitragus, posterior to intertragus and the lower edge of forehead	prosopantritis, eye disorders
Temple (AT2)	on the middle part of the lateral side of the antitragus, on the AT2	migraine, dizziness
Occiput (AT3)	on the posterior part of the lateral side of the antitragus, on the AT3	dizziness, headache, epilepsy, asthma, neurasthenia
Subcortex (AT4)	on the medial side of the antitragus, on AT4	pain, neurasthenia, pseudomyopia, insomnia,
Apex of the Antitragus (AT1, 2, 4 i)	at the free end of the apex of the antitragus, at the junction of AT1, AT2 and AT4	asthma, mumps, testitis, epididymitis, neurodermatitis,
Central Rim of the Antitragus (AT2, 3, 4 i)	on the free rim of the antitragus, at the midpoint of the apex of the antitragus and antihelix-antitragus notch at the juncture of AT2, AT3, and AT4	enuresis, aural vertigo, diabetes insipidus, functional uterine bleeding
Brain Stem (AT3, 4 i)	on the antihelix-antitragus notch at the junction of AT3 and AT4	dizziness, occipital headache, pseudomyopia

表 6-8　对耳屏穴位部位及主治

穴名	部位	主治
额	在对耳屏外侧面的前部，即对耳屏 1 区	前额痛、头晕、失眠、多梦
屏间后	在屏间切迹后方对耳屏前下部，即对耳屏 1 区下缘处	额窦炎、眼病
颞	在对耳屏外侧面的中部，即对耳屏 2 区	偏头痛、头晕
枕	在对耳屏外侧面的后部，即对耳屏 3 区	头晕、头痛、癫痫、哮喘、神经衰弱
皮质下	在对耳屏内侧面，即对耳屏 4 区	痛症、神经衰弱、假性近视、失眠
对屏尖	在对耳屏游离缘的尖端，即对耳屏 1、2、4 区交点处	哮喘、腮腺炎、睾丸炎、附睾炎、神经性皮炎
缘中	在对耳屏游离缘上，对屏尖与轮屏切迹之中点处，即对耳屏 2、3、4 区交点处	遗尿、内耳性眩晕、尿崩症、功能性子宫出血
脑干	在轮屏切迹处，即对耳屏 3、4 区之间	眩晕、后头痛、假性近视

middle and upper 1/3 of the line from the notch of helix crus and the inferior edge of the inferior antihelix crus. In the concha, draw a level line from the end of the helix crus to the concha edge of the helix. Point D is located at the cross point of the line with the edge of the antihelix. Point B is located at the junction of the middle and posterior 1/3 of the line extending from the end of the helix crus to Point D. Point C is located at the junction of the upper 1/4 and lower 3/4 of the posterior edge of the orifice of

水平线与对耳轮耳甲缘相交，设交点为 D 点；设耳轮脚消失处至 D 点连线中、后 1/3 交界处为 B 点；设外耳道口后缘上 1/4 与下 3/4 交界处为 C 点；从 A 点向 B 点作一条与对耳轮耳甲艇缘弧度大体相仿的曲线；从 B 点向 C 点作一条与耳轮脚下缘弧度大体相仿的曲线（图 6-11）。

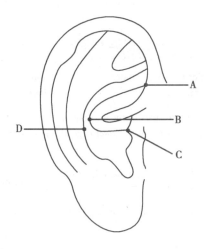

Fig. 6-11　Points on the Concha

图 6-11　耳郭标志点线示意图

the external auditory meatus. Draw a curved line similar to the concha edge of the antihelix from Point A to B. Draw a curved line similar to the inferior edge of the helix crus from Point B to C (Fig. 6-11).

　　Divide the part, formed by the inferior edge of the helix crus and its opposite BC line (the front part), into 3 equal areas. There is area 1, 2 and 3 counting from front to back. The fan-shaped area at the end of the helix crus is area 4. Divide the part, formed by the superior edge of the helix crus and its opposite AB line (the front part), into 3 equal areas. They are from the back to the front area 5, 6 and 7 respectively.

　　Connect Point A with the junction of the anterior 1/3 and the posterior 2/3 of the lower edge of the inferior crus of the antihelix. The concha anterior to this line is area 8. Divide the part posterior to area 8 and superior to area 6 and 7 into two areas. The anterior area is area 9 and posterior area id area 10. Divide the part posterior to area 10 and superior to line BD into 2 areas. The superior area is area 11 and the inferior area is area 12. Draw a line from the helix notch to point B. The area between this line and BD line is area 13. Take the middle point of cavum concha as the center of a circle. The circle with a radius of half the distance from the center to line BC is area 15. Make two tangents from the highest and lowest points to the office of the external auditory meatus, then the area with the lines is area 16. The area external to area 15 and 16 is area 14. Draw a line from the lowest point of the orifice of the external auditory meatus to the middle point of the concha edge of the antitragus, and then divide the part inferior to the line into 2 areas. The upper area is area 17 and lower is area 18 (Table 6-9).

　　将 BC 线前段与耳轮脚下缘间分成 3 等份，前 1/3 为耳甲 1 区，中 1/3 为耳甲 2 区，后 1/3 为耳甲 3 区。ABC 线前方，耳轮脚消失处为耳甲 4 区。将 AB 线前段与耳轮脚上缘及部分耳轮内缘间分成 3 等份，后 1/3 为 5 区，中 1/3 为 6 区，前 1/3 为 7 区。

　　将对耳轮下脚下缘前、中 1/3 交界处与 A 点连线，该线前方的耳甲艇部为耳甲 8 区。将 AB 线前段与对耳轮下脚下缘间耳甲 8 区以后的部分，分为前、后 2 等份，前 1/2 为耳甲 9 区，后 1/2 为耳甲 10 区。在 AB 线后段上方的耳甲艇部，将耳甲 10 区后缘与 BD 线之间分成上、下 2 等份，上 1/2 为耳甲 11 区，下 1/2 为耳甲 12 区。由轮屏切迹至 B 点作连线，该线后方、BD 线下方的耳甲腔部为耳甲 13 区。以耳甲腔中央为圆心，圆心与 BC 线间距离的 1/2 为半径作圆，该圆形区域为耳甲 15 区。过 15 区最高点及最低点分别向外耳门后壁作两条切线，切线间为耳甲 16 区。15、16 区周围为耳甲 14 区。将外耳门的最低点与对耳屏耳甲缘中点相连，再将该线以下的耳甲腔部分为上、下 2 等份，上 1/2 为耳甲 17 区，下 1/2 为耳甲 18 区（表 6-9）。

Table 6-9　Locations and Indications of Points on the Concha

Name	Location	Indications
Mouth (CO1)	on the anterior 1/3 of the area inferior to the crus of helix, on CO1	facial paralysis, stomatitis, cholecystitis, cholelithiasis, withdrawal syndrome, periodontitis, glossitis
Esophagus (CO2)	on the middle 1/3 of the area inferior to the crus of the helix, on CO2	esophagitis, esophagospasm
Cardia (CO3)	on the posterior 1/3 of the area inferior to the crus of the helix, on CO3	cardiospasm, nervous vomiting
Stomach (CO4)	on the terminus of the helix crus, on CO4	gastrospasm, gastritis, gastric ulcer, nausea and vomiting, insomnia, toothache, indigestion
Duodenum (CO5)	on the posterior 1/3 of the area superior to the helix crus, on CO5	duodenal ulcer, cholecystitis, cholelithiasis, pylorospasm, abdominal distension and pain, diarrhea
Small Intestine (CO6)	on the middle 1/3 of the area superior to the helix crus, on CO6	indigestion, abdominal pain and distension, tachycardia
Large Intestine (CO7)	on the anterior 1/3 of the area superior to the helix crus, on CO7	diarrhea, constipation, cough, toothache, acne
Appendix (CO6, 7i)	at the junction of CO6 and CO7	appendicitis, diarrhea
Angle of Superior Concha (CO8)	at the anterior part under the inferior antihelix crus, on CO8	prostatitis, urethritis
Bladder (CO9)	at the intermediate part under the inferior crus of antihelix, on CO9	cystitis, enuresis, retention of urine, lower back pain, sciatica, occipital headache
Kidney (CO10)	at the posterior part under the inferior crus of antihelix, on CO10	lower back pain, tinnitus, neurasthenia, pyelitis, asthma, nocturnal enuresis, irregular menstruation, seminal emission, premature ejaculation, impotence asthma, irregular menstruation
Ureter (CO9, 10i)	at the junction of Kidney (CO9) and Bladder (CO10)	urethral colic
Pancreas and Gallbladder (CO11)	at the posterior part of the cymba concha, on CO11	cholecystitis, cholelithiasis, biliary ascariasis, migraine, herpes zoster, otitis media, tinnitus, acute pancreatitis
Liver (CO12)	on the posteroinferior area of the superior cymba concha, on CO12	pain in the chest and rib-sides, dizziness, premenstrual syndrome, irregular menstruation, menopause syndrome, hypertension, myopia, simple glucoma
Center of Superior Concha (CO6, 10i)	in the center of the superior concha, at the junction of Small Intestine (CO6) and kidney (CO10)	abdominal pain or distension, biliary ascariasis
Spleen (CO13)	at the part inferior to BD line, posterosuperior part of the cavum concha, on CO13	diarrhea, constipation, poor appetite, dysfunctional uterine bleeding, leukorrhagia, Meniere's disease
Heart (CO15)	in the depression at the center of the cavum concha, on CO15	angina pectoris, aortic arch syndrome, neurasthenia, hysteria, oral ulcers
Trachea (CO16)	at the part between the Heart (CO15) and the orifice of the external auditory meatus, on CO16	asthma, bronchitis
Lung (CO14)	in the cavum concha around Heart (CO15) and Trachea (CO16), on CO14	cough, asthma, pain or fullness in the chest, loss of voice, acne, pruritus, urticaria, constipation, withdrawal syndrome
San Jiao (CO17)	at the part posteroinferior to the orifice of the external auditory meatus and between the Lung (CO14) and Endocrine (CO18), on CO17	constipation, abdominal distension, pain on the lateral side of the upper limb
Endocrine (CO18)	at the inside of the notch of the intertragus and anteroinferior part of cavum concha, on CO18	dysmenorrhea, irregular menstruation, menopausal syndrome, acne, hyperthyroidism or hypothyroidism

表 6-9　耳甲穴位部位及主治

穴名	部位	主治
口	在耳轮脚下方前 1/3 处，即耳甲 1 区	面瘫、口腔炎、胆囊炎、胆石症、戒断综合征、牙周炎、舌炎
食管	在耳轮脚下方中 1/3 处，即耳甲 2 区	食管炎、食管痉挛
贲门	在耳轮脚下方后 1/3 处，即耳甲 3 区	贲门痉挛、神经性呕吐
胃	在耳轮脚消失处，即耳甲 4 区	胃痉挛、胃炎、胃溃疡、消化不良、恶心呕吐、前额痛、牙痛、失眠
十二指肠	在耳轮脚及部分耳轮与 AB 线之间的后 1/3 处，即耳甲 5 区	十二指肠溃疡、胆囊炎、胆石症、幽门痉挛、腹胀、腹泻、腹痛
小肠	在耳轮脚及部分耳轮与 AB 线之间的中 1/3 处，即耳甲 6 区	消化不良、腹痛、腹胀、心动过速
大肠	在耳轮脚及部分耳轮与 AB 线之间的前 1/3 处，即耳甲 7 区	腹泻、便秘、咳嗽、牙痛、痤疮
阑尾	在小肠区与大肠区之间，即耳甲 6、7 区交界处	单纯性阑尾炎、腹泻
艇角	在对耳轮下脚下方前部，即耳甲 8 区	前列腺炎、尿道炎
膀胱	在对耳轮下脚下方中部，即耳甲 9 区	膀胱炎、遗尿、尿潴留、腰痛、坐骨神经痛、后头痛
肾	在对耳轮下脚下方后部，即耳甲 10 区	腰痛、耳鸣、神经衰弱、肾盂肾炎、遗尿、遗精、阳痿、早泄、哮喘、月经不调
输尿管	在肾区与膀胱区之间，即耳甲 9、10 区交界处	输尿管结石绞痛
胰胆	在耳甲艇的后上部，即耳甲 11 区	胆囊炎、胆石症、胆道蛔虫症、偏头痛、带状疱疹、中耳炎、耳鸣、急性胰腺炎
肝	在耳甲艇的后下部，即耳甲 12 区	胁痛、眩晕、经前期紧张症、月经不调、更年期综合征、高血压、近视、单纯性青光眼
艇中	在小肠区与肾区之间，即耳甲 6、10 区交界处	腹痛、腹胀、胆道蛔虫症
脾	在 BD 线下方，耳甲腔的后上部，即耳甲 13 区	腹胀、腹泻、便秘、食欲缺乏、功能性子宫出血、白带过多、内耳性眩晕
心	在耳甲腔正中凹陷处，即耳甲 15 区	心动过速、心律不齐、心绞痛、无脉症、神经衰弱、癔病、口生疮
气管	在心区与外耳门之间，即耳甲 16 区	哮喘、支气管炎
肺	在心、气管区周围处，即耳甲 14 区	咳嗽、胸闷、声音嘶哑、皮肤瘙痒症、荨麻疹、便秘、戒断综合征
三焦	在外耳门后下，肺与内分泌区之间，即耳甲 17 区	便秘、腹胀、上肢外侧疼痛
内分泌	在屏间切迹内，耳甲腔的前下部，即耳甲 18 区	痛经、月经不调、更年期综合征、痤疮、甲状腺功能减退或亢进

8. Point on the Earlobe (9 Areas, LO1-LO9)

A grid of 9 sections is delineated on the frontal surface of the earlobe by drawing three equidistant horizontal lines below the lower border of the cartilage of the notch between the tragus and the antitragus, and two equidistant vertical lines. From front to back, the upper 3 areas are LO1, LO2 and LO3. The middle areas are LO4, LO5 and LO6, and the lower areas are LO7, LO8 and LO9 (Table 6-10).

8. 耳垂穴位部位及主治 将耳垂分为9区。在耳垂上线至耳垂下缘最低点之间划两条等距离平行线,于上平行线上引两条垂直等份线,将耳垂分为9个区,上部由前到后依次为耳垂1、2、3区;中部由前到后依次为耳垂4、5、6区;下部由前到后依次为耳垂7、8、9区(表6-10)。

Table 6-10 Locations and Indications of Points on the Earlobe

Name	Location	Indications
Teeth (LO1)	on the anterosuperior area of the front surface of the earlobe, on LO1	toothache, periodontitis, hypotension
Tongue (LO2)	on the central superior area of the front surface of the earlobe, on LO2	glossitis, stomatitis
Jaw (LO3)	on the posterosuperior area of the front surface of the earlobe, on LO3	toothache, dysfunction of the temporomandibular joint
Anterior Ear Lobe (LO4)	on the anterior central area of the front surface of the earlobe, on LO4	neurathenia, toothache
Eye (LO5)	on the center of the front surface of the earlobe, on LO5	acute conjunctivitis, electric opthalmitis, stye, myopia
Internal Ear (LO6)	on the central posterior part of the front surface of the earlobe, on LO6	tinnitus, hearing impairment, otitis media, Meniere's disease
Cheek (LO5, 6 i)	on the central posterior part of the front surface of the earlobe, at the junction between LO5 and LO6	facial paralysis or spasm, trigeminal neuralgia, acne, verruca plana, mumps
Tonsil (LO7, 8, 9)	on the inferior part of the front surface of the earlobe, including LO7, 8, 9	tonsillitis, pharyngitis

表 6-10 耳垂穴位部位及主治

穴名	部位	主治
牙	在耳垂正面前上部,即耳垂 1 区	牙痛、牙周炎、低血压
舌	在耳垂正面中上部,即耳垂 2 区	舌炎、口腔炎
颌	在耳垂正面后上部,即耳垂 3 区	牙痛、颞颌关节功能紊乱症
垂前	在耳垂正面前中部,即耳垂 4 区	神经衰弱、牙痛
眼	在耳垂正面中央部,即耳垂 5 区	急性结膜炎、电光性眼炎、睑腺炎、近视
内耳	在耳垂正面后中部,即耳垂 6 区	内耳性眩晕症、耳鸣、听力减退、中耳炎
面颊	在耳垂正面与内耳区之间,即耳垂 5、6 区交界处	面瘫、三叉神经痛、痤疮、扁平疣、面肌痉挛、腮腺炎
扁桃体	在耳垂正面下部,即耳垂 7、8、9 区	扁桃体炎、咽炎

9. Point on the Posterior Surface of the Ear (5 Areas, P1-P5) The dorsal side of the ear is separated into 5 areas. Draw 2 horizontal lines passing through the back corresponding points of the bifurcation of the antihelix crura and helix notch, thus the posterior surface is thereby divided into 3 parts. The upper part is P1, and the lower part is P5. The middle part, once again, is divided equally into 3 equal areas. The medial area is P2. The middle area is P3 and the lateral area is P4 (Table 6-11).

10. Point on the Root of the Ear To see table 6-12.

9. 耳背穴位部位及主治 将耳背分为5区。分别过对耳轮上、下脚分叉处耳背对应点和轮屏切迹耳背对应点作两条水平线，将耳背分为上、中、下3部，上部为耳背1区，下部为耳背5区，再将中部分为内、中、外3等份，内1/3为耳背2区、中1/3为耳背3区、外1/3为耳背4区（表6-11）。

10. 耳根穴位部位及主治 见表6-12。

Table 6-11 Locations and Indications of Points on the Posterior Surface of the Ear

Name	Location	Indications
Heart of Posterior Surface (P1)	on the upper portion of the posterior surface of the auricle, on P1	palpitation, insomnia, dream-disturbed sleep
Lung of Posterior Surface (P2)	on the centromedial portion of the posterior surface of the auricle, on P2	cough, asthma, pruritus
Spleen of Posterior Surface (P3)	on the posterior surface of the auricle close to the terminus of the crus of the helix, on P3	gastric pain, indigestion, poor appetite
Liver of Posterior Surface (P4)	on the centrolateral portion of the posterior surface of the auricle, on P4	cholecystitis, cholelithiasis, pain in rib sides
Kidney of Posterior Surface (P5)	on the lower portion of the posterior surface of the auricle, on P5	dizziness, headache, neurasthenia
Groove of Posterior Surface (GPS)	on the posteromedial surface of the ear formed by the superior and inferior antihelix crura	hypertension, pruritus

表 6-11 耳背穴位部位及主治

穴名	部位	主治
耳背心	在耳背上部，即耳背1区	心悸、失眠、多梦
耳背肺	在耳背中内部，即耳背2区	哮喘、皮肤瘙痒症
耳背脾	在耳背中央部，即耳背3区	胃痛、消化不良、食欲缺乏
耳背肝	在耳背中外部，即耳背4区	胆囊炎、胆石症、肋痛
耳背肾	在耳背下部，即耳背5区	头痛、头晕、神经衰弱
耳背沟	在对耳轮沟和对耳轮上、下脚沟处	高血压、皮肤瘙痒症

Table 6-12 Locations and Indications of Points on the Root of the Ear

Name	Location	Indications
Upper Ear Root (R1)	at the top of the root of the ear	epitaxis
Root of Ear Vagus (R2)	at the ear root on the posterior groove of the helix crus	cholecystitis, cholelithiasis, abdominal pain, diarrhea, nasal congestion, tachycardia
Lower Ear Root (R1)	on the lowest part of the ear	hypotension, paralysis of the lower limbs, sequelae of infantile paralysis

表 6-12　耳根穴位部位及主治

穴名	部位	主治
上耳根	在耳根最上处	鼻衄
耳迷根	在耳轮脚后沟的耳根处	胆囊炎、胆石症、腹痛、腹泻、鼻塞、心动过速
下耳根	在耳根最下处	低血压、下肢瘫痪、小儿麻痹后遗症

v. Principle for Selecting Auricular Point

1. Choose Point Based on the Corresponding to the Location of the Disease Choose points which are corresponding to the location of the disease or affected part. There will be sensitive points on the ear when disease is present. For example, choose stomach (*wèi*) for the treatment of stomachache.

2. Choose Point Based on the Visceral Manifestation Theory According to the theory of visceral manifestation, select the point by pattern identification which depends on viscera physiological function and pathological reaction. For instance, choose kidney (*shèn*) for alopecia or lung (*fèi*) and large intestine (*dà cháng*) for skin disorders.

3. Choose point Based on the Channel Pattern Identification Select points according to the channel running route. For instance, choose bladder (*páng guāng*) for sciatica because the foot *taiyang* channel runs on the part. Choose large intestine (*dà cháng*) for toothache.

4. Choose Point as Instructed by Biomedical Principle

Some points are named according to biomedical principles, such as adrenal gland (*shèn shàng xiàn*), endocrine (*nèi fēn mì*). As their names imply, their functions are in accordance with modern medical theories. For example, we can choose adrenal gland (*shèn shàng xiàn*) point for inflammatory diseases, subcortex (*pí zhì xià*) point for pain, and endocrine (*nèi fēn mì*) point for irregular menstruation.

5. Choosing Point Based on Clinical Experience There are some effective points discovered in clinical practice, but they do not meet the criteria of the above principles. For example, choose external genital (*wài shēng zhí qì*) for pain in the lower back and legs, the ear apex (*ěr jiān*) for bloodletting and for red, swollen and painful eyes, shen men (*shén mén*) for pain.

Confirming the reasonable prescription of points should be considered comprehensively according to the patients' conditions and principles for selecting auricular points. First definite main points, then select matching points. The prescription of points should be concise. In general, the total number of points are 2-5, including 2-3

（五）选穴原则

1. **按相应部位取穴**　当机体患病时，在耳郭的相应部位上有一定的敏感点，它便是本病的首选穴位，如胃痛取"胃"穴等。

2. **按脏腑辨证取穴**　根据藏象学说的理论，按各脏腑的生理功能和病理反应进行辨证取穴。如脱发取"肾"穴；皮肤病取"肺""大肠"穴等。

3. **按经络学说取穴**　根据经络的循行部位取穴，如坐骨神经痛（后支），其部位属足太阳膀胱经的循行部位，即取耳穴的"膀胱"穴，又如牙痛，取耳穴"大肠"穴。

4. **按现代医学理论取穴**　在耳穴中有些穴位是根据现代医学理论命名的，如"肾上腺""内分泌"等，与现代医学理论所认识的功能基本上一致，如炎性疾病取"肾上腺"穴，疼痛取"皮质下"，月经不调可取"内分泌"穴。

5. **按临床经验取穴**　从临床实践中发现有些耳穴对某些疾病具有特异的治疗作用，如"外生殖器"穴可治疗腰腿痛，目赤肿痛取"耳尖"放血，"神门"穴可治疗痛证。

对于耳穴的确定，应根据病情的需要和取穴原则，全面考虑，合理组穴，先选定主穴，然后再定配穴。提倡少而精，一般 2~5 个穴位为宜，主穴 2-3 个，配穴 1~2 个。

main points and 1-2 matching points.

vi. Auricular Diagnostic Method

1. Inspection   Push the helix to back and upward side in order to expose auricle fully. Under natural light, observe from top to bottom whether auricle appears positive reaction with the naked eye or the aid of a magnifying glass from top to bottom.

2. Detection of the Tender Spot   Press and move on the surface of the ear gently and smoothly from around the center of point area with a probe, the head of an acupuncture needle handle, or the end of a match sticker. Find out the tender spot when the patients show the series of reactions including frown, blink of eyes, shouting pain or dodge and so on.

3. Measurement of Electrical Resistance This technique detects decreased electrical resistance in points with an electrical detector that has an indicator lamp or special sound.

vii. Indication of Auricular Acupuncture Therapy

1. Painful Disorders   Such as sprains, headaches, and neuropathic pains, *etc.*.

2. Inflammatory and Infectious Diseases Such as acute and chronic colitis, periodontitis, laryngopharyngitis, tonsillitis, cholecystitis, influenza, whooping cough, bacillary dysentery, mumps, *etc.*.

3. Functional Disorders and Allergic Diseases Such as dizziness, hypertension, arrhythmia, neurasthenia, hives, asthma, rhinitis, purpura, *etc.*.

4. Endocrinal and Metabolic Disorders   Such as hyperthyroidism, hypothyroidism, diabetes, obesity, menopausal symptoms, *etc.*.

5. Other Conditions   Such as anaphylactic reactions to transfusion and infusion, for beauty therapy, smoking and drug addictions, anti-aging and disease prevention , *etc.*.

viii. Procedure and Method of Auricular Acupuncture

1. Assessment   Check the doctor's prescription, and check the patient's name, bed number, patient's condition, skin condition of ear, tolerance to pain, psychological status and so on. Explain to the patients and get their cooperation.

2. Preparation   Prepare supplies which include 75% alcohol, 0.2% anerdian or 2% iodine, sterile swabs, sonde, electrical detector of auricular point, disposable and sterile auricular needle, bending plate, and hand sanitizers. Bring all materials to the patient's bedside. Patient's

（六）耳穴探查法

1. 观察法   用拇、示指将耳轮向后上方拉，充分暴露耳郭，在自然光线下，用肉眼或借助放大镜，从上至下，全面观察耳郭有无阳性反应点。

2. 按压法   用前端圆滑的金属探捧或火柴头等进行探压。探压时要轻、慢、均匀压力，从穴区周围向中间按压。当患者会出现皱眉、眨眼、呼痛或躲闪等反应，说明压迫到敏感点。

3. 电阻测定法   根据与疾病有关的耳穴电阻较低的原理，用耳穴探测仪进行探测，通过显示屏的指示灯、音响、仪表反映出来。

（七）耳针法的适应证

1. 疼痛性疾病   如各种扭挫伤、头痛和神经性疼痛等。

2. 炎性疾病及传染病   如急慢性结肠炎、牙周炎、咽喉炎、扁桃体炎、胆囊炎、流感、百日咳、菌痢、腮腺炎等。

3. 功能紊乱和变态反应性疾病   如眩晕综合征、高血压、心律不齐、神经衰弱、荨麻疹、哮喘、鼻炎、紫癜等。

4. 内分泌代谢紊乱性疾病   甲状腺功能亢进或低下、糖尿病、肥胖、更年期综合征等。

5. 其他   耳穴可以催乳、催产，预防和治疗输血、输液反应，同时还有美容、戒烟、戒毒、延缓衰老、预防保健等作用。

（八）操作程序

1. 评估   核对医嘱，床边核对患者姓名、床号，评估患者病情、耳部皮肤、疼痛的耐受程度、心理状态等，并做告知定穴时感觉等解释工作，以取得患者合作，必要时擦净双耳。

2. 准备   用物准备（75% 乙醇、0.2% 安尔碘或 2% 碘酒、棉签、镊子、探棒、耳穴电子测定仪、耳针、弯盘、洗手液），备齐用物，携至床旁；患者准备，取坐或卧舒适体位，

preparation: get sitting or lying position, and expose the operation site.

3. Location of Auricular Point　The patient selects a comfortable position. The operator hold the helix zone by one hand and observe where there is positive site. Of course, the operator can adopt the other two kinds of auricular diagnostic methods to detect by the other hand and confirm auricular points.

4. Disinfection　The auricular points should be swab with 0.2% anerdian or 2% iodine first and then disinfected with 75% alcohol as routine asepsis.

5. Manipulation　Filiform needles that are 0.5*cun* in length or specially-made thumbtack shape of needles are selected for auricular acupuncture therapy. To begin the procedure, stabilize the ear with the left hand and insert the needle with the right hand. For the intradermal insertion of the thumbtack needle, the needle should be fastened to the ear with a piece of adhesive tape and kept in place for 2-3 days.

6. Observation　There will be local pain or heat sensation in most of the patients after the needle insertion. They may experience soreness, heaviness, coldness or numbness due to the needing sensation traveling along certain channels. Generally speaking, patients who experience these sensations obtain a relatively better therapeutic outcome.

7. Retaining and Withdrawing of Needle　Filiform needles are allowed to be retained for 20 to 30 minutes. However, they may be prolonged by 1 to 2 hours or even longer for chronic conditions. During the needle retention, the needles should be rotated intermittently. When removing the needles, stabilize the ear with the left hand, and withdraw the needles with the right hand. Then press the needle pores quickly with dry cotton balls to avoid bleeding.

8. Tidy up　When the operation is end, tidy supplies, wash hands and conduct health education.

9. Evaluation　Evaluate whether the auricular point is accurate, technique is skillful, patient's symptoms are being improved or there is any other discomfort. Evaluate communication and humanistic care, and whether there is any acupuncture accident.

10. Record　Record the auricular points, method, time of needle retaining, efficacy and signature.

ix. Precaution

1. The ears should be disinfected carefully to prevent infection. Do not to adopt auricular acupuncture therapy in the situation of auricle with inflammatory lesions or frostbite.

暴露施术部位。

3. **定穴**　取舒适体位,术者一手持耳轮,观察有无阳性反应点,另一手持探棒在选区内找敏感点,或应用耳穴电子测定的仪器,正确取穴。

4. **消毒**　耳穴须先用 0.2% 安尔碘或 2% 碘酒,再用 75% 乙醇常规消毒。

5. **针刺**　根据治疗需要,选用 0.5 寸毫针或特殊的图钉形针。左手固定耳郭,右手持针将针刺入耳穴。如用图钉形针,针刺后用胶布将其固定,留针 2~3d。

6. **观察**　针刺后,多数患者针刺局部有疼痛或热感、胀痛,部分患者有酸、重、冷、麻感,或感觉循经络路线放射传导。一般来说,有这些感觉的患者可获得较满意的疗效。

7. **留针和出针**　一般留针 20~30min,慢性疾病可留针 1~2h,甚至更长,留针期间可捻针。出针时,术者左手托住耳郭,右手迅速将毫针垂直拔出;再用消毒干棉球压迫针眼片刻,以防出血。

8. **整理**　整理清理用物,健康宣教。

9. **评价**　选穴是否准确,操作方法是否正确、熟练,沟通是否到位,患者是否有得气感,症状是否缓解,是否发生针刺意外。

10. **记录**　洗手、记录施术的穴位、方法、时间、疗效、签名等。

(九)注意事项

1. 严格执行无菌技术操作原则,预防感染,耳郭皮肤有炎性病变、冻疮等不宜采用此法。

2. When treating a sprain or other soft tissue injuries, it is very beneficial to encourage the patient to move the affected part in order to increase the therapeutic outcome.

3. Auricular acupuncture therapy should be contraindicated for pregnant women or women who are prone to miscarriage. It is not recommended for patients with severe disease or severe anemia. In the treatment of severe heart disease or severe hypertension, strong stimulation should be avoided.

4. Acupuncture syncope should also be prevented during the treatment. Prompt intervention is needed if this happens.

III. Dermal Needling Therapy

Skin needle is used to prick the skin superficially with a specialized skin needle to free the meridians, dredge the collaterals, balance qi and blood and regulate the functions of *zang-fu* organs. It is also named the plum-blossom needle or seven-star needle, and is made of 5 to 7 short stainless steel needles which are bound together or is in the shape of a lotus seedpod to affix one end of the handle.

This therapy is in foundation of channel theory. Channel and collaterals are pathways that connect the internal *zang-fu* organs with the skin covering the body. Prick the body surface corresponding to the positive reactions of the visceral disease to treat visceral disease. It also treats superficial diseases by pricking local lesions.

i. Indication

This dermal needle therapy is indicated for a wide range of diseases such as in painful disorders including headache, lumbago, intercostal neuralgia, dysmenorrhea, neurodermatitis, alopecia, stubborn tinea, chronic gastritis, constipation, myopia, optic atrophy, and *etc.*.

ii. Procedure and Method of Dermal Needling Therapy

1. Assessment Patients' condition, skin condition of operated area, tolerance to pain, psychological status, environment, and so on.

2. Preparation

(1) Supplies preparation: Disinfect skin needle (disposable skin needle), skin disinfectant, disinfected dry cotton ball, bending plate. Check whether the needle tip is flush without hook, and whether the needle handle is connected to pinpoint firmly.

(2) Patients' preparation: Take comfortable

2. 对扭伤和有运动障碍的患者，进针后宜适当活动患部，有助于提高疗效。

3. 有习惯性流产的孕妇应禁针。患有严重器质性病变和伴有高度贫血患者不宜针刺。对患有严重心脏病、高血压的患者不宜强刺激。

4. 耳针治疗时亦应注意防止发生晕针，若发生应及时处理。

三、皮肤针法

皮肤针法是运用皮肤针叩刺人体一定部位或穴位，激发经络功能，调整脏腑气血，以达到防治疾病目的的方法。皮肤针又称梅花针、七星针，是用 5~7 枚短针集成一束，或如莲蓬形固定在富有弹性的针柄上而制成。

依据经络理论，认为经络是联系体表与内脏的通路。叩刺内脏疾病反映于体表的阳性部位治疗脏腑病证，也可叩刺局部病灶治疗浅表病证。

（一）适应证

皮肤针的适应范围很广，临床各种病证均可应用。如头痛、腰痛、肋间神经痛、痛经等各种痛证；神经性皮炎、斑秃、顽癣等皮肤疾患；慢性肠胃病、便秘，近视、视神经萎缩等。

（二）操作程序

1. 评估 患者病情、施术皮肤状况、对疼痛的耐受度、心理状况、环境等。

2. 准备

（1）用物准备：消毒的皮肤针（一次性皮肤针），皮肤消毒液，消毒干棉球、弯盘。检查针尖是否平齐无钩，针柄与针尖联结处是否牢固。

（2）患者准备：取舒适体位，松衣着、暴

postures, loose clothing, expose the operation site, choose acupuncture points or parts of operation, and clean local skin.

3. Part or Point Confirmation　According to patients' condition, confirm tapping-needling place or points (Fig. 6-12).

(1) Along meridian tapping-needling: This method is used along the meridians based on the meridian pattern or differentiation. The most commonly selected are the governor vessel and bladder meridian on the back along the spine. Tapping-needling these two meridians has many therapeutic effects, because the governor vessel may regulate yang qi all over the body, and the *back-shu* points which control the viscera are distributed along the bladder meridian on the back. Meridians in the area below the elbows and knees are also selected because the *yuan-source* points, *luo-connecting* points, *xi-cleft* points are all located there. Tapping-needling these areas are used to treat diseases of *zang-fu* organs and the corresponding meridians.

(2) Acupoint tapping-needling: This method is used to tap and needle points depending upon the condition to be treated. The commonly selected points in the clinic are specific points, EX-B2 (*Jiá jí*) and *ashi* points and several others.

(3) Local tapping-needling: This method is used to tap and needle the local affected area using needling accompanying circular or scattered tapping to treat swelling and pain caused by sprains or stubborn tinea.

4. Skin Disinfection　Disinfect patient's skin where tapping-needling with disinfectant.

5. Tapping-Needling　Hold the backend of needle handle with thumb, middle finger and ring finger of right hand. Make the index finger to straight press on the middle and lower section of needle handle. Prick the pinpoint at the point in operation site vertically and quickly bounce using wrist action, do it repeatedly. If there

露施术部位，清洁局部皮肤。

3. 定位　根据病情选择叩刺部位或穴位（图 6-12）。

（1）循经叩刺：是指循着经脉走行进行叩刺的一种方法，常用于项背腰骶部的督脉和足太阳膀胱经。督脉为阳脉之海，能调节一身之阳气；五脏六腑之背腧穴，皆分布于膀胱经，故其治疗范围广泛；其次是四肢肘膝以下经络，因其分布着各经原穴、络穴、郄穴等，可治疗各相应脏腑经络的疾病。

（2）穴位叩刺：是指在穴位上进行叩击的一种方法，主要是根据穴位的主治作用，选择适当的穴位予以叩刺治疗，临床常用的是各种特定穴、华佗夹脊穴、阿是穴等。

（3）局部叩刺：是指在患部进行叩刺的一种方法，如扭伤后局部的瘀肿、疼痛、顽癣等，可在局部进行叩刺。

4. 皮肤消毒　用 75% 乙醇消毒叩刺针具（或使用一次性叩刺针具）和叩刺部位。

5. 叩刺　以右手拇指、中指、无名指握住针柄，示指伸直压在针柄中下段处，针尖对准施术部位，使用腕力，将针尖垂直叩刺在皮肤上，并迅速弹起，反复叩击。局部如有出血，用消毒干棉球擦拭，无菌纱布包扎

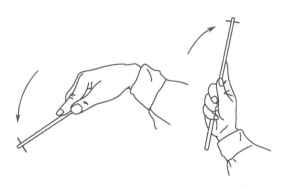

Fig. 6-12　Tapping-needling of Dermal Needling Therapy
图 6-12　皮肤针叩刺法

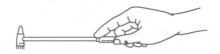

Fig. 6-13　Tapping-needling
图 6-13　皮肤针持针法

occurs bleeding, it should be wiped with disinfectant and dry cotton and bound up with sterile gauze (Fig. 6-13).

The tip of needle must be prependicular to the skin; the tapping must be accurate; the intensity of tapping must be even. According to the patient's constitution, condition and location for the treatment, the intensities are divided into mild, strong and moderate stimulation.

(1) Mild stimulation: Tap and needle the skin gently with the needle using wrist action until the area becomes red and slightly congested but the patient is painless. This is used for old and weak patients, in cases of facial illness, deficiency syndrome or protracted diseases.

(2) Moderate stimulation: Tap and needle the skin with a moderate force using wrist action until the area is congested but does not bleed and the patient feels a bit painful. The intensity of the tapping should be between mild and strong stimulations. This is used mainly for common illnesses or patients with normal constitutions.

(3) Strong stimulation: Tap needle the skin heavily with the needle using wrist action until the area bleeds slightly and the patient feels painful. This is applied to young patients with strong constitutions, suffered in the back and buttocks, young and strong patients, and for excess syndrome and new diseases.

6. Observation　Observe and ask the patients whether there is any uncomfortable feeling, such as pale complexion, pain, *etc.*, observe the change of the local skin.

7. Tidy　Assist patients to dress up, get comfortable lying position, tidy bed unit, and perform health education. Tidy supplies, and wash your hands.

8. Evaluation　Evaluate whether tapping place and/or tapping method is correct, whether patients feel any uncomfortable during the operation. Observe the change of the local skin, whether the change of local skin is normal.

9. Record　Record the operation place, thorn method, frequency, changes of skin, and then take signature.

iii. Precaution

1. Check the needle regularly, and keep the needle tips even and free from hooking.

2. Disinfect skin needle and patient's tapping place skin strictly.

3. When tapping, swiftly act and keep the needle tips

（图 6-13）。

叩击时针尖与皮肤必须垂直，叩刺要准确，强度要均匀，刺激的强度根据刺激的部位、患者的体质和病情的不同而决定，一般分轻、中、重三种。

（1）轻刺：用力较小，叩刺后皮肤仅出现潮红、充血，患者无疼痛感为度。适用于头面部、老弱妇女患者，以及病属虚证、久病者。

（2）中刺：介于轻刺和重刺之间，以局部有较明显潮红，但不出血为度，患者稍有疼痛感觉。适用于一般疾病和多数患者。

（3）重刺：用力较大，叩刺后皮肤有明显潮红、局部皮肤可见隐隐出血点，患者有疼痛感觉。适用于压痛点、背部、臀部、年轻体壮患者，以及病属实证、新病者。

6. 观察　患者面色、表情，探知疼痛情况，观察皮肤变化情况，询问有无不适。

7. 整理　协助患者着装，安排舒适体位，整理床单位，整理用物，洗手。做好健康教育。

8. 评价　叩刺部位及叩刺方法是否正确，叩刺过程中及叩刺后，患者有无不适。局部皮肤变化是否正常。

9. 记录　施术部位、叩刺方法、次数、皮肤变化情况、签名。

（三）注意事项

1. 针具要经常检查，注意针尖有无钩曲，针面是否平齐。

2. 针具及叩刺局部皮肤要严格消毒。

3. 叩刺时动作要轻捷，垂直无偏斜，以

vertical to the skin surface to reduce pain.

4. The area after tapping should be strictly cleaned and disinfected especially if bleeding occurs. The clinician should avoid contact with blood directly.

5. This therapy is not advisable for patients with local trauma, ulcers or acute infectious disease hemorrhagic diseases.

IV. Intradermal Needling Therapy

Intradermal needling therapy, also known as intradermal embedding of the needle, embedding specialized needles under skin for a period of time. It exerts lasting stimulation so as to regulate the functions of *zang-fu* organs and channels to prevent and treat diseases.

i. Type of Intradermal Needle

There are two types of intradermal needle. One is grain-like type. It is about 1 cm in length with a wheat grain sized ring handle. The handle and needle body are in the same plane. The other is thumbtack type. It is about 0.2-0.3 cm long. The handle is like ring. The needle body and the handle are perpendicular to each other like a thumbtack (Fig. 6-14).

This method is usually adapted to an area where is not inhibited by movement of the body, such as the *back-shu* points, ear points or some places on the arms and legs.

ii. Indication

This therapy is commonly used to treat chronic, stubborn and recurring repeatedly conditions, such as angioneurotic headache, lumbago, *bi*-syndrome, dysmenorrheal, trigeminal neuralgia, hypertension, asthma, infantile enuresis and so on.

iii. Manipulation

1. Grain-like Needle Fix the skin of treatment region with one hand, hold the needle body with a pair of tweezers and insert the needle transversely into the skin up to a depth of 0.5-0.8 cm by the other hand, and then affix the needle handle with a piece of adhesive plaster.

2. Thumbtack-like Needle Hold the ring

免造成患者疼痛。

4. 叩击局部和穴位，若手法重而出血者，应进行清洁和消毒，注意防止感染。医务工作人员勿直接接触患者血液。

5. 局部如有溃疡或损伤者不宜使用本法，急性传染病患者和有凝血功能障碍者也不宜使用本法。

四、皮内针法

皮内针法又称埋针法，是用特制的小型针具固定于腧穴部位的皮内，给腧穴以较长时间的刺激以治疗疾病的一种方法。

（一）针具

皮内针的针具有两种。一种是颗粒型，一般长1cm，针柄形似麦粒，针身与针柄成一直线；一种是图钉型，长0.2~0.3cm，针柄呈环形，针身与针柄呈垂直状（图6-14）。

针刺部位多以不妨碍正常的活动处腧穴为主，一般多选用背腧穴、四肢穴和耳穴等。

（二）适应证

皮内针法临床适用于需要久留针的疼痛性疾病和久治不愈的慢性病证，如神经性头痛、腰痛、痹证、痛经、三叉神经痛、高血压、哮喘、小儿遗尿等。

（三）操作方法

1. **麦粒型皮内针** 一手固定所刺部位的皮肤，另一手用镊子夹住针尾，对准腧穴，平刺于皮内，针柄留于皮外，用胶布顺着针身进入方向粘贴固定。

2. **图钉型皮内针** 用镊子夹住针尾，对

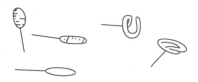

Fig. 6-14　Intradermal Needling Therapy
图6-14　皮内针

handle of the needle with a pair of tweezers, insert the needle into the point keeping the ring handle flat over the skin, and then affix it with a piece of adhesive plaster.

The retaining time depends on the condition. Generally speaking, the needle maybe retained for 3-5 days or even up to a week at most. In the summer or during hot weather, the retaining time should be shortened to 1-2 days to prevent infection. During the retaining needle period, the embedded needle should be pressed with finger for 1-2 minutes every 4 hours so as to intensify the stimulation and improve the therapeutic effects.

iv. Precaution

1. Avoid applying intradermal needles on joints because the movements of the joint will cause pain. It is also not advised to use this method on the chest and abdomen because respiratory movements will cause pain.

2. The needle should be taken out and reinserted, or choose other less painful place if it causes a great pain after insertion.

3. During the embedding period, keep the treated area clean and dry to prevent infection. In hot weather, the embedding time should be reduced in case of infection because of sweating.

4. Take out the needle and treat symptoms, if the embedding area occurs infection.

5. It is not advised to apply the embedding needle to area containing ulcers, infection, unexplained lump, to place where large vessels are distributed, or to the abdomen, waist and sacrum of pregnant women, or to patients who are allergic to metal.

V. Electro-Acupuncture Therapy

Electro-acupuncture is a therapy which combines needling and electric stimulation by applying a small amount of electric current on the inserted needles after the arrival of qi to prevent and treat diseases.

i. Indication

It is widely used in all kinds of pains, *bi*-syndrome, paralysis, disorders of heart, stomach, intestine, gallbladder, bladder, and uterus, traumatic diseases of muscle, ligament, and joints. It is used as an acupuncture anesthesia as well.

ii. Operating Procedure

1. Assessment　Besides adding to assess tolerance to electric current, the others refer to filiform needle therapy, chapter 6 section 1 part 1.

准腧穴，直刺皮内，再用胶布覆盖在针柄上。

皮内针可根据病情决定其留针时间的长短，一般为 3~5d，最长可达 1 周。若天气炎热，留针时间不宜过长，以 1~2d 为宜，以防感染。在留针期间，可每隔 4h 用手按压埋针处 1~2min，以强加刺激，提高疗效。

（四）注意事项

1. 关节附近因活动时会疼痛，不可埋针。胸腹部因呼吸时会活动，亦不宜埋针。

2. 埋针后，如患者感觉疼痛或妨碍肢体活动时，应将针取出，改选穴位重埋。

3. 埋针期间，针处不可着水，避免感染。热天出汗较多，埋针时间不宜过长。

4. 若发现埋针局部感染，应将针取出，并对症处理。

5. 溃疡、炎症、不明原因的肿块，体表大血管部位、孕妇下腹、腰骶部和金属过敏者禁止埋针。

五、电针法

电针是在针刺腧穴"得气"后，在针上通以接近人体生物电的微量电流，利用针和电两种刺激的结合，以防治疾病的一种操作方法。

（一）适应证

临床常用于各种痛证、痹证、痿证，心、胃、肠、胆、膀胱、子宫等器官的功能失调，肌肉、韧带、关节的损伤性疾病等，并可用于针刺麻醉。

（二）操作程序

1. **评估**　评估电流刺激的耐受度，余可参考第六章第一节第一部分毫针刺法。

2. Preparation　Besides adding electric stimulator, the others refer to filiform needle therapy, in part 1 of section 1, chapter 6 .

3. Locating Acupoint　Refer to filiform needle therapy, in part 1 of section 1, chapter 6.

4. Disinfecting　Refer to filiform needle therapy, in part 1 of section 1, chapter 6.

5. Selecting and Examining Filiform Needle Refer to filiform needle therapy, in part 1 of section 1, chapter 6.

6. Inserting Needle　Refer to filiform needle therapy, in part 1 of section 1, chapter 6.

7. Manipulating the Needle　Refer to filiform needle therapy, in part 1 of section 1, chapter 6.

8. Connecting Wire and Adjusting Current Connect the two wires of electric stimulator to the handle of two needles respectively after the arrival of qi. Turn on the electric stimulator, the waveform and frequency are selected and electric current is slowly increased to the required stimulation. It generally lasts for 10 to 30 minutes.

9. Observation　Observe whether there is rhythmic contraction and toleration in patients' local muscle, and if the wire leads off and there are any discomfortable feelings or fainting in patient.

10. Withdrawing Needle　After treatment, adjust the outlet potentiometer to "0" position, turn the power off, dismantle output wires and withdraw needles.

11. Tidying　Refer to filiform needle therapy, in part 1 of section 1, chapter 6.

12. Evaluation　Evaluate whether acupoint is accurate, patients have a sense of "*qi*", electric current stimulus is appropriate, symptoms are improved or patients have any other discomfort, technique is skilled, communication is good, there is a humanistic care, and there is acupuncture accident.

13. Recording　Record the acupoints, method, retaining needle time, current stimulus quantity, curative effect, signature, and so on.

iii. Precaution

1. The electric stimulator should be checked carefully whether the instrument performance is in good condition and all the switches should be turned off before operating.

2. The electric current should be increased gradually in order to prevent intense muscular contraction and the bending or breakage of the needle.

3. The maximum output voltage is over 40V for the electric stimulator, while the maximum output current

2. **准备**　电针仪，其余同毫针刺法。

3. **定位**　同毫针刺法。

4. **皮肤消毒**　同毫针刺法。

5. **选检毫针**　同毫针刺法。

6. **进针**　同毫针刺法。

7. **行针**　同毫针刺法。

8. **接电线、调电流**　针刺得气后，将输出电位器调至"0"位，将两根导线任意接在两个针柄上，然后打开电源开关，选好波形和频率，慢慢调高至患者能耐受的程度。通电时间一般在 10~30min。

9. **观察**　观察患者局部肌肉是否做节律性收缩及忍受程度，导线有无脱落，有无不适感、晕针现象等。

10. **起针**　治疗完毕，将电位器拨至"0"位，关闭电源，拆除输出导线，起针。

11. **整理**　同毫针刺法。

12. **评价**　选穴是否准确，操作方法是否正确、熟练，沟通是否到位，患者是否有得气感，电流刺激量是否合适，症状是否缓解，是否发生针刺意外。

13. **记录**　穴位、方法、留针时间、电流刺激量，疗效、签名。

（三）注意事项

1. 电针仪在使用前须检查性能是否完好，各开关应处于关闭状态。

2. 开机后输出强度应从零位开始，逐渐增强，不可突然增强，以防止引起肌肉强烈收缩，造成弯针或折针意外。

3. 电针仪最大输出电压在 40V 以上者，最大输出电流应限制在 1mA 以内，防止发生

should be under 1mA to prevent electric shock.

4. Usually a pair of outputs is connected with the handles of the two needles respectively which should be located on the same body side. It shouldn't be cross-over two sides of body, especially nearby the points which lie in the chest and back. Even current should be small. All of these are to avoid danger of current loop through the heart or central nervous system.

5. For patients with heart disease, it should avoid passing the electric current circuit through the heart. It should be inapplicable for the patients with cardiac pacemaker.

6. For patients with a weak constitution, strong electric stimulation should be avoided since it may induce fainting.

7. For pregnant women, the electro-acupuncture should be used with great caution.

VI. Hydro-Acupuncture Therapy

Hydro-acupuncture therapy also is known as point injection. It is a therapy that drug is injected into the points to prevent from and treat diseases.

i. Instrument and Commonly Used Drug

1. Instrument　It should choose the different types of disposable sterile injection syringes according to the patients' condition and injection site. In general, lml, 2ml, 5ml, 10ml, and 20ml injectors are recommended. Long needles of size 9 are used for deep points, and needles of size 5 and 7 are used for common points.

2. Commonly Used Drug

(1) The kinds of drugs: The drugs for muscular injection can be adopted in hydro-acupuncture, such as the herbal injection: *dāng guī, hóng huā, bǎn lán gēn chái hú, yú xīng cǎo, dān shēn, chuān xiōng*, and western drug injection: 25% magnesium sulfate, Vitamin B1, Vitamin B_{12}, Vitamin C, 0.25%-2% procaine hydrochloride, atropine, reserpine, ephedrine, antibiotics, normal saline, and so on.

(2) Dosage of injection: According to the instruction of the injection, overdose should be avoided, 1/5-1/2 of the original dosage is better for a small dosage. Dosage in hydro-acupuncture depends on the location of injection. The points on the head, face may be injected with 0.3ml to 0.5ml per point. The points at the auricle may be injected with 0.1ml per point. The locations on the four limbs,

触电。

4. 通常与毫针连接的一对输出电极，应安排在身体同侧。在靠近延髓、脊髓等胸、背部的穴位上使用针时，不可将两个电极跨接在身体两侧，且电流宜小，避免电流回路经过心脏和中枢神经系统出现危险。

5. 对心脏病患者，应避免电流回路通过心脏，安装起搏器者禁用电针。

6. 体质弱者，电流不宜过大，以防晕针。

7. 孕妇慎用电针。

六、水针法

水针法又称为穴位注射，以中西医理论为指导，依据穴位作用与药物的性能，将注射液注入穴位以防治疾病的一种疗法。

（一）用具及常用药物

1. **针具**　根据病情和注射部位的需要选择不同型号的一次性无菌注射器。一般可选 1ml、2ml、5ml 注射器，若肌肉肥厚可使用 10ml、20ml 注射器。针头一般选用 5 号或 7 号，深部穴位可用 9 号长针头。

2. **药物**

（1）药物种类：凡可供肌内注射用的药物，都可供水针使用。常用的中药注射液有当归、红花、板蓝根、柴胡、鱼腥草、复方丹参、川芎等；西药有 25% 硫酸镁、维生素 B_1、维生素 C、0.25%~2% 盐酸普鲁卡因、阿托品、利血平、麻黄碱、抗生素、生理盐水等。

（2）药物剂量：应根据药物说明书规定的剂量，不能过量，小剂量注射时，可用原药物剂量的 1/5~1/2。一般以穴位部位来分，头面部可注射 0.3~0.5ml；耳穴可注射 0.1ml；四肢部可注射 1~2ml；胸背部可注射 0.5~1ml；腰臀部可注射 2~5ml；如用 5%~10% 葡萄糖液

chest and back, waist and buttocks where the muscles are abundant can be injected with a little larger dosage, which is 1-2ml, 0.5-1ml, and 2-5ml respectively. 5%-10% glucose can be injected 5-20ml per point.

ii. Course of Treatment

Hydro-acupuncture therapy is applied once or twice daily for the acute disease, and once a day or every other day for the chronic diseases. One treatment course consists of 6-10 times of operations.

iii. Operating Procedure

1. Assessment It includes patients' condition, skin condition of operated area, past medical history, history of drug allergy, psychological status, environment and so on.

2. Preparation

(1) Supplies preparation: Treatment plate, bending plate, drugs, skin disinfectant, sterile syringes, grinding wheel, cotton swabs.

(2) Patients' preparation: Get comfortable postures, loose clothing, expose the operation site, choose acupuncture point and keep warm.

3. Locating Acupoint Help patient to take an appropriate posture, and select an effective acupoints in fleshy area according to patient's condition. The acupoints might be *ashi* or positive reacted points which be felt like nodule or funicular *etc.*. Expose acupoints, then, press the acupoints along the meridians with thumb and/or index finger, in the meantime ask patients' feeling, and determine the injection acupoint at last.

4. Drawing Drug Following the principle of "three inspections and seven verifications" strictly, select the appropriate and disinfected syringe to draw the drug according to the aseptic operation and operation procedures of suction liquid.

5. Skin Disinfection Regular disinfect the skin of acupoints.

6. Injection Hold the syringe with right hand and expel any excess air. Tense point skin with left hand, rapidly insert the pinhead into the acupoint or positive reacted point with the right hand, then gradually insert the needle by lifting and thrusting syringe until the qi arrives. Withdraw the handle of the syringe a little to observe whether blood is withdrawn into to the tube. If not, inject the solution into the point. In general, moderate speed of injection is adopted according to medical requirement. For excess-heat syndrome, rapid injection is indicated and for deficiency-cold syndrome, the injection should be slow.

可注射 10~20ml。

（二）疗程

急证每日 1~2 次；慢性病一般每日或隔日 1 次，6~10 次为一疗程。

（三）操作程序

1. **评估** 患者病情、施术皮肤状况、既往史、药物过敏史、心理状况、环境等。

2. **准备**

（1）用物准备：治疗盘、弯盘、药物、皮肤消毒液、无菌注射器、砂轮、棉签、无菌持物镊。

（2）患者准备：取舒适体位，松衣着、暴露施术部位，保暖，选穴。

3. **确定穴位** 取合适体位，根据病情选择有效的、肌肉较丰满处的穴位。也可选择阿是穴，或检查时触到的呈结节、条索状等阳性反应点。暴露腧穴，拇（示）指循位按压腧穴，询问患者感觉，确定注射穴位。

4. **抽取药液** 严格执行查对制度，按无菌操作与操作规程抽吸药液。

5. **消毒皮肤** 常规消毒穴位局部皮肤。

6. **穴位注射** 右手持注射器（排出空气），左手绷紧穴位皮肤，对准穴位或阳性反应点，快速刺入皮下，然后缓慢进针，得气后，回抽无血，即可将药液注入。注入的速度可根据治疗需求进行调节，实热证，注入宜速；虚寒证，注入宜缓。

7. Observation　To observe whether there occurs acupuncture syncope, bent needle, stuck needle or drug allergy reaction, and ask patients whether they have any discomfort.

8. Withdrawal of Needle　After all liquid was injected, quickly pull out the needle, and press with sterile swabs on pinholes for a moment.

9. Tidy　Assist patients to dress up, get comfortable position, tidy bed unit, and perform health education. Tidy supplies and wash hands.

10. Evaluation　To evaluate whether the acupoint is accurate, whether patients have a sense of "*de* qi" or have any other discomfort, whether symptoms have been improved, whether the manipulation is skilled, whether the communication is good, whether there occurs acupuncture accident, and whether there is drug allergy.

11. Record　Record points, medicines, dose, concentration, reaction of patients, then take signature and so on.

iv. Precaution

1. Following the principle of "three inspections and seven verifications" strictly, great attention should be paid to the pharmacological property, action, dosage, quality, validity, contraindications, side effects and allergic reaction. Since the injection may cause allergic reaction to some patients, skin test should be done before the treatment. The injection with serious side effects should be avoided, and that with relatively strong stimulation should be used very cautiously.

2. Deep injection is not allowed on the points at the neck, chest and back. The dosage should be carefully controlled and injection should be applied slowly.

3. The solution in general should not be injected into the vessels, the joint cavity, and the spinal cord cavity. The intra-vascular injection should be prevented if the blood is withdrawn in the treatment, and the improper injection of the solution into the joint cavity may lead to redness and swelling of the joint or fever and pain. Improper injection into the spinal cord cavity may impair the spinal cord.

4. For pregnant women, the low abdomen, the lumbar and sacral places as well as the points of LI 4 (*hé gǔ*) and SP 6 (*sān yīn jiāo*) should be avoided.

5. For the elder and the weak, patients receiving treatment first time for the one should select few points and decrease the dosage.

6. Syringes and locations of injection should be strictly disinfected. Sterilized procedure should be followed.

7. It should pay attention to prevent fainting, bending or breaking of the needles in the treatment. If the accident

7. **观察**　观察有无晕针、弯针、滞针及药物过敏反应，询问有无不适感。

8. **出针**　药液注完，迅速拔针，用无菌棉签按针孔片刻。

9. **整理**　协助患者着装，安排舒适体位，整理床单位，整理用物，健康教育。

10. **评价**　选穴是否准确，操作方法是否正确、熟练，沟通是否到位，是否做到人文关怀。患者是否有"得气"感，症状是否缓解。是否发生针刺意外。是否发生药物过敏。

11. **记录**　穴位，药名，剂量，浓度，患者反应，签名等。

（四）注意事项

1. 严格三查七对，必须注意药物的性能、药理作用、剂量、药物的质量、有效期、配伍禁忌、副作用和过敏反应。凡能引起过敏反应的药物必须先做皮试。副作用较严重的药物，不宜采用。刺激作用较强的药物，应谨慎使用。

2. 项、颈、胸背部注射时，切勿过深，药物也必须控制剂量，宜缓慢注射。

3. 药液不宜注入血管内，注射时如回抽有血，必须避开血管后再注射。一般药物不能注入关节腔、脊髓腔。如误入关节腔可引起关节红肿热痛等反应；如误入脊髓腔，会损害脊髓。

4. 孕妇的下腹、腰骶部和三阴交、合谷等孕妇禁针穴位，不宜使用水针。

5. 年老体弱者、初次治疗者，选穴须少，药液剂量须酌减。

6. 注射器、注射部位必须严格消毒，注射时严格执行无菌技术操作。

7. 须注意预防晕针、弯针和断针，如果发生晕针等情况，处理方法同毫针刺法。

such as acupuncture syncope occurs, one should deal with it quickly following the same rules of filiform needling.

(Yang Liu)

（杨柳）

Section 2 Tuina

第二节 推拿法

Manipulations of tuina is one of external treatments in TCM performed by the operator with hands or other parts of the body to stimulate the treated areas and activate the limbs, for preventing or treating diseases. There are different types of manipulations with different operation methods of stimulation, intensity and time, such as pushing manipulation, pressing manipulation, kneading manipulation and so on. They are essential contents of manipulations of tuina. The combination of two more basic manipulations is called compound manipulation, such as pressing and kneading manipulation, pushing and rubbing manipulation and so on. These manipulations have effects of dredging channels, promoting qi and blood circulation, lubricating joints, regulating *zang-fu* organs, *etc.*.

推拿法是操作者用手或肢体的其他部分刺激患者需治疗的部位和辅助其活动肢体，以达到为其防病治病目的的一种中医外治法。由于刺激方式、强度、时间的不同，形成了不同的手法，如推法、按法、揉法等，这些基本手法是推拿手法的主要组成部分。将两个以上基本手法结合起来的操作形成复合手法，如按揉法、推摩法等。推拿法具有疏通经络、行气活血、滑利关节、调节脏腑功能等作用。

I. Indication

一、适应证

Tuina manipulations for adults are indicated for disorders of orthopedics and traumatism, such as stiff neck, cervical spondylopathy, acute lumbar sprain, chronic lumbar muscle strain, scapulohumeral periarthritis, prolapse of lumbar intervertebral disc, chronic strain of soft tissues, acute soft tissue injury, *etc.*. Tuina manipulations are used for treating the diseases of internal medicine, such as constipation, diarrhea, hypertension, headache *etc.*, diseases of gynaecology such as dysmenorrheal, irregular menstruation, and diseases of otolaryngology such as toothache, deafness. Tuina manipulations for infants are indicated for cough, fever, asthma, vomiting, anorexia, constipation, *etc.*.

成人推拿手法适用于骨伤科病证，如落枕、颈椎病、急性腰扭伤、慢性腰肌劳损、肩周炎、腰椎间盘突出症、慢性软组织劳损、急性软组织损伤等；同时，对于内科病证如便秘、腹泻、高血压、头痛等；妇科病证如痛经、月经不调；五官科病证如牙痛、耳聋等亦有疗效；儿科推拿手法适用于咳嗽、发热、哮喘、呕吐、厌食、便秘等病证。

II. Basic Requirement

二、基本要求

The basic requirements of manipulation are being persistent and forceful with even speed and rhythm, soft and deep penetration. "Being persistent" means that the manipulation should be performed for a continuous

推拿手法的基本要求是持久、有力、均匀、柔和、深透。"持久"要求手法操作能持续一定的时间，且动作规范不变形；"有力"

period of time without any deformation. "Being forceful" means the manipulation must be performed with moderate force, which should be adjusted according to the patient's constitution, state of illness and the difference of treated areas. Do not perform with clumsy strength and force. "Evenness" means that the manipulation should be rhythmical with appropriate speed and steady force. "Gentleness" means that the manipulation is operated gently and carefully, light but not superficial, heavy but not unsmooth, while operations are with nature and smooth shift of movements. "Deep penetration" means that the stimulation must be penetrated deeply into the deep tissues. Only when the manipulation is operated persistently, forcefully, evenly and softly can the purpose of deep penetration be achieved.

III. Commonly Used Manipulation for Adult

i. One-Finger Pushing Manipulation

The operator exerts force by swinging the forearm and directs it to the treated areas or points continuously with the tip or the whorled surface of the thumb. This is the so-called one-finger pushing manipulation.

1. Operation Method　The operator grasps a hollow fist with suspended and flexed wrist and palm, relaxing the muscles of upper limb. Exert force on the surface of the client's body with the tip or whorled surface of the thumb. The operator should lower the shoulder, drop the elbow and suspend the wrist. And then, the operator swings the forearm initiatively to drive the wrist swinging transversely while flexing and extending the thumb joint to make the force on the channels and points continuously with the light and heavy force alternately. The frequency is 120-160 times *per* minute.

2. Essential for Operation

(1) Lowering shoulders: Relax the shoulder joints with the scapulas dropping naturally; keep the armpit free with the space of a fist; avoid shrugging shoulders to exert strength.

(2) Dropping the elbow: Drop the elbow joint naturally and make a little lower than the wrist. Do not extend the elbow outwards or adduct excessively.

(3) Suspending the wrist: Flex the wrist joint and naturally suspend it; get the wrist relax and try best to flex to 90°.

(4) Exerting force to the thumb: Fix the tip or the whorled surface of the thumb on the treated area or points, avoid pressing forcefully.

要求手法必须具有恰当的力量,力量的大小应根据患者的体质、病情和治疗部位的不同进行调整,切忌使用拙力、暴力;"均匀"要求手法动作有节奏性,速度不能时快时慢,压力不能时轻时重;"柔和"要求手法轻柔缓和,用力轻而不浮,重而不滞,变换手法动作要自然;"深透"要求手法作用达到组织深层。只有符合持久、有力、均匀、柔和要求的手法才能深透。

三、成人常用推拿手法

(一)一指禅推法

以拇指指端或罗纹面着力,前臂摆动,使所产生的力通过拇指持续不断的作用于施术部位或穴位上,称为一指禅推法。

1. 操作方法　术者手握空拳,腕掌悬屈,拇指端自然着力,用拇指指端或末节罗纹面着力于体表上,沉肩、垂肘、悬腕,运用前臂的主动摆动带动腕部的横向摆动及拇指关节的屈伸活动,使力轻重交替、持续不断地作用于经络穴位上,频率每分钟120~160次。

2. 动作要领

(1)沉肩:肩关节放松,肩胛骨自然下沉,保持腋下空松,能容纳一拳的距离,不要耸肩用力。

(2)垂肘:肘关节自然下垂,略低于腕部,肘部不要向外支起,亦不宜过度内收。

(3)悬腕:腕关节屈曲,自然悬垂,在保持腕关节放松的基础上,尽可能屈腕至90°。

(4)指实:拇指指端或罗纹面自然着实,吸定于施术部位或穴位上,但不可拙力下压。

(5) Emptying the palm: Keep the palm and other four fingers except the thumb relaxed and grasp an empty fist; accumulate the strength in the palm and send it from the fingers.

(6) Pushing fast and shifting slowly: Pushing fast refers to swing quickly with the speed of 120-160 times *per* minute; shifting slowly refers to fix on the surface of the skin with the tip or the whorled surface of the thumb and shift slowly along the channels or a special path. Don't slip or rub.

3. Precaution

(1) There are two methods in performing one-finger pushing manipulation, to be performed either with the thumb joint flexed or not flexed. If the operator's interphalangeal joint of thumb is stiff with the small activity range or soft stimulation is needed in the treatment, the manipulation can be done with the thumb joint flexed and extended. If the operator's interphalangeal joint of thumb is flexible, it is favorable to do the manipulation with straight thumb joint.

(2) The treatment site for thumb should be relatively fixed. The flexion and extension of finger joint and the swing of wrist joint should be coordinated.

ii. Rolling Manipulation

The operator takes the ulnar side of opisthenar as the contact surface, swings the forearm to drive the wrist to flex, extend and roll the opisthenar on the treated areas. This is the so-called rolling manipulation.

1. Operation Method　The operator keeps the thumb straight naturally, grasps an empty fist, naturally flexes the metacarpophalangeal joints of the little finger and the ring finger to about 90°. The flexed angles of the metacarpophalangeal joints of other fingers should be gradually reduced to make the palm round along the palm surface. Press the treated area with the dorsum of the hand closed to the little finger. Swing the forearm initiatively to flex and extend the wrist in large amplitude and rotate the forearm as well. Roll the ulnar side of the opisthenar on the treated areas continuously. The swinging frequency is about 120 times *per* minute.

2. Essential for Operation

(1) Lower the shoulders and drop the elbow with the elbow joint flexed naturally 140° to keep a space of a fist to the chest. Relax the wrist and grasp an empty fist. The angle of the metacarpophalangeal joints from the little finger to the ring finger should become small one by one, enable the back of hand to be an arch and fix on the treated area.

(2) The wrist joint flexes and extends about

（5）掌虚：除拇指外的其余四指及手掌放松，握虚拳，做到蓄力于掌，发力于指。

（6）紧推慢移：紧推是一指禅推法的摆动频率相对较快，维持在每分钟120~160次；慢移是拇指指端或罗纹面在吸定于体表的基础上，可沿经络或特定的路径缓慢移动，同时不可滑动或摩擦。

3. 注意事项

（1）一指禅推法有拇指指间关节屈伸和不屈伸两种不同术式。若术者拇指指间关节较僵硬，活动范围较小或治疗时需要较柔和的刺激，可采用屈伸拇指指间关节的操作；若术者拇指指间关节较柔软，宜选用不屈伸拇指指间关节的操作。

（2）拇指的治疗部位要相对固定；指尖关节的屈伸和腕关节的摆动要协调一致。

（二）揉法

以尺侧手背为接触面，前臂摆动带动腕关节屈伸，手背在体表施术部位滚动，称为揉法。

1. 操作方法　术者拇指自然伸直，手握空拳，小指、无名指的掌指关节自然屈曲约90°，其余手指掌指关节屈曲角度依次减小，使手背沿掌横弓排列成弧面，以手掌背部近小指侧部分贴附于治疗部位上，前臂主动摆动，带动腕关节较大幅度的屈伸和前臂旋转的协同运动，使手背尺侧在治疗部位上做持续不断地来回滚动，摆动频率为每分钟约120次。

2. 动作要领

（1）沉肩，垂肘，肘关节自然屈曲140°，距胸壁约一拳，松腕，手握空拳，小指至示指掌指关节屈曲角度依次减小，手背呈弧形，吸定于患者需治疗的部位。

（2）腕关节屈伸幅度约120°，即外摆时

120°, that is to say, the opertator flexes the wrist about 80° when the arm swings outward, while extends the wrist about 40° when the arm swings backward. The operator should enable the hypothenar area to the third metacarpophalangeal joint (occupies 1/3 to 1/2 of opisthenar) to touch the treated area. The forearm rotates outward while swaying externally, and inwards while swaying backward.

(3) The stimulation should be changed with light and heavy force in turn. The ratio of heaviness and lightness for rolling forth and rolling back is 3 ： 1, which is "rolling forward three times and rolling back once".

(4) The frequency should be fixed when applying the rolling manipulation. The shifting speed should not be too fast.

3. Precaution

(1) The flexing-extending movement of the wrist joint should be maximized when performing the rolling manipulations. Avoid rotating the forearm mainly or flexing and extending the wrist joints insufficiently.

(2) It is favorable to fix on the surface of client's body for performing the rolling manipulation. The dragging, jumping or rotating-swinging are allowed. Bumping between the opisthenar and body surface should be avoided.

(3) Avoid operating on the apophysial points of vertebral spinous process and other joints because it may cause discomfort.

iii. Kneading Manipulation

Fix on the body surface of clients with the certain part of major thenar or hypothenar, palmar base or whorl surfaces of the fingers to rotate the subcutaneous tissues gently and softly, which is the so-called kneading manipulation. According to the different contacting surfaces during the operation, it can be divided into the palm base kneading manipulation, major thenar kneading manipulation and finger kneading manipulation.

1. Operation Method

(1) Palm-base kneading manipulation: Exert the force with the palm base; flex the fingers naturally and extend the wrist joint slightly backwards; crook the elbow joint slightly as a fulcrum, and swing the forearm initiatively to drive the palm base to knead on the treated area with the frequency of about 120-160 times *per* minute.

(2) Major thenar kneading manipulation: Exert the force with the major thenar and crook the wrist joint slightly to an angle of 120°-140°; use the elbow joint as a pivot and swing the forearm initiatively to knead with

屈腕约 80°，回摆时伸腕约 40°，使小鱼际掌背侧至第 3 掌指关节（占掌背的 1/3~1/2）作用于治疗部位。外摆的同时前臂外旋，回摆时前臂内旋。

（3）刺激轻重交替，前滚同回滚时着力重轻之比为 3：1，即"滚三回一"。

（4）滚法在体表移动时应在吸定的基础上，保持手法的固有频率，移动速度不宜过快。

3. 注意事项

（1）滚法操作应尽量做到腕关节最大幅度的屈伸，避免出现前臂旋转为主、腕关节屈伸幅度不足的错误方式。

（2）滚法宜吸定，不宜拖动、跳动或旋转摆动，避免出现手背与体表的撞击感。

（3）避免在脊椎棘突或其他各部位关节的骨突处施术，以免给患者带来不适感。

（三）揉法

以手掌的大小鱼际、掌根部或指端螺纹面吸定于患者体表，带动该处的皮下组织做轻柔缓和的环旋揉动，称为揉法。根据操作时接触面的不同又可分将揉法为掌根揉法、大鱼际揉法和指揉法。

1. 操作方法

（1）掌根揉法：术者以掌根部分着力，手指自然弯曲，腕关节略背伸，肘关节微屈作为支点，前臂做主动摆动，带动掌根在治疗部位揉动，频率为每分钟 120~160 次。

（2）大鱼际揉法：术者以手掌大鱼际部着力，腕关节微屈 120°~140°，以肘关节为支点，前臂做主动摆动，带动大鱼际在治疗部位揉

the major thenar on the treated area with the frequency of about 120-160 times *per* minute.

(3) Thumb kneading manipulation: Exert the force with the whorled surface of the thumb while the other four fingers supporting on a suitable position; flex the wrist joint slightly or straighten; swing the forearm in small amplitude and drive the thumb to rotate on the treated area. The frequency is about 120-160 times *per* minute.

(4) Middle finger kneading manipulation: Exert the force with the whorled surface of the middle finger, extend straight the interphalangeal joint of the middle finger and slightly bend the metacarpophalangeal joints. Take the elbow joint as a fulcrum, swing the forearm initiatively in small amplitude and drive the whorled surface of the middle finger to rotate on the treated area. The frequency is 120-160 times *per* minute.

Kneading with the index finger or the juxtaposed index finger, middle finger and ring finger is called "index finger kneading manipulation" or "three fingers kneading manipulation" respectively. The operation essentials are the same as those of middle finger kneading manipulation.

2. Essential for Operation

(1) In performing, the operator should lower the shoulders, drop the elbow and relax the wrist joint. Swing the forearm in small amplitude to rotate the contacting parts with force from the wrist joint.

(2) The subcutaneous tissues should be activated to move together. The movement should be flexible and rhythmic.

(3) The pressure should be moderate, making the patient feel comfortable.

3. Precaution

(1) Avoid rubbing or slipping between the treated part and the body surface during the manipulation.

(2) The force should be passed through the relaxed wrist joint. When performing this manipulation, the wrist joint should be kept in certain intensity, and excessive stiffness of the wrist joint should be avoided.

iv. Circular Rubbing Manipulation

Using the finger or palm surface as the touching part to make rhythmic and circular rubbing movement of the client's body surface is the so-called circular rubbing manipulation, which is the gentlest tuina manipulation.

1. Operation Method

(1) Palm-rubbing manipulation: Press on the client's body surface with the fingers juxtaposed, the palm straightened naturally and the wrist joint stretched slightly;

动摆动，频率为每分钟 120~160 次。

（3）拇指揉法：以拇指罗纹面着力，其余手指扶持于合适部位，腕关节微屈或伸直，前臂做小幅度摆动，带动拇指在施术部位上做环转运动，频率为每分钟 120~160 次。

（4）中指揉法：以中指罗纹面着力，中指指间关节伸直，掌指关节微屈，以肘关节为支点，前臂做小幅度主动运动，带动中指罗纹面在施术部位做环转运动，频率为每分钟 120~160 次。

以示指或示、中、无名指并拢做指揉法分称为示指揉法和三指揉法，操作要领同中指揉法。

2. 动作要领

（1）要做到沉肩、垂肘、腕关节放松，以前臂小幅度的主动摆动，通过腕关节传递，带动接触部位回转运动。

（2）操作时要带动皮下组织一起运动，动作要灵活协调而有节律。

（3）所施压力要适中，以受术者感到舒适为度。

3. 注意事项

（1）操作时，术者的接触部位不可和患者的体表之间有相对摩擦运动。

（2）功力要通过放松的腕关节传递，注意在做指揉法的时候，腕关节应在放松的基础上，保持一定的紧张度，不可使腕关节过分僵硬。

（四）摩法

以指、掌面为接触部位，在受术者体表做环形而有节奏的摩擦运动，称为摩法，是推拿手法中最轻柔的一种手法。

1. 操作方法

（1）掌摩法：术者手指并拢，手掌自然伸直，腕关节微伸，将手掌平放在患者的体表

use the elbow joint as a fulcrum; then move the forearm actively to rub in circles with the palm on the treated areas. It can be performed either clockwise or counter-clockwise with the frequency of 100-120 times *per* minute.

(2) Finger-rubbing manipulation: Take the surface of the index finger, middle finger, ring finger and little finger as the contacting surface with the fingers juxtaposed, the palm straightened naturally and the wrist joint flexed slightly; use the elbow as a pivot and moving the forearm actively to drive the surface of the four fingers to rub in circles on the treated area. It can be performed either clockwise or counter-clockwise with the frequency of 100-120 times *per* minute.

2. Essential for Operation

(1) Relax the shoulder joints, and actively swing the forearm to drive the relaxed wrist joint to do the circular movement. When operating the finger-rubbing manipulation, the wrist joints should be kept in certain intensity and avoid being stiff.

(2) The force should be moderate and the speed should be even. Finger-rubbing manipulation should be performed with lighter force and faster speed while palm-rubbing manipulation is performed with heavier force and slower speed.

3. Precaution

(1) The direction of the manipulation should be chosen according to the deficiency and excess syndrome of the illness. TCM supposes that clock-wise circular-rubbing manipulation is suitable for deficiency syndrome while counter-clockwise circular-rubbing manipulation is indicated for excess syndrome. In clinic, different directions of the rubbing manipulation are selected according to the anatomical structure of the treated areas and pathological conditions.

(2) When performing the rubbing manipulation, ointments with different kinds of function can be smeared according to the disease condition. Scallion and ginger juice, as well as turpentine can also be smeared to enhance the effect.

(3) Pay attention to the difference between kneading manipulation and circular rubbing manipulation: When performing kneading manipulation, the operator should fix the fingers and palm on the treated area to drive the subcutaneous tissues to move with a relatively stronger force. Remember not to rub on the body surface. When performing circular rubbing manipulation, the fingers and palm make circular rubbing with a relatively lighter force on the body surface without moving the subcutaneous

上，术者以肘关节为支点，前臂做主动运动，带动手掌在患者体表施术部位做环旋摩擦运动。频率为每分钟 100~120 次，顺时针逆时针均可。

（2）指摩法：以示、中、无名、小指末节指面为接触部位，四指并拢，手掌自然伸直，腕关节微屈，以肘关节为支点，前臂做主动运动，带动四指指面在患者受术部位做环形摩擦运动，频率为每分钟 100~120 次，顺时针逆时针均可。

2. 动作要领

（1）肩关节应放松，以前臂主动摆动为主，带动放松的腕关节做环转运动。指摩法时腕关节在放松的基础上可保持一定的紧张度，但要紧而不僵。

（2）用力要轻重得宜，速度均衡。指摩法较轻快，掌摩法稍重缓。

3. 注意事项

（1）根据病情的虚实决定手法的方向。传统认为虚证宜用顺时针方向的摩法，实证宜用逆时针方向的摩法，临床还应结合施术部位的解剖结构和病理状况选择使用不同方向的摩法。

（2）应用摩法时，常根据病情，涂以各种性能的药膏。也可涂以葱姜汁、松节油等推拿介质，以加强摩法的作用。

（3）注意揉法和摩法的区别：揉法着力较重，操作时指掌吸定患者的一个受术部位，带动其皮下组织，和患者的体表没有摩擦动作；摩法则着力较轻，操作时指掌在患者的体表做环旋摩擦，而不带动其皮下组织。临床上两者常结合使用。

tissues. The two manipulations are often used together in clinic.

v. To-and-fro Rubbing Manipulation

Exert force on the treated areas with the major thenar, the palm base and the hypothenar to do the linear rubbing movements back and forth, so that the heat generated by the rubbing can penetrate the body surface into the deeper layer. This is the so-called to-and-fro rubbing manipulation. It can be divided into to-and-fro rubbing with palm, to-and-fro rubbing with major thenar and scrubbing with hypothenar.

1. Operation Method

(1) To-and-fro rubbing with the palm: Exert force on the treated body with the surface of the palm and extend the wrist joint straight; take the shoulder joint as the fulcrum and move the upper arm actively with the surface of the palm scrubbing the body surface along a straight line back and forth. The frequency is 100-120 times *per* minute and it is mostly used in the chest and hypochondrium as well as in the abdomen.

(2) To-and-fro rubbing with the major thenar: Exert force on the body surface of clients with the major thenar and extend the wrist joint straight, take the shoulder joint as the fulcrum and move the upper arm actively with the major thenar scrubbing on the body surface along a straight line back and forth. The frequency is 100-120 times *per* minute and it is mostly used in the chest and abdomen, waist and back and four limbs.

(3) To-and-fro rubbing with the hypothenar: Exert force on the body surface of clients with the hypothenar, keep the palm vertical to the body surface and extend the wrist joint straight; take the shoulder joint as the fulcrum and move the upper arm actively with the hypothenar scrubbing on the body surface along a straight line back and forth. The frequency is 100-120 times *per* minute and it is mostly used on the shoulder and back, waist and buttocks and lower limbs.

2. Essential for Operation

(1) The route should be kept straight whether the scrubbing is from top to down or from left to right. Moreover, the distance of moving back and forth should be long and continuous without pause.

(2) The palm should be kept close to the treated area. The pressing force should be kept even. It is noticed that the treated skin should not be fold during scrubbing. The frequency should also be even.

3. Precaution

(1) When operating to-and-fro rubbing, it should smear some lubricant on the treated areas, which not only

（五）擦法

术者以手掌的大鱼际、掌根或小鱼际着力于施术部位，做直线往返摩擦运动，使摩擦产生的热量透过体表渗透至深层，称为擦法。可分为掌擦法、大鱼际擦法和小鱼际擦法。

1. 操作方法

（1）掌擦法：术者腕关节平直，以肩关节为支点，以手掌的掌面紧贴于患者的皮肤，上臂做主动运动，使手掌的掌面在其体表做直线往返的摩擦运动，频率为每分钟100~120次，多用于给予患者胸胁及腹部的推拿。

（2）大鱼际擦法：术者腕关节平直，以肩关节为支点，以大鱼际着力贴于患者体表，上臂做主动运动，使大鱼际在患者的体表做直线往返的摩擦运动。频率为每分钟100~120次，多用于胸腹、腰背和四肢部的推拿。

（3）小鱼际擦法：术者腕关节平直，以肩关节为支点，以小鱼际着力贴于体表，立掌，上臂做主动运动，使小鱼际在患者体表做直线往返的摩擦运动。频率为每分钟100~120次，多用于肩背、腰臀及下肢部的推拿。

2. 动作要领

（1）无论是上下或左右摩擦，都要直线往返，不可歪斜，而且往返距离要拉长且连续，不能间歇停顿。

（2）术者的手掌应与受术者体表接触平实，向下的压力要保持均匀，以摩擦时不使其皮肤起皱为度，动作频率也应均匀。

3. 注意事项

（1）操作时，可在施术的部位涂些润滑剂，既可保护受术者的皮肤，又有利于热量

protects the skin, but also facilitates the heat permeating into the body.

(2) Since to-and-fro rubbing is operated directly on the body surface, it should pay attention to keep the operating room warm.

(3) After operating to-and-fro rubbing generally, it is inadvisable to use other manipulations on the treated areas to avoid injuring the skin.

vi. Pushing Manipulation

It is called pushing manipulation for exerting force on certain parts or points of the human body with fingers and palm or other parts of the body to make linear or arc movement in one direction. It can be divided into flat pushing manipulation, straight pushing manipulation, spiral pushing manipulation, separate pushing manipulation and coalescent pushing manipulation.

1. Operation Method

(1) Flat pushing manipulation: According to the difference of force exerting parts, there are flat pushing manipulations with the thumb, palm and elbow. Exert force on the body surface with the thumb, palm and elbow. Push heavily and slowly in a one-way direction along the channels or the direction of muscle fibers. Press and knead on the major areas or points where need to be treated.

(2) Straight pushing manipulation: Exert force on certain parts or points of the body with the radial surface of the thumb or the whorled surfaces of the index finger and middle finger; push straightly in one way direction.

(3) Spiral pushing manipulation: Push spirally on the points by the whorled surface of the thumb.

(4) Separate pushing manipulation: Keep the whorled surfaces of the thumb or the palm of both hands close to the body surface; push from the center part to the left or right side separately in a one-way direction.

(5) Coalescent pushing manipulation: Keep the whorled surfaces of the thumb or the palm of both hands close to the body surface; push from either side of the points to the center of the points.

2. Essential for Operation

(1) Flat pushing manipulation can exert comparatively stronger force among pushing manipulations. When operating, it is better to push with steady force and slow speed along straight line in one way direction.

(2) To operate the straight pushing manipulation, the wrist, palm and fingers should be moved straightly forwards in one direction with the elbow joint flexed and extended. The pressure used is lighter than that of the flat pushing manipulation. The movements should be light

渗透到其体内。临床使用擦法宜使患者自觉透热为度。

（2）需直接在受术者的体表操作，应注意室内保暖。

（3）操作后，一般不宜在该施术部位再使用其他手法，避免损伤受术者的皮肤。

（六）推法

用指、掌或其他部位着力于人体一定部位或穴位上，做单方向直线或弧线的移动，称为推法。可分为平推法、直推法、旋推法、分推法和合推法等。

1. 操作方法

（1）平推法：根据着力部位的不同，有拇指平推法、掌平推法和肘平推法三种。用拇指面着力紧贴受术者的体表，按经络循行或肌纤维平行方向做单方向沉缓推动。在推进过程中，可在重点治疗的部位或穴位上做按揉动作。

（2）直推法：术者用拇指桡侧面或示、中两指罗纹面着力于一定部位或穴位上，做单方向的直线推动。

（3）旋推法：术者用拇指罗纹面在受术的穴位上做螺旋形推动。

（4）分推法：术者用双手拇指罗纹面或掌面紧贴在受术的体表上，自中心部位分别向左右两侧单方向推开。

（5）合推法：术者用双手拇指罗纹面或掌面紧贴受术的体表上，自穴位两旁推向穴位中间。

2. 动作要领

（1）平推法是推法中着力较大的一种，推的时候需用一定的压力，用力要平稳，推进速度要缓慢，要沿直线做单方向运动。

（2）直推法以肘关节的伸屈带动腕、掌、指，做单方向的直线运动，所用压力较平推法为轻，动作要求轻快连续，以推后受术处的皮肤不发红为佳。

and continuous. It is appropriate to prevent the skin of the treated area from redness after the manipulation.

(3) When operating the spiral pushing manipulation, it should relax the elbow joint and wrist joint, and make the spiral movement in small amplitude by the thumb without the subcutaneous tissue movement. It is similar to the finger-rubbing manipulation.

(4) During the operation of separate pushing manipulation, it is required that the strength of the two hands should be even, and the movement should be soft and consonant. The pushing movement to both sides can be operated in a straight line or in a curved line.

(5) The operation essentials of coalescent pushing manipulation are the same as that of the separate pushing manipulation. But the operation should be done in the opposite direction.

3. Precaution

(1) Pushing manipulation should be performed along a straight line or a curved line in one direction, and rubbing back and forth should be avoided.

(2) During the operation, the operating part should stick tightly on the body surface of clients. The strength should be stable, even and moderate while the speed of pushing should not be fast.

(3) When pushing manipulation is operated on the body surface, talcum powder or the scallion and ginger juice can be smeared on the treated areas.

vii. Wiping Manipulation

The whorled surface of thumb is tightly close to the skin of treated area, pushing up and down, left to right or along a curved path, which is called the wiping manipulation. It can be divided into wiping manipulation with fingers and wiping manipulation with the palm.

1. Operation Method

(1) Wiping manipulation with fingers: Exert force on the body surface with the whorled surface of one thumb or two thumbs and support with the other four fingers; slightly exert force with the thumb and slowly shift up to down, left to right or along a curved line.

(2) Wiping manipulation with the palm: Exert force with one or two palms on the body surface and relax the wrist joint. The forearm and upper arm exert force cooperatively to drive the palm to move up and down, left to right, or along a curved line.

2. Essential for Operation

(1) During the operation of wiping manipulation, the whorled surface of thumb or the palm should stick tightly on the body surface.

(2) When wiping, the strength should be even and

（3）旋推法要求肘、腕关节放松，仅靠拇指作小幅度的环旋运动，不带动皮下组织运动，与指摩法类似。

（4）分推法操作时，要求两手用力均匀，动作柔和协调一致，向两旁分推时既可做直线推动，又可沿弧形推动。

（5）合推法的操作要领同分推法，但是方向相反。

3. 注意事项

（1）推法是单方向的直线或弧线运动，忌往返摩擦。

（2）操作时应贴紧体表，用力平稳，均匀适中，推动的速度不宜过快。

（3）在受术者的体表操作时，可在施术部位涂滑石粉或葱姜汁等推拿介质。

（七）抹法

以拇指罗纹面贴紧皮肤，沿上下、左右或弧形路径往返推动，称为抹法。抹法分为指抹法和掌抹法两种。

1. 操作方法

（1）指抹法：术者用单手或双手拇指罗纹面着力于受术处的体表，其余四指扶持助力，拇指略用力，缓慢地做上下、左右或直线或弧线的往返移动。

（2）掌抹法：术者用单手或双手掌面着力于受术处的体表，腕关节放松，前臂与上臂协调用力，带动手掌掌面在体表做上下、左右或直线或弧线的往返移动。

2. 动作要领

（1）操作时，拇指罗纹面或手掌的掌面应贴紧于受术处的体表。

（2）用力要均匀，动作要和缓，在施术区

the movement should be soft and mild. While the distance of wiping back and forth in the treated area should be long as far as possible.

3. Precaution

(1) The stimulation of wiping manipulation is superficial. Do not affect the subcutaneous tissues in deep layer when wiping.

(2) It is easy to confuse wiping manipulation with pushing manipulation. Pushing manipulation is linear movement in one direction. Whereas, wiping manipulation can be done up and down, in a straight line, or in a curved line, which is more flexible.

viii. Scattering Manipulation

Scattering manipulation means to push and rub back and forth along the channel of *shaoyang* over the temporal region with the radial surface of thumb and the tips of the other four fingers.

1. Operation Method　The operator holds the patient's head with one hand and keeps close to the temple of the head with the radial surface of thumb and the tips of the other four fingers. Then it should push and rub back and forth behind the ear along the *shaoyang* channel with slight force. The frequency is about 250 times *per* minute.

2. Essential for Operation

(1) The operator should lower the shoulder, drop the elbow and bend the elbow joint with the angle of 90°-120°, while keep the wrist joint relaxed.

(2) Take the elbow joint as the fulcrum, actively swing the forearm to drive the wrist joint to swing, while push and rub on the temple back and forth with the operating hand.

3. Precaution

(1) During the operation, the exerting parts of the fingers should stick tightly on the scalp with slight strength. When pushing and rubbing forward, the strength should be heavier. While pushing and rubbing backward, the strength should be lighter.

(2) When operating scattering manipulation, the holding hand should fix the patient's head to avoid shaking and generating discomfort.

(3) The scattering manipulation should be operated along the channel forward and backward, and the distance of movement should not be too long.

ix. Palm-twisting Manipulation

Clipping a certain part of the body or limbs of clients with both palms, and twisting alternatively or quickly back and forth. As a supplementary manipulation, this is often used on the shoulders and the upper limbs.

域内来回抹动的距离应尽量拉长。

3. 注意事项

（1）刺激较表浅，操作时不宜带动皮下深部组织。

（2）注意不要将抹法与推法相混淆。推法是单向、直线的运动，而抹法可上可下，或直线往来，或曲线运转，应用较灵活。

（八）扫散法

用拇指桡侧和示、中、无名、小指的指端在患者颞部沿少阳经自前向后，做来回推擦运动，称为扫散法。

1. 操作方法　术者以一手扶患者头部，一手的拇指桡侧面及其余四指端，同时贴于头颞侧部，稍用力向耳后沿少阳经循行路线做快速来回抹动。频率为每分钟250次左右。

2. 动作要领

（1）术者应沉肩、垂肘、肘关节屈曲90°~120°，腕关节放松。

（2）以肘关节为支点，前臂作主动摆动，带动腕关节摆动，使着力手指在受术者的颞侧来回推擦。

3. 注意事项

（1）扫散法操作时，术者手指着力部位稍用力紧贴于受术处的头皮，向前推擦时用力稍重，回返时用力稍轻。

（2）扫散时，扶持手应固定好患者的头部，避免其晃动产生不适。

（3）扫散法应自前向后循经操作，每次推擦的距离不应太长。

（九）搓法

用双手掌面夹住受术者的躯干或肢体的一定部位，相对用力交替或往返快速搓动，称为搓法。搓法是一种辅助手法，常用于肩及上肢部。

1. Operation Method

(1) Palm-twisting on the shoulders and upper limbs: Help the patient to take a sitting position with shoulders and arms relaxed and dropped naturally. The operator stands by the patient with the upper body slightly inclining forward. Clip the front and back of the patient's shoulder with both palms. The operation is done from upper limb to the wrist for 3-5 times.

(2) Palm-twisting on the hypochondria: Assist the patient in taking a sitting position and slightly extends the two arms outside. The operator stands behind the patient and clamps the two hypochondriac regions of the patient with the two palms. Twist from armpits to waist for several times at the two sides.

(3) Palm-twisting on the lower limbs: Help the patient take the supine position and bend knees with an angle about 60°. The operator stands beside the bed, and clamps the two sides of the patient's thigh with two palms from the upper down to the crus.

2. Essential for Operation

(1) The operator should exert force symmetrically with the palms, and the patient should relax the limbs.

(2) It is better to twist quickly while shifting up and down slowly.

3. Precaution

(1) The strength used should not be too heavy.

(2) Palm-twisting manipulation is mainly used when the tuina treatment goes to the end.

x. Shaking Manipulation

It is called shaking manipulation to hold the distal end of the treated limbs with both hands or one hand to shake continuously up and down or from left to right in a small amplitude.

1. Operation Method The operator holds the distal end of the patient's upper or lower limbs (wrist or ankle) by hand, and lifts the treated limbs to a certain angle (the upper limbs should be extended about 60° outside in the sitting position, and the lower limbs should be lifted to form an angle about 30° between the extremity and the bed in the supine position). When pulling with slight strength, it should continuously shake up and down in small amplitude to make the parenchyma of the treated limbs generate the vibration and convey to the proximal end of the limbs.

2. Essential for Operation

(1) The treated limbs of the patient should naturally extend straight and relax. The operator should breathe naturally and do not hold breath.

1. 操作方法

（1）肩及上肢部搓法：协助患者取坐位，肩臂放松，自然下垂，术者站于其后侧，上身略前倾，双手掌分别夹其肩前后部，相对用力快速搓揉，同时自上而下沿上肢移动至腕部，往返 3~5 遍。

（2）胁肋部搓法：协助患者取坐位，嘱其两臂略外展，术者站其身后，以两掌分别夹其两胁肋，自腋下搓向腰部两侧数遍。

（3）下肢搓法：协助患者取仰卧位，嘱其双腿屈膝约 60°，术者站于床侧，以双手掌夹其大腿两侧，自上而下搓揉至小腿部。

2. 动作要领

（1）操作者应双掌对称用力，患者肢体宜放松。

（2）搓动要快，上下移动要慢。

3. 注意事项

（1）用力不可过重。

（2）多在推拿治疗结束时使用。

（十）抖法

以双手或单手握住患肢远端，做小幅度的上下或左右的连续抖动，称为抖法。

1. 操作方法 术者用手握住受术者上肢或下肢的远端（腕部或踝部），肢体抬高一定的角度（上肢在坐位下外展约 60°，下肢在仰卧位下抬离床面约 30°），在稍用力牵引状态下，做小幅度、连续的上下抖动，使患者肢体的软组织产生颤动并传达到肢体近端。

2. 动作要领

（1）患者被抖动肢体要自然伸直放松，术者呼吸自然，不可屏气。

(2) The amplitude of shaking should be small and the frequency should be fast.

3. Precaution

(1) When shaking the patient's lower limbs, the amplitude of shaking can be larger than that of the upper limbs, and the frequency should be lower because the lower limbs are heavier.

(2) The shaking manipulation is usually used as an ending of manipulation, while the shaking manipulation of the upper extremities is commonly used.

xi. Pressing Manipulation

It is called pressing manipulation to exert force on the particular point or part of the treated body surface with the fingers or the palm, and pressing down gradually.

1. Operation Method

(1) Pressing manipulation with fingers: Extend the thumb straight, and press on the channels and points of the body surface with the tip or the whorled surface of the thumb supported by the other extended four fingers. If the strength is not enough for one hand, it should overlap the other thumb on it to press down heavily with the surface of the thumb.

(2) Pressing manipulation with the palm: Press on the body surface with the palm root, the thenar or the whole palm. If the strength is not enough for one hand, it should overlap the two hands to press.

2. Essential for Operation

(1) The direction of pressing should be vertical. The strength used should be from light to heavy, stable and lasting to make the stimulation fully penetrate into the deep layer of the body tissue. And then it should decrease the pressure gradually. The principle "light-heavy-light" should be followed.

(2) If the bigger stimulation is needed in the pressing manipulation, the operator can slightly incline his upper body forward to increase the stimulation by his own gravity.

3. Precaution

(1) It should avoid using the sudden violent force to prevent the adverse effect.

(2) The force should be changed rhythmically in operation. Pay attention to the difference between the constinuous-pressing manipulation and pressing manipulation. In clinic, it is commonly used to combine the pressing with the kneading manipulation, forming the compound manipulation of pressing and kneading.

xii. Continuous Pressing Manipulation

It is called continuous pressing manipulation to exert force on the special point or part of the body surface

（2）抖动的幅度要小，频率要快。

3. 注意事项

（1）因下肢较重，抖动下肢的幅度可比上肢大些，频率低些。

（2）抖法常用作结束手法，上肢抖法较为常用。

（十一）按法

用手指或手掌面着力于受术处体表特定的穴位或部位上，逐渐用力下压，称为按法。

1. 操作方法

（1）指按法：拇指伸直，用拇指指端或罗纹面按压在受术处体表的经络穴位上，其余四指张开，扶持在旁相应位置上以助力，单手指力不足时可用另一手拇指重叠按压其上，使拇指指面用力向下按压。

（2）掌按法：用掌根、鱼际或全掌着力按压体表，单手力量不足时，可用双手掌重叠按压。

2. 动作要领

（1）按压方向要垂直，用力要由轻到重，稳而持续，使刺激充分透达机体组织的深部，之后逐渐减轻压力，遵循从轻到重再到轻的原则。

（2）按法如需较大刺激时，可略前倾身体，借助躯干的力量增加刺激。

3. 注意事项

（1）切忌用迅猛的爆发力，以免产生不良反应。

（2）用力应有节律变化。注意和较长时间持续用力的压法区别。按法在临床上常和揉法结合使用，形成复合手法按揉法。

（十二）压法

用拇指面、掌面或肘关节鹰嘴突起部着

with the thumb, palm or the olecranon of the elbow and pressing downwards continuously.

1. Operation Method The operator presses the body surface vertically with the whorled surface of the thumb, palm or the upper part of the forearm of the flexed elbow. Gradual slipping on the body surface can also be done during the pressing. Pressing with the upper part of the forearm is also called continuous pressing manipulation with elbow.

2. Essential for Operation The method of pressing manipulation is similar to continuous pressing manipulation, so they are always collectively called "pressure manipulation". If distinguished strictly, the former is more dynamic while the latter is more static. The lasting time of pressing manipulation is short while the continuous pressing manipulation is long. The force of pressing manipulation is small and the stimulation is light, whereas, the force of continuous pressing manipulation is great and the stimulation is strong.

3. Precaution

(1) When continuous pressing is used on the back and waist, the force should be controlled to prevent the adverse effects.

(2) The stimulation of the continuous pressing manipulation with elbow is stronger, so it is mostly used on the waist and buttocks of the strong people where there are thick muscles.

xiii. Pointing Manipulation

Pressing on the certain point or part of the treated body with the tip of finger or the articular protrusion is called pointing manipulation. It can be divided into pointing with fingers and pointing with elbow in clinic.

1. Operation Method

(1) Pointing manipulation with fingers: The operator makes an empty fist, extends the thumb straight and makes it close to the middle interphalangeal joint of the middle finger. Exert force with the tip of the thumb or the interphalangeal joint of the thumb, or the tip of the middle finger supported by overlapping the index finger on the back of the middle finger. Press on a certain point or part of clients with a steady force.

(2) Pointing manipulation with the elbow: The operator bends the elbow, exerts force with the olecranon, slightly inclines his body and presses continuously with the elbow. The pressure from the operator's own gravity is transmitted through the shoulder joint and upper arm to the elbow.

2. Essential for Operation

The pointing manipulation is developed from the

力于受术处体表特定的穴位或部位上，持续用力下按，称为压法。

1. **操作方法** 术者用拇指罗纹面、手掌或屈肘以肘部前臂上段垂直向下按压受术处的体表，按压时也可在体表上逐渐滑动。肘部前臂上段按压又称为肘压法。

2. **动作要领** 按法和压法两者动作相似，故常混称为"按压法"。若严格区分，按法偏动，压法偏静；按法持续时间短，压法持续时间长；按法压力小、刺激轻，压法压力大、刺激强。

3. **注意事项**

（1）在背腰部使用时，注意控制用力大小，避免产生不良反应。

（2）肘压法的刺激较强，多用于体格健壮者的腰臀部肌肉丰厚处。

（十三）点法

以指端或关节突起部点压一定的穴位或部位，称为点法，临床上可分为指点法和肘点法。

1. **操作方法**

（1）指点法：术者手握空拳，拇指伸直并靠近示指中节，以拇指端着力或拇指屈曲，以拇指指间关节背侧着力或以中指端着力，示指末节叠压于中指背侧助力，由轻而重，平稳施力，按压一定的穴位或部位。

（2）肘点法：术者屈肘，以尺骨鹰嘴突起部着力，身体略前倾，用身体上半身的重量通过肩关节、上臂传递至肘部，持续点压。

2. **动作要领** 点法是由按法衍化而来，要领基本相同，只不过接触面积较小，刺激

pressing manipulation. The essentials are basically the same, but the touching area is smaller and the stimulation is stronger.

3. Precaution

(1) In operating the pointing manipulation, the touching area is small, the stimulation intensity is big and the stimulation time is short. It is often used to relieve pain, which is also called "finger needle". After the pointing manipulation, kneading manipulation can be used to prevent.

(2) It should be carefully applied to people who are old, weak and frail.

(3) It is different in the position of exerting force between the methods of "pointing manipulation with the elbow" and "pressing manipulation with the elbow". The former exerts force with the sharp olecranon while the latter exerts force with the blunt upper part of the forearm.

xiv. Pinching Manipulation

Exerting force symmetrically with the thumb and other fingers and extruding the treated area is called pinching manipulation. The manipulation used to treat the spine is called spine pinching manipulation, which is usually used for children.

1. Operation Method　Clamp the treated area with the thumb, index finger and middle finger or the thumb and the other four fingers, and then extrude symmetrically and loosen at once. Repeat the manipulation mentioned above and shift gradually.

2. Essential for Operation　The force should be exerted with the thumb and other four fingers symmetrically, evenly and softly. The movement should be consecutive and rhythmic.

3. Precaution

(1) The force should be exerted with the palm rather than the tip of the finger.

(2) The force of the fingers is highly required, especially the combined force of the thumb with other four fingers. The operator can adopt the relative exercise for basic training to improve the finger force.

xv. Grasping Manipulation

It is called grasping manipulation to exert force symmetrically with the thumb and the other four fingers to lift and pinch or clamp the limbs or skin.

1. Operation Method　The operator relaxes the wrist joint and clamps the treated area symmetrically with the whorled surface of thumb and index finger, middle finger or other fingers to lift the skin and continuously do the kneading and pinching movement alternately with light and heavy strength.

较强。

3. 注意事项

（1）点法接触面较小，刺激强度大，刺激时间短，多用于止痛，又称"指针"。点按后应用揉法可避免局部软组织损伤。

（2）年老体弱、久病虚衰者慎用点法。

（3）肘点法和肘压法的施力部位不同，前者用尖锐的尺骨鹰嘴突起部着力，后者以肘部平钝的前臂上段着力。

（十四）捏法

用拇指和其他手指对称用力，挤压施术部位，称为捏法。用以脊柱的捏法称为"捏脊"，多用于小儿推拿。

1. 操作方法　用拇指与示、中指的指面或拇指与其余四指指面夹住施术部位，相对用力挤压，随即放松，重复上述动作并循序移动。

2. 动作要领　拇指与其余手指用力要对称，均匀柔和，动作连贯，富有节奏。

3. 注意事项

（1）以手指掌面着力，不可用指端着力。

（2）捏法对指力要求较高，尤其是拇指与其他四指的对合力，可采用相应功法练习以提高指力。

（十五）拿法

用拇指与其他四指相对用力，提捏或夹持肢体或肌肤，称为拿法。

1. 操作方法　术者腕关节放松，以拇指与示、中指或其余手指的罗纹面相对用力夹紧需治疗的部位，将肌肤提起，并做轻重交替而连续的揉捏动作。

2. Essential for Operation

(1) Relax the wrist joint, extend the fingers straightly, exert force with the flat finger pulp to clamp the treated area, bend the metacarpophalangeal joints that is opposite to the thumb, lift and pinch the skin and the subcutaneous parenchyma symmetrically, which seems to be a scissor type.

(2) The strength should be slow, gentle and even, from light to heavy and then from heavy to light. The kneading and pinching movement should be continuous.

3. Precaution

(1) In the operation of grasping manipulation, it should avoid bending the interphalangeal joint of the fingers to form the action of pinching the skin by the tip of fingers or nipping with the fingernails.

(2) During the operation of grasping manipulation, it should pinch the subcutaneous parenchyma as much as possible according to the clinical needs and avoid the fingers slipping on the body surface.

(3) After the grasping manipulation, kneading and rubbing manipulation can be used to ease local discomfort.

xvi. Twiddling Manipulation

It is called twiddling manipulation to clamping the treated area with the thumb and index finger, and twiddling with kneading and pinching symmetrically.

1. Operation Method　Exert force symmetrically, clamp the treated area with the whorled surface of thumb and the radial surface of the index finger, and make a quicker twisting with slight force like twiddling a thread. Twiddling is a supplementary manipulation, and it is mostly used for the joints of fingers and toes.

2. Essential for Operation

(1) It is required that the movement is continuous and flexible when performing the twiddling manipulation and the sluggish operation should be avoided.

(2) The speed of the twiddling is quick, but the shift speed on the treated area should be slow.

3. Precaution

When applying the twiddling manipulation, it should pay attention to twist fast while move slowly.

xvii. Plucking Manipulation

Pressing on the treated area with the thumb and plucking back and forth along the direction that is perpendicular to the direction of the tendons and muscles. The method is called plucking manipulation.

1. Operation Method　Straighten the thumb and exert strength with the tip or the whorled surface of the thumb with the assistance of the other four fingers.

2. 动作要领

（1）腕关节放松，手指伸直，以平坦的指腹着力挟住需治疗的部位，与拇指相对手指掌指关节屈曲，做类似剪刀式、相对用力提捏受术处皮肤及皮下软组织。

（2）用力缓慢柔和而均匀，由轻到重，再由重到轻，揉捏动作连贯。

3. 注意事项

（1）操作时，应避免手指的指间关节屈曲，形成指端夹持肌肤或指甲抠掐的动作。

（2）操作时，应根据临床需要尽可能多地捏拿皮下软组织，避免手指在体表滑移。

（3）操作后，可用轻柔的揉摩法以缓解局部不适。

（十六）捻法

用拇指和示指以指面相对夹住施术部位，做对称式的揉捏捻动，称为捻法。

1. 操作方法　术者用拇指的罗纹面及示指桡侧面相对用力，夹住治疗部位，拇指与示指稍用力作较快速的揉捏捻动，如捻线状。捻法为辅助手法，多用于指、趾关节部。

2. 动作要领

（1）动作要连贯灵活，用劲不可呆滞。

（2）速度稍快，在施术部位上的移动速度宜慢。

3. 注意事项　施用捻法时，注意捻动要快，移动要慢。

（十七）拨法

以拇指的指腹深按于施术部位，做与筋腱、肌肉等组织走行相垂直地来回拨动，称为拨法，又称"弹拨法"。

1. 操作方法　拇指伸直，以拇指指端或罗纹面着力，其余四指置于相应的位置以助

Press deeply with the thumb until the patient feels aching and distending. Then pluck back and forth in a direction perpendicular to the direction of the muscle fiber and tendon. If the force of one finger is not enough, it can be operated by two thumbs overlapped.

2. Essential for Operation

(1) In the operation of plucking manipulation, the thumb should pluck with the subcutaneous muscle fiber or tendon and ligament together rather than move on the body skin.

(2) When plucking, the strength should be increased gradually according to the patient's endurance.

3. Precaution

(1) Plucking manipulation is usually operated on the tenderness point.

(2) The stimulation of plucking manipulation is stronger, so it is better to use kneading and rubbing manipulation to ease local discomfort after operating this manipulation.

xviii.Patting Manipulation

Patting in rhythm on the body surface with the hollow palm is called patting manipulation.

1. Operation Method　The operator juxtaposes the fingers and thumb together, flexes the metacarpophalangeal joints slightly so as to form an empty palm, and then pats the treated parts in rhythm at a frequency of 100-120 times *per* minute.

2. Essential for Operation

(1) The shoulder joint and wrist of operator should be relaxed and dropped. The wrist joint should be relaxed. The patting should be light and steady. The palm should rise up as soon as patting the treated area. It should pat in rhythm until the skin turns to reddish with congestion.

(2) The manipulation can be operated by one hand or both hands.

3. Precaution

(1) The palm that pats on the body surface should be steady and avoid dragging on the body surface.

(2) Avoid using the patting manipulation for the patient who suffers from tuberculosis, serious osteoporosis, bone tumor, and coronary heart disease.

xix. Striking Manipulation

It is called striking manipulation to strike the treated parts in rhythm with the palm base, the lateral side of palm, fingertip or the stick made of mulberry twigs is called striking manipulation.

1. Operation Method

(1) Striking manipulation with the palm base:

力，用拇指深按至患者局部有酸胀感后，再做与肌纤维或筋腱走行方向垂直的来回拨动。单手指力不足时，可双手拇指叠加操作。

2. 动作要领

（1）操作时，拇指不能和体表皮肤有相对摩擦移动，应带动皮下肌纤维或筋腱韧带一起拨动。

（2）用力宜由轻渐重，以患者能忍受为度。

3. 注意事项

（1）常用在压痛点上操作。

（2）因刺激较强，操作后宜用轻柔的揉摩法以缓解局部的不适。

（十八）拍法

用虚掌在体表有节律地拍打，称为拍法。

1. 操作方法　术者五指并拢，掌指关节微屈，掌心凹陷呈虚掌，有节奏地拍打需治疗的部位。击打频率为每分钟 100~120 次。

2. 动作要领

（1）操作时，术者肩关节宜松沉，腕关节放松，击打要轻快而平稳，手掌着实后即抬起，动作富有节律，拍打次数以受术者的皮肤出现微红充血为度。

（2）可用单手或双手操作。

3. 注意事项

（1）手掌落在受术者的体表上应平实，不能在体表有拖抽的动作。

（2）对结核、严重的骨质疏松、骨肿瘤、冠心病的患者禁用拍法。

（十九）击法

用掌根、掌侧小鱼际、拳背、指尖或桑枝棒等有节奏地击打需治疗的部位，称为击法。

1. 操作方法

（1）掌根击法：手指自然伸展，腕关节略

Fingers stretch naturally, while the wrist joint stretches slightly backward and tap the body surface with the palm root.

(2) Striking manipulation with the lateral side of palm: Fingers stretch naturally, while the wrist joint stretches slightly backward and then strike the body surface with the hypothenars of both hands alternately.

(3) Striking manipulation with fist: Hold a fist and keep the wrist joint straight, and then strike the body surface with the back of fist. The frequency is 3-5 times *per* time.

(4) Striking manipulation with the finger-tips: Strike the treated parts lightly and quickly with the five finger-tips juxtaposed together.

(5) Striking manipulation with a stick: Strike the body surface with the upper half of the stick made of mulberry twigs.

2. Essential for Operation

(1) The force should be quick with a short duration. Strike vertically to the body surface with an even and rhythm frequency.

(2) When operating striking manipulation with palm base, the operator takes the palm base as the force origin and strikes with the strength from the forearm. The arms can be flirted in great amplitude. The frequency is 3-5 times *per* time.

(3) Striking manipulation with the lateral side of palm can be operated with one hand or both hands. Take the elbow joint as the supporting point and make the forearm move actively. When operating, the lateral side of palm should be perpendicular to the direction of the muscle fiber and the movement should be rhythmic and rapid.

(4) When operating striking manipulation with the fist, take the elbow joint as the supporting point and strike with the force from the flexion and extension of the elbow joint and the forearm. The force should be steady.

(5) When operating striking manipulation with fingertips, relax the wrist joint and flex and extend the elbow joint in small amplitude. Strike the body surface with the finger tips lightly at a rapid speed just like rain drops.

(6) When operating striking manipulation with stick, hold the 1/3 part of the lower part of the mulberry stick, move the forearm actively and strike the treated part with the upper part of the stick in rhythm.

3. Precaution

(1) When operating striking manipulation, pay attention to the rebounding. The stick should bounce up once it touches the treated parts. Do not pause or drag on

背伸，以掌根部击打受术者的体表。

（2）侧击法：手指自然伸直，腕关节略背伸，以双手手掌小鱼际部交替击打受术者的体表。

（3）拳击法：术者手握拳，腕关节平直，以拳背平击受术者的体表，一般每次击打3~5下。

（4）指尖击法：以手之五指指端合拢轻快敲击需治疗的部位。

（5）棒击法：用特制的桑枝棒前段约1/2部着力，击打受术者的体表。

2. 动作要领

（1）击法用力要快速而短暂，垂直叩击体表，频率均匀有节奏。

（2）掌根击法以掌根为着力点，运用前臂的力量击打，手臂挥动的幅度可较大，每次击打3~5下。

（3）侧击法可单手或双手合掌操作，以肘关节为支点，前臂主动运动，击打时手掌小鱼际应与肌纤维方向垂直，动作轻快有节奏。

（4）拳击法以肘关节为支点，运用肘关节的屈伸和前臂的力量击打，着力宜平稳。

（5）指尖击法操作时，腕关节放松，运用腕关节的小幅度屈伸，以指端轻击受术者的体表，频率快如雨点落下。

（6）棒击法以手握桑枝棒下段的1/3，前臂做主动运动，使桑枝棒前段有节奏地击打施术部位。

3. 注意事项

（1）击法操作时，应注意击打的反弹感，一触施术部位即弹起，不可在体表停顿

the body surface.

(2) Strictly grasp the treated parts and indications of different striking manipulations, and avoid striking violently.

(3) Striking manipulation with the palm base in mainly indicated for DU 14 (*dà zhuī*), lumbosacral region. Striking manipulation with a stick can be used on DU 20 (*bái huì*), GB 30 (*huán tiào*). Striking manipulation with the finger tips is usually used on the head. In operating with a stick, the body of the stick rather than the tip should be used. The ordinate axis of the stick body should be parallel with the direction of the muscle fiber except for the lumbosacral parts.

xx. Flicking Manipulation

Pressing the back side of the index finger tightly with the middle finger and springing swiftly to flick the part or the point of the body, which is called flicking manipulation.

1. Operation Method　Flex the forefinger, press the back side of the forefinger with the whorled surface of middle finger and then flick the treated parts rapidly. The frequency is 120-160 times *per* minute. The manipulation is usually used as a supplementary manipulation on the head face.

2. Essential for Operation　This manipulation should be slight, swift, gentle, flexible and rhythmic. The intensity of stimulation should be controlled without causing pain.

3. Precaution　The manipulation should be slight, swift, and flexible.

xxi. Nipping Manipulation

Nipping is a method that is done by the finger nails to irritate the acupuncture points forcefully without injury of the skin.

1. Operation Method　Nip the points by nails of thumb or index finger forcefully without injury of the skin.

2. Essential for Operation

(1) The nipping direction should be perpendicular. The strength should be started from gentle to strong. Do not dig with the finger to avoid damaging the skin of the treated points.

(2) Kneading with the belly of thumb gently to the treated points after nipping can be used to relieve the pain.

3. Precaution　In operating, the force should be gradually given until it penetrates into the deep part and be sure not to injure the skin.

或拖抽。

（2）严格掌握各种击法的适应部位和病证，忌暴力击打。

（3）拳击法主要用于大椎、腰骶部；掌击法可用于百会、环跳；指尖击法常用于头部；桑枝棒击法击打时要用棒体平击，不用棒尖。除腰骶部外，其他部位应用顺棒（棒体纵轴与肌纤维方向平行）击打。

（二十）弹法

用中指的指腹紧压示指背侧，用力快速弹出，连续弹击受术处的某一部位或穴位，称为弹法。

1. **操作方法**　将示指屈曲，以中指罗纹面紧压示指背侧，然后迅速弹出，击打患处，频率为每分钟 120~160 次。本法常作为头面部操作的辅助手法使用。

2. **动作要领**　动作要轻快、柔和、有弹性、有节律。

3. **注意事项**　操作要轻快而有弹性，刺激强度以不引起疼痛为度。

（二十一）掐法

用指甲缘重按穴位而不损伤治疗部位皮肤的方法，称为掐法。

1. **操作方法**　用拇指或示指的指端甲缘重按穴位，而不损伤治疗部位皮肤。

2. **动作要领**

（1）要垂直向下用力，力量逐渐加大，不可抠动，以免损伤治疗部位的皮肤。

（2）掐后可在治疗部位上用拇指罗纹面轻揉以缓解疼痛。

3. **注意事项**　操作时应逐渐用力达渗透为止，注意不要掐破皮肤。

IV. Self-Massage for Healthcare

Self-massage for healthcare based upon the theories of TCM means that people may use some basic manipulations to work on certain parts or acupuncture points of the body in order to regulate the channels, activate and promote transportation and circulation of qi and blood, and balance yin and yang in this way, so as to achieve the purpose of strengthening body constitution, preventing and treating diseases, as well as preserving health and prolonging life.

i. Practical Manipulation

1. General Self-Massage Self-massage is a common therapy of health cultivation and health care. People can use manipulations to work on the skin or acupoints of their own body in order to prevent and treat diseases, as well as improve and strengthen body constitution. It should be operated flexibly, step by step according to individual conditions and in accordance with the passage of the channels and collaterals of the five viscera. One can also do the general self-massage for health care from the head to foot. Good effects will be obtained if self-massage is done properly as follows:

Tapping the teeth→ cleaning the mouth→ wiping the face→ kneading the eyes→ press BL 1 (*jíng míng*) points→ brushing the LI 20 (*yíng xiāng*) points→ pressing the temples→ making sounds in the ears (Mingtiangu) → combing the hair→ kneading the neck→ pinching the shoulder→ swing the hands→ broadening the chest→ kneading the abdomen→ beating the back→ rubbing the waist→ pressing the GB 30 (*huán tiào*) → rubbing the thigh→ kneading the calf→ rubbing the KI 1 (*yǒng quán*) points.

2. Broadening the Chest The normal physiological function of the lung is to ensure normal respiration, nutrition and water metabolism. If the function of the lung is abnormal, it will lead to difficulty in breath, stuffiness in the chest, cough, asthmatic breath, and even edema. Thus, the manipulation of broadening the chest may effectively prevent and treat diseases of the lung.

(1) Kneading the breast: Use the middle finger to press and knead below the collarbone and between the ribs from inside to outside, and then the operator should keep the middle finger moveing from upper to lower, from one side to another until aching or bulging feeling is present.

(2) Vibrating the chest: Hold greater pectoral muscle of the left side, grasp with the right hand for 9 times, and repeat the same manipulation on the right side with the left hand. Then, cross the fingers and hold the nape with

四、实用自我推拿保健调护

自我推拿保健调护法是指在中医基础理论的指导下，运用推拿的一些基本手法，在体表一定部位或穴位进行主动推拿，或配合一定的肢体活动，以调整经络，激发营卫气血的运行，平衡阴阳，达到增强体质、防病治病的目的。

（一）实用自我推拿保健调护手法

1. 全身自我推拿保健法 成人在自身体表部位或穴位进行推拿手法操作，以舒缓疲劳、愉悦心情，并达到强身健体、防病治病的目的，也是保健养生调护的常用方法。具体操作依自身状况而灵活掌握，可以结合五脏循经进行，亦可形成从头到脚连续的动作完成全身自我推拿，施之有法，行之有效。

可遵循如下顺序：叩齿→净口→摩面→熨目→点睛明→擦迎香→按太阳→鸣天鼓→梳头→拿颈项→捏肩→甩手→揉胸→摩腹→捶背→搓腰→点环跳→擦大腿→抓小腿→摩涌泉。

2. 宽胸法 肺的正常生理功能可使人体的呼吸、营养、水液代谢保持良好的状态，反之则出现呼吸不利、胸闷、咳喘，甚至水肿等病证。采用宽胸法对肺系疾患可起到防治作用。

（1）揉胸部：以一手中指罗纹面沿锁骨下、肋间隙，由内向外，由上而下，用力按揉，以感觉酸胀为宜。

（2）拿胸膺：先用右手从腋下捏拿左侧胸大肌约9次，再换左手如法操作。然后双手十指交叉抱持于后枕部，双肘相平，尽力向后扩展，同时吸气，向前内收肘呼气，一呼一

the elbow flexed horizontally; try to extend the elbow backward as much as possible when breathing out; repeat the same procedure for 9 times, and relax it from inner to forth and inside to outside.

(3) Tapping the chest: Put the right hollow palm over the right breast, pat with proper force and move to the left horizontally, as well as back and forth for 9 times until it is warm in the local area.

(4) Rubbing the chest: Cross the hands with fingers and put them on the chest. Transversely rub back and forth forcefully for 36 times until it is warm in the local area.

(5) Pushing the RN 17 (*dàn zhōng*): Put one hand over the other hand at RN 17 (*dàn zhōng*) between the nipples, and rub from up to down for 36 times.

(6) Kneading LU 1 (*zhōng fǔ*): Cross the both of two forearms in front of the chest. Put the tips of middle fingers at LU 1 (*zhōng fǔ*) on both sides. Knead the point with slightly forceful strength clockwise and counterclockwise for 36 times, respectively.

(7) Hooking RN 22 (*tiān tū*): Hook RN 22 (*tiān tū*) with the tip of the index finger and knead for 1 minute.

(8) Removing obstruction from the lung channel: Take a sitting or standing position, put the right hand above the left breast and rub in circles till it is warm in the local area. Then rub backward and forward along the front of the shoulder, anterior border of medial aspect of the arm, radial side of the wrist and dorsum of the index finger (the route of the lung channel) for 36 times. Then repeat the same procedure with the left hand on the right side.

3. Strengthening the Spleen　When the spleen is functioning well in transportation and transformation, the food nutrient is absorbed continuously, qi and blood are constantly produced, the body is well nourished, and the lips are red and lustrous. On the contrary, it will cause emaciation, muscular atrophy and weakness, tastelessness or abnormal taste in the mouth, and pale lips without luster. The manipulation for strengthening the spleen and regulating the stomach can effectively prevent and treat disorders of the spleen and stomach.

(1) Rubbing RN 12 (*zhōng wǎn*): The operator puts the left or the right hand on RN 12 (*zhōng wǎn*), rubs the epigastric region counterclockwise in circles for 36 times from small to large circles, and then performs the same rubbing movement clockwise for 36 times from big to small circles.

(2) Kneading ST 25 (*tiān shū*): Take a sitting position or lie down on the back, press and knead ST 25 (*tiān shū*) with the index and middle fingers simultaneously clockwise and counterclockwise for 36 times, respectively.

吸，操作 9 次。一呼一吸，一提一拿，慢慢由里向外松之。

（3）拍胸：用右手虚掌置于右乳上方，适当用力拍击并渐横向左侧移动，来回 9 次，以热为度。

（4）擦胸：以两手掌交叉紧贴胸部体表，横向用力往返擦动 36 次，以热为度。

（5）推膻中：双手手掌相叠，置于两乳中间的膻中穴，上下推擦 36 次。

（6）揉中府：两手掌交叉抱于胸前，用两手中指指端置于两侧的中府穴，稍用力作顺时针、逆时针方向的揉动，各 36 次。

（7）勾天突：用示指指尖置于天突穴处，向下勾点，揉动 1min。

（8）疏肺经：坐位或立位，右掌先置左乳上，环摩至热后，以掌沿着肩前、上臂内侧前上方、前臂桡侧至腕、拇指、示指背侧（肺经的循行路线），做往返推擦 36 次，然后换左手操作右侧。

3. **健脾法**　脾的生理功能健运则饮食精微不断吸收，化生气血，营养充足，口唇红润光泽；反之则形体消瘦，肌肉痿软，口淡无味或异味，口唇淡白无光泽。采用此保健推拿法可对脾胃疾患起防治作用。

（1）摩中脘：用左手或右手手掌置于中脘部，先逆时针，从小到大摩脘腹 36 圈，然手再顺时针，从大到小摩 36 圈。

（2）揉天枢：坐位或仰卧位，用双手的示、中指同时按揉天枢穴，顺、逆时针各 36 次。

(3) Pressing epigastric region: Juxtaposing the four fingers of the left or the right hand and put them on RN 12 (*zhōng wǎn*), and the operator takes abdominal respiration and presses downward when breathing in, and kneads in circles when breathing out. Repeat the whole procedure for 36 times.

(4) Separating yin and yang: Put hands on the xiphoid process with fingers pointing to each other, perform pulling manipulation from the front midline to the hypochondriac regions along the rib arcs and shift to the lower abdomen, and repeat the whole procedure for 9 times.

(5) Rubbing the navel: Put the palm center of one hand on the navel, press the back of the hand with another hand, and circle-rub clockwise for 3-5 minutes.

(6) Pressing ST 36 (*zú sān lǐ*): Put the thumbs, index or middle finger on ST 36 (*zú sān lǐ*), and press and knead with slight strength for about 3 minutes until there is aching and distending pain.

(7) Kneading SP 10 (*xuè hǎi*): Take a sitting position, and knead SP 10 with the thumbs clockwise and counterclockwise for 36 times, respectively.

(8) Pinching LI 4 (*hé gǔ*): Press LI 4 (*hé gǔ*) with the thumb and index finger of the right hand for about 1 minute. Then perform the same procedure with the left hand on the other side.

4. Calming the Mind The normal function of the heart is manifested as vigorous spirit, sound mental activities, agile movement, moderate and forceful pulse as well as light reddish tongue with moist coating. Insufficient heart qi may cause low spirit, slow reaction, irregular pulse, and dark purple or pale tongue property. Thus, the manipulation for tranquilizing the heart and calming the mind can effectively prevent and treat heart disease.

(1) Rubbing the chest: The operator puts the right hand on the area between the breasts with fingers pointing downward to the side of the abdomen. Firstly, push downward to the area below the left breast and rub the heart area, then return in the initial position. Secondly, withdraw the hand to the area below the right breast to repeat rubbing in circles, and the last, push and rub in this way to form a figure of "∞"(horizontal 8) for 36 times.

(2) Patting the calvaria: Use the palm to pat the calvaria with rhythm. It should be gently done at the beginning. Then strengthen gradually when there is no bad reaction, and tap about 10 times each procedure.

(3) Grasping the heart channel: Put the thumb of the right hand under the left armpit and the rest other four fingers on the medial aspect of the upper arm, grasp, press

（3）按脘腹：左手或右手并拢四指放置于中脘穴上，采用顺腹式呼吸，吸气时稍用力下按，呼气时做轻柔的环形揉动，如此操作36次。

（4）分阴阳：两手相对，全掌置于剑突下，稍稍用力从内向外沿肋弓向胁肋处分推，并逐渐向小腹移动，操作9次。

（5）摩脐：一手掌心贴脐部，另一手按手背，顺时针方向旋转摩动3~5min。

（6）按足三里：双手拇指或示、中指置于足三里穴位上，稍用力做按揉，使局部有酸胀感，约3min。

（7）点血海：取坐位，两手分别置于大腿部，拇指点按于血海穴，再作顺、逆时针方向的揉动各36次。

（8）捏合谷：右手拇、示指相对捏、拿左侧合谷穴1min，再换左手操作右侧。

4. 安神法 心的生理功能正常，可见人精神振奋，思维敏捷，动作灵活，脉搏和缓有力，舌质淡红润泽；反之则见精神萎靡，反应迟钝以及脉涩不畅，节律不整，舌质紫暗或苍白等。经常采用安神法的保健推拿法可对心系疾病有防治作用。

（1）摩胸：右掌按置两乳正中，指尖斜向前下方，先从左乳下环行推摩心区复原，再以掌根在前，沿右乳下环行推摩，如此连续呈"∞"（横8字）形，操作36次。

（2）拍头顶：用手掌心有节律地拍击头顶，初做时，拍击力量宜轻，若无不适反应，力量可适当加重，每次拍击10次左右。

（3）拿心经：右手拇指置于左侧腋下，其余四指置上臂内上侧，边做拿捏，边做按揉，沿上臂内侧渐次向下操作到腕部神门穴，如

and knead simultaneously. Then shift the hands bit by bit to HT 7 (*shén mén*). Repeat the same procedure up and down for 9 times. Then change the hand to perform the same procedure on the right arm.

(4) Kneading HT 7 (*shén mén*): Take a sitting position, and put the middle finger over the index finger of the right hand to knead HT 7 (*shén mén*) on the left hand for about l minute. Then change the hand and repeat the same procedure on the opposite side.

(5) Squeezing PC 6 (*nèi guān*): Take a sitting position, and press PC 6 (*nèi guān*) on the left side with the thumb of the right hand with the other four fingers assisting to squeeze the point from the back of the wrist. Press and squeeze for 9 times. Then change the hand and perform the same manipulation on the right side.

(6) Making sounds in the ears (*míng tiān gǔ*: Press the hands on the ears with the bottom of the palms pointing to the front with the five fingers pointing to the back. Hit the occiput region with the index, middle and ring fingers for 3 times, and then move the hands away suddenly. Repeat the same procedure for 9 times.

(7) Stirring the tongue in the mouth (*jiǎo cāng hǎi*): Rotate the tongue to rub the outside and inside of the gums from the right to the left, and then the left to the right for 9 times, respectively. Swallow the excreted saliva in three divided times.

5. Soothing the Liver If liver qi is sufficient, the tendons will be strong, the nails will be firm and the eyes will be bright. Deficiency of liver qi will result in soft and weak tendons and blurred vision. Thus, frequently application of the manipulations for soothing the liver and smoothing the gallbladder is an effective way to prevent and treat the diseases of the liver.

(1) Kneading RN 17 (*dàn zhōng*): Take a sitting position, juxtapose the four fingers and put them on RN 17 (*dàn zhōng*), and knead clockwise and counterclockwise for 36 times respectively with relatively forceful strength.

(2) Rubbing the hypochondriac region: Take a sitting position, put the hands over the chest at the sides of the nipples with the left hand over the right hand, rub horizontally along the ribs and gradually shift downward to the floating ribs, then put the right hand over the left side and perform the same movement again. Repeat the same process until it is warm in the hypochondriac region.

(3) Rubbing the lower abdomen: Take a sitting or supine position, put the hands below the hypochondriac regions, and rub forcefully along an oblique line to the lower abdomen and pubis for 36 times.

(4) Pointing and pressing LV 13 (*zhāng mén*): Put the tips of the middle fingers on LV 13 (*zhāng mén*), and

此往返操作 9 次，再换左手操作右侧。

（4）揉神门：坐位，用右手示、中指相叠，示指按压在左手的神门穴，按揉 1min，换手操作。

（5）挤内关：坐位，用右手拇指按压在左手的内关穴位上，其余四指在腕背侧起到辅助作用，稍用力用拇指指端向上、下挤按内关穴 9 次。再换左手如法操作右侧。

（6）鸣天鼓：双手掌分按于两耳上，掌根向前，五指向后，以示、中、环指叩击枕部 3 次，双手掌骤离耳部 1 次，如此重复 9 次。

（7）搅沧海：舌在口腔上、下牙龈外周从左向右，从右向左各转 9 次，产生津液分 3 口缓缓咽下。

5. **疏肝法** 肝的生理功能正常者筋强力壮，爪甲坚韧，眼睛明亮；否则可有筋软弛缩，视物不清。经常施行疏肝法进行保健推拿，对于防治肝胆病变具有积极的作用。

（1）揉膻中：坐位，用左手，四指并拢置于膻中穴，稍用力做顺时针、逆时针方向的揉动各 36 次。

（2）擦胁肋：坐位，两手五指并拢置于胸前乳头，左手在上，右手在下，从胸前横向沿肋骨方向擦动并逐渐下移至浮肋，然后换右手在上，左手在下操作，以胁肋部有透热感为度。

（3）擦少腹：坐或卧位，双手掌分置于两胁肋下，同时用力斜向少腹推擦至耻骨，往返 36 次。

（4）点章门：用两手的中指指尖分别置于两侧的章门穴上，稍用力点按，约 1min，以

press the point for about 1 minute with slightly strong force till there is aching and numb feeling.

(5) Kneading LV 14 (*qī mén*): Take a sitting or supine position, put the palm root of the left hand on the right LV 14 (*qī mén*), knead it forcefully clockwise and counterclockwise for 36 times respectively, and then change the other hand to repeat the same manipulation.

(6) Nailing LV 3 (*tài chōng*): Take a sitting position, press LV 3 (*tài chōng*) with the tips of thumbs forcefully for about 1 minute till aching and numb feeling is felt, and then knead the point gently with the whorl surface of the thumbs.

6. Strengthening the Kidney The kidney is considered as "the foundation of congenital constitution" and is the energy source of human life. The major function of the kidney is to store essence, control reproduction and development and regulate metabolism of body fluid. In addition, its role in accepting qi is of great importance to respiration. This manipulation can help strengthen and consolidate kidney function, prevent and cure disorders of the kidney system.

(1) Rubbing RN 4 (*guān yuán*): Take RN 4 (*guān yuán*) as the center of a circle, and rub in circles clockwise or counterclockwise with the left and right hands for 36 times, respectively. Then press RN 4 (*guān yuán*) inward and downward for 3 minutes with the rhythm of respiration.

(2) Rubbing the lower abdomen: From the area below hypochondriac regions to the pubis, two hands push and rub repeatedly along an oblique course until it is warm in the local area.

(3) Rubbing the lumbosacral region: Lean the body forward slightly, flex the elbow, and put two palms on the sides of the lower back. Then rub the sacral region up and down with the whole palm or hypothenar until it is warm in the local area.

(4) Rubbing kidney regions: Put the hands over BL 23 (*shèn shū*), rub and turn for 36 times in circles with both hands simultaneously [Rubbing clockwise is reinforcing and counterclockwise is reducing. It is not advisable to apply reducing method on BL 23 (*shèn shū*)]. If one has the problems of kidney deficiency or lumbago, it is necessary to increase the times of turning activity.

(5) Kneading DU 4 (*mìng mén*): Put the index finger and middle finger on DU 4 (*mìng mén*) and knead the point in circles clockwise and counterclockwise for 36 times respectively.

(6) Rubbing KI 1 (*yǒng quán*): Take a sitting position with the legs crossed, rub both hands till they are hot, and then rub back and forth from SP 6 (*sān yīn jiāo*) to the toe until the skin is hot. Rub KI 1 (*yǒng quán*) with both hands respectively until it is warm inside. The rubbing

酸胀为度。

（5）揉期门：坐或卧位，用左手的掌根置于右侧的期门穴位上，用力沿顺时针、逆时针方向，各揉动36次，再换右手操作左侧，动作相同。

（6）掐太冲：坐位，用两手拇指的指尖置于两侧太冲穴上，稍用力按掐，以酸麻为度，约1min，换用拇指的罗纹面轻揉该穴位。

6. 固肾法 肾为先天之本，是人体生命的动力源泉。主要功能是贮藏人体精气，主管人体生殖与发育，并可调节人体水液代谢，肾的纳气功能对人体呼吸亦有重要意义。选用固肾法推拿保健可对肾系疾病有防治作用。

（1）摩关元：用左或右掌以关元穴为圆心，做逆时针和顺时针方向摩动各36次，然后随呼吸向内向下按压关元3min。

（2）擦少腹：双手掌分置两胁肋下，同时用力斜向少腹部推擦至耻骨，往返操作以透热为度。

（3）擦腰骶：身体微前倾，屈肘，两手掌尽量置于两侧腰背部，以全掌或小鱼际着力，向下至骶尾骶部快速来回擦动，以透热为度。

（4）摩肾府：两手掌紧贴肾腧穴，双手同时按由外向里的方向做环形转动按摩，共转动36次（此为顺转，为补法，反之为泻，肾腧穴宜补不宜泻，转动时要注意顺逆），如有肾虚、腰痛诸病者，可以增加转动次数。

（5）揉命门：以两手的示、中两指点按在命门穴上，稍用力做环形的揉动，顺、逆各36次。

（6）搓涌泉：盘膝而坐，双手掌对搓至发热后，沿足三阴经并过内踝关节至足大趾根，往返摩擦至透热为止，然后左右手分别搓涌泉穴至局部发热。搓揉时要不缓不急，略有

movement should be done in proper rhythm.

(7) Contracting the anus and perineum: Relax the body in a quiet environment, and take abdominal respiration (breathe in with the abdomen protruded and breathe out with the abdomen contracted). During the expiration, slightly contract the anus and perineum. During inspiration, relax the abdomen. Repeat the whole procedure for 36 times.

ii. Precaution

1. Self-massage or family-massage should be done based on definite diagnosis. Please go to see the doctor in time if one feels uncomfortable.

2. Keep moderate temperature and humidity to prevent cold. Select comfortable position and lay some skin lubricant such as massage paste on the exposed skin.

3. Manipulations of self-massage should be harmonious and tender, while energize moderately from gently to strongly, from shallowly to deeply. It can last 20-30 minutes every time according to different conditions. Self-massage should be done step by step, and the time, frequency and intensity of application should be carefully monitored for permanent impact.

4. Do not choose parts in the lower abdominal and lumbar region for pregnant women or some acupuncture points such as LI 4 (*hé gǔ*), SP 6 (*sān yīn jiāo*), *etc.*. Do not do massage when one exercises excessively, feels fatigue or nervous. Neither the one is too full, famished, drunken nor is during the menstruation period. Do not apply self-massage if one is seriously ill, or suffers from trauma and infectious disease.

(Wang Yun-cui)

Section 3　Moxibustion

Moxibustion is a therapy that utilizes cauterization or heating with ignited flammable material and drug to stimulate the acupuncture points or certain areas of the body in order to treat and prevent diseases. It has effects of warming channels and expelling coldness, supporting yang and rescuing collapse, removing swells and lumps, disease prevention and health maintenance. Moxibustion originates from the primitive society. When the hominids started to use fire, they found out that physical pain can

节奏感。

（7）缩二阴：处于安静状态下，全身放松，用顺腹式呼吸法（即吸气时腹部隆起，呼气时腹部收缩），并在呼气时稍用力收缩前后二阴，吸气时放松，重复36次。

（二）实用自我推拿保健调护的注意事项

1. 自我推拿或家庭推拿宜在明确诊断的基础上进行，若有病患应及时就诊，以免延误病情。

2. 推拿时保持环境温湿度适宜，防止外感。取舒适体位，于推拿部位暴露的皮肤施以适量皮肤润滑剂，如按摩膏等。

3. 推拿手法应协调柔和，用力适中，先轻后重，由浅入深。每次以20~30min为宜，因人而异，以舒适愉快为佳。自我推拿应持之以恒、循序渐进方显持久效果。

4. 孕妇腹部、腰骶部及有些穴位如合谷、三阴交等一般慎用推拿手法。在剧烈运动、极度疲劳、情绪不稳、过饱、饥饿、酒醉、在妇女经期等情况下不宜实施推拿。对病情严重、有外伤及传染病患者禁忌推拿。

（王云翠）

第三节　灸法

灸法是指以艾绒或其他物质为主要灸材，通过烧灼、温熨或熏烤人体体表一定部位，借用灸火的热力以及药物的作用，达到防治疾病和保健目的的一种操作方法。具有温经散寒、扶阳固脱、消肿散结、防病保健等作用。灸法起源于原始社会，当人类学会用火以后，随着身体某一部位的病痛在受到火的

be relieved by the toasting. Then people have gradually cognized that moxibustion has effects on treating diseases. Afterwards the materials in moxibustion have developed from branches and leaves to moxa-wool. Moxibustion plays an important role in maintaining body health.

There are lots of materials to be used for moxibustion, such as moxa-wool, *bái jiè zǐ*, *dēng xīn cǎo*, etc.. Among these materials, the moxa-wool is the most common material which is made of dry mugwort leaves that are purified and formed into fine and soft fibers. Mugwort leaves are fragrant, warm and pungent in nature, and bitter in flavor. They are combustible and of mild firepower, so it could be used in moxibustion to treat lots of illnesses.

烘烤而感到缓解或舒适的同时，逐渐认识到灸熨可以治疗疾病，继而从以各种树枝、树叶施灸发展到用艾叶施灸，最终形成现代灸法，为维护人类健康发挥着重要的作用。

用于施灸的原料较多，有艾绒、白芥子、灯心草等，其中以艾绒最为常用。将干燥的艾叶经过反复捣碎，去除杂质，留取纯净细软的部分，即为艾绒。艾叶气味芳香、辛温味苦，易于燃烧，火力温和，主灸百病。

I. Indication

Fuanctiona and indications of moxibustion are listed as follows (Table 6-13).

一、适应证

灸法的主治作用、适应证见表 6-13。

II. Contraindication

1. Avoid using moxibustion to treat the patients with excess-heat syndrome and fever due to yin deficiency.

二、禁忌证

1. 阴虚发热、实热证者禁灸。

Table 6-13　Fuanctiona and indications of moxibustion

Function	Indication
warming channels and dispersing the coldness	diseases which are due to wind-cold-dampness pathogen and/or cold syndromes, such as join pain, abdominal pain, diarrhea or dysentery
removing blood stasis and stagnation	diseases which caused by stagnation of qi and blood stasis, such as the initial stage mammary abscess, scrofula, goiter and many other diseases
supporting yang to rescue collapse	deficient cold syndromes (enuresis, rectocele) and impotence caused by insufficiency in the middle qi and the sinking or collapsing of the yang qi
drawing the internal heating out	heat syndrome such as furuncle, herpes zoster, erysipelas and so on
preventing disease and maintaining healt	prevention and health care for healthy and sub-healthy person

表 6-13　灸法的主治作用、适应证

主治作用	适应证
温经散寒	治疗风寒湿痹和寒邪所致关节痛、胃脘痛、腹痛、泄泻、痢疾等
消瘀散结	常用于气血凝滞所致的乳痈初起、瘰疬、瘿瘤等
扶阳固脱	常用于虚寒证和中气不足、阳气下陷而引起的遗尿、脱肛、阴挺、崩漏、带下等
引热外行	常用于某些热性病，如疖肿、带状疱疹、丹毒、甲沟炎等
防病保健	无病时施灸有防病保健

2. Avoid using moxibustion in cardiac apex area, places with main vessels and joints. Avoid using moxibustion in the abdominal and lumbosacral region of pregnant women.

3. Do not do moxibustion immediately when a patient who is in a state of famine, tiredness, extremely thirst, drunkenness, nervousness and so on.

2. 心前区、大血管部和关节部位；孕妇的小腹部、腰骶部不宜施灸。

3. 一般空腹、过饱、过饥、醉酒、大渴、极度疲劳、对灸法恐惧者，应慎灸。

III. Classification of Moxibustion

There are many kinds of moxibustion. The most commoly used mosxbustion are listed in Fig. 6-15.

三、灸法的种类

灸法的种类很多，根据用物不同，临床常用的灸法见图6-15。

IV. Commonly Used Manipulation

四、常用灸法操作

i. Moxibustion with Moxa Cone

This is a method that moxa cone which is formed by shaping a small amount of moxa-wool tightly into a cone is put on a selected area of the body and ignited to treat diseases. The size of a moxa varies depending on the conditions and the locations of treatment regions. A small sized cone is like a wheat grain shape. A middle one is like a half of the kernel of Chinese date, and a big one is like a half of an olive. Every cone after burning is called one "*zhuang*" in TCM term. Moxibustion with moxa cone is divided into direct moxibustion and indirect moxibustion.

1. Direct Moxibustion　Direct moxibustion: It is a method that an ignited cone with appropriate size is put

（一）艾炷灸

艾炷灸是用手工或器具把艾绒搓捏成规格大小不同的圆锥形艾炷，置于施灸部位，点燃灼烧而治病的方法。艾炷大小可根据患者病情及施灸部位而定，小者如麦粒大，中者如半截枣核大，大者如半截橄榄大。每燃烧一个艾炷，称为一壮。施灸时，艾炷灸可分为直接灸和间接灸。

1. **直接灸**　又称为"着肤灸"和"明灸"。即选择大小合适的艾炷，直接放在所选部位

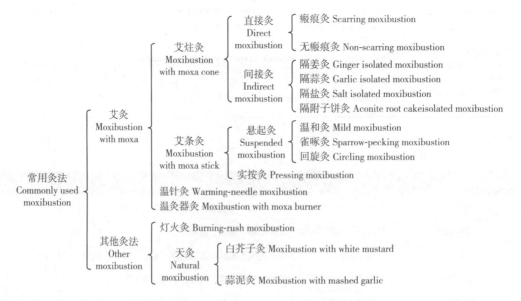

Fig. 6-15　Classifications of Moxibustion

图6-15　灸法种类

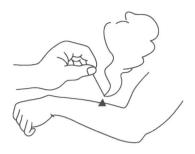

Fig. 6-16　Direct Moxibustion
图 6-16　直接灸

directly on the skin (Fig. 6-16). It can be further divided into scarring moxibustion and non-scarring moxibustion according to whether there are scars on the skin after moxibustion. Because scarring moxibustion makes the patient feel painful badly, it is rarely used in clinical practice. Therefore, only non-scarring moxibustion is introduced here.

Non-scarring moxibustion: It is also known as non-pustulating moxibustion. It is a method that there will be no any scars on the skin. It is indicated for pain syndrome caused by wind-cold pathogen, and abdominal pain, diarrhea and dysmenorrhea due to deficiency-cold. Smear a bit Vaseline on the selected point. Put the moxa cone on the point and ignite it. When 3/5 of the cone is burnt and the patient feels a slight pain, take it off with a forceps, place a new one and ignite it again for the second cone or *Zhuang*. Three to seven cones or *Zhuang* are needed for each point until the local skin becomes congested and reddish without blister.

2. Indirect Moxibustion　It is also known as material isolated moxibustion or namely a method that the ignited moxa cone is isolated with some materials from contacting the skin directly (Fig. 6-17). Generally speaking, ginger isolated moxibustion, garlic isolated moxibustion, salt isolated moxibustion and aconite root cake isolated moxibustion are commonly used.

(1) Ginger isolated moxibustion: This method is indicated for deficiency-cold syndrome such as abdominal pain, diarrhea, vomiting, dysmenorrheal and so on. Cut ginger into a slice 2-3cm in diameter and 0.2-0.3cm in thickness, and puncture some holes in it. Smear a bit Vaseline on the selected point and put ginger slice on the point. Then put the moxa cone on it and ignite the cone. When the first cone completely burns out, replace a new one and ignite it again for the second cone or *Zhuang*. Five to ten cones or *Zhuang* are needed for each point until the local skin becomes reddish without blister.

(2) Garlic isolated moxibustion: This method is

的皮肤上施灸的方法（图 6-16）。根据灸后皮肤是否留有瘢痕，又分为瘢痕灸和无瘢痕灸两种。因瘢痕灸给患者带来的痛苦较大，目前临床已很少使用，在此仅介绍无瘢痕灸。

无瘢痕灸，又称为非化脓灸，即灸后不留有瘢痕的治疗方法。临床常用于治疗风寒痹痛以及虚寒性的腹痛、泄泻和痛经等。治疗时在所选部位的皮肤上涂少量凡士林，再放置艾炷点燃，当艾炷燃剩 2/5 左右，患者感觉疼痛时，用镊子将燃剩的艾炷夹去，置于污物盘内，换炷再灸。一般连续灸 3~7 壮，以患者局部皮肤充血、红晕，但以不起疱为度。

2. 间接灸　又称隔物灸，即在艾炷与施灸部位的皮肤之间，隔垫上某种物品而施灸的一种方法（图 6-17）。一般常用的有隔姜灸、隔蒜灸、隔盐灸和隔附子饼灸等。

（1）隔姜灸：是以生姜为间隔物而施灸的一种方法。临床常用于治疗虚寒性病证，如腹痛、泄泻、呕吐及痛经等。将生姜切成直径为 2~3cm，厚约 0.2~0.3cm 的薄片，中间以针刺上数孔。在所选部位的皮肤上涂少许凡士林，放上姜片，再将艾炷置于姜片上，点燃施灸。待艾炷燃尽后，除去灰烬，换炷再灸。一般灸 5~10 壮，以局部皮肤红晕，但以不起疱为度。

（2）隔蒜灸：是以大蒜片为间隔物而施

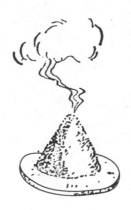

Fig. 6-17　Indirect Moxibustion
图 6-17　间接灸

mainly used to treat pulmonary tuberculosis and abscesses at the initial stage. Cut a slice of the garlic about 0.2-0.3cm thick, and puncture some holes in it. Smear a bit Vaseline on the selected point, and put garlic slice on the point. Then put the moxa cone on it and ignite the cone. When the first cone completely burns out, replace a new one and ignite it again for the second cone or *Zhuang*. Five to seven cones or *Zhuang* are needed for each point until the local skin becomes reddish without blister.

(3) Salt isolated moxibustion: This method is used to treat acute abdominal pain due to cold pathogen, vomiting, diarrhea, dysentery and flaccid pattern of stroke. RN 8 (shén què) is frequently used. Fill the umbilicus with salt, and put a piece of ginger with holes on the salt to prevent burning the patient. Then put the moxa cone on the ginger and ignite it. Replace a new one and ignite it again for the second cone or *Zhuang* when the first cone completely burns out. Continue to operate until symptoms are relieved. The number of cones or *Zhuang* is not limited.

(4) Aconite root cake isolated moxibustion: This method is used to treat diseases due to insufficiency of vital essence such as impotence, premature ejaculation and a ruptured abscess which are not healed for a long time. Grind a piece of aconite root into a fine powder, mix the powder with yellow rice wine into the paste, shape it into a cake 3cm in diameter and 0.8cm in thickness, and puncture some holes in it. Put a moxa cone on the aconite cake and ignite it. Replace a new one and ignite it again for the second cone or *Zhuang* when the first cone completely burns out and the ashes are removed. Five to seven cones or *Zhuang* are used per point.

ii. Moxibustion with Moxa Stick

A moxa stick is prepared by wrapping moxa-wool with a piece of Cortex Mori paper and shaping it into a cylinder. Ignite one end of the moxa stick and point it at the point or the diseased area. It can be divided into

灸的一种治疗方法。临床主要用于治疗肺结核及疮疡初期等病证。将大蒜头切成 0.2~0.3cm 的薄片，中间以针穿刺数孔。在所选部位的皮肤上涂少许凡士林，放上大蒜片，再将艾炷置于蒜片上，点燃施灸。待艾炷燃尽后，除去灰烬，换炷再灸。一般灸 5~7 壮，以局部皮肤红晕，但以不起疱为度。

（3）隔盐灸：是以盐为间隔物而施灸的一种治疗方法，常用于急性寒性腹痛、吐泻、痢疾以及中风脱证等证。一般多选用神阙穴。先用精盐将肚脐填平，在盐上放一中间刺数孔的姜片，以防食盐受热爆起而引起烫伤，再将艾炷置于姜片之上，点燃施灸。燃尽后，除去灰烬，易炷再灸，壮数不拘，直至病情缓解。

（4）隔附子饼灸：是以附子片或附子饼为间隔物而施灸的一种治疗方法，常用于治疗因命门火衰引起的阳痿、早泄、疮疡久溃不愈等证。将附子研成细末，用黄酒调合，制成直径为 3cm，厚约 0.8cm 的附子饼，中间用粗针刺数孔，上置艾炷，放于施灸部位上，点燃施灸。燃尽后，除去灰烬，易炷再灸，一般灸 5~7 壮。

（二）艾条灸

艾条灸是指用桑皮纸将纯净的艾绒（或加入中药）卷成圆柱形艾条，将其一端点燃，对准腧穴或患处施灸的一种方法。按照施灸

suspending moxibustion and pressing moxibustion.

1. Suspending Moxibustion　It can be further divided into mild moxibustion, sparrow-pecking moxibustion and circling moxibustion based on the ways of operation. Preparation includes treatment plate, moxa stick, lighter, tweezer, curve tray.

(1) Mild moxibustion: Prepare all materials for the patient, assist the patient to make the comfortable post and expose the operate region according to needed points which is based on the disease condition. Ignite one end of the moxa stick and keep it 2-3cm away from the skin. Patient should feel warm but without causalgia (Fig. 6-18). Each point should usually be heated for 10-15 minutes until the skin becomes reddish. The method is used to treat chronic diseases due to deficiency-cold, such as abdominal pain, dysmenorrhea and so on.

(2) Sparrow-pecking moxibustion: Prepare all materials for the patient, assist the patient to make the comfortable post and expose the operate region according to needed points which is based on the disease condition. Ignite one end of the moxa stick to warm the area. Move the ignited end up and down between 2 and 5cm as if a bird is pecking. Each point should usually be heated about 5 minutes (Fig. 6-19). This method is often used to treat acute diseases because the patient will have a stronger feeling of warmth.

时操作手法的不同，可分为悬起灸和实按灸。

1. **悬起灸**　按其操作方法又可分为温和灸、雀啄灸、回旋灸。用物包括治疗盘、艾条、打火机、镊子、清洁弯盘。

（1）温和灸：备齐用物，根据病情选取穴位，协助患者取合理舒适体位，暴露治疗部位，点燃艾条一端，一手持艾条与施灸部位皮肤保持 2~3cm 的距离进行持续熏灸，以患者局部皮肤有温热感而无灼痛感为宜（图 6-18）。一般每个部位灸 10~15min，直至局部皮肤红晕为度。临床常用于治疗慢性虚寒性疾病，如腹痛、痛经等。

（2）雀啄灸：备齐用物，根据病情选取穴位，协助患者取合理舒适体位，暴露治疗部位，点燃艾条一端，一手持艾条与施灸部位皮肤保持 2~5cm，像鸟雀啄食般一上一下不停移动，进行反复熏灸，一般每个部位灸 5min 左右（图 6-19）。此法温热感较强烈，常用于治疗急性病证。

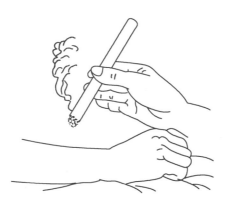

Fig. 6-18　Mild Moxibustion
图 6-18　温和灸

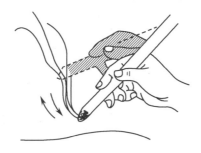

Fig. 6-19　Sparrow-pecking Moxibustion
图 6-19　雀啄灸

(3) Circling moxibustion: Prepare all materials for the patient, assistant the patient to make the comfortable post and expose the operate region according to needed points which is based on the disease condition. Ignite one end of the moxa stick, keep it about 3cm away from the skin and move it left and right or in a circular motion to warm the area. Each point should usually be heated for 20-30 minutes (Fig. 6-20). This method is often used to treat acute diseases.

These three methods mentioned above can be used alone or together.

2. Pressing Moxibustion　Place a piece of cloth or several layers of paper on the selected point, and then press the ignited end of the moxa stick onto the cloth or paper tightly until it is extinguished. Ignite and press it again (Fig. 6-21). This method is indicated for dual syndrome of wind-cold-dampness and deficiency-cold.

iii. Warming-needle Moxibustion

It is a method that combines acupuncture with moxibustion and conducts the heat from the ignited moxa into the body through the needle body to strengthen the curative effect of acupuncture (Fig. 6-22). It is usually used to treat diseases that need stimulation of both needle and moxibustion, such as rheumatism and pain syndrome due to wind-cold pathogen.

（3）回旋灸：备齐用物，根据病情选取穴位，协助患者取合理舒适体位，暴露治疗部位，点燃艾条一端，在距离施灸部位皮肤约3cm处，左右来回或旋转移动，进行反复熏灸，一般每个部位可灸20~30min。临床常用于治疗急性病证（图6-20）。

以上三种方法，可单独使用，亦可混合使用。

2. 实按灸　施灸时，先在施灸腧穴或患处垫上布或纸数层。然后将艾条的一端点燃后按到施术部位上，使热力透达深部。若艾火熄灭，再点再按（图6-21）。其适用于风寒湿痹和虚寒证。

（三）温针灸

温针灸是将毫针刺法与灸法相结合的一种治疗方法，使艾绒燃烧的热力，通过毫针针身传入患者体内而增加针刺的疗效。临床常用于治疗风湿、风寒痹痛等证（图6-22）。

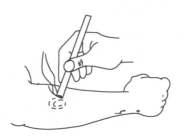

Fig. 6-20　Circling Moxibustion
图6-20　回旋灸

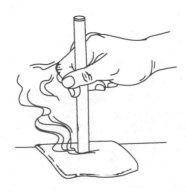

Fig. 6-21　Pressing Moxibustion
图6-21　实按灸

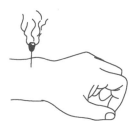

Fig. 6-22 Warming-needle Moxibustion
图 6-22 温针灸

1. Preparation sterile needles, sterile swabs, skin disinfectant short moxa strick or moxa cone, lighter, tweezer, paper, *etc.*.

2. Manipulation Selection of points is according to disease condition. And then, assist the patient to make a comfortable and reasonable position and expose the treatment region. Finally, implement acupuncture until the patient get the arrival of qi. During the retaining of the needle with needling sensation, affix a 3-5cm moxa stick to the needle handle or place a little moxa-wool onto the needle handle and ignite it. Put paper on the patient's skin around the needle to prevent scalding. Replace a new one and ignite it again for the second cone when the first cone completely burns out. Two to five cones are used per point. After the moxa cone burns out and the ashes are removed, withdraw the needle and press the pinhole with the sterile cotton swab for a while.

iv. Moxibustion with Moxa Burner

The moxa burner is a kind of moxibustion that utilizes a special utensil (such as moxibustion box, moxibustion frame, moxibustion cylinder) to implement operation. The moxa or moxa stick is ignited and put into the moxa burner. Then place the burner on the selected point until the local skin becomes congested and reddish and the patient feel warm but without causalgia (Fig. 6-23). The operation is so easy to be done alone.

v. Natural Moxibustion

It is also known as drug moxibustion or vesiculate moxibustion. It is a sort of moxibustion therapy that spreads some irritant herbs on the selected point to induce blisters and inflammation, so that it adjusts qi and blood to prevent diseases. There are several tens species herbs to be used, of which some are single herbs or combination drugs, such as mustard seed, asarum, Rhizoma Arisaematis, garlic, *etc.*. Moxibustion with mashed garlic and *bái jiè zǐ* seed are commonly used.

1. Moxibustion with Mashed Garlic Take 3-5g of mashed garlic and apply it on the selected point for 1-3 hours until the local skin is itching, flushed and

1. 用物准备 治疗盘内备无菌毫针、无菌棉签、皮肤消毒液、短艾条或艾炷、打火机、清洁弯盘、镊子、纸片等。

2. 操作方法 根据病情选取穴位，协助患者取舒适合理体位，暴露治疗部位，按毫针刺法进行针刺，得气后将事先准备好的艾条（将艾条剪成 3~5cm）插在针柄上，或将艾炷捏在针柄上点燃，直到燃尽为止。根据具体情况，易炷再灸。一般可连续灸 2~5 壮。施灸完毕，除去艾灰，起出毫针，用无菌棉签轻按针孔片刻。注意在治疗期间，可将大小合适较厚的纸片剪至中心，夹在毫针周围，以接住脱落的艾灰，避免烫伤患者。

（四）温灸器灸

温灸器灸是借用施灸的特制器具，实施灸法。临床常用的有灸盒灸、灸架灸、灸筒灸。操作时，将点燃艾条段或艾绒置于器具中，灸至患者有温热舒适无灼痛的感觉，皮肤稍有红晕为度，使用方便，可独自一人操作（图 6-23 ）。

（五）天灸

天灸又称药物灸、发泡灸。即将一些具有刺激性的药物，涂敷于穴位或患处，使局部皮肤发红充血，甚至起疱，以激发经络、调整气血而防治疾病的一种灸疗法。所用药物多是单味中药，也有用复方，其常用的有白芥子灸、细辛灸、天南星灸、蒜泥灸等数十种。常用的有蒜泥灸和白芥子灸等。

1. 蒜泥灸 将大蒜捣烂如泥，取 3~5g 贴敷于穴位上，敷灸 1~3min，以局部皮肤发痒

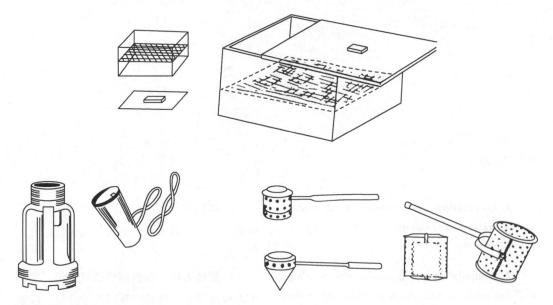

Fig. 6-23   Moxibustion with Moxa Burner
图 6-23   温灸器灸

blistered. This moxibustion on KI 1 (*yǒng quán*) and LI 4 (*hé gǔ*) can respectively treat hemoptysis and tonsillitis.

2. Moxibustion with White Mustard Seed

Grind a certain amount of white mustard seed into fine powder and mix it with water to make a paste. Then apply it on the selected point, cover it with oiled paper and affix it with adhesive plaster. This method is usually used to treat arthralgia. It can be combined with other medication to treat asthma as well.

Natural moxibustion has better curative effect, but it is avoided using to treat pregnant woman, elderly and weak patients, patients whose skin is easy to be allergic. Because all of medicines have strong stimulation to the skin, even some toxic effects. The patients feel mild causalgia in the local area which is normal after pasting medicines. Remove the medicines after one to three hours. If the patients feel serious causalgia, remove it immediately. If the local skin becomes blister, burn ointment should be smeared. During the day of receiving treatment, one should not eat the food which is coldness in property and pungent in flavor, and should take bath with warm water, avoid touching cold water and using cold compress.

Box 6-3 Learning more

San Fu Tian Jiu, San Jiu Tian Jiu

San Fu Tian Jiu means natural moxibustion in dog days, namely, on the hottest summer days. San Jiu Tian Jiu means nature moxibustion in the coldest days of winter, namely, the third nine-day period after the winter solstice. It is recorded in the The Yellow Emperor's Inner Classic that

发红起疱为度。如敷涌泉穴可治疗咯血，敷合谷穴可治疗扁桃体炎等。

2. 白芥子灸 将适量白芥子研成细末，用水调和成糊状，贴敷于腧穴或患处，敷以油纸，胶布固定。一般可用于治疗关节痹痛，或配合其他药物治疗哮喘等证。

天灸疗法有较好的效果，但所用中药有些为有毒之品，对皮肤有强烈的刺激作用，故孕妇、年老体弱、皮肤过敏者等应慎用或禁用。另外，贴药处避免挤压，贴药后局部皮肤有轻度灼热感，属正常现象，一般1~3min后可将药物自行除去，切忌贴药时间过长。如贴药后，局部灼热难受，可提前除去。贴药后局部起水疱可涂烫伤软膏、万花油。贴药当日禁食生冷、寒凉、辛辣之物，并用温水洗澡，忌用冷水、冷敷。

知识拓展 6-3

三伏天灸，三九天灸

三伏天灸是利用一年中阳气最盛的三伏天，人体内阳气也相对充沛，应用具有温经、散寒、补虚、助阳的中药，通过辨证分析后，选择相应的穴位进行贴敷治疗，可祛除体内

yang qi is the strongest in the dog days and is weakest in the third nine-day period after the winter solstice in nature. Yin-yang in human body rise and fall corresponding to changes of nature. In order to reinforce yang qi and dispel wind-cold-dampness pathogen, it applies some traditional Chinese medicines which have the characteristics of warming channels, dispersing the coldness, supporting yang, reinforcing deficiency on the selected points by differentiation of syndrome in the periods. San Jiu Tian Jiu can consolidate and complement effects of San Fu Tian Jiu. They are the most representative methods that are based on the principle of "nourishing yang in spring and summer while nourishing yin in autumn and winter".

风寒湿邪。

三九天灸是利用一年中最冷的时候，此时进行贴敷穴位，起到温阳益气，祛风散寒的功效。因此冬天进行三九天灸巩固三伏天灸疗效，是对三伏天灸的有效延续和补充。

"三伏天灸，三九天灸"是运用"春夏养阳，冬病夏治"理论最具代表性的方法。

V. Sequence of Moxibustion

In general, the order of moxibustion is supposed to follow the principle to operate as below: the upper first and then lowers of body part, from the yang meridians to the yin meridians, back and waist first, and then chest and abdomen, head and trunk, and limbs finally. The amount of moxa cones is at first few and then gradually increased. The size of moxa cone is small at first and then large step by step. The use is adjustable in case of special clinical situation.

五、施灸的先后顺序

施灸顺序一般是先上后下，先灸背部，后灸胸腹部，先灸头、躯干部，后灸四肢。临床上如遇特殊情况也应灵活变用，应因人因病而宜。

VI. Precaution

1. Make explanation to the patient before treatment and help the patient to take a comfortable posture to prevent scalding due to change of posture during the treatment.

2. Pay attention to ask and observe the patient's feeling and reaction during the treatment. Once the moxibustion syncope happened, the operation should be stopped immediately and it should let the patient lie down with head down. Mild cases will get well after taking a break or drinking warm water. Serious cases can be administrated by pinching strong certain points such as DU 26 (*shuǐ gōu*, also called *rén zhōng*), PC 6 (*nèi guān*) and ST 36 (*zú sān lǐ*). Other first-aid methods should be applied as occasion requires.

3. When moxibustion with moxa stick is operated on the elderly, infants and patients with sensation disorder, the operator should use his index and middle fingers to put both sides of the point respectively to feel the temperature and adjust the distance between the burning moxa and the patient's skin in time in order to avoid scalding. During

六、注意事项

1. 施灸前应向患者做好解释，并协助患者摆好体位，避免患者因疲劳而移动体位，造成烫伤。

2. 施灸过程中要密切观察患者的病情及对施灸的反应。若发生晕灸应立即停止艾灸，使患者头低位平卧，注意保暖，轻者一般休息片刻，或饮温开水后即可恢复；重者可掐按人中、内关、足三里即可恢复；严重时按晕厥处理。

3. 施灸的患者如是皮肤感觉迟钝或小儿、老年人等，施术者可将拇、示二指或示、中二指，置于施灸部位两侧，通过施术者的手指来感知患者局部的受热程度，以便及时调节施灸距离，防止烫伤皮肤。如是隔姜灸时，

indirect moxibustion, it should raise or move the isolator such as ginger and garlic, when patients have intolerable causalgia.

4. Remove the ashes in time to prevent scalding. Put the ash in the disc where there is some water to avoid burning again.

5. If the patient's skin appears to be red or the patient feels a little burning pain, it is normal and it does not need to be managed. The liquid in small blisters can be absorbed by the body. If the blister is large, the liquid can be suck out by a sterile syringe. The area needs to be covered with sterile gauze to prevent infection.

(Yang Liu)

Section 4   Cupping Therapy

Cupping is a kind of therapy that a jar is attached to the skin surface using negative pressure brought by means of suction or inducing a flame into the cup so as to form a local congestion or blood stagnation to prevent or treat diseases. It is also called "horn" method, for the buffalo horn is most used as a cup in the ancient time. Cupping therapy is time-honored. It is recorded in the *Formulas for Fifty-two Diseases* (*Wǔ Shí èr Bìng Fāng*, 五十二病方), one of the silk books excavated from the Han Tombs of *Ma Wang Dui* of Changsha in China. Cupping therapy is widely used in clinic and community due to its simple administration and prominent effects.

I. Indication

Cupping therapy can free channels and collaterals, dispel wind and scatter cold, relieve swelling and pain, suck toxin and evacuate purulence. It is often used in clinical practice to treat headache, dizziness and general discomfort caused by wind and cold pathogen, arthralgia, limb numbness and ache on the waist and back due to wind-cold-dampness pathogen, cough, asthma, acute sprains, snakebite, *etc.*.

II. Contraindication

1. Don't do cupping for the patient with severe heart

患者感觉灼热不可忍受时，可将姜片向上提起，或缓慢移动姜片。

4. 及时除去灰烬，防止烫伤皮肤。污物盘内可盛少许水，将燃剩的艾灰放入，以防复燃。

5. 施灸后如局部皮肤出现潮红或有灼热感，属正常现象，无须处理。如灸后局部起疱，小者可自行吸收，较大的水疱可用无菌注射器抽出液体，用无菌纱布覆盖，防止感染。

（杨柳）

第四节　拔罐法

拔罐法是指以罐为工具，借助抽吸或燃烧热力，排除罐内空气，使之形成负压，将罐吸附于需施治部位的体表或腧穴上，使局部皮肤充血、瘀血，以达到防治疾病目的的一种方法，亦称"吸筒法"。因古时多用牛角作为拔罐工具，故又称"角法"。拔罐法历史悠久，早在马王堆汉墓出土之帛书《五十二病方》中就有记载。因其操作简单、疗效显著，目前被临床和社区广泛使用。

一、适应证

拔罐法具有通经活络、祛风散寒、消肿止痛、吸毒排脓等功效。临床常用于治疗外感风寒之头痛、头晕、全身不适等，风寒湿痹导致的关节疼痛、腰背酸痛、四肢麻木等，虚寒性咳喘，胃肠功能失调，亦可用于处理软组织的闪挫扭伤以及毒蛇咬伤等。

二、禁忌证

1. 严重心脏病、心力衰竭、呼吸衰竭、

disease, heart failure, respiratory failure or severe edema.

2. Don't do cupping for the patient with clotting disorder, spontaneous bleeding tendency or bleeding after injury, such as hemophilia, purpura, leukemia, *etc.*.

3. Don't do cupping in the abdominal or lumbosacral region, or breasts of the pregnant women. The manipulation should also be gentle when cupping for the patients.

4. Don't apply cupping to the areas containing an allergic reaction, ulcers, edema or the regions where large blood vessels are distributed.

5. Don't apply cupping to the part that is uneven or hairy, .the facial parts, the genitalia or the anus.

6. Don't do cupping for the one with severe nervousness, after drinking, extreme tired, excessive eating, over-thirst or defatigation.

7. Don't do cupping for the patient with active pulmonary tuberculosis, or the women in their menstrual period.

III. Type of the Cup

At present, bamboo cup, pottery cup, glass cup and piston air-sucking cup are mainly used in clinical practice. The glass cup is the most commonly used. The advantages and disadvantages of these four types of cup are described in table 6-14.

1. Bamboo Cup　It is a cup made of a jointed section of bamboo. The bamboo cup is 3-5cm in diameter, and 6-10cm in length. The rim of the cup should be smooth and polished. It is suitable for boiling in a medicinal liquid. It can be disinfected by boiling.

2. Pottery Cup　It is made from pottery. The characteristics of the pottery cup are following: large belly, a slightly small mouth, and the bottom looks like a drum. The pottery cup can be disinfected by boiling or soaking in disinfector.

3. Glass Cup　Glass cup is the most commonly used in clinical practice. It's made of glass, and looks like a ball with smooth opening. It has a variety of sizes. It can be disinfected by boiling or soaking in disinfector.

4. Sucking Cup　It is made of transparent plastic with a piston inside. The suction is created for drawing the air out by moving the piston upwards. It can be disinfected by soaking in disinfector.

重度水肿者不宜拔罐。

2. 高热抽搐及凝血机制障碍，有自发性出血倾向或损伤后出血不止的患者，如血友病、紫癜、白血病等，不宜拔罐。

3. 经期妇女、孕妇腹部和腰骶部及乳部均不宜拔罐，拔其他部位时，手法也应轻柔。

4. 治疗局部的皮肤如有过敏、溃疡不宜拔罐。

5. 骨骼凹凸不平、毛发较多、有大血管的分布的部位，以及五官和前后二阴部位不宜拔罐。

6. 精神紧张、疲劳、饮酒后，以及过饥、过饱、烦渴、过劳时不宜拔罐。

7. 活动性肺结核患者不宜拔罐。

三、罐的种类

目前临床使用的罐具主要有竹罐、陶罐、玻璃罐及抽气罐，其中以玻璃罐最为常用。四种罐具的优、缺点见表6-14。

1. **竹罐**　竹罐是用直径为3~5cm、坚固无损的竹子，截成6~10cm不同长度，一端留节作底，另一端作罐口，并用砂纸磨光而成。适于水（药）煮，用后可煮沸消毒。

2. **陶罐**　陶罐是用陶土烧制而成，罐的两端较小，中间略向外凸出，状如腰鼓，底平，口径大小不一。用后可煮沸消毒或用消毒剂浸泡消毒。

3. **玻璃罐**　玻璃罐是临床较为常用的拔罐器具，用玻璃制成，形如球状，罐口平滑，有大、中、小三种类型。用后煮沸或用消毒剂浸泡消毒。

4. **抽气罐**　用透明塑料制成，顶部设置活塞，便于抽气。用后可用消毒液浸泡消毒。

Table 6-14　Comparison of the Four Types of Cup

Types of cup	Advantages	Disadvantages
Bamboo cup	Easily-made, light, cheap and durable	Crack and leak the air out easily, weak suction, opaque and skin reactions can not be observed
Pottery cup	strong suction, economical and easy to keep	Heavier and easily broken
Glass cup	Transparent, skin reactions can be observed and the time during which the cup is retained can be controlled	Fast heat conduction causing the possibility of scalding and easily broken
Sucking cup	Convenient and safe, difficult to break, suction can be adjusted, skin reactions can be observed and the time during which the cup is retained can be controlled	No warm feeling and can not be used in sliding cupping

表 6-14　四种罐具的比较

罐的种类	优点	缺点
竹罐	取材容易，制作简单，轻巧价廉，不易破碎	易爆裂、漏气、吸附力不大，不透明，无法观察罐内皮肤的变化
陶罐	吸附力强，造价低，容易保管	较重，易碎，不透明，无法观察罐内皮肤的变化
玻璃罐	质地透明，使用时可直接观察局部皮肤的变化情况，便于掌握留罐时间	传热较快而易烫伤，易破碎
抽气罐	使用方便安全且不易破碎，可随意调节吸附力，便于观察吸附部位皮肤的充血情况，便于掌握拔罐时间	无温热感，不能用于走罐等手法

IV. Cup-Sucking Method

Cup-sucking method means adopting a certain way to expel air in the cup to create negative pressure, so that the cup is attached tightly to the skin. The common methods used to attach the cup onto the body are fire cupping, water cupping and sucking cupping.

i. Fire Cupping

Fire cupping is used to expel air in the cup by a flame to create suction and attach the cup to the skin. The methods include flash-flame cupping, flame-casting cupping, cotton-sticking cupping and alcohol-dripping cupping.

1. Flash-flame Cupping　Hold a cup with appropriate size by one hand, and ignite a 95% alcohol-soaked cotton ball held with forceps by the other hand. Put the flame quickly into the cup and take it out after circling it inside once or twice. Place the cup on the patient's skin quickly (Fig. 6-24). This is a safe and the most common way. Do not keep the flame at the opening of the cup and avoid heating the opening of the cup, which is leading to

四、罐的吸附方法

罐的吸附方法是指采用一定的方法排除罐内空气，使之形成负压，吸附于需拔罐局部的方法。目前常用的有火吸法、水吸法和抽气吸法三种。

（一）火吸法

火吸法是指利用燃烧时火的热力排除罐内空气，形成负压，将罐吸附于治疗部位的皮肤上。吸附方法有闪火法、投火法、贴棉法和滴酒法。

1. **闪火法**　操作者一手持大小适宜的罐具，另一手用止血钳夹紧 95% 的乙醇棉球，点燃后尽快伸入罐内，在罐壁中段绕 1~2 圈后立即退出，同时迅速将罐扣在所拔部位的皮肤上（图 6-24）。此种点火方法比较安全，也是临床最常用的点火方法。需要注意的是点

the burns of skin.

2. Flame-casting Cupping   Put an ignited 95% alcohol-soaked cotton ball into the cup, and then place the cup on to the skin. This method is suitable for transverse cupping (Fig. 6-25).

3. Cotton-sticking cupping   Stick a piece of 95% alcohol-soaked cotton ball onto the lower inner wall of the cup, ignite it and place the cup rapidly onto the skin.

4. Alcohol-dripping cupping   Drip 1-3 drops of 95% alcohol into the cup, shake the cup in order to make the alcohol spread evenly along the wall of the cup, ignite the alcohol, and then swiftly place the cup onto the skin.

ii. Water Cupping

Water cupping is used to expel air inside the cup by the water vapor with high temperature to create suction, and attach the cup to the skin. It is also named cup-boiling method. Boil the bamboo cup in boiling water or medicinal water for 5-10 minutes. Take it out with a long forceps and pour the excess liquid out with the opening of the cup downward. Cover the opening with a cold wet towel and place the cup on the skin.

燃的乙醇棉球应尽快伸入罐内中部，不要在罐口停留，以免将罐口烧热，引起烫伤。

2. 投火法   将 95% 的乙醇棉球或纸片点燃后投入罐内，迅速将罐扣在应拔部位。此法适用于身体侧面横位拔罐（图 6-25）。

3. 贴棉法   用浸有 95% 乙醇的一小块棉花，平贴于罐内壁的上中段，点燃后迅速扣在需拔罐的部位。

4. 滴酒法   在火罐内滴入 95% 的乙醇 1~3 滴，使其均匀地布于罐壁，点燃后迅速扣在需拔罐的部位。

（二）水吸法

水吸法又称煮罐法，是指利用高温的水排出罐内空气，使之形成负压，并将罐吸附于局部皮肤的一种方法。可以用水，亦可以用中药汤剂煮罐，临床多用竹罐。将大小适宜的竹罐投入沸水或药液中煮 5~10min，用长镊子夹住罐底，使罐口朝下，甩去罐内剩余的水分，立即用湿冷毛巾紧扣罐口，再迅速

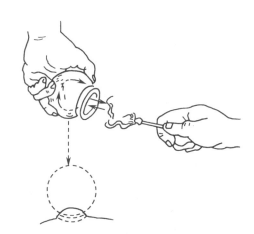

Fig. 6-24   Flash-flame Cupping
图 6-24   闪火法

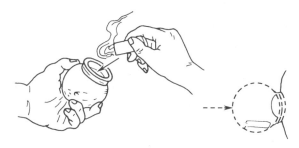

Fig. 6-25   Flame-casting Cupping
图 6-25   投火法

iii. Sucking Cupping

Place the cup tightly on the skin, and draw out the air by pulling the piston so as to form the negative pressure in the cup. After firmly absorbed, the smoke vent of the cup can be taken out and the valve should be closed. The cup can be attached onto the skin.

V. Method for Removing Cup

When local skin of cupping turns red or ecchymosis appears after certain time of cupping, the cups can be removed. The attached cup should be removed by holding it aslant with one hand and pressing the skin around the cup with the thumb or index finger of the other hand to let air in (Fig. 6-26). When the attached cup is removed automatically, remove the screw cap on the gas-mouth first, and then pull out the valve core to let air in. Do not remove the cup with force, which may cause pain or local skin injury.

VI. Manipulation

Here, take flash-fire cupping as an example to introduce preparation and process of operation.

i. Preparation

1. Patient Preparation Check the patients' name, bed number and the area needed cupping. Assess the patient's condition, medical history, hypoesthesia or obstacles, tolerance to pain, psychological status and local skin conditions. Explain the purpose, the main steps, key points and related matters, the effects and adverse reactions of cupping to the patient, in order to obtain consents of the patient and/or their families. Help the patient to apply

将罐扣在需拔罐的部位上。

（三）抽气吸法

此法是指将负压吸引罐扣于局部皮肤上，将抽气筒连接罐顶部抽气活塞，抽出罐内的空气，使之形成负压，待吸牢后，将抽气筒取下，关闭气门，使罐吸附于需施治的部位上。

五、起罐方法

待拔罐局部皮肤出现明显瘀斑或留罐时间已到，即可起罐。手工起罐时，操作者先用一手提罐使其稍倾斜，另一手的拇指或示指按压罐口皮肤，待空气进入罐内，即可取下（图6-26）。自动起罐时，先卸掉气嘴上的螺丝帽，再抽气门芯，使空气进入罐内，把罐拿下即可。不可强行上提或旋转提拔，以免引起疼痛或损伤局部的皮肤。

六、火罐操作法

（一）操作前准备

1. **患者准备** 核对患者姓名、床号、拔罐部位等；评估患者的病情、既往史、有无感觉迟钝或障碍、对疼痛的耐受程度及心理状况、局部皮肤情况；向患者解释操作目的、主要步骤、配合要点以及相关事项，说明拔罐的作用及可能出现的不良反应，以取得患者和/或家

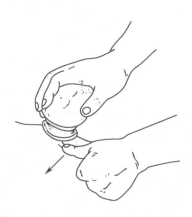

Fig. 6-26　Method for Removing Cups
图6-26　起罐方法

a safe and comfortable position according to their disease. Ask the patient to empty stool and urine.

2. Material Preparation Prepare cups, 95% ethanol immersed swab, lighter, forceps, clean disc, large towel and screens. Prepare Vaseline when planning to use the method of moving cupping.

3. Environment Preparation Environment should be well-lit, quiet and clean. Suitable temperature. Non-flammable materials.

4. Operator Preparation The operator should be well-groomed, hand washed and wear masks.

ii. Procedure of Operation

1. Explain the purpose and notice of the operation. Check medical order again.

2. Choose points according to patient condition. Help the patient to apply a comfortable position, expose the area where needs treatment, and keep warm for patients.

3. Choose a suitable cup. Check whether the edge of the opening is smooth.

4. Choose the method to fire and attach the cup against the skin. The operation should be done steadily, correctly and swiftly to prevent burns.

5. Retain the cup for 10-15 minutes. Pay attention to the adsorption of the cup, condition of the skin and general condition of the patient while retaining the cup.

6. Remove cup, wipe off the dirty, help the patient get dressed, and apply a comfortable position.

7. Tidy up, wash the hands, and take a record.

VII. Clinical Application

i. Retaining Cupping

Attach the cup onto the skin and retain it for 10-15 minutes. Remove the cup when the local skin becomes reddish or forms blood stagnation. If the cup is large and the suction is strong, the time of retaining cupping should be properly shortened to avoid forming blisters. This method can be applied to all kinds of diseases. Retaining cupping can be divided into a single-cup or multi-cup retaining based on the number of cups. This method is suitable for a variety of ailments, mainly for diseases caused

属对执行该操作的知情同意；根据病情协助患者取安全舒适的体位；嘱患者排空大、小便。

2. 用物准备 治疗盘内放罐具（根据所拔部位选择大、中、小罐具及数量，并检查罐口边缘是否光滑、有无裂缝）、95% 乙醇棉球或纸片、打火机、止血钳、小口瓶（内盛少许水）、大毛巾、屏风等，如为走罐，则需另备凡士林或按摩乳。

3. 环境准备 环境应光线充足、安静整洁、温度适宜，无易燃物品。

4. 操作者准备 操作者应仪表整洁，洗手，戴口罩。

（二）操作步骤

1. 备齐用物，携至患者床旁，解释操作时注意事项，再次核对医嘱。

2. 根据病情，协助患者取合理舒适体位，暴露拔罐部位，注意保暖。

3. 选择大小合适的罐具，再次检查罐口边缘是否光滑。

4. 用闪火法将罐吸附于局部皮肤上，动作要稳、准、轻、快，防止烫伤。

5. 留罐 10~15min。留罐过程中，注意观察火罐吸附情况、局部皮肤颜色变化及患者的全身情况。

6. 起罐，擦去污渍，协助患者穿衣，取舒适体位。

7. 整理用物，洗手，记录。

七、拔罐法的临床应用

（一）留罐

留罐是指待罐吸牢后，将罐留置 10~15min，待被拔部位出现潮红，皮下出现瘀血时即可起罐。如果罐体较大，吸附力较强时，可适当缩短留罐时间，以免局部皮肤起疱。此法较为常用，一般疾病均可使用。留罐法又根据罐具多少分为单罐留罐法和多罐留罐法。留罐法主要用于寒邪引发的疾患及脏腑

by pathogenic cold and visceral lesions, such as pathogenic factors invading in meridian, blood stasis, exogenous cold, numbness, indigestion and so on.

ii. Flashing Cupping

It refers to attach and remove the cup quickly and repeatedly until the skin turns reddish, congested or stagnated. It has a certain excitatory effect on the nerves. This method is usually indicated for local numbness and pain, and used on patients with the symptoms such as muscle atrophy, skin numbness, hypothyroidism weakness and stroke sequelae, who cannot accept retaining cupping.

iii. Moving Cupping

Smear some unguent or Vaseline to the treated area, and attach the cup onto the skin. Hold the body of the cup with one hand. Move it up and down or left and right. Remove the cup when the skin becomes reddish, congested and stagnated (Fig. 6-27). This method is suitable for the places of large area and the regions with thick muscles, such as the back, waist, buttocks and thighs. Select the cup whose opening is large, smooth and polished. Moving cupping is mainly used for acute heat syndromes, paralysis, numbness, *Bi* syndrome due to wind-cold-dampness, muscular atrophy, *etc.*.

iv. Pricking and Cupping

This method is a combination of pricking to bleed and cupping. Firstly, carefully disinfect the area to be treated. Prick the points with a three-edged needle to induce bleeding, and then attach the cup to the appropriate points. This is a way to strengthen the effects of the blood-letting. The standards of light, moderate and heavy prick are that the skin becomes reddish, minor bleeding or spot bleeding, respectively. It is indicated for acute or chronic soft tissue injury, neurodermatitis, pruritus, erysipelas, neurasthenia, gastrointestinal neurosis, and so on.

的病变，如经络受邪、气血瘀滞、外感风寒、肢体麻木和消化不良等。

（二）闪罐

闪罐是指将罐拔住后立即起下，反复多次地拔上、起下，直至皮肤潮红为度，为"留 - 拔 - 留"的循环手法。闪罐法对神经有一定的兴奋作用，多适用于局部麻木、疼痛等证或不易留罐的患者，如肌肉痿软、皮肤麻木、功能减退的虚弱病证及中风后遗症等。

（三）走罐

走罐是指先在罐口或预拔部位涂一些润滑油或凡士林，再将罐拔住，用手握住罐体，进行上下或左右往返推移，直至所拔部位皮肤出现红润、充血或瘀血时，将罐起下（图6-27）。一般适用于面积较大、肌肉丰厚的部位，如背部、腰臀部以及大腿部等。常选用罐口口径较大，且罐口较圆滑的玻璃罐。可用于治疗急性热病、瘫痪麻木、风湿痹证及肌肉萎缩等病证。

（四）刺血拔罐

此法是将拔罐与刺血疗法配合应用的一种方法。将应拔罐部位的皮肤消毒后，用三棱针点刺出血或用皮肤针叩打后，再将火罐吸拔于点刺的部位上，使之出血，以加强放血治疗的作用。针刺的力度是：轻刺以皮肤出现红晕为标准；中刺是以轻微出血为准；重刺以点状出血为准。刺血拔罐多用于治疗急、慢性软组织损伤、神经性皮炎、皮肤瘙

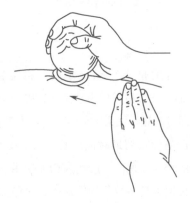
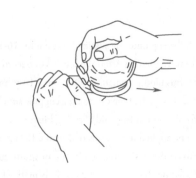

Fig. 6-27 Moving Cupping
图6-27 走罐

v. Needle-Retaining Cupping

This method is a combination of acupuncture and cupping. Insert the needles into the selected acupoints, and then attach a cup to the area around one or more of the retained needles and keep the needles inside the cup. Remove the cup and needles after 5-10 minutes, or when the localized skin becomes reddish, congested or extravasated (Fig. 6-28).

VIII. Precaution

1. Cupping should be applied to the areas with thick muscles. Help the patient to take a comfortable posture.

2. Select the cup with proper size according to the treated area. Equipment needs to be disinfected. Pay attention to examine whether the opening of the cup is smooth and whether there are cracks.

3. The operation should be done steadily, correctly and swiftly in order to attach the cup tightly.

4. Pay attention to ask the feeling of the patient, and observe the reaction of the local skin during the treatment. Remove and attach the cup again when the patient has the feeling of heat, tightness, ache, pain in the treated area.

5. Help the patient to cover the cloth and quilt to keep warm during the retaining cupping. Do not remove the cup with force, which may cause local skin injury.

6. The cupping procedure should be done with great care in order to avoid burning the skin. If a few small blisters appear due to excessive burning or prolonged cup retention, it should cover them with sterilized gauze to protect the area and avoid infection. If the blisters are large, they may be pricked. The liquid in the blisters can be drawn out by syringe, and the local position should be covered with sterilized gauze to avoid infection.

7. Observe whether the patient has the reaction of cupping syncope. When the patient suddenly presents symptoms of dizziness, nausea, pale complexion, *etc.*, it should stop cupping immediately, and remove all the cups.

痒、丹毒、神经衰弱、胃肠神经官能症等。

（五）留针拔罐

此法是将针刺与拔罐相结合应用的一种方法。即先选定穴位、然后对其进行针刺，待得气后留针时，将罐拔在以针为中心的部位上，留置 10~15min，待皮肤红润、充血或瘀血时，起罐、起针（图 6-28）。

八、拔罐法的注意事项

1. 拔罐时要选择肌肉丰厚的部位和舒适合理的体位。

2. 根据所拔部位选择大小适宜的罐，器具均需消毒，注意检查罐口是否边缘平滑、无裂缝。

3. 拔罐时动作要稳、准、快，才能使罐拔紧，吸附有力。

4. 拔罐过程中注意询问患者的感觉，观察局部皮肤情况。当患者感觉所拔部位发热、发紧、发酸、疼痛、灼热时，应取下重拔。

5. 留罐时应帮助患者盖好衣被以保暖，起罐时切勿强拉或扭转，以免损伤皮肤。

6. 拔火罐或水罐时要避免灼伤或烫伤皮肤。若烫伤或留罐时间过长而皮肤出现小水疱时，可外敷无菌纱布加以保护，防止水疱被擦破感染；水疱较大时应经消毒后用无菌注射器将渗液抽出，再用无菌纱布覆盖以防感染。

7. 注意有无晕罐先兆。当患者出现头晕、恶心、面色苍白等晕罐反应时，应立即停止拔罐，将罐具全部起下。使患者平卧，注意

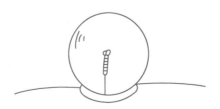

Fig. 6-28　Needle-Retaining Cupping
图 6-28　留针拔罐

Help the patient to lie on supine posture and keep his or her body warm. In minor cases, ask the patient to have a rest, and give him or her some warm water or sugar water to drink. The symptoms will be removed shortly. For severe cases, inform the doctor and give remedy to the patient according to the symptoms.

(Yang Jin-hua)

保暖，待轻者仰卧片刻，饮温开水或糖水后，即可恢复正常。重者可通知医生并对症处理。

（杨金花）

Section 5　Scraping Therapy

Scraping therapy is a method to scrape repeatedly on the skin of certain parts of the human body with the dull and smoothly edged instrument so as to form a local congestion or blood stagnation to prevent or treat diseases. Through scrapping, interstices can be free. The evil qi of viscera can be easily expelled from the skin and muscles. The blood and qi of the whole body can be quickly free-flowing, so that the therapeutic effects can be obtained. Furthermore, scraping therapy can dredge the meridians, reestablish the harmony of nutritive qi and defensive qi, and harmonize *zang-fu* organs, so as to achieve the purpose of health care.

I. Indication

1. Exogenous diseases　Such as high fever, headache, nausea, vomiting due to exogenous dampness pathogen, and heatstroke, bellyache, diarrhea caused by exogenous summer-dampness pathogen.

2. Internal diseases　Such as stomach pain, headache, dizziness, insomnia, constipation, cough, rheumatism, *etc.*.

3. Surgical diseases　Such as pain in waist and lower limbs, stiff neck, cervical disease, *etc.*.

4. Gynecological Diseases　Such as irregular menstruation, dysmenorrhea, amenorrhea, breast hyperplasia, postpartum hypogalactia, *etc.*.

5. Pediatric disease　Such as malnutrition, indigestion, colds, fever, diarrhea, *etc.*.

6. Ears, nose and throat diseases　Such as toothache, sore throat, sinusitis, myopia, deafness, tinnitus, *etc.*.

7. Others　Such as beauty the features and skin care, *etc.*.

第五节　刮痧法

刮痧法是指用边缘钝滑的器具，在人体一定部位的皮肤上反复刮动，使局部皮下出现痧斑或痧痕，以达到防治疾病目的的一种方法。通过刮痧，一方面可疏通腠理，使脏腑秽浊之气通达于外，促使周身气血流畅，逐邪外出，达到治病的目的；另一方面疏通经络，通调营卫，和谐脏腑，从而达到保健的目的。

一、适应证

1. **外感疾病**　外感湿邪所致的高热、头痛、恶心、呕吐及外感暑湿所致的中暑、腹痛、腹泻等证。

2. **内科疾病**　胃痛、头痛、眩晕、失眠、便秘、咳嗽、风湿痹痛等。

3. **外科疾病**　腰腿痛、落枕、颈椎病等。

4. **妇科疾病**　月经不调、痛经、闭经、乳腺增生、产后缺乳等。

5. **儿科疾病**　疳证、积滞、小儿感冒发热、腹泻等。

6. **五官科疾病**　牙痛、咽喉肿痛、鼻渊、近视、耳聋、耳鸣等。

7. **其他**　用于养颜美容、消斑除痘。

II. Contraindication

1. Avoid using scraping for the patients with severe or life-threatening diseases, such as acute infectious disease, severe heart disease or liver and kidney dysfunction, *etc.*.

2. Avoid using scraping for the patients with bleeding tendency, such as thrombopenia or dysfunction of coagulation, *etc.*.

3. Avoid using scraping at areas with skin ulcers, sores, scalding, acute sprain, recent fracture, or skin masses due to unclear reason.

4. Avoid using scraping for people with excessive hunger, overeat, fatigue or nervousness.

5. Avoid using scraping among the old, or people with weak constitution, or the excessively thin people.

6. Avoid using scraping on the abdomen, lumbosacral region and certain acupuncture points of pregnant women, such as SP 6 (*sān yīn jiāo*), LI 4 (*hé gǔ*), GB 21 (*jiān jǐng*), BL 60 (*kūn lún*), *etc.*.

7. Avoid using scraping on eyes, ears, nose, tongue, lips, genitalia and anus, navel (RN 8, *shén quē*). Do not use scraping on the crown of the head of an infant since his or her fontanelle has not closed yet.

III. Scraping Instrument

Select suitable instrument according to the patient's condition. At present, scrapping board made by buffalo horn is the most commonly used instrument for scrapping (Fig. 6-29). The standard buffalo horn scraping board is rectangular, 10cm in length, 6cm in wide, 0.2cm in the thick side. The edges of board are smooth and without breakage, and the wide side is concave. Use the thick side for health care, and the thin side for treating disease. Spoon, buttons, coins, porcelain wine cup, tender bamboo

二、禁忌证

1. 凡危重病证，如急性传染病、严重的心脑血管疾病、肝肾功能不全等禁止刮痧。

2. 有出血倾向的疾病，如血小板减少症、凝血功能障碍等禁用刮痧。

3. 各种皮肤溃疡、疮疡、烫伤、急性扭伤或外伤骨折处及皮肤有不明病因的包块等禁止直接在病灶部位刮拭。

4. 过饥、过饱、过度疲劳或过度紧张者禁用刮痧。

5. 形体过于消瘦者或久病体弱者不宜刮痧。

6. 妊娠妇女的腹部、腰骶部及身体的一些穴位，如三阴交、合谷、肩井、昆仑等禁用刮痧。

7. 眼睛、耳孔、鼻孔、舌、口唇、前后二阴、肚脐（神阙穴）处禁止刮痧；囟门未闭合的小儿头部禁用刮痧。

三、刮痧工具

根据病情选择合适的刮具。刮痧板是目前最常用的刮痧工具，临床使用最多的是水牛角刮痧板（图 6-29）。标准的水牛角刮痧板呈长方形：长 10cm，宽 6cm，厚的一边为 0.2cm；四角钝圆，宽的一侧呈凹形，保健刮痧时用厚的一边，治疗病证时用薄的一侧。日常刮痧用具可用边缘钝圆光滑的瓷匙、

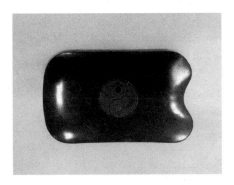

Fig. 6-29　Scrapping Board Made by Buffalo Horn
图 6-29　水牛角刮痧板

or small clam with smooth edges and without breakage can also be selected for the scraping instrument.

纽扣、铜钱、硬币、瓷酒盅、嫩竹板和小蚌壳等。

IV. Part for Scraping

1. Head　Usually scrape the part between the eyebrows and temples, bridge of the nose.

2. Neck and nape　Scrape the neck part, the two sides of the nape part.

3. Chest　Scrape the intercostal spaces and the sternum. The nipples are forbidden to be scrapped.

4. Shoulder and back　Shoulders and the two sides of vertebral column are the parts that are most commonly used.

5. Upper and lower limbs　The medial side of the upper limb, elbow fossa, the medial side of the thigh, and the popliteal fossa are mainly used for scraping.

V. Manipulation

i. Preparation

1. Patient Preparation　Check the patient's name, bed number, and the regions for scraping. Assess the patient's condition, medical history, hypoesthesia or obstacles, tolerance to pain, psychological status and local skin conditions. Explain the purpose, the main steps, key points and related matters, the discomfort and complications of scraping to the patient, in order to obtain consent of the patient and/or their families. Ask the patient to have a rest for 1 or 2 hours after a meal, and tell the patient to empty stool and urine in advance.

2. Material Preparation　Prepare plate, scrapping instrument (check the integrity and smoothness of the edges of the instrument), lubricant in bowl such as scraping oil, sesame oil or clean water, a piece of cloth or paper. Prepare a large towel, screen, warm water, *etc.* if necessary.

3. Environment Preparation　Environment should be well-lit, quiet and clean, and temperature should be suitable.

4. Operator Preparation　The operator should be well-groomed. Wash the hands and wear mask before performance.

ii. Procedure of Operation

1. Take the materials that have been prepared to the ward. Check the patient again and make an explanation to the patient to get his or her cooperation.

四、常用刮痧部位

1. **头部**　常取眉心、太阳穴、鼻梁处。

2. **颈项部**　取后项、颈部两侧。

3. **胸部**　包括各肋间隙、胸骨中线，注意乳头处禁止刮痧。

4. **肩背部**　两肩部、背部脊柱两侧为最常用的刮痧部位。

5. **上下肢**　上臂内侧、肘窝、下肢大腿内侧及腘窝。

五、刮痧法的操作

（一）操作前准备

1. **患者准备**　核对患者姓名、床号、刮痧的部位；评估患者的临床表现、既往史、对疼痛的耐受程度及心理状况、有无感觉迟钝或障碍、局部皮肤的情况；向患者解释操作目的、主要步骤、配合要点以及相关事项，说明可能出现的不适及并发症，以取得患者和/或家属对执行该操作的知情同意；嘱患者餐后 1~2h 才能刮痧，并排空大小便。

2. **用物准备**　治疗盘，刮具（检查刮具边缘的完整性和圆滑性），治疗碗内放润滑剂（可用专业刮痧油、香油或温开水等）、治疗巾或纸巾，必要时备大毛巾、屏风、温开水等。

3. **环境准备**　环境应光线充足、安静整洁、温度适宜。

4. **操作者准备**　操作者应仪表整洁，洗手，戴口罩。

（二）操作步骤

1. 根据刮痧部位备齐用物，携至床旁，再次核对，并向患者做好解释，取得合作。

2. Help the patient to select a comfortable posture according to the disease. Supine position or the position of leaning on one's back is normally chosen when scraping the chest, the abdomen, inside and front side of the lower limbs. Ventricumbent or sitting position is normally chosen for scraping the head, neck, back, lateral of the upper and lower limbs .

3. Expose the selected parts. Cover a large towel or small blanket to the non-scraping sites. Use screen if necessary.

4. Examine the edge of the instrument and make sure it is smooth and integrity.

5. Hold the instrument with hands and dip the lubricant to scrape gently on the selected parts. Keep an angle at 45°-90° between the instrument and the skin. Scrap the neck and two sides of vertebral column from top to bottom, while scraping the chest and the back from inside to outside. Scrape along one direction. The strength should be even and moderate. Don't scrape forcibly. Keep the instrument wet during the operation. Scrape until the skin appears red or mauve blood stagnation.

6. Determining the strip number of scrapping depends on the disease condition. Generally, 8-10 strips should be scrapped at one time, 6-15cm long every strip, and 20 times per strip.

7. Ask whether the patient feel discomfort at any time during the process of scrapping and observe color changes of the local skin that is being scrapped.

8. Wipe the oil or the water after scrapping finished. Assist the patient to put on clothes, and tidy up bed for the patient. Give the patient a cup of warm water (preferably light sugar brine) to drink, and let him or her take a rest for 15-20 minutes.

9. Tidy up. Instrument should be cleaned and sterilized. Wash the hands, and take a record.

VI. Precaution

1. Keep the fresh air circulating in the room, avoiding the patient being blown directly.

2. The scrapping board should be cleaned after using and be disinfected with 75% alcohol. It is recommended to prepare the individual scrapping board for each person.

3. Any part of the scraping therapy should firstly scrap the neck. The orders of general principle of scraping therapy are as follows: first neck, then back and waist, chest and abdomen, and finally limbs and joints. Scrapping yang

2. 根据病证协助患者取舒适、合理体位。如胸腹、下肢内侧、前侧部多选用仰卧位或仰靠坐位；头部、颈部、背部、上肢和下肢外侧部多选用俯卧位或俯伏坐位及坐位。

3. 暴露刮痧部位，非刮痧部位盖上大毛巾或小棉被，必要时屏风遮挡。

4. 检查刮具边缘，确定光滑无缺损。

5. 手持刮具，蘸润滑剂，在选定部位施刮。刮具与刮拭方向皮肤保持45°~90°角。颈部、脊柱旁从上至下，胸背部从内向外，单一方向刮拭皮肤，不可来回刮拭。用力应均匀，力度适中，禁用暴力。刮痧过程中，应保持刮具边缘湿润。一般刮至局部皮下出现红色或紫红色痧痕为度。

6. 刮痧的条数应视具体情况而定。一般每次刮8~10条，每条刮6~15cm，每条刮20次左右。

7. 刮痧过程中随时询问患者有无不适，注意观察病情及局部皮肤颜色的变化。

8. 刮痧结束后，擦干油或水渍，协助患者穿好衣裤，整理床单位。刮痧出痧后嘱患者饮一杯温开水（最好为淡糖盐水），并休息15~20min。

9. 整理用物，使用过的刮具应清洁消毒后备用。洗手，记录并签名。

六、刮痧法的注意事项

1. 保持室内空气新鲜、流通，避免直接吹风。

2. 刮痧用具一定要注意清洁，用后清洗并用75%的乙醇消毒。最好专人专板，固定使用。

3. 任何部位刮痧治疗宜先刮拭颈部，一般原则是先颈部、再背腰部、胸腹部，最后刮四肢和关节部，每个部位一般先刮阳经，

meridians first, and then yin meridians, from the left side to the right side of the body.

4. The force should be moderate and even during scrapping, which is decided by the tolerance of the patient. Scrape no more than 10 minutes in each area, or stop when the red spots under the skin appeared. Red spots should not be importuned though there is no or little.

5. Pay attention to observe the color change of the local skin and ask patient's feeling. Stop scrapping immediately when the patient has the symptoms of abnormal pain, cold sweating, chest discomfort and dysphoria.

6. Tell the patient to take a rest, keep good mood, take the light and digestive food, avoid eating cold and greasy food and prevent from catching cold after the treatment.

7. Generally, the interval between two scrapping is about 3-6 days until the blood stagnation disappears, and a treatment course consists of 3-5 sessions.

8. The lateral of instrument is appropriate to be used for the body parts where the muscles are fullness such as the back and the buttocks. The edges and corners of the scrapping instrument are appropriate to be used for the parts with fewer muscles.

(Yang Jin-hua)

Section 6　Acupressure

Acupressure is a healing technique using fingers, palms, knuckles and elbows to apply pressure at acupuncture points so as to inspire qi of the channels, and regulate yin and yang according to the basic theory of TCM.

I. Indication

Acupressure has the effects of releasing tension, relaxing the sinews and alleviating pain, invigorating blood and dissolving stasis, and dredging the channels and collaterals. Therefore, acupressure has extensive indications and can be used for nursing various diseases involving internal medicine, gynecology, surgery, pediatric, and

后刮阴经，先刮拭身体的左侧，再刮拭身体的右侧。

4. 刮痧时用力应均匀，力度适中，以患者能耐受为宜。每次每个部位刮拭不超过10min为宜，或以出痧为度，对不出痧或出痧少者不可强求出痧。

5. 操作中注意观察患者局部皮肤颜色的变化，随时询问其感觉。如患者出现异常疼痛、冷汗不止、胸闷烦躁等，应停止刮痧。

6. 嘱患者在刮治期间注意休息，保持心情愉快；饮食宜清淡易消化，禁食生冷油腻之品；出痧后避免受凉，一般刮痧后不洗澡，尤其是不要洗凉水澡。

7. 两次刮痧时间一般间隔3~6d，以皮肤痧退为准，3~5次为一疗程。

8. 凡肌肉丰满处（如背部、臀部）宜用刮痧板的横面刮拭；对一些关节部位、肌肉较少、凸凹较多处，宜用刮痧板的棱角刮拭。

（杨金花）

第六节　穴位按压法

穴位按压法，是指在中医理论指导下，运用手指、手掌、指间关节、肘等部位按压刺激穴位，以激发经络之气，调整阴阳，从而达到防病治病目的的方法。

一、适应证

穴位按压法具有缓解紧张、舒筋止痛、活血化瘀、疏通经络等作用，适用范围广泛，可用于内、妇、外、儿、伤科等多种病证的护理，尤其适用于疼痛性疾病、软组织损伤、情绪紧张、脏腑功能失调等病证的护理和

traumatology, especially for pain, injury of parenchyma, emotional tension, and functional disorders of *zang-fu* organs.

1. Traumatological Disease　Fibromyalgia, lumbago, cervical spondylopathy, periarthritis of shoulder, chronic muscular strain, ankle and knee sprain, *etc.*.

2. Internal Disease　The common cold, headache, dizziness, insomnia, cough, asthma, stomachache, diarrhea, constipation, impotence, hypertension, coronary heart disease, sequelae of wind stroke, chronic fatigue syndrome, depression, *etc.*.

3. Surgical Disease　Hyperplasia of the mammary gland, postoperative gastrointestinal dysfunction, adverse reactions of chemotherapy and radiotherapy, *etc.*.

4. Gynecological Disease　Irregular menstruation, dysmenorrhea, menopausal syndrome, *etc.*.

5. Ophthalmological and Otorhinolaryngological Disease　Myopia, tinnitus, rhinitis, *etc.*.

II. Contraindication

1. Surgery diseases such as acute peritonitis, enterobrosis, acute appendicitis, fracture.

2. Various acute and chronic infectious diseases such as typhoid, epidemic cerebrospinal meningitis, epidemic encephalitis B, hepatitis, tuberculosis, syphilis, gonorrhea, AIDS.

3. Various acute poisoning, such as food poisoning, gas poisoning, drug poisoning, alcoholism, venomous snake bites.

4. Various severe hemorrhagic conditions, such as cerebral hemorrhage, gastrorrhagia, metrorrhagia, hematochezia, hematuria, traumatic bleeding.

5. Various life-threatening diseases and serious medical problems, such as acute myocardial infarction, renal failure, heart failure.

III. Manipulation and Point of Acupressure

The majority of tuina manipulations can be used in acupressure, especially those techniques using fingers and palms to apply certain pressure at acupuncture points. The essentials of acupressure techniques are steady, forceful and soft with even speed and rhythm, and penetration. In general, gradual, steady and penetrating pressure on each point for approximately three minutes is ideal. How much pressure to apply to any point depends on the physique of

康复。

1. **伤科病证**　肌筋膜炎、腰痛、颈椎病、肩周炎、慢性肌肉劳损、踝关节扭伤和膝关节扭伤等。

2. **内科病证**　感冒、头痛、眩晕、失眠、咳嗽、哮喘、胃痛、泄泻、便秘、阳痿、高血压、冠心病、中风后遗症、慢性疲劳综合征、抑郁症等。

3. **外科病证**　乳腺增生、术后胃肠功能紊乱等。

4. **妇科病证**　月经不调、痛经、更年期综合征等。

5. **五官科病证**　近视、耳鸣、鼻炎等。

二、禁忌证

1. 某些外科疾病如急性腹膜炎、肠穿孔、急性阑尾炎、骨折等。

2. 各种急慢性传染病如伤寒、流行性脑脊髓膜炎、乙脑、肝炎、结核、梅毒、淋病、艾滋病等。

3. 急性中毒，如食物中毒、煤气中毒、药物中毒、酒精中毒、毒蛇咬伤等。

4. 各种严重出血性疾病如脑出血、胃出血、子宫出血、便血、尿血、外伤出血等。

5. 各种严重的、危及生命的疾病，如急性心肌梗死、严重肾衰竭、心力衰竭等。

三、常用手法及穴位

大部分推拿手法均可用于穴位按压，尤其是以手指、手掌等部位作用于穴位的推拿手法。持久、有力、均匀、柔和、渗透，也是穴位按压手法的基本要求。一般而言，持久而有渗透力的压力宜缓慢施加于穴位，每穴持续按压大约 3min。按压穴位的力度取决

the patient and the location of the point. Different amount of pressure is required according to different patients and areas. The area being pressed may be caused aching, numbness, heavy, distention and pain sensations. If it hurts a great deal, light touch should be used instead of pressure. The calves, the face, and genital areas are sensitive and need gentle pressure. The back, buttocks, and shoulders with thick musculature usually need deeper and firmer pressure.

The common used acupressure techniques include one-finger pushing, kneading, rubbing, scrubbing, wipping, pressing, continuous pressing, pointing, grasping, plucking, nipping, *etc.*. For the details of operation methods, essentials and precautions of those techniques, please refer to the "Tuina" part in Section 2 of Chapter 6.

For the frequently used acupressure points and its techniques, please refer to Table 2-7 in "Channels, Collaterals and Acupuncture Point", Section 6 of Chapter 2.

IV. Precaution

1. Maintain an appropriate room temperature and good ventilation prior to acupressure.

2. In order to make the patient comfortable and facilitate location of points, the patient should be placed in a posture according to the condition of disease, the constitution, age and gender of the patient, and the position should be suitable to the selected points.

3. Apply finger pressure in a slow and rhythmic manner to enable the layers of tissue and the internal organs to respond. Never press any area in an abrupt, forceful, or jarring way.

4. Do not do acupressure immediately when a patient is famished, tired, or in extreme nervous. Avoid practicing acupressure right after a big meal or on a full stomach. Wait until at least an hour after a meal.

5. Do not choose points in the lower abdominal region for pregnant women in the first trimester. For pregnant women over 3 months, acupuncturing points on the abdominal and lumbosacral areas should be avoided. Certain points including SP 6 (*sān yīn jiāo*), LI 4 (*hé gǔ*), BL 60 (*kūn lún*) and BL 67 (*zhì yīn*), which intensively promote blood circulation, are contraindicated during the entire pregnancy. Acupressure should not be applied to women during their menstrual periods, unless they are treated for irregular menstrual periods.

于患者的体型及穴位所在的部位。不同患者及不同部位所需的按压力度不同，按压局部可出现酸、麻、重、胀、痛等感觉。如果疼痛明显，则应减少按压力度，以更轻柔的手法代替。小腿部、面部以及外阴部穴位较为敏感，一般按压力度较轻。背部、臀部、肩部等肌肉丰厚部位可采用较大力度、更为深透的按压力度。

常用的穴位按压手法有一指禅推法、揉法、摩法、擦法、抹法、按法、压法、点法、拿法、拨法、掐法等。这些手法的具体操作方法、动作要领及注意事项见本书第六章第二节推拿法部分。

穴位按压的常用穴位及按压手法详见本书第二章第六节经络腧穴部分表2-7。

四、注意事项

1. 穴位按压前，操作室要保持适宜的温度和空气流通。

2. 根据受术者的病情、体质、年龄、性别及操作部位等情况，选择适当的治疗体位，务使受术者感到舒适。

3. 穴位按压时动作应缓慢、有节奏，以使身体不同组织及内脏对刺激产生适宜的反应。切忌生硬、暴力按压方式。

4. 患者在过于饥饿、疲劳、精神过度紧张时，不宜立即进行穴位按压；避免饭后立即进行穴位按压，一般可在餐后1h左右再进行穴位按压为宜。

5. 妇女怀孕3个月以内者，小腹部的腧穴不宜穴位按压。对怀孕3个月以上的妇女者，不宜对其腹部、腰骶部腧穴进行穴位按压。三阴交、合谷、昆仑、至阴等通经活血的腧穴，在怀孕期间禁忌穴位按压。在妇女行经期，若非为了调经，亦不应进行穴位按压。

6. Acupressure should not be applied to the infected, ulcerated or scarred skin or tumors.

7. Lymph areas, such as the groin, the area of the throat just below the ears, and the outer breast near the armpits, are very sensitive. These areas should be touched only lightly, and not be pressed.

(Wang Yun-cui)

Section 7　Auricular Seed Taping Therapy

Auricular seeds taping therapy is taping small, round, hard and smooth objects such as *wáng bù liú xíng* seed and small magnetic beads to particular auricular points. The taped objects are then pressed in order to stimulate the auricular points and attain therapeutic effect. This method has been widely used because of its wide range of indications, convenient for use, safety, and lack of side effects.

I. Indication

Refer to Part 2, Section 1, Chapter 6: auricular acupuncture.

II. Manipulation

1. Selecting Auricular Point　After making clear diagnosis, proper auricular points are selected according to principles which are mentioned in auricular acupuncture or positive reaction spots detected by diagnostic methods which are referred to in auricular acupuncture can be used.

2. Disinfection　The auricular points should be disinfected with 75% alcohol.

3. Manipulation　The *wáng bù liú xíng* seed and small magnetic beads are mainly used for auricular seeds taping. Tapping the seeds to a piece of adhesive tape sized in 0.5cm square, is named auricular plaste or ear acupoint application. Hold the auricle to expose auricular points as far as possible with one hand. Use tweezer to stick ear acupoint application to on auricular points with the other hand. Then press on the auricular points and give appropriate pressure with thumb and index fingers

6. 皮肤有感染、溃疡、瘢痕或肿瘤的部位，不宜进行穴位按压。

7. 淋巴结部位，如腹股沟、耳后、颌下、乳腺外上侧靠近腋窝部等只能轻用摩法，不能按压。

（王云翠）

第七节　耳穴埋豆法

耳穴埋豆法是在耳穴表面贴敷圆形、坚硬而表面光滑的小颗粒，如王不留行籽、小磁珠等，通过在敷贴处按压耳穴以加强刺激来防治疾病的一种方法。其治疗范围较广，操作简便安全，副作用少，运用非常广泛。

一、适应证

同耳针法（参考第六章第一节第二部分）。

二、操作方法

1. **选穴**　诊断明确后，根据耳穴的选穴原则或用耳穴探查方法在耳郭上所获得阳性反应点，确立处方。

2. **消毒**　耳穴用 75% 乙醇常规消毒。

3. **压丸**　压丸所选材料多用王不留行籽、小磁珠等。先将其贴在 0.5cm×0.5cm 小方块胶布中央即形成耳穴贴。一手捏住耳郭，充分暴露耳穴，另一手用摄子将耳穴贴敷于耳穴上贴按压在耳穴，并给予适当按压，使耳郭有发热、胀痛感。主要贴压患病侧耳穴，也可双侧同时贴压或交替贴压。一般每天患者

until a feeling of local heat or distending pain is achieved. Mainly tape the auricular points of the affected side. Bilateral auricular may be taped simultaneously or during alternate treatment sessions. The patient is asked to press the selected points 2-4 times a day. The seeds can be kept in place for 3-5 days. Remove the tape and seeds before the next treatment and modify the points according to the condition of the disease.

可自行按压 2~4 次，贴好的耳豆可保留 3~5d，复诊时按病情酌情增减或更换穴位。

III. Precaution

1. Smooth and hard seeds of appropriate size should be chosen. Seeds with rough surface should be avoided in case of causing injury. If soft seeds were used, therapeutic effect is difficult to be achieved due to weak stimulation.

2. Avoid exposure of the adhesive tape to moisture or contamination.

3. The patient who is allergic to adhesive should shorten the time to press and especially press auricular points adrenal gland (shèn shàng xiàn) and wind stream (fēng xī), or switch to adhesive paper.

4. In order to prevent the auricle from injury, do not rub in a sideways or circular motion while pressing the taped auricular points.

5. Stimulus intensity depends on the patients' situation. In generally, children, the aged and frail people should only accept light stimulation, while the patient who has acute pain should be stimulated heavily.

6. When treating a sprain or other soft tissue injuries, it should encourage the patient to move the affected part, apply massage or moxibustion in the affected area in order to increase the therapeutic effect.

(Yang Liu)

三、注意事项

1. 耳穴埋豆法的材料应选用光滑、大小和硬度适宜的种籽，不宜选用粗糙的种籽，以免按压时损伤皮肤。如选用质软的种籽，按压作用较小。

2. 防止胶布潮湿或污染。

3. 对胶布过敏者，可缩短贴压时间并加压肾上腺，风溪穴，或改用黏合纸代之。

4. 为避免耳郭皮肤损伤，不宜上下或环形揉动贴压的耳穴。

5. 刺激强度视患者情况而定，一般儿童、年迈体弱者用轻刺激法；急性疼痛性病证宜用强刺激法。

6. 有运动障碍的患者，按压埋籽后耳郭充血发热时，宜适当活动患部，并在患部按摩、艾灸等，以提高疗效。

（杨柳）

Section 8　Hot Compress Therapy

Hot compress therapy is a method to put the heated medicine into a cloth bag and move them back and forth or circularly on the certain part or point of the human body so as to promote qi and blood circulation, dispel cold and relieve pain, dispel blood stagnation and swelling, warm channels and free collaterals by means of heat and

第八节　热熨法

热熨法是将药物加热后，装入布袋内，在人体局部或特定穴位来回移动或回旋运转，利用温热及药物的共同作用，以达到行气活血、散寒止痛、祛瘀消肿、温经通络等作用的一种治疗方法。常用的热熨法包括药熨法、

medicine. It includes hot medicinal compress, hot Kanlisha compress, hot scallion compress, hot salt compress, hot vinegar compress, and hot soybean compress.

坎离砂熨法、葱熨法、盐熨法、醋熨法、大豆熨法。

I. Indication

1. Stomachache, abdominal pain, diarrhea due to deficiency cold of spleen and stomach.

2. Difficulty in urinating and uroschesis.

3. Cold pain or numbness of joints caused by wind-dampness pathogen.

4. Swelling and painful joints due to local blood stagnation from falls, soreness of lower back and knees.

5. Dysmenorrhea due to deficiency cold.

一、适应证

1. 脾胃虚寒引起的脘腹冷痛、泄泻、呕吐等症状。

2. 小便不利、癃闭。

3. 风湿痹引起的关节冷痛、麻木、沉重、酸胀。

4. 跌打扭伤引起的局部瘀血、肿痛、腰背不适等。

5. 阳虚内寒之痛经。

II. Contraindication

1. Avoid using this method to treat the patients with excess-heat syndrome or the patients who haven't awaken from anesthesia.

2. Don't use it in the abdomen where the patient has mass with uncertain character or in the abdominal and lumbosacral region of pregnant women.

3. Don't use it in the places with large vessels, on the injured skin and in the insentient parts.

二、禁忌证

1. 各种实热证或麻醉未清醒者禁用。

2. 腹部包块性质不明者的腹部，孕妇腹部及腰骶部禁用。

3. 身体大血管处、皮肤有破损及局部无知觉处禁用。

III. Manipulation and Precaution

i. Hot Medicinal Compress

It is a method to mix the herbs with white spirit or vinegar, heat up it, and put them into a bag, then move them back and forth or circularly on the certain part or point of the patient.

1. Indication Stomachache, diarrhea due to deficiency cold of spleen and stomach, local blood stagnation due to injuries from falls, cold pain or numbness of joints caused by wind-dampness pathogen.

2. Preparation It includes treatment plate, medicine (prepare according to the doctor's advice), white spirit or vinegar, treatment bowl, cotton swab, Vaseline, 2 double-layer bags, big towel, wok, electric cooker, bamboo spade or bamboo chopsticks. Prepare screen if it is necessary.

3. Procedure of Operation

(1) Wash hands and wear a mask. According to the

三、各类热熨法的操作方法及注意事项

（一）药熨法

药熨法是将中药用白酒或食醋搅拌后炒热，装入布袋中，在患者患处或某个穴位上来回移动滚熨。

1. 适应证 适用于脾胃虚寒引起的胃脘疼痛、泄泻；跌打损伤等引起的局部瘀血；风湿痹痛引起的关节冷痛、麻木等。

2. 用物准备 治疗盘、药物（根据医嘱准备）、白酒或醋、治疗碗、棉签、凡士林、双层纱布袋2个，另备大毛巾、炒锅、电炉、竹铲或竹筷，必要时备屏风。

3. 操作步骤

（1）洗手、戴口罩；根据医嘱，将药物倒

doctor's advice, put the medicine into the wok, then add moderate white spirit or vinegar and mix them. Saute them to 60℃ or 70℃ by slow fire and put them into the bag, wrapped by the big towel to keep warm.

(2) After the materials are prepared, take them to the ward and check again. Explain the purposes and ways of the operation to the patient in order to get his/her cooperation. Assist the patient to take a comfortable posture according to the disease condition and expose the parts to be treated. Pay attention to keep the patient warm, and use the screen based on the situation.

(3) After smearing a little Vaseline on the selected skin, move the medicinal bag on the part or point back and forth with the even force. At the beginning, the force should be small but the speed could be a little quicker. The force can be greater gradually but the speed can be slower with the fall of the temperature. When the medicinal bag's temperature is too low, change the medicinal bag in time to keep warm and enhance the effects. During the compress, pay attention to observe the skin to prevent scalding.

(4) The operation usually lasts for 15-30 minutes, once or twice a day.

(5) After finishing the operation, clean the local skin, assist the patient to put on the clothes and take a comfortable lying posture.

(6) Clean up the materials, wash hands, record and sign name.

4. Precaution

(1) Before the operation, make a full explanation to the patient and tell him/her to empty the urine.

(2) Pay attention to keep warm in winter. The temperature in the room should be comfortable and the air should be fresh.

(3) The temperature of the medicinal bag is inadvisably higher than 70℃. For the old, infants, children and the patients with sensation disorder, the temperature of the medicinal bag shouldn't be higher than 50℃ in order to prevent scalding.

(4) During the operation, keep the medicinal bag warm, change or heat the bag in time. If the patient feels uncomfortable, the compress should be stopped.

(5) Pay attention to keep safety during sauting the herbs. When adding the white spirit to the herbs, take the wok away from the fire to prevent danger.

ii. Hot Kanlisha Compress

It is a kind of therapy that one puts the Kanlisha into the bowl, adds moderate mature vinegar and mixes them, puts them into the cloth bag and uses the heat caused by

入锅中，用适量白酒或食醋搅拌均匀后，用文火炒至 60~70℃，装入布袋中，用大毛巾裹好，保温、备用。

（2）备齐用物，携至床旁，再次核对；解释治疗目的、方法，以取得患者的配合；根据病情协助患者取舒适、合理的体位，并暴露药熨部位；注意保暖，视情况使用屏风。

（3）局部皮肤涂一层凡士林后，将药袋放在患处或相应穴位处用力来回推熨，力量要均匀。开始时用力要轻，速度可稍快，待药袋温度逐渐下降时用力可逐渐增大，速度可减慢。药袋温度过低时，及时更换药袋，以保持温度，加强效果；药熨过程中应随时注意观察局部皮肤情况，防止烫伤。

（4）药熨时间一般为 15~30min，每日 1~2次。

（5）药熨后擦净局部皮肤，协助患者穿好衣服，取舒适卧位。

（6）整理用物，洗手，记录，并签名。

4. 注意事项

（1）药熨前向患者做好解释，嘱患者排空小便。

（2）冬季注意保暖，注意室内温度要适宜、空气新鲜。

（3）药熨温度不宜超过 70℃，年老、婴幼儿及感觉障碍者，药袋温度不宜超过 50℃，以免烫伤。

（4）操作过程中应保持药袋温度，保证及时更换或加热。如患者感到不适，应停止操作。

（5）炒药过程中要注意安全，中途加入白酒时要将炒锅离开热源，以免发生危险。

（二）坎离砂熨法

坎离砂熨法是将坎离砂放入治疗碗内加入适量陈醋，搅拌均匀，装入布袋中，利用铁和醋酸的化学反应所产生的热在患处进行

the chemical reaction of iron and acetic acid to do the hot compress on the affected part.

1. Indication It is indicated for joint and muscle ache, limb numbness and bellyache caused by wind-cold pathogen.

2. Preparation It includes treatment plate, treatment bowl, wooden stick or bamboo chopsticks, mature vinegar, 2 double-layer cloth bags, Vaseline, Kanlisha. Prepare bath towel if it is necessary.

3. Procedure of Operation

(1) Put 250g Kanlisha into the treatment bowl, add 50-100ml mature vinegar into the bowl, and mix them with wooden stick or bamboo chopsticks until Kanlisha becomes moist. Put them into the double-layer cloth bag. It will become hot after a while.

(2) Smear a little Vaseline on the selected skin, put the bag on the skin and then move it by hand back and forth.

(3) The operation lasts for 20-30 minutes each time, once or twice a day. When Kanlisha is used every time, add the mature vinegar into it which can be used repeatedly. Change it until the Kanlisha can't become hot.

iii. Hot Scallion Compress

It is a kind of therapy that hot compress is applied on the patient's abdomen using the scallion that is sauted to heat, putting the white spirit into it, then putting it into the cloth bag, which achieves the effect of ascending the clear and descending the turbid.

1. Indication It is commonly used for eliminating ascites, inducing urination, releasing urine retention, relieving flaccidity syndrome, paralysis and so on.

2. Preparation This includes treatment bowl, 200-250g fresh scallion stalk (cut into 2-3cm segments), and 30ml white spirit, bamboo chopsticks, cloth bag, Vaseline, electric cooker and fry wok.

3. Procedure of Operation

(1) Put the scallion stalks into the wok and heat them. When the scallion stalk becomes half-cooked, take the wok away from the electric cooker and add 30ml white spirit into the wok. After mixing the white spirit with scallion stalk, put the wok on the electric cooker again to continuously heat.

(2) Put the scallion stalk into the cloth bag by bamboo chopsticks, do the hot compress when the temperature falls to 50-60℃.

(3) Smear Vaseline on the patient's abdomen, move the scallion bag up and down from the right side of peripheral umbilicus to the left side, which can achieve the effect of right ascending and left descending, discharging

热熨的一种治疗方法。

1. 适应证 适用于感受风寒所致的关节肌肉酸痛，以及肢体麻木、阴寒腹痛等证。

2. 用物准备 治疗盘、治疗碗、木棒或竹筷、陈醋、双层纱布袋、凡士林、坎离砂。必要时备浴巾。

3. 操作步骤

（1）将坎离砂 250g 放在治疗碗中，倒入陈醋 50~100ml，用木棒或竹筷拌匀，以坎离砂湿润为宜，然后装入双层纱布袋中，稍等片刻即发热。

（2）局部涂一层凡士林，将坎离砂袋放在患处皮肤上，用手来回推熨。

（3）每次可熨 20~30min，每日 1~2 次。坎离砂可反复使用，每次用时加入陈醋，直至不能发热时再更换。

（三）葱熨法

葱熨法是将大葱炒热加入白酒，装入布袋中，在患者腹部热熨，达到升清降浊之功效的一种治疗方法。

1. 适应证 临床常用于消除腹水，通利小便，解除癃闭，以及缓解痿证、瘫痪等症状。

2. 用物准备 治疗盘内放新鲜大葱白 200~250g（切成 2~3cm 长），白酒 30ml、竹筷、纱布袋、凡士林，另备电炉、炒锅。

3. 操作步骤

（1）将葱段放入锅内炒至半熟时，将炒锅移开电炉，倒入 30ml 白酒，搅拌均匀后再放到电炉上炒热。

（2）用竹筷把葱段挟入纱布袋内，待温度为 50~60℃时才可热熨。

（3）患者腹部涂适量凡士林，用葱熨袋从脐周右侧向左侧进行上下滚熨，以达到右升左降，排出腹内腹水、积气，通利大小便的作用。

ascites and accumulation of qi, and inducing urination as well as stool.

(4) The operation takes about 20 minutes, twice a day.

(5) After the operation, the abdomen should be kept warm.

iv. Hot Salt Compress

It is a kind of therapy that one puts the heated sea salt with the similar size into the cloth bag, and moves it on the affected parts or special parts repeatedly when the bag's temperature is appropriate. It is applied to the gastric or abdominal region of the patient with chronic stomachache and diarrhea due to deficiency cold. If the patient suffers from arthralgia syndrome, flaccidity syndrome, paralysis or pain of muscles and bones, directly compress on the painful parts. For the patient with urine retention, compress RN 8 (*shén què*) or the lower abdomen. The salt bag can be put under the head as a pillow if the patient has dizziness and tinnitus. It can be applied on the center of the thenar for the patient with kidney yang deficiency. This operation lasts for 20-30 minutes each time, twice a day.

v. Hot Vinegar Compress

It is a kind of therapy that one adds 50-100ml vinegar into the salt, puts them into the cloth bag and does compress. It is used to treat injuries from falls, pain syndrome due to wind-dampness, paralysis, contraction of muscle, cold pain of lower abdomen, and urine retention. Especially, it has better effect of relieving cicatricle contracture caused by scalding or burning.

vi. Hot Soybean Compress

Put the heated 500g soybean into the cloth bag and compress on the affected parts. It can be used to treat lumbago due to deficiency cold, arthralgia caused by cold-dampness pathogen or flaccidity syndrome. It is indicated for headache, pain of the nape or tinnitus.

(Xu Dong-ying)

Section 9　Fumigating and Steaming Therapy

This is an external approach to prevent or treat diseases by fumigating or steaming the body surface or local focus, or through direct action of the vapor from the

（4）每次葱熨时间为 20min 左右，每日 2 次。

（5）操作结束后腹部应注意保暖。

（四）盐熨法

盐熨法是将颗粒大小均匀的大青盐或海盐炒热，装入纱布袋中，待温度适宜时，在患处或特定部位来回运转的一种方法。慢性虚寒性胃痛、腹泻可在胃脘部或腹部滚熨。痹证、痿证、瘫痪、筋骨疼痛直接熨患处。癃闭者熨神阙或小腹。耳鸣头晕者可将盐熨袋枕于头下。肾阳不足者熨足心。每次熨 20~30min，每日 2 次。

（五）醋熨法

在盐熨的基础上加醋热熨。即在炒盐时将陈醋 50~100ml 洒入盐内炒匀，装入布袋中外熨。其适应证包括跌扑损伤、风湿痹痛、瘫痪、肌肉拘急、少腹冷痛、癃闭。尤其对烫伤或烧伤后瘢痕挛缩的缓解效果更好。

（六）大豆熨法

将大豆 500g，炒热装布袋中敷熨患处。适用于虚寒性腰痛或寒湿痹痛、痿证。把大豆熨袋枕于头项下可治疗头项痛证或耳鸣等病证。

（徐冬英）

第九节　熏洗法

熏洗法是根据中医辨证选用相应的方药经过煎煮加热产生温热药气，利用中草药剂

boiling herbs on the human body so as to warm meridians and collaterals, promote blood circulation and relieve pain, dispel wind and cold, expel wind and dampness, kill parasites and relieve itching, remove swelling and stagnation, regulate function of the viscera, and support the vital and eliminate the pathogenic. Common methods are fumigating therapy, steaming therapy, macerating therapy, washing with herbal bag, sitz bath and body bathing therapy.

I. Fumigating Therapy

i. Definition

It is an external approach to prevent and treat diseases by fumigating the body surface with prepared herbal smoke.

ii. Indication

It is commonly used for skin disease, rheumatic arthralgia and air sterilization.

iii. Preparation

This needs container resistant to high temperature, match, 95% alcohol, drugs, and cotton paper.

iv. Operation Method

1. Treatment for Skin Disease Process the medicinal herbs into rough powder and then wrap them into medicated stick with cotton paper. Light the stick to fumigate the local area, 10-30 minutes each time and once a day. The treatment will not be stopped until the local affected skin heals. It is used for chronic eczema, tinea manuum as well as various types of tinea.

2. Air Sterilization Close the windows and door with nobody in, and get *cāng zhú* ($1g/m^3$) and *huò xiāng* ($1g/m^3$) permeated by 95% alcohol into a container. Light it up until the herbs burn out. Open the windows and door 2 hours later when the air is clear. Do the air bacteria culture. Keep away from the combustible when air sterilization is on going.

II. Steaming Therapy

i. Definition

It is an external method that medicinal vapor of boiling herbs penetrates into the skin and deep tissues of the body to dispel wind and eliminate dampness, relax and activate the tendons, promote blood circulation, remove

的热力或蒸汽渗透入人体皮肤毛窍、经络，达到温经通络、活血止痛、疏风散寒、祛风除湿、杀虫止痒、消肿祛瘀、协调脏腑功能、扶正祛邪的功效。常用的熏洗法包括熏法、蒸法、溻渍法、腾洗法、坐浴法和全身药浴法。

一、熏法

（一）概念

熏法是选用一定的药物燃烧后产生的烟雾，借着药力与热力的作用达到防治疾病目的的一种方法。

（二）适应证

常用于皮肤病的治疗或室内空气消毒。

（三）用物准备

耐高温容器，火柴，95%乙醇，药物，棉纸。

（四）操作方法

1. 皮肤疾患治疗 把药物卷入棉纸内，点燃后吹灭火焰，以烟火熏患处，每次熏10~30min，每日一次，至症状消失为止。用于慢性湿疹、鹅掌风和皮肤癣症。

2. 空气消毒 室内不留人，门窗关闭；将药物（常用苍术 $1g/m^3$，藿香 $1g/m^3$ 混合）放置在容器中，加入95%乙醇浸透，用火柴点燃，烧至产生烟雾，直至药物燃尽；药物燃2h后打开门窗，将烟雾散尽；按常规作空气细菌培养。注意防火，燃烧药物时要远离易燃物。

二、蒸法

（一）概念

蒸法是利用各种中草药加热后产生的蒸汽渗透入人体皮肤、深层组织，以祛风除湿、舒筋活络、活血祛瘀和温经止痛的一种治疗

stasis, as well as warm channels and relieve pain.

ii. Indication

It is commonly used in arthralgia syndrome due to wind-cold, hemiplegia, injuries from fall, gout, dysmenorrheal, dermatosis, edema, common cold due to pathogenic wind, and myasthenia gravis as well.

iii. Preparation

Herbal therapeutic machine, herbs, towel, sterile liquid and cold water are needed.

iv. Operation Method

1. The operator needs to dress clean, wear face mask and wash the hands.

2. Soak herbs in cold water for 20-60 minutes, and put them into the therapeutic machine. The machine is preheated for 15 minutes in summer and 20 minutes in winter.

3. The temperature of the machine should be adjusted to 32℃ in spring and summer while 32 to 35℃ in autumn and winter.

4. Check the patients' name, help them take off clothes and ask them to sit down or lie on the treated bed. Steam for 20-30 minutes each time, once or twice a day.

5. After steaming, turn off the power switch. Make the patients' skin dry, help them wear clothes, and ask them to take a rest about 30 minutes in the room before going back to the ward.

v. Precaution

1. Explain to the patients before operation in order to make them understand and get their cooperation.

2. Check the machine carefully before operation to prevent leakage of electricity and possible accident.

3. Drinking 500ml of glucose and sodium chloride solution is necessary for patients to prevent collapse from heavy sweating.

4. To sweat slightly is good for patients.

5. It is necessary to observe patients' condition during the operation. The therapy should be stopped immediately when the patient feels palpitation, rapidness of breath, red or pale complexion and heavy sweating. Ask the patient to take a rest and keep warm, and give him or her some warm salt water to drink. Inform the doctor for assistance if the symptoms have not been relieved.

6. The therapy should be inapplicable for the patients with fever, coma, malignant tumor, jaundice, hemorrhagic tendency, severe heart diseases, asthma attack, deficiency of qi

方法。

（二）适应证

常用于风寒痹证、半身不遂、跌打损伤、痛风、妇科痛经、各种皮肤病、水肿、风寒感冒、重症肌无力等。

（三）用物准备

中药草药治疗机，备用的中草药、毛巾、消毒液和冷水。

（四）操作方法

1. 操作者衣帽整洁，戴好口罩，洗净双手。

2. 将中草药用冷水浸泡20~60min后，放入中草药熏蒸机器的贮药机里，通电煮沸预热机器，夏天需要15min，冬天20min。

3. 机身内的温度春夏季可调至32℃左右，秋冬季可调至32~35℃。

4. 核对患者姓名，协助患者脱去衣裤，坐在椅子或卧于治疗床上。每次蒸20~30min，每日1~2次。

5. 熏蒸完后，关闭电源，操作者用毛巾擦干患者皮肤上的汗液，并协助其穿好衣服，嘱患者在治疗室内休息30min，汗止后回病房。

（五）注意事项

1. 在操作前向患者做好解释工作。

2. 在操作前应仔细检查机器是否正常、有无漏电，以防意外的发生。

3. 嘱患者喝500ml糖盐水，以防出汗太多出现虚脱。

4. 在熏蒸过程中注意皮肤微微出汗为宜，汗出太多易耗伤阴津。

5. 熏蒸过程中时刻关注患者情况，如出现心慌、气促、面色赤红或苍白、大汗不止等状况应立即关机，嘱其卧床休息，注意保暖，并给予盐开水。如不见缓解，请医生诊治。

6. 有以下情况者禁止使用蒸法：发热、昏迷、恶性肿瘤、黄疸、有出血倾向、严重

and blood, as well as woman in pregnant or menstrual period.

心脏病、哮喘发作、孕妇及经期妇女。

III. Macerating Therapy

i. Definition

It is an external therapy to bathe, soak or damply compress with the hot herbal decoction to clean open wounds and remove toxic substances. It has the effect of promoting blood circulation, removing swelling and relieving pain, clearing heat and detoxifying heat poison.

ii. Indication

It is mainly indicated for erysipelas, sores and ulceration, acute eczema, dermatitis, burns, tinea, chilblains, trauma, heat stroke and high fever.

iii. Preparation

Prepare herbal decoction, basin, towel, Vaseline, compress, gauze, bandage, adhesive plaster, rubber sheet, middle-size sheet and tray. Add blanket, folding screen, two oval forceps, curve tray, if they are necessary.

iv. Operation Method

1. The operator dresses clean, washes hands and wears face mask.

2. Check the patient's name, and close door and windows or put the folding screen beside the bed.

3. Help the patient to select a comfortable posture and expose the treated parts. Put the rubber sheet and middle-size sheet above the bed, and then put the curve tray on the middle-size sheet. Smear Vaseline on the local skin.

4. Soak the compress in the hot herbal decoction, and then wring out with forceps until there is no water drop. Fold and compress on the affected areas after the compress is not hot tested with the palm.

5. Change the compress for every 5-10minutes to keep it moist and warm. The treatment lasts for 30-60minutes each time. The compress can be changed once every 3 to 4 hours for the ulcer with little exudation.

6. Dry the local skin. Take away the tray, rubber sheet and middle-size sheet. Assist the patient to wear clothes, make the bed. Sterilize the used materials and record the procedure when the treatment has been finished.

v. Precaution

1. Explain the purposes and ways of the therapy to the patients before the operation in order to make them understand and get their cooperation.

三、溻渍法

（一）概念

溻渍法是用中草药煎汤趁热在身体局部淋洗、浸泡、湿敷，以洁净创口，祛除毒邪，温通经脉、消肿止痛的一种外治方法。

（二）适应证

多用于丹毒、疮疡肿痛、急性湿疹、皮炎、烧伤、皮肤癣症、冻疮、外伤、中暑、高热等。

（三）用物准备

药液、盆、毛巾、凡士林、敷布、纱布、绷带、胶布、橡胶单、中单、治疗盘，必要时备毛毯、屏风、卵圆钳 2 把、弯盘。

（四）操作方法

1. 操作者衣帽整洁，洗手，戴口罩。

2. 核对患者姓名，关闭门窗，或用屏风遮挡。

3. 协助患者取适合体位并暴露溻渍部位，下垫橡胶单、中单，置弯盘于中单上，局部涂凡士林。

4. 将药液倒入盆内，置敷布于药液中浸湿，用钳子拧干，以不滴水为度；抖开，用前臂掌测试温度，以不烫手为度，折叠后敷于患处。

5. 每隔 5~10min 用卵圆钳夹纱布浸药后淋药液于敷布上，保持敷布的湿度及温度，以发挥药效，每次溻渍约 30~60min。如果皮肤溃疡渗液不多，可 3~4h 换药一次。

6. 擦干局部药液，取下弯盘、中单、橡胶单，协助患者穿好衣裤，整理床单。对已用的物品进行消毒清洗处理后，做好有关局部情况、效果、溻渍时间等记录。

（五）注意事项

1. 操作前向患者解释溻渍的目的、方法，以取得患者合作。

2. The comfortable temperature of the herbal decoction is not more than 50℃ for the old and children to avoid burning.

3. Remove compress from the local enswathed areas. Change the compress and wrap the local areas with sterilized compress after the operation.

4. Sterile operation is necessary for the wound requiring the macerating therapy.

5. Different ways can be used for different parts. Bathing is good for extremities, soaking for acra, and damp compress for the waist and back.

6. All the used materials should be disinfected to avoid cross-infection.

IV. Washing with Herbal Bag

i. Definition

It is an external therapy to wash the local skin with gauze bag in appropriate temperature filled with herbs in order to invigorate blood flow and remove stasis, dispel wind and eliminate dampness, warm channels and collaterals, release swelling and relieve pain.

ii. Indication

It is commonly used for blood stagnation, swelling and pain of joints, soreness of bones and muscles, and injuries due to falls.

iii. Preparation

Prepare tray, wok, electric stove, rubber sheet, therapeutic towel, herbal decoction, dual-layer gauze bag and forceps.

iv. Operation Method

1. Soak the dual-layer gauze bag filled with herbs in water for 30 minutes and then decoct for 30 minutes with electric stove or steam in wok for 40 minutes.

2. Help the patient to expose the local skin and keep a comfortable posture.

3. Put the rubber sheet and towel under the local area. Take out the bag with forceps and compress the skin when the bag is not very hot.

4. Soak the limbs in herbal decoction of suitable temperature. Steaming method is available for the back. Put the bag on the back covered with the towel. Keep the patient warm with cotton quilt in winter.

5. The operation lasts for 30-60 minutes each time, twice a day. Wipe and clean the patient's skin and help him

2. 药液温度不宜过热，避免烫伤，老年、儿童药液不得超过 50℃。

3. 包扎部位湿渍时，应揭去敷料。湿渍完后，更换敷料，重新包扎。

4. 伤口部位进行湿渍疗法，应按无菌操作进行，操作后按换药法处理伤口。

5. 患部不同可采用不同的方法，四肢宜淋洗法，肢端宜浸泡法，腰背部宜湿敷法。

6. 所用物品须消毒，避免交叉感染。

四、腾洗法

（一）概念

腾洗法是将中药装在纱布袋内，经过蒸或煮后使药性透出，温度适宜时直接在局部腾洗，以达到活血祛瘀、祛风除湿、温经通络、消肿止痛等功效的一种方法。

（二）适应证

适用于瘀血不散、关节肿痛、筋骨疼痛、跌打损伤等。

（三）用物准备

治疗盘、蒸锅或煮锅、电炉、橡胶单、治疗巾、腾洗药、双层纱布袋和镊子。

（四）操作方法

1. 将腾洗的药装入纱布袋里，扎紧或缝好袋口，用水浸 30min，使药物充分浸湿后，电炉上煮 30min 或蒸锅蒸 40min。

2. 帮助患者暴露腾洗部位，取舒适体位。

3. 铺橡胶单和治疗巾于腾洗部位下面，用镊子钳取出药袋，用前臂掌侧测试药液温度，不烫手时方可腾洗。

4. 腾洗四肢待温度适宜时将肢体浸泡药液中，边泡边用药袋腾洗。腾洗腰背部用蒸法，将蒸热的药袋放在腰背部，上盖治疗巾，冬季用棉被盖好保温。

5. 每次腾洗 30~60min，每日 2 次。腾洗完后擦干局部，协助患者穿好衣裤。嘱患者休

to wear clothes. Tell the patient to take a rest in ward for 30minutes.

v. Precaution

1. The bag can be used for 3 days in summer and for 5 days in winter. The bag should be steamed each time before operation.

2. Prevent burning and accident.

3. Keep patients warm and away from cold.

4. Make patients stay indoors to prevent the joints from attacking cold pathogen.

V. Sitz Bath

i. Definition

Sitz bath is an external approach to fumigate and wash the perineum or anus with hot herbal decoction or melted medicine with boiled water in order to kill parasites and relieve itching, reduce swelling and relieve pain, promote blood circulation and dissipate blood stasis.

ii. Indication

It is commonly used for anus diseases including external hemorrhoid, perianal abscess, prolapse of internal hemorrhoid, hemorrhoid infection, and gynecological diseases such as pruritus of vulva, excessive leucorrhea, wound in perineal region.

iii. Preparation

Drugs, boiled water, bidet, chair, sterile gauze, tray, medicine, folding screen are needed.

iv. Operation Method

1. Put the hot herbal decoction into the chair, help the patient to expose the buttocks and sit above the bidet to fumigate. Wash the local region with the soaked sterile gauze until the temperature of herbal solution is appropriate. Finally, make the buttocks dry with the sterile gauze.

2. Do sitz bath once a day, 20-30 minutes for each time. The bidet and medicinal solution should be sterile and routinely change medicine for the case with wound.

v. Precaution

1. Keep the temperature of medicinal solution at 50-70℃ for fumigating. The temperature of medicinal solution for washing is advisable at 38-43℃.

2. Observe the patient's condition during the treatment. Sitz bath should be stopped if patients feel uncomfortable, and the nurse should inform the doctor at once.

息半小时后方可离开病室。

（五）注意事项

1. 腾洗药袋夏季每袋可连续使用 3d，冬季可连续使用 5d，每次用时都应重新煮或蒸。

2. 药袋不要过热，防止烫伤，使用电炉加热时注意防止意外发生。

3. 注意给患者保暖，防止风寒侵袭而感冒。

4. 腾洗结束后不要让患者立即外出活动，防止关节再次受凉而降低腾洗疗效。

五、坐浴法

（一）概念

坐浴法指将药物煎汤或开水冲化后趁热熏洗会阴部或肛门部。利用药物加热后产生的热力和药力共同对局部起到杀虫止痒、消肿止痛、活血化瘀的作用。

（二）适应证

常用于肛肠科疾病如外痔肿痛、肛周脓肿、内痔脱出、痔疮发炎等；妇科疾病如外阴瘙痒、带下过多、会阴部手术后等。

（三）用物准备

坐浴用药、开水、坐浴盆或椅、无菌纱布、治疗盘、准备换用的药物及屏风。

（四）操作方法

1. 将煎好或开水冲溶的坐浴药液趁热放在坐浴椅上，协助患者暴露臀部，坐在坐浴椅上熏蒸，待温度下降至不烫手时再用纱布浸湿药液，洗涤局部，最后用纱布擦干臀部。

2. 坐浴时间为每次 20~30min，每日 1 次。如有伤口时，浴盆及溶液应为无菌，坐浴后按常规给伤口换药。

（五）注意事项

1. 熏患处时药液温度应保持在 50~70℃，洗患处时药液温度应保持在 38~43℃。

2. 患者坐浴时应观察其病情有无异常变化，如发现异常，即刻停止坐浴，将患者扶

3. One patient has his own bidet to prevent cross-infection. The bidet must be sterilized after use.

4. Sitz bath is not allowed for female patients in menstrual period or in late pregnancy or with vaginal hemorrhage and acute pelvic infections.

VI. Body Bathing Therapy

i. Definition

It is an external approach to treat diseases by washing and bathing the body with hot herbal decoction in order to relax and activate the tendons, remove swelling and relieve pain, dispel wind and eliminate dampness, and clear heat and detoxify heat poison.

ii. Indication

It is used commonly for skin disease, sore and ulceration, soft tissue injury, and hemiplegia.

iii. Preparation

Prepare bathtub, thermometer, boiled water, herbal decoction, tressel, pants, trousers, slippers, and towel.

iv. Operation Method

1. The operator dresses clean and tidy, prepares the materials and checks the patients' name.

2. Adjust the bathroom's temperature ranging from 20-22℃. Make the medicinal solution range from 50-70℃.

3. Help the patient to take off clothes and sit on the tressel for bathing and steaming the body.

4. Soak the patient's body and four limbs in medicinal solution when it is in suitable temperature. The bath lasts for 40 minutes.

5. Wash the body with warm water when it is finished and cover the patient with bath towel. Then help patient to dress up and go back to the ward.

6. Sterilize the bathtub and bathroom, put everything in order and make record.

v. Precaution

1. It is important to explain the therapy to the patients before bath in order to make them understand and get their cooperation. Keep the patient's privacy.

2. The bath room should be kept in suitable temperature to prevent collapse because of excessive sweat in summer and avoid common cold in winter. The temperature of medicinal

回病室休息，同时报告医生处理。

3. 坐浴盆应每人一个，用后注意清洗消毒，避免交叉感染。

4. 女患者在月经期或阴道出血、妊娠后期忌用坐浴，盆腔器官急性炎症期也不宜坐浴。

六、全身药浴法

（一）概念

全身药浴法指将中药煎成汤液，进行全身性熏洗、浸渍，以达到舒筋活络、消肿止痛、祛风除湿、清热解毒目的的一种治疗方法。

（二）适应证

适用于皮肤病、疮疡、伤筋挫骨、肢体偏瘫等。

（三）用物准备

浴盆、温度计、开水、汤药、活动架、备好患者更换的衣裤、拖鞋、毛巾。

（四）操作方法

1. 操作者衣帽整洁，准备好所有物品后，核对患者姓名。

2. 调节浴室的温度在 20~22℃，将药液倒入浴盆内加开水调温度至 50~70℃。

3. 必要时协助患者脱去衣裤，扶入浴盆内坐在活动架上，先使药液蒸气熏蒸全身。

4. 药液温度下降到能浸入四肢时，将躯体及四肢全部浸泡于药液中，必要时协助患者擦洗患处。药浴时间控制在 40min 为宜，以免其疲劳。

5. 药浴结束后，用温水冲去患者皮肤上的药液，帮其擦干后披上浴巾，扶出浴盆，待其穿好衣裤后送回病室休息。

6. 消毒浴盆、浴室，整理用物，并做好相关记录。

（五）注意事项

1. 操作前要做好患者的思想工作，争取获得合作，注意患者的隐私保护。

2. 浴室内温度适宜，夏季防止出汗过多而虚脱，冬季预防受凉感冒。药液的温度，

solution should also be adjusted to be appropriate.

3. Help and observe the old, the weak, children and patients who move inconveniently.

4. Observe the patient's complexion and breath. The bath should be stopped when patient feels uncomfortable, keep him in lying posture and give him warm water. In a serious case, inform the doctor immediately.

5. The body bathing therapy is not allowed for female patients in menstrual period or pregnancy.

(Xu Dong-ying)

Section 10　Wet Compress Therapy

Wet compress therapy is a method to put the sterile gauze that has been soaked in liquid medicine in the local part or point of the human body so as to clear the striae, detoxicate toxic heat, reduce swelling, promote blood circulation and relieve pain.

I. Indication

Facial acne, eczema, erysipelas, gangrene, arthritis, tinea, kibe and other surgical and skin disease.

II. Contraindication

Avoid using this method to treat the patients with bullous skin diseases, serious sores abscess, skin broken serious collapse, and the patients who are allergic to wet compress drug.

III. Preparation

This includes herbal decoction, fresh herbal juice, rubber sheet, curve tray, sterile gauze, Vaseline and sterile forceps.

以不烫伤为度。

3. 对年老体弱者、儿童及活动不便者必须给予帮助，并严密观察。

4. 在药浴过程中要随时观察患者的面色、呼吸等是否有异常，如有异常应立即停止药浴，将其扶出浴盆，平卧休息，必要时给予温开水，严重的应及时通知医生。

5. 孕妇和经期患者禁用此法。

（徐冬英）

第十节　湿敷法

中药湿敷法是根据患者病情采用中草药煎汤或取汁后，用浸透药液的无菌纱布直接敷于局部的一种治疗方法，此法可达到疏通腠理、清热解毒、消肿散结、活血止痛的作用。

一、适应证

多用于面部痤疮、湿疹、丹毒、脱疽、关节炎、手足癣等外科疮疡及皮肤病。

二、禁忌证

大疱性皮肤病、疮疡脓肿急速扩散者、皮肤破溃严重者以及对湿敷药物过敏者。

三、用物准备

中药液、中药汁、橡胶单、中单、弯盘、无菌纱布、凡士林、无菌钳。

IV. Manipulation

1. After the materials are prepared, take them to the ward and check again. Explain the purposes and process of the operation to the patient in order to get his cooperation. Pay attention to keep the patient warm. Use the screen based on the situation.

2. Assist the patient to take a state and comfortable posture, and expose the treatment parts. Put the rubber sheet, middle-size sheet and curve tray beside the treated part. Keep warm in winter and keep the patient's privacy. Put Vaseline on local skin (avoid eye area).

3. Measure the medical liquid temperature. The appropriate temperature should be 38-40℃.

4. Soak the compress in the medical liquid and squeeze it with sterile forceps.

5. Shake off the compress, and put it on the exposed part closely. The size of the wet compress should be appropriate to the size of the exposed part.

6. Observe skin changes of the patients. Stop treatment immediately and report to doctors when some conditions appear such as blisters, local pale, rash, itching and pain or breaking. Keep the compress moist, and replace the dressing once for every 5-10 minutes. In general, the treatment can be applied 2-3 times a day and 30-60 minutes each time.

7. By the end of the treatment, take off the dressing and deposit them to the curve tray. Clean the skin with sterile gauze and observe the skin condition again.

8. Clean up the materials, inform the attention, and check the doctor's advice again.

9. Clean up the materials, wash hands, and record.

V. Precaution

1. Keep operator's hat clean, prepare all items, and check the patient's name.

2. Explain the process to the patient before operating for cooperation.

3. Prepare the herbal decoction or fresh herbal juice before operating in order to get good therapeutic effect.

4. Operate wet dressing according to the sterile operation of the wound, and deal with the wound according to the dressing method after the operating.

5. Pay attention to the disinfection and isolation of

四、操作方法

1. 备齐用物携至患者床旁，核对患者并做好解释，以取得患者和家属对执行该操作的知情同意及配合。

2. 协助患者取安全舒适体位，暴露湿敷部位，下垫橡胶单、中单，弯盘置于湿敷部位旁。冬季注意保暖，保护患者隐私。局部涂以凡士林（眼部勿涂凡士林）。

3. 测量药液温度，温度以 38~40℃为宜。

4. 置敷布于药液中浸湿，用无菌钳拧干至不滴药液为度。

5. 抖开敷布，覆盖于湿敷部位，整理敷布，使之平整并紧贴于皮肤，敷布大小应与湿敷部位大小适宜。

6. 注意观察患者湿敷部位的皮肤变化，如出现水疱、局部苍白、皮疹痒痛或破溃等症状时，应立即停止操作，报告医生，配合处理。敷布要保持湿润，每 5~10min 更换敷布一次。一般每日湿敷 2~3 次，每次 30~60min。

7. 湿敷结束后，取下敷布置于弯盘内，用无菌纱布擦干局部皮肤，再次观察局部皮肤情况。

8. 协助患者整理好衣物，整理床单，告知注意事项，再次核对医嘱。

9. 整理用物，归还原处，洗手并记录。

五、注意事项

1. 操作者衣帽整洁，准备好所有物品后，核对患者姓名。

2. 操作前应对患者做好解释，以取得其配合作。

3. 湿敷液应新鲜配制，防止因溶液变质影响效果。

4. 按无菌操作对伤口部位湿敷，操作后按换药法处理伤口。

5. 所用物品注意消毒隔离，避免交叉感染。

the waste so as to avoid cross infection.

6. Keep the temperature of herbal decoction being 38-40℃.The low temperature easily causes cold because of compensatory vasodilation and the high temperature may cause burning.

7. Tell the patients to avoid outdoor activities after wet compress therapy completed in case catching cold which could affect the therapeutic effect.

8. Keep warm in winter and prevent catching cold.

(Xu Dong-ying)

6. 湿敷的药液温度以 38~40℃为宜，温度过低易引起代偿性的血管扩张而致感冒；温度过高可能导致烫伤。

7. 湿敷结束后，嘱患者不要立即外出活动，防止湿敷部位受凉而降低湿敷效果。

8. 冬天注意保暖，防止受凉。

（徐冬英）

Section 11　Drug Smearing Therapy

Drug smearing therapy is a method to smear drugs in the local part or point of the human body. The dosage forms often used include water, tincture, ointment *etc.*.

I. Indication

Sores, bruises, insect bites, burns, hemorrhoids and other diseases.

II. Contraindication

Avoid smearing the drugs in the face of infants and young children.

III. Preparation

This includes treatment disc, drug (according to the doctor's orders to prepare), curve tray, cotton sign, tweezers, saline cotton ball, dry cotton ball, gauze, adhesive tape, bandages, rubber sheet, screen.

IV. Manipulation

1. After the materials are prepared, take them to the ward and check again. Explain the purposes and ways of

第十一节　涂药法

涂药法是将各种外用药物直接涂于患处或穴位的一种外治方法。其剂型有水剂、酊剂、油剂、膏剂等。

一、适应证

多用于疮疡、跌打损伤、虫咬伤、烫伤、烧伤、痔瘘等病证。

二、禁忌证

婴幼儿颜面部禁用。

三、用物准备

治疗盘、外用药物（根据医嘱准备）、弯盘、棉签、镊子、盐水、棉球、干棉球、纱布、胶布、绷带、橡胶单、中单，必要时备屏风。

四、操作方法

1. 备齐用物，携至床旁，核对医嘱；解释治疗目的、方法，以取得患者配合；根据

the operation to the patient in order to get the cooperation. Assist the patient to take a comfortable posture according to the disease condition, then expose the parts to be treated and put rubber sheet above the bed. Pay attention to keep the patient warm. Use the screen based on the situation.

2. Clean the skin, smear drug on to the exposed part with a cotton swab evenly or a cotton ball fixed with tweezers for a large affected area. Suitable humidity and good uniformity of coating is very important for good operating. When necessary the area can be covered with the appropriate size of gauze, and fixed with adhesive tape.

3. When the operation is completed, assist the patient to take a comfortable posture. Clean the sheet and check doctor's order again.

4. Clean up items, wash hands, push medical trolley cart back to the therapeutic room, clean medical waste according to the requirements, and record if necessary.

V. Precaution

1. Clean the local skin before applying the medicine.

2. The times of smearing drug are decided according to the character of medicine and illness. Cream can be smeared with the palm of your hand or fingers on the site repeatedly for good drug infiltration of the skin. Shake the suspension agent well before application. The cap of tincture or other liquid medicine should be promptly put tightly to prevent the volatilization of drugs after use.

3. After applying the medicine, observe the local skin closely. The treatment should be immediately discontinued when some allergic reactions happen, such as a rash, itching or local swelling and other allergic phenomena and the drug should be wiped clean if necessary. Take anti allergic drugs according to doctor's advice for oral or topical use.

4. The drug should not be applied too much or too thick, so as not to block the pores.

5. Strong irritant drugs can not apply to the face, and cannot be used for infants and young children.

(Xu Dong-ying)

病情协助患者取舒适、合理体位，并暴露用药部位，患处酌情铺橡胶单或中单；注意保暖，视情况使用屏风。

2. 清洁皮肤，用棉签蘸配制的药液、均匀地涂于患处。涂搽面积较大时，可用镊子夹棉球蘸药物涂布，蘸药干湿度适宜，涂药厚薄均匀。必要时用大小合适的纱布覆盖，用胶布固定，松紧适宜。

3. 涂药完毕，协助患者穿戴好衣物，安排舒适体位，整理床单，再次核对医嘱。

4. 清理物品，洗手，推车回治疗室，按要求处理医疗废物，必要时记录。

五、注意事项

1. 涂药前应清洁局部皮肤。

2. 涂药次数依病情、药物而定；使用霜剂可用手掌或手指在涂药部位反复轻揉，使药物渗入肌肤；混悬液使用前须摇均匀后再涂搽；水剂、酊剂用后及时将瓶盖盖紧，防止药物挥发。

3. 涂药后密切观察局部皮肤，如有丘疹、奇痒或局部肿胀等过敏现象，应立即停用，并将药物拭净或清洗，必要时遵医嘱内服或外用抗过敏药物。

4. 涂搽药物不宜过多、过厚，以免阻塞毛孔。

5. 不可将刺激性强的药物涂搽于面部，且禁用于婴幼儿。

（徐冬英）

Section 12　Acupoint Application

Acupoints application method refers to chop and mash the fresh herbs or grind Chinese herbal medicine into a fine powder, and add right amount of excipients to tune them into a paste, and then spread them to acupoints or affected area (*ashi* points). It can adjust the predominance or decline yin and yang of *zang-fu* organs, and improve the circulation of qi and blood through the interaction of the herbs and acupoints to prevent or treat diseases. Common excipients are water, wine, vinegar, honey, caramel, vegetable oil, egg white onion juice, ginger, garlic, tea, Vaseline, *etc.*.

I. Indication

Indications of acupoints application are quite extensive including a variety of acute and chronic diseases. Acupoints application can also be used to prevent diseases and help people to stay healthy.

1. Internal Disease　Common cold, cough, asthma, spontaneous sweating, night sweating, insomnia, headache, epigastralgia, diarrhea, constipation, vomiting, dyspepsia, diabetes, *etc.*.

2. Surgical Disease　swollen and sore, joint pains, traumatic injury, *etc.*.

3. Andrological and Gynecological Disease Nocturnal emission, impotence, irregular menstruation, dysmenorrhea, uterine prolapse, acute suppurative mastitis, hyperplasia of mammary glands, *etc.*.

4. Pediatric Disease　Infantile crying at night, anorexia, nocturnal enuresis, salivation, *etc.*.

5. Ophthalmological and Otorhinolaryngological Disease　Inflammation of the throat, toothache, oral sores, *etc.*.

II. Contraindication

1. Eyes and lips should be applied with caution.

2. Patients who are prone to drug allergy, rush pimples, blisters should be applied with caution.

III. Manipulation

1. Check medical order, gather equipment, and

第十二节　穴位贴敷法

穴位贴敷法，是指将新鲜的中药切碎、捣烂，或将中药研成细末，加适量赋形剂调成糊状后，敷布于腧穴或患处（阿是穴），通过药物和穴位的共同作用纠正脏腑阴阳的偏胜或偏衰，改善经络的气血运行，以达到防病治病的目的。常用的赋形剂有水、酒、醋、蜂蜜、饴糖、植物油、鸡蛋清、葱汁、姜汁、蒜汁、茶汁和凡士林等。

一、适应证

穴位贴敷法的适应证相当广泛，包括多种临床急、慢性疾患，还可以用于防病保健。

1. **内科病证**　感冒、咳嗽、哮喘、自汗、盗汗、不寐、胃脘痛、泄泻、呕吐、便秘、食积、消渴等。

2. **外科病证**　疮疡肿毒、关节疼痛、跌打损伤等。

3. **男科及妇科病证**　遗精、阳痿、月经不调、痛经、子宫脱垂、乳痈、乳核等。

4. **儿科病证**　夜啼、厌食、遗尿、流涎等。

5. **五官科病证**　喉痹、牙痛、口疮等。

二、禁忌证

1. 患者的眼部、唇部等处慎用。

2. 有药物过敏史或者皮肤容易起丘疹、水疱的患者慎用。

三、操作方法

1. 核对医嘱，备齐用物，携至床旁，做

then bring them to bedside. Identify the patient and give appropriate explanation to him/her so as to get cooperation.

2. Assist the patient to a comfortable position according to the selected acupoints. Expose the treated parts, find the right acupoints, keep the patient warm and protect his or her privacy.

3. If it is the first time to apply acupoints application for the patient, use cotton balls filled with saline solution to clean skin as needed. If apply dressing change, remove the old site dressing and discard, and then apply cotton balls with saline solution to clean traces of drugs on the skin. Observe the skin and therapeutic effect.

4. Apply well prepared liniment or rubbed fresh herbs to the appropriate acupoints, and then cover it with gauze sponge (or special application). Fix it well with adhesive tape or bandage, neither too loosely nor too tightly, preventing clothing being contaminated from overflows of heated medicine.

5. When finishing the process above, assist patient to get dressed and take a comfortable position. Make beds and then address tailored health education to the patient.

6. Clear up equipment, perform hand hygiene, and remember documentation and signature.

IV. Precaution

1. When applying medicine mixed with solvent, one should prepare it well and use it timely.

2. If apply plaster, pay attention to the appropriate temperature so as to avoid being burnt, and to keep adhere securely.

3. Fix the application securely to avoid shifting or falling off. If patient is allergy to adhesive tape, fix the medicine with other methods.

4. When use medicine with strong irritant and toxicant, patched acupoints should not be too much, treated area should not be too large, and time should not be too long so as to avoid causing too large vesiculation or being poisoned.

5. Do not use large dose of medicine or apply too long time for patients with chronic or serious physical illnesses. During the application period, one should pay close attention to the patient's condition and adverse reactions.

6. Pregnant women and young children should avoid being patched medicine with strong irritant and toxicant.

7. Do not use gasoline or irritating soap to wipe residual ointment on the skin.

(Wang Yun-cui)

好核对解释，取得合作。

2. 根据所选穴位协助患者取舒适体位，暴露敷药部位，定准穴位，注意保暖和遮挡。

3. 首次贴敷者，必要时用生理盐水棉球清洁局部皮肤；更换敷贴者，取下原敷贴，用生理盐水棉球擦洗皮肤上的用药痕迹，观察皮肤情况及敷药效果。

4. 将制好的敷药或研好的新鲜草药准确地贴敷于相应穴位，以纱布（或专用敷贴）覆盖，胶布固定或绷带包扎，松紧适宜，防止药物受热后溢出而污染衣被。

5. 敷药完毕，协助患者着衣，安排舒适体位，整理床单位，针对性地进行健康教育。

6. 整理用物、洗手，做好记录并签名。

四、注意事项

1. 凡用溶剂调敷药物时，需现调现用。

2. 若用膏药贴敷，应掌握好温度，以免烫伤或者粘不住。

3. 应固定稳妥，以免移动或脱落，对胶布过敏者可用其他的方法固定。

4. 对刺激性强、毒性大的药物，贴敷穴位不宜过多，面积不宜过大，时间不宜过长，以免发疱过大或引起药物中毒。

5. 对久病体弱或有严重身体疾病时，使用药量不宜过大，贴敷时间不宜过久，并在贴敷期间密切观察患者的病情变化和有无药物不良反应的发生。

6. 对于孕妇、幼儿，应避免为其贴敷刺激性强、毒性大的药物。

7. 对于残留在皮肤上的药膏等，不可用汽油或肥皂等有刺激性的物品擦拭。

（王云翠）

Section 13   Medical Wax Therapy

Medical wax therapy is an external treatment of TCM referring to apply heated medical wax on the surface of skin or the corresponding acupoints to cure diseases through the thermal stimulation, mechanical pressure and moisturizing effects. Medical wax can be applied to all parts of the body, especially the joints because of its plasticity, viscosity and ductility. Wax is solid at room temperature with larger thermal storage, small thermal conductivity, slow heat elimination and durable treat time. Therefore, medical wax therapy has the effects of warming middle and dissipating cold, and reliving swelling and pain. Common medical wax therapies include yellow wax therapy, paraffin therapy, and ozokerite therapy.

Contemporary studies have found that applying heated medical wax on the surface of skin can cause irritation or warming effect, which dilate local blood vessels, accelerate blood flow to improve the nutrition of the surrounding tissue and promote tissue healing. Meanwhile, the volume of hot wax is gradually reduced during the cooling process, resulting in a soft mechanical pressure effect to prevent blood and lymph oozing from tissues, or promoting the absorption of exudate, so as to relieve swelling and pain and improve motor function of joints.

I. Indication

1. Diseases of Joints   Joints stiffness and contractures, chronic non-specific arthritis, frozen shoulder, tenosynovitis, bursitis, *etc.*.

2. Various Injury and Strain   Bruise, sprains, muscle strains, *etc.*.

3. Trauma or Surgery Complication   Postoperative scar and adhesion, invasion or poor healing of wounds or chronic ulcers, *etc.*.

4. Various Inflammations   Neuritis, myositis, osteomyelitis, neuralgia, *etc.*.

5. Dermatological Disease   Eczema, scabies, skin sclerosis, neurodermatitis, *etc.*.

6. Internal Disease   Epigastralgia, abdominal pain, deficiency-cold diarrhea, gastrointestinal neurosis, gastritis, cholecystitis, *etc.*.

7. Gynecological Disease   Chronic pelvic inflammatory disease, infertility, *etc.*.

第十三节   蜡疗法

蜡疗法是指将加热的医用蜡贴敷于患处或者相应穴位上，利用蜡的温热刺激、机械压迫及滋润作用以治疗疾病的一种中医外治法。蜡具有可塑性、黏稠性、延展性，适用于人体各个部位，尤其是关节部位。在常温下，蜡为固体，有较大的蓄热性，且导热系数小，散热慢，治疗时间持久，故蜡疗法具有温中散寒、消肿定痛之功效。常用的蜡疗法包括黄蜡疗法、石蜡疗法、地蜡疗法。

现代研究发现，利用加热的医用蜡贴敷在体表，可产生刺激或温热作用，使局部血管扩张，血流加快从而改善周围组织的营养，促进组织愈合；另一方面，热蜡在冷却过程中，体积逐渐缩小，产生柔和的机械压迫作用，能防止组织内的淋巴液和血液的渗出，或促进渗出液的吸收，从而达到消肿止痛、改善运动功能的作用。

一、适应证

1. **关节病证**   关节强直、挛缩、慢性非特异性关节炎、肩周炎、腱鞘炎、滑囊炎等。

2. **各种损伤及劳损**   挫伤、扭伤、肌肉劳损等。

3. **外伤或手术后遗症**   术后瘢痕、粘连、浸润或愈合不良的伤口或慢性溃疡等。

4. **各种炎症**   神经炎、肌炎、骨髓炎、神经痛等。

5. **皮肤病证**   湿疹、疥疮、皮肤硬化症、神经性皮炎等。

6. **内科病证**   胃脘痛、腹痛、虚寒泄泻、胃肠神经官能症、胃炎、胆囊炎等。

7. **妇科病证**   慢性盆腔炎、不孕症等。

II. Contraindication

Medical wax therapy can not be used for treating sensory impairment, heart and kidney failure, malignant tumors, tuberculosis, bleeding tendency, purulent infection and infants.

III. Manipulation

1. Check medical order, gather equipment, and then bring them to bedside. Identify the patient and give appropriate explanation to him so as to get cooperation.

2. Assist the patient to a comfortable position and then expose the treated parts.

3. Select the type and method of medical max therapy according to the medical order.

(1) Yellow wax therapy

1) Carbon wax therapy: Expose the affected area, make paste mud with flour and water, knead them into thin strips about 1cm in diameter, and place it around the affected area. Sprinkle powdered yellow wax about 1cm thick in the paste circle, cover the skin out of the paste circle with clothes or other things to prevent healthy skin being burned. Then filled copper spoon with charcoal to bake the wax, add wax while it is melting until the height is as tall as the paste circle. Remove the wax when it is cold. Repeat once every other day.

2) Artemisia-wax therapy: The manipulation is the same as carbon wax therapy, but spread moxa on the yellow wax in order to melt wax by burning the moxa.

(2) Paraffin therapy

1) Paraffin cloth sticking: Dip sterile gauze pad with hot wax, cool it until the patient can tolerate the temperature, and paste the gauze pad on treated area. Then cover the first piece of paraffin cloth with another smaller one (60-65℃). At last put blankets, large towels or other items on them to preserve heat. Apply this therapy daily or every other day for 30 minutes *per* treatment, 15 times as a period of treatment.

2) Paraffin pie sticking: The appropriate amount of paraffin is heated to melt, and then pour it into a porcelain dish covered with a layer of tape (The thickness of paraffin is about 2-3cm).When the surface temperature of paraffin drops to about 50℃, take it out together with tape, and then stick it on the surface of the skin. One can also pour paraffin into the porcelain dish without tape. When paraffin is cooled into a pie, and isolated by knife, place the appropriate blocks on the affected area, and wrap up with thermal insulation 30

二、禁忌证

感觉障碍、心力衰竭、肾功能衰竭、恶性肿瘤、结核、有出血倾向、化脓性感染者及婴幼儿禁用此法。

三、操作方法

1. 核对医嘱，备齐用物，携至床旁，做好核对解释，取得合作。

2. 协助患者取得舒适卧位，暴露治疗部位。

3. 按医嘱选择蜡疗的种类和方法。

（1）黄蜡疗法

1）碳蜡法：暴露患处，用白面和水揉成面泥，搓成直径为 1cm 左右的细条状，围放在患部周围，面圈内撒上黄蜡末或贴敷黄蜡饼约 1cm 厚，面圈外皮肤以物覆盖，以防灼伤周围部位的皮肤。用铜勺盛炭火，置蜡上烘烤，随化随添蜡末，直至蜡与所围面圈高度相平为止，蜡冷后去掉，隔日一次。

2）艾蜡法：操作方法同碳蜡法，需要在蜡末上铺撒艾绒，以点燃的艾绒使蜡熔化。

（2）石蜡疗法

1）蜡布贴敷法：用无菌纱布垫浸蘸热蜡液，待冷却至患者能耐受之温度，贴敷于治疗部位上，用另一块较小的 60~65℃ 的高温热蜡布盖在第一块蜡布上，用棉被、大毛巾等物品覆盖保温。每日或隔日 1 次，每次治疗 30min，15 次为一个疗程。

2）蜡饼贴敷法：将适量石蜡加热熔化，倒入一个盘底内铺有一层胶布的瓷盘中，厚度约 2~3cm。当蜡层表面温度降至 50℃ 左右时，连同胶布一同起出，贴敷于患处；也可直接倾蜡入盘，待盘中石蜡冷却成饼后，用刀分离，切成适当块状放置患处，保温包扎。每次治疗 30min，15 次为一个疗程。

minutes *per* treatment, 15 times as a period of treatment.

3) Paraffin bags sticking: Put the melted paraffin into a rubber bag, or put the paraffin into the bag first and then melt the paraffin. The melted paraffin should be account to 1/3 volume of the bag. When surface temperature of the paraffin is suitable to treatment, apply it on the treated area.

4) Coating paste therapy with liquid paraffin: Paraffin is heated to 100℃. After sterilized for 15 minutes, the paraffin is cooled to 50-60℃, and then is applied to the treated area with a sterile brush. When the first layer of paraffin is applied, try to make a uniform thickness and bigger area to form a protective film. There after spread liquid paraffin with slightly higher temperature, but make sure it will not scald the skin. All of the layers are applied as soon as possible, until the thickness is 1cm. Finally, wrap up and keep warm with insulation materials (such as pad).

5) Liquid paraffin immersion: The medical paraffin is melted indirectly and placed into the insulation vessel. The appropriate temperature is controlled at 55.5-57.5℃. The affected area is immersed into liquid paraffin (Starting time is from forming a thick layer of paraffin).The treated area is out of the liquid paraffin and it should remove the layer of the paraffin 15 minutes later. 1 or 2 times a day, 15 times as a period. This therapy is fit for limbs disorders.

There are also pouring paraffin therapies, spraying paraffin therapy, eye or facial spreading paraffin therapy, vaginal paraffin embolism therapy, *etc.*.

(3) Ozocerite therapy: The melting point of ozocerite is 52-55℃. Its nature and functions are similar to paraffin, and manipulation is also roughly same with paraffin therapy.

4. Observe local and general condition of the patient at any time during the procedure.

5. When finishing the process above, assist patient take to a comfortable position, address tailored health education to the patient, and then ask patients to have a 30-minute break.

6. Clear up equipment, perform hand hygiene, and remember documentation and signature.

IV. Precaution

1. Medical wax should be heated through water-heating to prevent it from being scorched or burned.

2. Interrupt procedure immediately if the patient indicates allergy during the process.

3. The performance (plasticity and viscosity) of used wax (except for the parts of the body cavity and the

3）蜡袋贴敷法：将石蜡熔化后装入橡皮袋内，或将石蜡装入袋内再行熔化，蜡液应占袋装容积约 1/3，待蜡袋表面温度达到治疗之需时，即可贴敷于患处。

4）蜡液涂贴法：将石蜡加热到 100℃，经 15min 消毒后，冷却到 50~60℃，用无菌毛刷向患处涂抹。在涂抹第一层蜡液时，要尽量做到厚薄均匀，面积大些，以形成保护膜。此后可涂抹温度稍高一些的石蜡液，但不可烫伤皮肤。各层尽快涂抹，厚度达 1cm 为止，最后以保温物品（如棉垫）包裹。

5）蜡液浸泡法：将医用石蜡间接熔化，放入保温器皿中，温度控制在 55.5~57.5℃为宜，将患部浸入蜡液之中（形成较厚蜡层时开始计算浸入蜡液的时间），15min 后抽出，脱去蜡层。每日 1~2 次，15 次为一个疗程。本法以四肢疾患为宜。此外还有浇蜡法、喷雾法、面部或眼部涂蜡法，阴道石蜡栓塞法等。

（3）地蜡疗法：地蜡的熔点为 52~55℃，其性质和作用与石蜡相似，使用方法大致相同。

4. 操作过程中随时观察患者的局部和全身情况。

5. 操作结束后置患者于舒适的体位，嘱患者休息 30min，并有针对性地给予健康教育。

6. 整理用物，洗手，做好记录并签名。

四、注意事项

1. 加热医用蜡时，要采用隔水加热法，以防烧焦或燃烧。

2. 蜡疗过程中，若患者出现过敏现象要立即停止操作。

3. 用过的蜡（用于创面和体腔部位的除外），其性能（可塑性及黏滞性）降低，在重

wound) decreases, so when using them repeatedly, one need to add 15%-25% of new wax each time.

4. The temperature of medical wax therapy should vary from person to person due to illness. Make sure that the temperature is neither too low to reduce effects, nor too high to scald the skin.

(Wang Yun-cui)

Section 14   Foot Bath Therapy

Foot bath therapy is a kind of method that can make medicaments ion enter the affected part of the body *via* the approaches of warm, mechanical, and chemical reaction of medical solution. Through the drug steam and fumigation, the therapeutic effects of the medical solution quickly are distributed to the whole body with the blood circulation. This therapy could keep *zang-fu* organs fit, promote the circulation of qi and blood, regulate yin and yang, dredge the meridians, improve blood circulation, accelerate the discharge of metabolism product, and thus prevent and cure diseases and enhance the physical fitness.

I. Indication

Foot bath therapy is often used in clinical practice to treat internal medicine, surgery, gynecology, pediatrics, dermatology and other diseases, and is a kind of adjuvant therapy for some acute and difficult diseases, such as diabetes and neuropathy. In addition, foot bath therapy is useful for the rehabilitation of disease.

II. Contraindication

1. Avoid using foot bath for patients with serious illnesses such as heart, lung, brain and mental disorders.

2. Avoid using foot bath at the areas with burns, scald, impetigo or skin diseases, skin damage or infection on the foot.

3. Avoid using foot bath for patients with gastrointestinal bleeding, menorrhagia, and bleeding tendency.

4. Avoid using foot bath for the one with temperature sensors unconscious, such as extreme fatigue, severe

复使用时，每次需要加入 15%~25% 的新蜡。

4. 蜡疗的温度要因人、因病而异，既不能温度过低而影响疗效，又要防止温度过高而烫伤皮肤。

（王云翠）

第十四节   足浴疗法

足浴疗法是通过药液的温热、机械、化学作用及借助药物蒸汽和药液的熏洗和治疗作用使药物离子通过各种途径进入患部，并随血液循环快速输送到全身，从而起到颐养脏腑、促进气血运行、调理阴阳平衡、疏通经脉、改善血液循环、加速体内新陈代谢产物排出的功效，进而达到防病治病、增强体质的目的。

一、适应证

足浴疗法临床广泛适用于内、外、妇、儿及皮肤科等多种疾患，急性病、慢性病及某些疑难病的辅助治疗，如糖尿病、神经病变等，还可用于疾病康复治疗。

二、禁忌证

1. 患有心、肺、脑及精神障碍等严重疾病的患者禁用。

2. 凡足部有烧伤、烫伤、脓疱疮或皮肤病、皮肤破损或感染者禁用。

3. 消化道出血及月经过多者、有出血倾向者禁用。

4. 对温度感应失去知觉者，如极度疲劳、

drunk.

5. Avoid using foot bath for people with fasting or within half an hour after a meal.

III. Preparation

Prepare the foot bath device (check whether the performance is intact and safe), decoction of Chinese medicine, disposable bag for foot bath, water temperature meter, container pot, hot water, cold water, towels, *etc.*.

IV. Manipulation

1. Prepare all the materials and take them to the ward. Make explanation to the patient to get his or her cooperation.

2. Help the patient select a comfortable posture according to the disease. Expose the selected parts and keep warm.

3. Pour the decoction of Chinese medicine into the container pot and add hot water. Adjust the water temperature to 38-42℃. Take a constant foot bath device, put a disposable bag on it, and then pour the prepared foot bath liquid into the constant foot bath device.

4. Assist patient's feet immersed in the foot bath liquid. Appropriately, let the patient's ankle be immersed in the liquid more than 10cm. Connect the power of the device, select the foot mode and adjust the time. 20-30 minutes each time, 1 or 2 times a day are usually selected.

5. Massage the feet during the process of foot bath. The acupuncture points such as KI 1 (*yǒng quán*), KI 2 (*rán gǔ*) and *ashi* points are often chosen to be massaged , and the bottom of the heel is as well.

6. Maintain the temperature of the liquid. Enquire whether the patient feels discomfort at any time of the foot bath process.

7. Clean the local skin after the procedure finished, assist the patients to tidy up clothes and place them in the comfortable position.

8. Tidy up the materials, wash the hands, and take a record.

V. Precaution

1. Do not use the foot bath container made of metal, which is prone to react with the tannic acid, generate

严重醉酒者禁用。

5. 空腹、饭后半小时内不宜足浴。

三、用物准备

足浴器（检查其性能是否完好、安全），中药煎剂或中药免煎颗粒、一次性足浴袋、水温计、容器盆、热水、冷水、毛巾等。

四、操作方法

1. 备齐用物，携至患者床旁，向患者做好解释，取得合作。

2. 协助患者取合适体位，暴露足浴部位，注意保暖。

3. 将中药煎剂或中药免煎颗粒倒入容器盆中加热水，调节水温至 38~42℃，取恒温足浴器，套上一次性足浴袋，将已配好的足浴药液倒入足浴器中。

4. 协助患者双足浸入足浴药液中，足浴液的量以能浸没脚踝以上 10cm 为宜，接上电源，选择足浴模式，调节时间。一般每次 20~30min，每日 1~2 次。

5. 足浴过程中可多按摩双足的足趾和足心，常选的穴位有然谷、涌泉、阿是穴及足跟底部。

6. 保持药液温度，询问患者有无不适。

7. 操作完毕，清洁局部皮肤，协助患者整理衣着并为其安置舒适卧位。

8. 整理用物，洗手，记录并签名。

五、注意事项

1. 足部药浴的容器不要用金属盆，因金属容易与中药中的鞣酸发生反应，生成鞣酸

iron and other harmful substances. It is best to use the specialized foot bath device sold in the market. If not, the tub, wood bucket or enamel pots can also be used.

2. It is not suitable to do foot bath 30 minutes before or after a meal. Bath foot before meals may inhibit the secretion of gastric juice, affecting digestion. Bath foot after meals could dilate foot blood vessels, resulting in the decreases of blood in gastrointestinal tract and viscera, and affecting the gastrointestinal digestive function.

3. Observe the patient's condition during the process of foot bath. Stop the foot bath, and report to a doctor immediately when patients feel dizzy, fatigue, palpitation or in other symptoms. Observe whether there are allergic reactions such as redness, itching, *etc.* on the skin.

4. Liquid temperature should be appropriate, which is generally at 38-42℃. Liquid temperature for patients with diabetes, chapped feet or lower extremity sensory disorders should be reduced to avoid scalding.

5. The dose of external treatment drugs used for medicated foot bath is large, and some are toxic, thus they are not suitable for oral administration.

6. Do well in the disinfection and isolation to the patient with infectious skin diseases, such as tinea pedis, so as to prevent cross-infection.

(Yang Jin-hua)

铁等有害物质，最好用市面上卖的专用足浴器，也可以用木盆、木桶或搪瓷盆。

2. 饭前、饭后30min内不宜进行足部药浴，饭前足部药浴可抑制胃液分泌，影响消化；饭后足部药浴使血管扩张，造成胃肠及内脏血液减少，影响胃肠的消化功能。

3. 足浴过程中严密观察患者的病情变化。注意观察皮肤情况，有无发红、瘙痒等皮肤过敏反应。如患者出现头晕、乏力、心慌等症状，应立即停止足浴，并报告医生，配合处理。

4. 药液温度适宜，一般以38~42℃为宜，糖尿病患者、足部皲裂患者、下肢感觉障碍患者，应适当降低药液温度，慎防烫伤。

5. 足部药浴所用的外治药物，因剂量较大，而且有些药物尚有毒性，不宜入口。

6. 对有传染性皮肤疾病者，如足癣患者，应做好消毒隔离预防交叉感染。

（杨金花）

Section 15　Chinese Medicine Ion Introduction Therapy

Chinese medicine ion introduction therapy is a method to cause the ionic drug to enter the body through intact skin or mucous membranes according to the principle of the electrical repulsion and attraction, so as to dissipate blood stasis, eliminate stasis, soften hard masses and achieve the functions of anti-inflammation and analgesia. According to different disease symptoms, traditional Chinese medicine formula can be modified in different ways.

I. Indication

Periarthritis humeroscapularis (periarthritis of shoulder), cervical spondylosis, rheumatism arthritis,

第十五节　中药离子导入法

中药离子导入法是用直流电电场（或低频脉冲电场）的作用，将中药液中的分子电解为离子，根据同性相斥、异性相吸的原理，使药物离子通过完整的皮肤或黏膜导入人体，以达到治疗目的的一种方法。具有活血化瘀、软坚散结、抗炎镇痛等作用。根据不同的病证，可选用不同的中药配方。

一、适应证

肩周炎、颈椎病、风湿性关节炎、急性乳腺炎、带状疱疹、跌打损伤、腰肌劳损、

acute mastitis, herpes zoster, traumatic injury, waist muscle strain, lumbar intervertebral disc herniation, pelvic inflammatory disease and bone hyperplasia.

II. Contraindication

Avoid using this method to treat the patients with some diseases or in special condition, such as high fever, active pulmonary tuberculosis, bleeding, severe cardiac insufficiency, women's pregnancy, and patients having a metal foreign body in treatment sites or a cardiac pacemaker.

III. Preparation

It includes Chinese medicine ion introduction therapy apparatus, herbal decoction, cotton cushion, treatment bowls, tweezers, sandbag, plastic film, bandage, gauze or toilet paper.

IV. Manipulation

1. After the materials are prepared, take them to the ward and check again. Explain the purposes and ways of the operation to the patient in order to get his/her cooperation.

2. Help the patient to select a comfortable posture and expose the treated parts, and protect the privacy of the patient with the screen. Tell the patient not to move the body during the treatment so as to avoid accident.

3. Check each wire connection of treatment instrument to make sure they are closely connected, set the output adjustment in the "0" position, turn on the power supply, and adjust the electric current. Set the treatment time to 20-30 minutes.

4. Drop the herbal decoction into the plaster on the cotton cushion to make it soaked sufficiently, and place the cushion in the corresponding parts of the body, then place the electrode plate of the treatment instrument in the cotton cushion.

5. In the treatment process, keep patient warm, observe the patient's response, assess the patient's tolerance level, and make the appropriate adjustments in time. Stop the treatment immediately if the patient complains of discomfort.

6. After the treatment is completed, the output is adjusted to "0". Shut off the power supply, and take off the electrode plate from the therapeutic instrument.

腰椎间盘突出症、盆腔炎、骨质增生等。

二、禁忌证

高热、活动性肺结核、出血、妇女妊娠期、治疗部位有金属异物、严重心功能不全，以及带有心脏起搏器者。

三、用物准备

中药离子导入治疗仪、中药液，衬垫，治疗碗，镊子，纱包，塑料薄膜，绷带，纱布或卫生纸。

四、操作方法

1. 备齐用物，携至床旁，核对医嘱；解释治疗目的、方法，以取得患者的配合。

2. 协助患者取舒适、合理的体位，充分暴露治疗部位，必要时遮挡患者，告知患者在治疗过程中不要移动体位，以免发生意外。

3. 检查治疗仪各导线连接是否紧密，设置输出调节在"0"位置，接通电源，开启仪器，调节电流量。设置治疗时间为20~30min。

4. 将中药液滴在药贴棉垫上，充分浸润，以不外溢为宜，然后将其置于相应部位，再将治疗仪的电极板放置在贴片上。

5. 治疗过程中注意保暖，观察患者治疗反应，评估患者的耐受程度，及时做出相应的调整。若有不适感，立即停止治疗。

6. 治疗完毕后，先将输出调节至"0"，再关闭电源，取下治疗仪的电极板。

7. Take off the patch, and clean the local skin with gauze. Assist the patient to get dressed and take a comfortable position. Clean bed sheets, inform the attention, and check the doctor's advice once again. Manage the medical waste according to the classification.

8. Wash hands, record the time and observe the response of the patient's skin.

V. Precaution

1. Explain the mechanism of Chinese medicine ion therapy to patients and their family members. Let them understand the treatment process in order to obtain their informed consent and cooperation.

2. The concentration of the decoction on the cotton cushion is generally about 5%, but the concentration of the decoction applied in the mucosa and body cavity can be lowered, and the pH of the drug solution is adjusted so as to reduce the irritation of the skin and mucous membranes.

3. One kind of ionic liquid is used for each treatment, and each cotton cushion is only for one drug use in order to avoid or reduce the impact of parasitic ions. Use clean water to clean and disinfect each pad. Detergent should not be used.

4. Stay with the patient, observe the response in the process of treatment, control the electric current, and adjust the appropriate current to avoid electrical burns.

5. The treatment should be stopped and the nurse should notify the doctor if the patient has allergic reactions such as itching skin, while symptomatic treatment will be applied.

(Xu Dong-ying)

Section 16　Retention Enema with Chinese Herb

Retention enema with Chinese herbs is a method to pour herbal decoction into and retained in the rectum or colon through the anus so as to detoxicate heat toxicity, soften hard masses and invigorate blood and promoting

7. 拿下药物贴片，用纱布清洁局部皮肤。协助患者穿衣，取舒适体位，整理床单，告知注意事项，再次核对医嘱。按规定分类处理用物。

8. 洗手，记录治疗时间，观察局部皮肤情况。

五、注意事项

1. 向患者及家属宣传中药离子导入的作用机理，让其了解离子导入的治疗过程及注意事项，取得患者和家属对执行该操作的知情同意及配合。

2. 衬垫上药物的浓度一般为 5% 左右，用于黏膜和体腔内导入的药物浓度可以低些，注意药物溶液的 pH，以减少对皮肤黏膜的刺激性。

3. 每次治疗最好使用一种离子导入液，每张衬垫只供一种药物使用，以避免或减少寄生离子的影响。用洁净水分别清洁消毒每张衬垫，不宜使用洗涤剂。

4. 治疗过程中应留在患者身边，密切观察患者的反应，控制好电流量、及时调节合适的电流以避免电灼伤。

5. 患者出现局部瘙痒等皮肤过敏反应时，应停止治疗，对症处理。

（徐冬英）

第十六节　中药保留灌肠法

中药保留灌肠法是将中药煎剂经肛门灌入，保留在直肠或结肠内，通过肠黏膜充分吸收，以治疗疾病的一种方法。该法可起到

blood circulation.

I. Indication

Chronic colitis, chronic kidney dysfunction, fever, leucorrhea, chronic pelvic inflammation, pelvic masses, chronic dysentery and other diseases.

II. Contraindication

1. Avoid using this method to treat the patients with some diseases, such as abscess of anus, operation around anus, rectum, and colon, fecal incontinence.

2. Avoid using this method to treat the patients with hemorrhage of digestive tract, pregnancy, acute abdominal disease, as well as the advanced patient with serious disease.

III. Preparation

It includes herbal decoction, rubber sheet, therapeutic towel or disposable diaper, toilet paper, therapeutic bowl, curve tray, medical anal tube, hemostatic forceps, paraffin oil, cotton swab, thermometer, enema barrel, rubber tube, tweezers, bedpan, transfusion rack and screen.

IV. Manipulation

1. After the materials are prepared, take them to the ward and check again. Explain the purposes and ways of the operation to the patient in order to get his/her cooperation.

2. Make preparation and check the doctor's advice. Instruct patient have defecation and urination before operating and protect the privacy of the patient with the screen.

3. The supine position is determined according to the location of the lesion. Generally the left side of the bed is used. The patient lies in his/her left side, keep two knees flexion, loosen the underwear, and take pants off to the thigh 1/2. Move the patient's buttocks to the side of the bed, and put the rubber cloth and the treatment towel (or disposable diaper) or the toilet paper pad under the buttocks and put curve tray beside the buttocks. Keep the patient warm.

清热解毒、软坚散结、活血化瘀等作用。

一、适应证

慢性结肠炎、慢性肾功能不全、发热、带下病、慢性盆腔炎、盆腔包块、慢性痢疾等疾病。

二、禁忌证

1. 肛周脓肿，肛门、直肠和结肠等手术或大便失禁的患者。

2. 消化道出血，妊娠，急腹症，以及各种严重疾病晚期患者。

三、用物准备

中药灌肠液，橡胶单，治疗巾（或一次性尿布），卫生纸，治疗碗，弯盘，肛管，止血钳，石蜡油，棉签，水温计，灌肠桶，橡胶管，镊子，便盆，输液架，屏风。

四、操作方法

1. 评估患者，做好核对解释工作，嘱患者排二便，遮挡患者。

2. 备齐用物，携至床旁，核对医嘱；解释治疗目的、方法，以取得患者的配合。

3. 卧位选择根据病变部位而定，一般多采用左侧卧位。协助患者取左侧卧位，两膝屈曲，松开衣裤，将裤脱至大腿上 1/2 处。臀部移至床边，将橡胶布和治疗巾（或一次性尿布）或卫生纸垫于臀下，弯盘置臀边。注意保暖。

4. Put a small pillow under the buttocks 10cm height in order to keep the retention of liquid. Pad on the rubber sheet and the treatment of towels under the buttocks.

5. Take the enema liquid about 200ml with temperature of 39-40℃, and pour into the enema barrel with closed tweezer.

6. The enema barrel is hung on a transfusion stand and carried to a patient's bedside (The distance between the liquid level and anus is 40-50cm).

7. The operator lubricates the front end of medical anal tube with paraffin oil, exit gas, and clamp water clamp, hold the buttocks with left hand, expose anal and insert the medical anal tube into the anal canal about 15-20cm deep. Wait a moment until it is fixed. Loosen the water clip, let the decoction drop in and adjust the dropping speed. Let the herbal decoction flow slowly for retention into the colon. The flow rate of herbal decoction should be kept slow, and the pressure must be low in order to facilitate the liquid retention.

8. Observe and inquire the patient's response to the decoction.

9. When the operation is finished, the medical anal tube should be taken off from colon and put in curve tray. Clean the patient's anus and keep him/her in bed about 1 hour.

10. Clean up the materials, wash hands, record and sign the name.

V. Precaution

1. Before the retention enema operation, the operator should determine the site of lesion in order to understand the enema position and insertion depth of medical anal tube.

2. Instruct patient to defecate before enema, operate cleaning enema if necessary. The medical anal tube should be thin and inserted deeply, with low pressure and less dosage.

3. It is better to have enema in the evening before going to bed with less activity for the patients with intestinal lesions.

4. The temperature of the decoction should be appropriate, which is generally 39-40℃. Because too low temperature can lead to intestinal peristalsis strengthening with the manifestation of abdominal pain, and high temperature can cause intestinal mucosa empyrosis or bowel dilatation, resulting in defecation and shortening the residence time of liquid in the intestines, so as to reduce the efficacy.

4. 用小枕垫高臀下 10cm，利于药液保留，垫上橡胶单及治疗巾。

5. 灌肠液去渣，温度适宜。一般以 39~41℃为宜。取灌肠液约 200ml，倒入灌肠桶内。

6. 将灌肠桶挂在输液架上，携至患者床旁（液面离肛门 40~50cm）。

7. 润滑肛管前段，排气，夹紧水夹。左手分开臀部，右手持肛管插入，入肛管要深，约 15~20cm，溶液流速宜慢，压力要低，以便于药液保留。稍等片刻后固定。松开水夹，滴入通畅，调整滴速。

8. 询问患者对药液滴入的反应。

9. 药液滴完后，用止血钳夹紧肛管缓缓拔出，置弯盘内。分离肛管，用卫生纸轻轻按压肛门。嘱患者平卧 1h。

10. 整理、洗净灌肠用物，并消毒备用。洗手，做好操作记录并签名。

五、注意事项

1. 在保留灌肠操作前，应明确病变的部位，以便掌握灌肠的卧位和肛管内插入的深度。

2. 灌肠前应嘱患者先排空大便，必要时可先行清洁灌肠。肛管要细，插入要深，压力要低，药量要少。

3. 肠道病变患者在夜间睡前灌入为宜，并减少活动。

4. 药液温度要适宜，一般为 39~41℃，虚症可为 40~44℃。温度过低可导致肠蠕动加强，引起腹痛，过高可引起肠黏膜烫伤或肠管扩张，产生便意，使药液在肠管内停留时间缩短而降低疗效。

5. Observe the patient's response in the process of enema. The enema should be stopped and the nurse should notify the doctor if the patient has some signs and symptoms such as pale, cold sweats, severe abdominal pain, rapid pulse, palpitation, as well as shortness of breath.

6. To avoid cross infection, disposable medical anal tube is recommended according to the administration of medical waste. Clean and sterilize the enema barrel after operating.

7. In order to keep long retention of decoction in colon for good effect, it is better to have enema in the evening before going to bed with dose of less than 200ml and keep in bed with fewer activities.

(Xu Dong-ying)

Key Points

1. When learning the tuina manipulation, the essential requirements of tuina manipulations must be understood and remembered. The manipulation should meet the essential technical requirements of being enduring, forceful, even, gentle, deep and penetrative. "Being during" means that the manipulation should be performed for a continuous period of time without any deformation. "Being forceful" means the manipulation must be performed with moderate force and it should not perform with clumsy strength and force. "Being even" means that the manipulation should be rhythmical with appropriate speed and steady force. "Being gentle" means that the manipulation is operated gently and carefully, light but not superficial, heavy but not unsmooth operations with nature and smooth shift of movements. "Being deep and pentrative" means that the stimulation must be penetrated deeply into the deep tissues.

2. Pay attention to the difference between kneading manipulation and circular rubbing manipulation: when performing kneading manipulation, fix the fingers or palm on a certain part of the body surface to drive the subcutaneous tissues to move with a relatively stronger force without rubbing movement with the body surface. When performing circular rubbing manipulation, the fingers or palm make circular rubbing with a relatively lighter force on the body surface without moving the subcutaneous tissues.

3. When pushing is performed, the palm base or the hypothenar implements the linear rubbing movements back and forth, so that the heat generated by the rubbing

5. 灌肠过程中注意观察患者的反应，若出现面色苍白、出冷汗、剧烈腹痛、脉数速、心慌气急，应立即停止灌肠，通知医生进行处理。

6. 建议用一次性的肛管，一人用一管，不能合用，以免交叉感染，用后按《医疗废物管理条例》规定处理，灌肠桶要清洁消毒处理。

7. 为延长药液在肠道内的保留时间，可在夜间睡前灌肠，药液一次不宜超过200ml，灌肠后不宜再下床活动，以提高疗效。

（徐冬英）

要点

1. 推拿操作的基本要求，即持久、有力、均匀、柔和和深透。"持久"是指操作应在动作不变形的情况下持续一定时间。"有力"是指操作手法要有一定的力度，但是要避免使用蛮力。"均匀"是指操作手法应有节律，速度适当，力量稳定。"柔和"是指动作轻柔，但轻而不浮，重而不滞，手法变换自然流畅。"深透"是指手法刺激应该深入到深层组织。

2. 揉法与摩法的区别：揉法是指操作时将手指和手掌固定在身体表面的某个部位，用力带动皮下组织运动但皮肤表面不发生摩擦运动。摩法是指手指或手掌在身体表面以相对较轻的力度进行圆形摩擦，但不带动皮下组织。

3. 推法是掌根和小鱼际在身体表面进行单方向的线性运动，以便摩擦产生的热量能穿透

can penetrate the body surface into the deeper layer. The route should be kept straight whether the scrubbing is from top to down or from left to right. Moreover, the distance of moving back and forth should be long and continuous without pause. Pushing manipulation should be performed along a straight line or a curved line in one direction. And rubbing back and forth should be avoided, and the speed of pushing should not be fast.

身体表面到达深层组织。无论操作是上下还是左右运动，都要保持直线，而且前后移动的距离尽可能长，并持续不停止。推法一定是单方向的直线或曲线运动，不能做往返摩擦运动，推的速度也不可过快。

Appendix 1 Name of Chinese Herb

附录 1 中药名称

Pīn yīn	Chinese	Pharmaceutical
guā lóu	瓜蒌	Fructus Trichosanthis
shēng dì huáng	生地黄	Radix Rehmanniae
huáng lián	黄连	Rhizoma Coptidis
rén shēn	人参	Radix et Rhizoma Ginseng
lù róng	鹿茸	Cornu Cervi Pantotrichum
fù zǐ	附子	Radix Aconiti Lateralis Praeparata
huáng qí	黄芪	Radix Astragali
jīng jiè	荆芥	Herba Schizonepetae
zǐ sū yè	紫苏叶	Folium Perillae
ē jiāo	阿胶	Colla Corii Asini
dōng chóng xià cǎo	冬虫夏草	Cordyceps
dāng guī	当归	Radix Angelicae Sinensis
dǎng shēn	党参	Radix Codonopsis
qiàn shí	芡实	Semen Euryales
pī shuāng	砒霜	Arsenicum
xióng huáng	雄黄	Realgar
mǎ qián zǐ	马钱子	Semen Strychni
bā dòu	巴豆	Fructus Crotonis
chán chú	蟾蜍	Bufonid
bān máo	斑蝥	Mylabris
shēng cǎo wū	生草乌	Unprocessed Radix Aconiti Kusnezoffii
tiān nán xīng	天南星	Rhizoma Arisaematis
wū tóu	乌头	Aconite
guā dì	瓜蒂	Pedicellus Melo
cháng shān	常山	Radix Dichroae
gān cǎo	甘草	Radix et Rhizoma Glycyrrhizae
gān suì	甘遂	Radix Kansui
léi gōng téng	雷公藤	Radix Tripterygii Wilfordii

Pīn yīn	Chinese	Pharmaceutical
fān xiè yè	番泻叶	Folium Sennae
lù jiǎo jiāo	鹿角胶	Colla Cornus Cervi
bàn xià	半夏	Rhizoma Pinelliae
bèi mǔ	贝母	Bulbus Fritillariae
bái liǎn	白蔹	Radix Ampelopsis
bái jí	白及	Rhizoma Bletillae
hǎi zǎo	海藻	Sargassum
dà jǐ	大戟	Radix Euphorbiae Pekinensis
yuán huā	芫花	Flos Genkwa
lí lú	藜芦	Radix et Rhizoma Veratri Nigri
xuán shēn	玄参	Radix Scrophulariae
shā shēn	沙参	Radix Adenophorae seu Glehniae
dān shēn	丹参	Radix et Rhizoma Salviae Miltiorrhizae
kǔ shēn	苦参	Radix Sophorae Flavescentis
xì xīn	细辛	Radix et Rhizoma Asari
sháo yào	芍药	Radix Paeoniae Alba seu Rubra
liú huáng	硫黄	Sulphur
pò xiāo	朴硝	Mirabilitum
shuǐ yín	水银	Hydrargyrum
láng dú	狼毒	Radix Euphorbiae Fischerianae
mì tuó sēng	密陀僧	Lithargyrum
qiān niú zǐ	牵牛子	Semen Pharbitidis
dīng xiāng	丁香	Flos Caryophylli
yù jīn	郁金	Radix Curcumae
yá xiāo	牙硝	Natrii Sulfas
sān léng	三棱	Rhizoma Sparganii
chuān wū	川乌	Radix Aconiti
cǎo wū	草乌	Radix Aconiti Kusnezoffii
xī jiǎo	犀角	Cornu Rhinocerotis
wǔ líng zhī	五灵脂	Faeces Trogopterori
guān guì	官桂	Cortex Cinnamomi
chì shí zhī	赤石脂	Halloysitum Rubrum
niú xī	牛膝	Radix Achyranthis Bidentatae
chuān xiōng	川芎	Rhizoma Chuanxiong
hóng huā	红花	Flos Carthami
táo rén	桃仁	Semen Persicae
jiāng huáng	姜黄	Rhizoma Curcumae Longae

Pīn yīn	Chinese	Pharmaceutical
mǔ dān pí	牡丹皮	Cortex Moutan
zhǐ shí	枳实	Fructus Aurantii Immaturus
zhǐ qiào	枳壳	Fructus Aurantii
dà huáng	大黄	Radix et Rhizoma Rhei
lú huì	芦荟	Aloe
máng xiāo	芒硝	Natrii Sulfas
qīng fěn	轻粉	Calomelas
shāng lù	商陆	Radix Phytolaccae
dǎn fán	胆矾	Chalcanthitum
gān qī	干漆	Resina Toxicodendri
é zhú	莪术	Rhizoma Curcumae
shè xiāng	麝香	Moschus
fú líng	茯苓	Poria
hé shǒu wū	何首乌	Radix Polygoni Multiflori
hòu pò	厚朴	Cortex Magnoliae Officinalis
wáng bù liú xíng	王不留行	Semen Vaccariae
cāng zhú	苍术	Rhizoma Atractylodis
huò xiāng	藿香	Herba Agastachis
bǎn lán gēn	板蓝根	Radix Isatidis
chái hú	柴胡	Radix Bupleuri
yú xīng cǎo	鱼腥草	Herba Houttuyniae
dēng xīn cǎo	灯心草	Medulla Junci
bái jiè zǐ	白芥子	Semen Sinapis

Appendix 2　Formulas

附录 2　方剂名

Pīn yīn	Chinese	English Name
Dà Qīng Lóng Tāng	大青龙汤	Major Green Dragon Decoction
Wǔ Líng Sǎn	五苓散	Five Substances Powder with Poria
Shí Zǎo Tāng	十枣汤	Ten Jujubes Decoction
Dà Chéng Qì Tāng	大承气汤	Major Purgative Decoction
Gān Cǎo Fù Zǐ Tāng	甘草附子汤	Licorice and Aconite Decoction
Fáng Jǐ Huáng Qí Tāng	防己黄芪汤	Stephania Root and Astragalus Decoction
Guì Zhī Tāng	桂枝汤	Cinnamon Twig Decoction
Kǔ Dòu Tāng	苦豆汤	Sophora Alopecuroides Decoction
Tú Sū Jiǔ	屠苏酒	Tusu Liquor
Xī Huáng Wán	犀黄丸	Rhinoceros Bezoar Pill
Gān Cǎo Liú Jìn Gāo	甘草流浸膏	Extractum Glycyrrhizae Liquidum
Yì Mǔ Cǎo Liú Jìn Gāo	益母草流浸膏	Extractum Leonuri Sibirici Liquidum
Pí Pá Gāo	枇杷膏	Loquat Extract
Sān Huáng Ruǎn Gāo	三黄软膏	Ointment of Three Yellow Drugs
Gǒu Pí Gāo	狗皮膏	Dog-skin Plaster
Shāng Shī Zhǐ Tòng Gāo	伤湿止痛膏	Rheumatic Analgesic Plaster
Shí Quán Dà Bǔ Jiǔ	十全大补酒	Perfect Great Tonic Liquor
Fēng Shī Yào Jiǔ	风湿药酒	Medicated Wine for Rheumatism
Jīn Yín Huā Lù	金银花露	Distillate of Honeysuckle
Sāng Jú Gǎn Mào Piàn	桑菊感冒片	Mulberry Leaf and Chrysanthemum Tablet for Cold
Yín Qiào Jiě Dú Piàn	银翘解毒片	Fructus Forsythiae Antidotal Tablet
Bǎn Lán Gēn Chōng Jì	板蓝根冲剂	Radix Isatidis Granules
Gǎn Mào Líng Chōng Jì	感冒灵冲剂	Infusion Granules for Reducing Fever Due to Common Cold
Fù Fāng Dān Shēn Zhù Shè Yè	复方丹参注射液	Compound Salvia miltiorrhiza injection
Sān Huáng Shuān	三黄栓	Three Yellow Suppository
Yún Nán Bái Yào Jiāo Náng	云南白药胶囊	Yúnnán White Capsule
Huò Xiāng Zhèng Qì Ruǎn Jiāo Náng	藿香正气软胶囊	Agastache Qi-Correcting Capsule

Pīn yīn	Chinese	English Name
Dà Huáng Fù Zǐ Tāng	大黄附子汤	Rhubarb and Aconite Decoction
Wēn Pí Tāng	温脾汤	Spleen-Warming Decoction
Wǔ Rén Tāng	五仁汤	Decoction of Kernels of five drugs
Má Zǐ Rén Wán	麻子仁丸	Cannabis Fruit Pill
Dāng Guī Sì Nì Tāng	当归四逆汤	Chinese Angelica Frigid Extremities Decoction
Bái Hǔ Tāng	白虎汤	White Tiger Decoction
Pǔ Jì Xiāo Dú Yǐn	普济消毒饮	Universal Relief Toxin-Removing Beverage
Zhǐ Shí Dǎo Zhì Wán	枳实导滞丸	Immature Bitter Orange Stagnation-Moving Pill
Xiǎo Qīng Lóng Hé Jì	小青龙合剂	Minor Green Dragon Mixture

References

参考文献

1 ••••••• 郝玉芳，陈锋.中医护理学基础：双语 [M].北京：人民卫生出版社，2009.

2 ••••••• 沈雪勇.针灸学 [M].第 2 版 .北京：人民卫生出版社，2007.

3 ••••••• 徐桂华，刘虹.中医护理学基础 [M].北京：中国中医药出版社，2012.

4 ••••••• 陈佩仪.中医护理学基础：中医特色 [M].北京：人民卫生出版社，2012.

5 ••••••• 孙秋华，孟繁洁.中医护理学 [M].北京：人民卫生出版社，2012.

6 ••••••• 孙秋华.中医护理学 [M].北京：人民卫生出版社，2012.

7 ••••••• 徐桂华，李佃贵.中医护理学 [M].北京：人民卫生出版社，2009.

8 ••••••• 刘虹.中医护理学基础 [M].北京：中国中医药出版社，2005.

9 ••••••• 成肇智.中医药英语 [M].北京：人民卫生出版社，1999.

10 ••••••• 郝玉芳，马良宵.中医护理学：双语 [M].北京：人民卫生出版社，2015.

11 ••••••• 梁传荣.实用中医护理常规与操作技能 [M].北京：军事医学科学出版社，2008.

12 ••••••• 王虹.实用中医专科护理常规及操作规程 [M].北京：中国医药科技出版社，2012.

13 ••••••• 陈建章，顾红卫.中医护理学基础 [M].北京：中国中医药出版社，2013.

14 ••••••• 陈岩.中医养生与食疗 [M].北京：人民卫生出版社，2012.

15 ••••••• 中华中医药学会.中医体质分类与判定 [M].北京：中国中医药出版社，2009.

16 ••••••• 刘占文.中医养生学 [M].北京：人民卫生出版社，2007.

17 ••••••• 王鲁芬，李照国，鲍白.中医诊断学 [M].上海：上海浦江教育出版社，2002.

18 ••••••• 孙秋华.中医护理学概要 [M].北京：北京大学医学出版社，2015.

19 ••••••• 柴可夫.中医基础理论 [M].第 2 版 .北京：人民卫生出版社，1998.

20 ••••••• 刘昭纯.中医基础理论：双语 [M].北京：高等教育出版社，2007.

21 ••••••• 柴可夫.中医基础理论：双语 [M].北京：人民卫生出版社，2007.

22 ••••••• 龙致贤.中医基础理论：双语 [M].北京：学苑出版社，2004.

23 ••••••• 刘明军.针灸推拿与护理 [M].北京：人民卫生出版社，2012.

24 ••••••• 沈雪勇，许能贵.经络腧穴学 [M].北京：人民卫生出版社，2012.

06